BASIC CONCEPTS OF
PSYCHIATRIC–MENTAL
HEALTH NURSING

FOURTH EDITION

BASIC CONCEPTS OF PSYCHIATRIC–MENTAL HEALTH NURSING

FOURTH EDITION

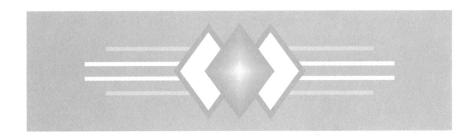

Louise Rebraca Shives
MSN, ARNP, CNS

Private Practice in Psychiatric–Mental Health Nursing
Consultant in Long-Term Care
Orlando, Florida

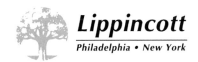

Lippincott

Philadelphia • New York

Acquisitions Editor: Margaret Zuccarini
Editorial Assistant: Emily Cotlier
Production Editor: Virginia Barishek
Production Manager: Helen Ewan
Production Service: P.M. Gordon
  Associates, Inc.

Compositor: Circle Graphics
Printer/Binder: R. R. Donnelley & Sons
  Company/Crawfordsville
Cover Designer: William T. Donnelly
Cover Printer: Lehigh Press

Fourth Edition

9 8 7 6 5 4 3 2 1

Library of Congress Cataloging-in-Publication Data

Shives, Louise Rebraca.
    Basic concepts in psychiatric–mental health nursing / Louise
Rebraca Shives.—4th ed.
        p.   cm.
    Includes bibliographical references and index.
    ISBN 0-397-55457-5
    1. Psychiatric nursing.   I. Title.
    [DNLM: 1. Psychiatric Nursing.   WY 160 S558b 1998]
RC440.S487   1998
610.73′68—dc21
DNLM/DLC   97-12761
                                                                CIP

Care has been taken to confirm the accuracy of the information presented and to describe generally accepted practices. However, the authors, editors, and publisher are not responsible for errors or omissions or for any consequences from application of the information in this book and make no warranty, express or implied, with respect to the contents of the publication.

The authors, editors and publisher have exerted every effort to ensure that drug selection and dosage set forth in this text are in accordance with current recommendations and practice at the time of publication. However, in view of ongoing research, changes in government regulations, and the constant flow of information relating to drug therapy and drug reactions, the reader is urged to check the package insert for each drug for any change in indications and dosage and for added warnings and precautions. This is particularly important when the recommended agent is a new or infrequently employed drug.

Some drugs and medical devices presented in this publication have Food and Drug Administration (FDA) clearance for limited use in restricted research settings. It is the responsibility of the health care provider to ascertain the FDA status of each drug or device planned for use in their clinical practice.

This book is dedicated to my daughters,
Terri Spence, Lorrie Shives, and Debbie
Moore; to my father, Pete
Rebraca; and to my grandchildren,
Jeffray, Jennifer, and Zachary.

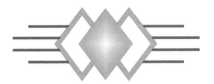

PREFACE

Dramatic changes continue to occur in the nature and availability of settings for student clinical experiences. The publication of the fourth edition of the *Diagnostic and Statistical Manual of Mental Disorders* (DSM-IV), the proliferation of community-based outpatient mental health services, and limited insurance coverage for inpatient psychiatric care are factors that are reflected in the preparation of this fourth edition of **Basic Concepts of Psychiatric–Mental Health Nursing**.

As with all editions of this text, the goal is to present the concepts used in psychiatric–mental health nursing briefly and succinctly so that this "core" textbook can also be used by practicing nurses and other mental health professionals.

Text Organization

The text is organized into seven Units:

Unit I, **Psychiatric–Mental Health Nursing**, presents basic concepts. It includes four chapters that present an overview and address pertinent history and developing trends, the increasing importance of community mental health and community-based care delivery sites as well as important legal issues related to the practice of psychiatric nursing.

Unit II, **Components of Psychiatric–Mental Health Nursing**, includes two chapters on applying the nursing process in psychiatric nursing and six chapters that focus on the range of interventions that are crucial for delivering therapeutic nursing care to the patient with a psychiatric disorder. These interventions include the Therapeutic Milieu, Crisis Intervention, Group Therapy, Family Therapy, and Psychopharmacology.

Unit III explores **The Patient as a Person**. Its three chapters focus on theories of personality development, emotional responses to illness and hospitalization, and the nature and impact of loss and grief.

Unit IV presents eight chapters that focus on **Nursing Interventions for Persons with Psychiatric Disorders**. These include Anxiety and Anxiety-Related Disorders, Sexual Disorders, Mood Disorders, Suicide, Delusional and Paranoid Disorders, Schizophrenic Disorders, and Cognitive Disorders.

Unit V presents four chapters on **Special Populations in Psychiatric–Mental Health Nursing**. This unit includes two chapters on Disorders of Infancy, Childhood, and Adolescence and Eating Disorders, as well as two chapters on Alcoholism and Psychoactive Substance Abuse Disorders.

Unit VI addresses **Relational Problems** prevalent in our society. It includes three chapters: Child Abuse and Neglect, The Abused Adult Within the Family Unit, and Rape and Sexual Assault.

Unit VII presents three chapters on **Populations with Special Needs** including people with AIDS, Psychosocial Aspects of Aging, and Psychiatric Patients with Medical Problems/Syndromes. This chapter content is daily becoming more important as more patients with psychiatric disorders are being cared for in community and home care settings.

Features

The format and strong pedagogical features of the previous edition have been preserved, including:

- Learning Objectives
- Use of the American Psychiatric Association's DSM-IV and other current references to describe psychiatric disorders
- Discussion of Transcultural Considerations
- Use of references to cite Diagnostic Criteria and Symptoms
- Research
- Examples of the nursing process including Nursing Diagnosis, Goals, Nursing Interventions, and Outcome Criteria
- Clinical Examples of psychiatric disorders
- End-of-chapter summaries
- Learning Activities
- Critical Thinking Questions
- Self-Tests
- Glossary of terms

Examples of student reactions to various experiences and conditions in the clinical setting continue to provide a means of encouragement and support for the novice student.

As in previous editions, tables or boxes are used throughout the text to provide clear summaries of complex information. They include the characteristics of mental health and mental illness, milestones influencing psychiatric–mental health nursing, therapeutic communication techniques, the stages of various theories of personality development, descriptions of various disciplines composing the mental health team, a summary of neurologic side effects of psychotropic drugs, and the daily dosage of commonly used psychotropic drugs. Psychotropic drugs approved by the Food and Drug Administration within the past four years are discussed in the appropriate chapters.

New Content

Content within the text was rewritten to reflect current statistics and is now consistent with the DSM-IV classification of psychiatric disorders. Important new and revised content in this edition includes:

- Managed care
- Role of independent mental-health nurse practitioners
- Transcultural Considerations as they apply to the nursing process and treatment of specific psychiatric disorders
- Psychiatric nursing models
- Classification of crises according to severity
- Role of the nurse and patient in group therapy
- Psychopharmacologic guidelines when medicating a patient with a psychiatric disorder
- Medication Alerts discussing drug–drug interactions, unusual side effects, and monitoring of laboratory values
- Living wills
- Research regarding anxiety, sexual orientation, herbal medicine for psychiatric disorders, bipolar disorder, schizophrenia, Alzheimer's disease, and attention deficit/hyperactivity disorder
- Patient Teaching Checklists
- Culture-bound syndromes
- Suicide lexicon
- Behaviors due to specific central nervous system pathology
- Action Plan to Avert Violence
- Myths about aging

New Features

- Patient Teaching Checklists
- Medication Alerts
- Assessment Tools

New Assessment Tools

- Basic Sexual Assessment
- Positive and Negative Syndrome Scale
- Functional Assessment Staging Test for Alzheimer's
- CAGE Test for Alcoholism
- Domestic Abuse Assessment Screen
- Geropsychiatric Assessment Tool
- Family Assessment Guide

Ancillary and Teaching Support Materials

- **Instructor's Manual and Test Bank:** This valuable adjunct to teaching the basic psychiatric nursing course includes: key terms, classroom teaching strategies, and an NCLEX-style test bank.
- **Basic Mental Status Examination** video series: This four-video series, designed for in-classroom use, assists students in understanding how to conduct *and interpret* the basic mental-status examination. The series includes:
  Video I: Conducting the Patient Interview
  Video II: Evaluating Aspects of Appearance and Mood
  Video III: Evaluating Language and Thought Patterns
  Video IV: Evaluating Intellectual and Cognitive Function

Study and Review Materials

- **Lippincott's Self-Study:** This *Mental-Health and Psychiatric Nursing* computer disk contains 350 NCLEX-style questions with rationale.
- **Lippincott's Listen and Learn:** These two *Mental Health and Psychiatric Nursing* 50-minute audio cassettes provide content overviews of key psychiatric nursing concepts, presented in live-action, real-life scenarios followed by review questions. Includes answers with rationale.
- **Lippincott's Review Series:** *Mental Health and Psychiatric Nursing* is a comprehensive outline review and self-test for course or NCLEX review.

I would like to take this opportunity to extend my thanks to the nursing instructors, students, practicing nurses, and other mental health professionals who continue to use this textbook, now in its fourth edition. Your comments and suggestions have been incorporated into the text.

Louise Rebraca Shives, MSN, ARNP, CNS

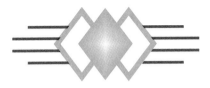

ACKNOWLEDGMENTS

The following individuals were supportive, both professionally and personally, during the development of this fourth edition: Dr. Shahedra Akhtar, board-certified child, adolescent, and adult psychiatrist, who specializes in the treatment of children and adolescents and who provided current information on the treatment of disorders of childhood and adolescence; Dr. Sardar Aziz, board-certified psychiatrist and geropsychiatrist, who also provided current treatment to update various chapters; Darlene Barrett, Licensed Clinical Psychologist and associate, who provided information in the clinical setting; Elizabeth Koon, Licensed Clinical Social Worker, NASW Diplomat in Clinical Social Work, and former associate, who provided supportive adjunctive therapy to clients and kept this clinician informed about the legal aspects of psychiatric treatment in the state of Florida; Marie Magnuson, RNC, BSN, former contributor, and present unit manager of a sub-acute unit in the long-term care setting, who provided information regarding the frequency and types of psychiatric disorders treated on sub-acute units; Helene K. Nawrocki, RN, MSN, CNA, a nurse educator, editor, and management consultant in Roslyn, Pennsylvania, who prepared the critical thinking questions; Dr. Katy R. Reynolds, RN, MSN, MA, who prepared the Instructor's Manual; and Emily Cotlier, Editorial Assistant, and Margaret Belcher Zuccarini, Editor, of the Nursing Division of Lippincott–Raven Publishers, who offered professional editorial guidance throughout the development of this edition.

CONTENTS

Unit II
Components of Psychiatric–Mental Health Nursing

◈ UNIT VI
Relational Problems

BASIC CONCEPTS OF PSYCHIATRIC–MENTAL HEALTH NURSING

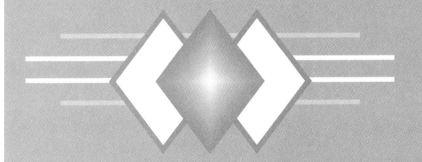

Psychiatric–Mental Health Nursing

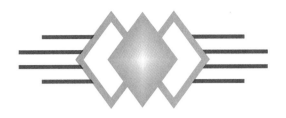

CHAPTER 1

MENTAL HEALTH AND MENTAL ILLNESS

M ental health is like a violin with strings of interaction, behavior, affect and intellect. All these together may produce a pleasant or stimulating melody or they may be discordant and irritating. The tune continually changes. No one is entirely mentally unhealthy and no one is fully healthy at all times.

Ebersole and Hess, 1985

1 Define mental health.

2 Differentiate between mental health and mental illness.

3 State factors that influence the development of mental health.

4 Cite misconceptions or myths about mental illness.

5 Explain how one maintains mental health.

6 Describe the levels of communication by which a person communicates with others.

7 State positive ways of dealing with one's emotions.

8 Define *ego defense mechanism.*

9 Cite examples of defense mechanisms and the purpose that each serves.

10 Explain the role of a significant other or support person in maintaining mental health.

Introduction

The concepts of mental health and mental illness are discussed in psychological, sociologic, and psychiatric nursing texts under various headings, including the health–illness continuum, stress and mental health, and aspects of mental health.

Best-selling books have been written focusing on self-awareness, personal growth, and interpersonal communication. These dynamics play an important part in the development of emotional maturity and mental health.

Defining Mental Health

Although there is no universal definition of mental health, people in the helping professions seem to agree that mental health is a positive state in which one is responsible, displays self-awareness, is self-directive, is reasonably worry-free, and can cope with usual daily tensions. Such individuals function well in society, are accepted within a group, and are generally satisfied with their lives.

Other definitions refer to the ability to (1) solve problems; (2) fulfill one's capacity for love and work; (3) cope with crises without assistance beyond the support of family or friends; and (4) maintain a state of well-being by enjoying life, setting goals and realistic limits, and becoming independent, interdependent, or dependent as the need arises without permanently losing one's independence.

Factors Influencing Mental Health

Three factors influence the development of mental health: inherited characteristics, nurturing during childhood, and life circumstances. Some theorists believe that no one is completely normal and that the ability to maintain a mentally healthy outlook on life is, in part, due to one's genes, just as genetic defects may predispose a person to cognitive disability, schizophrenia, or bipolar disorder. Such people have innate differences in sensitivity and temperament that prompt various responses to their environment. Nurturing during childhood refers to parent–child interactions, which also affect the development of mental health. Positive nurturing starts with bonding at childbirth and includes feelings of love, security, and acceptance. The child experiences positive interactions with parents and siblings. Negative nurturing includes circumstances such as maternal deprivation, parental rejection, sibling rivalry, and early communication failures. Life circumstances can influence one's mental health from birth. Examples of positive circumstances are success in school, financial security, good physical health, an enjoyable occupation, and a successful marriage. Negative circumstances include poverty, poor physical health, unemployment, or an unsuccessful marriage.

Defining Mental Illness

Like diabetes or cerebral palsy, mental illness is no one person's fault. It can be caused by chemical imbalances in the brain, by transfer of drugs across the placental barrier, or by organic changes within the brain. If a person is unsuccessful in dealing with environmental stresses because of faulty inherited characteristics, poor nurturing during childhood, or negative life circumstances, mental illness may develop. The American Psychiatric Association's definition of mental illness or a mental disorder is an "illness with psychologic or behavioral manifestations and/or impairment in functioning due to a social, psychologic, genetic, physical/chemical, or biologic disturbance. The disorder is not limited to relations between the person and society. The illness is characterized by symptoms and/or impairment in functioning" (1980, p. 89). Other definitions refer to mental illness as (1) a disorder causing people to display abnormal behavior more consistently than most people; (2) a psychopathology exhibiting frequent irresponsibility, the inability to cope, frequently being at odds with society, and an inaccurate perception of reality; and (3) the absolute absence or constant presence of a specific behavior that has a socially acceptable range of occurrences.

Characteristics of Mental Health

Maslow (1954), an eminent psychologist and writer, developed the following ideas about mentally healthy people:

1. They possess the ability to accept themselves, others, and nature. Stated another way, they have positive self-concepts and relate well to people and their environment.
2. They are able to form close relationships with others and display kindness, patience, and compassion for others.
3. They perceive the world as it really is and people as they really are. Problem solving occurs because these people are able to make decisions pertaining to reality rather than fantasy.
4. They are able to appreciate and enjoy life. Optimism prevails as they respond to people, places, and things in daily encounters.
5. They are independent or autonomous in thought and action and rely on personal standards of behavior and values. Such people are able to face with relative serenity and happiness circumstances that would drive other people to self-destructive behavior.
6. They are creative, using a variety of approaches as they perform tasks or solve problems.
7. Their behavior is consistent as they appreciate and respect the rights of others, display a willingness to listen and learn from others, and show reverence for the uniqueness of and difference in others.

A comparison of some of the characteristics of mental health and mental illness is found in Box 1-1.

People who are mentally healthy do not necessarily possess all the characteristics listed. Under stress they may exhibit transitory traits of mental illness but are able to respond to the stress with automatic, unconscious behavior that serves to satisfy their basic needs in a socially acceptable way.

 Misconceptions About Mental Illness

Altrocchi (1980) lists several misconceptions about abnormal behavior and mental illness. Summarized, they are as follows:

1. *Abnormal behavior is different or odd, easily recognized.* We all are irrational at times and behave in an unusual or different manner. Such behavior may occur in the privacy of one's home, at work, or even in a public place, and

BOX 1-1   Comparison of Mental Health and Mental Illness

Mental Health	Mental Illness
Accepts self and others	Feels inadequate
	Has poor self-concept
Is able to cope with or tolerate stress. Can return to normal functioning if temporarily disturbed	Is unable to cope
	Exhibits maladaptive behavior
Is able to form close and lasting relationships	Is unable to establish a meaningful relationship
Uses sound judgment to make decisions	Displays poor judgment
Accepts responsibility for actions	Is irresponsible or unable to accept responsibility for actions
Is optimistic	Is pessimistic
Recognizes limitations (abilities and deficiencies)	Does not recognize limitations (abilities and deficiencies)
Can function effectively and independently	Exhibits dependency needs because of feelings of inadequacy
Is able to distinguish imagined circumstances from reality	Is unable to perceive reality
Is able to develop potential and talents to fullest extent	Does not recognize potential and talents because of poor self-concept
Is able to solve problems	Avoids problems rather than coping with them or attempting to solve them
Can delay gratification	Desires or demands immediate gratification
Mental health reflects a person's approach to life by communicating emotions, giving and receiving, working alone as well as with others, accepting authority, displaying a sense of humor, and coping successfully with emotional conflict.	Mental illness reflects a person's inability to cope with stress, resulting in disruption, disorganization, inappropriate reactions, unacceptable behavior, and the inability to respond according to the person's expectations and the demands of society.

still may go unnoticed by others. Maladaptive behavior can occur subtly; for example, individuals may be suspicious of everyone and avoid contact with people. Unless they voice their concerns, their thoughts and behavior may go unnoticed. Depressed individuals who are diagnosed as mentally ill may appear quiet, sullen, or distracted but don't necessarily exhibit abnormal or bizarre behavior.

2. *Abnormal behavior can be predicted and evaluated.* Newspaper articles and television newscasts prove otherwise. A candidate for the Florida House of Representatives fired five shots into the home of his opponent a few days before the primary elections. He was described by family and friends as a nice, smart, quiet guy with a pleasant face. No motive was given for his sudden unpredictable behavior.

3. *Internal forces are responsible for abnormal behavior.* Although internal forces may cause abnormal behavior, other factors (*e.g.*, people, culture, and environment) can influence one's behavior. Consider a couple having marital problems. Individually they may be mature, independent people who are unable to live together owing to differences of opinion, values, or priorities. Stress and conflict from marital discord may result in abnormal or maladaptive behavior, such as regression, hostility, or even a suicide attempt.

4. *People who exhibit abnormal behavior are dangerous.* According to statistics provided by the National Institute of Mental Health (NIMH) in 1990, more than 40 million Americans have a psychiatric diagnosis at any given time. Approximately 60% to 65% of those individuals who are hospitalized for psychiatric treatment are discharged and live with their families. Such illnesses include autism, depression, panic attacks or anxiety disorders, substance abuse, and schizophrenia. Many of these people function to some extent in society and are not considered dangerous. They turn to others for help in an attempt to cope with their problems.

5. *Maladaptive behavior is inherited.* Heredity may play a part in the development of some types of abnormal behavior; however, learning influences behavior. Children learn early in life how to satisfy their needs. They may cry excessively, become stubborn, have temper tantrums, or manipulate a parent to achieve immediate gratification. Children as well as adults may observe specific behaviors used by others to meet their needs. As a result, they imitate behavior that they believe to be acceptable to others.

6. *Mental illness is incurable.* Much progress has occurred in the diagnosis and treatment of mental illness. Early detection and treatment may alleviate symptoms and allow the person to function normally in society. People with a chronic mental disorder may receive maintenance doses of medication, attend various therapies, or care for themselves with minimal supervision. The current trend toward deinstitutionalization emphasizes returning the

patient to the community as a functioning person under the supervision of community mental health workers.

Maintaining Mental Health

"A growing person is self-renewing . . . as new as each day. . . . Study his face and hands, listen to his voice . . . look for change. . . . it is certain he has changed" (Powell, 1969, p. 28). *Emotional maturity, fully functioning, growing personally, fully human,* and *self-actualizing* are all terms used to describe the person who achieves and maintains mental health. Characteristics of mental health have already been discussed, but how does one maintain mental health? Harry Stack Sullivan, an eminent psychiatrist, states that people mistakenly believe that they can solve their own problems and maintain control of their lives without assistance from anyone or anything. The truth is that those who attempt to solve problems by themselves may become consumed by their problems and suffer some type of mental disorder or illness. Mental health is in part determined by relationships between those who either love or refuse to love one another.

Factors that influence the ability to achieve and maintain emotional maturity include interpersonal communication, dealing directly with one's emotions, and resorting to "human hiding places," or ego defense mechanisms (Powell, 1969).

Interpersonal Communication

Interpersonal communication is discussed at length in the chapter on therapeutic interactions. A relationship is only as good as the interaction that occurs. Powell (1969) discusses five levels of communication that affect an individual's personal growth and maturity during interpersonal encounters. He refers to them as "the five degrees of willingness to go outside of himself, to communicate himself to others" (p. 50). A discussion of these levels of communication enables one to understand one method of maintaining mental health. They are presented in order from the least willingness to communicate with others to the most healthy response:

Level 5: Cliché Conversation No sharing of oneself occurs during this interaction. Comments such as "How are you doing?" "How's your new job?" or "Talk to you later" are empty, superficial statements in which no answers are expected. No personal growth can occur at this level.

Level 4: Reporting Facts Communicating at this level reveals very little about oneself, and minimal or no interaction is expected from others. No personal interaction occurs at this level.

Level 3: Revealing Ideas and Judgments Such communication occurs under strict censorship by the speaker, who is watching the listener's response for an indication of acceptance or approval. If the speaker is unable to read the reactions of the listener, the speaker may revert to safer topics or even say what he or she thinks the listener would like to hear rather than face disapproval or rejection.

Level 2: Spontaneous, Here-and-Now Emotions Revealing one's feelings or emotions takes courage because one faces the possibility of rejection by the listener. Powell (1969) states that if one reveals the contents of the mind and heart, one may fear that such emotional honesty will not be tolerated by another. As a result, the speaker may resort to dishonesty and superficial conversation to maintain contact with another person.

Level 1: Open, Honest Communication When this type of communication occurs, two people share emotions. They are in tune with each other, capable of experiencing or duplicating each other's reactions, as individual sopranos in a choir sing the same notes and sound as one voice. Such an interaction is termed complete emotional and personal communication and helps one maintain emotional maturity. Open communication may not occur until people relate to each other over a period of time, getting to know and trust each other.

As people respond to various stressors in their environment or within themselves, they may fluctuate from one level of communication to another in an attempt to alleviate tension or anxiety. Examine your own levels of communication. Which level do you use during most interactions? Do the levels differ with friends, families, coworkers, or patients?

Facing Emotions

People handle their innermost thoughts and feelings in various ways. A comparison of healthy and unhealthy ways to deal with one's emotions during an interaction is included in Box 1-2.

Defense Mechanisms

Defense mechanisms, also referred to as ego defense mechanisms, are mental processes first described by Sigmund Freud (1946). He identified them as usually unconscious, protective barriers that are used to manage instinct and affect in the presence of stressful situations. Depending on their use, they can be therapeutic or they can be pathologic, because all defense mechanisms include a distortion of reality, some degree of self-deception, and what appears to be irra-

BOX 1-2 Comparison of Healthy and Unhealthy Reactions

Healthy Reactions	Unhealthy Reactions
Be aware of any emotional response or feeling during an interaction with your environment or with another person. Try to identify what you are feeling.	Ignore any emotional response on your part. Bottle it up inside so that your mind is not aware of the response. Your body may feel the effects in the form of a headache or chest pain.
Admit that you are capable of experiencing various emotions, including anger, hostility, frustration, or disappointment.	Deny your true feelings by ignoring them or telling yourself they do not really exist. You are not the type of person who becomes angry or bitter.
Examine the intensity of each emotion you feel. What caused such a reaction? How is it affecting your relationship with others?	Let the emotion rule as you become defensive during an interaction. It's not you; it's the other guy who is at fault.
Share your emotional response. For example, saying "I need time to cool off. I'm too angry to think straight" is a healthy way of avoiding an unnecessary confrontation.	Allow yourself to lose control and become argumentative, incoherent, or disorganized. Blame your reaction on the other person or thing.
Let your mind tell you what is the correct approach to a specific interaction. Think before you act.	Let your emotions rule your actions. Act without thinking and be impulsive.

tional behavior. Such mechanisms are supposedly in action by 10 years of age. Following is an explanation of the uses of defense mechanisms:

1. *To resolve a mental conflict.* For example, you are scheduled to work Friday night but have been invited to a concert you want to attend. How would you handle this mental conflict? Tell yourself you have a good work record so it is okay to miss one night of work? Convince yourself that other people miss work for less significant reasons? Suddenly develop a headache Friday, preventing you from going to work or attending the concert? These are just a few options available to resolve your conflict.

2. *To reduce anxiety or fear.* Anxiety is an unexplained feeling of apprehension, tension, or uneasiness. The statement "I feel jittery, as if something terrible is about to happen" denotes anxiety. Fear is an emotional response to a recognizable object or threat; it decreases when the danger or threat subsides. How do you think you would react if you were suddenly hospitalized to undergo tests to rule out the diagnosis of cancer? Would you deny the possibility, rationally discuss the possibility with your doctor, or elect not to think about the possibility? In any event, your defense mechanisms would be called into action to reduce any anxiety or fear you experience.

3. *To protect one's self-esteem.* After you have worked for the same employer for 3 years, your immediate supervisor resigns to accept another position. Although you have received satisfactory periodic evaluations and yearly increases in salary, and have indicated an interest in the job, you are not offered the position. Such a decision would affect almost anyone's self-esteem. How would you protect yours? Would you believe that the incoming employee is much better qualified, or would you blame your employer for showing favoritism toward the new employee? Perhaps you would elect not to talk about the situation because it upsets you too much. Your ego defenses are attempting to protect your self-esteem.

4. *To protect one's sense of security. Webster's* defines "security" as safety or freedom from worry or uncertainty. Has your security ever been threatened? Suppose you were confronted by a robber while in a bank. How do you think you would react? Would you blame the security officer for allowing the robber to follow through with his intent? You might decide to comply with his demands, thinking no harm will come if you follow his directions. On the other hand, you may begin to hyperventilate and experience tachycardia as your emotions are expressed in physical symptoms.

Approximately 20 different defense mechanisms have been identified. Depending on their use, defense mechanisms are considered healthy or pathologic (characteristic of a mental disorder). The mechanisms are as follows:

1. *Suppression:* willfully or voluntarily putting an unacceptable thought or feeling out of one's mind with the ability to recall the thought or feeling at will. A deliberate, intentional exclusion from the conscious mind is referred to as "voluntary forgetting." Examples of suppression are "I'd rather not talk about it right now," "Let's talk about my accident later," or "I'm taking a vacation. My problems will still be here when I get back." This mechanism generally is used to protect one's self-esteem.

2. *Repression:* one of the most common defense mechanisms, referred to as the "burying alive mechanism." The person is unable to recall painful or unpleasant thoughts or feelings because they are automatically and invol-

untarily pushed into one's unconsciousness. The inability to remember the reason for an argument or recall feelings of fear after an automobile accident are examples of repression.

3. *Rationalization:* the most common ego defense mechanism, referred to as "self-deception at its subtle best." Rationalization is used unconsciously to justify ideas, actions, or feelings with good, acceptable reasons or explanations. Generally it is used to maintain self-respect, prevent guilt feelings, and obtain social approval or acceptance. For example, a teenaged girl who was not asked to the junior prom tells her friend, "John really wanted to date me but felt sorry for Sue and took her to the prom." A golfer overdrives the green by about 100 yards and states: "The wind really carried my golf ball. I didn't hit it that hard."

4. *Identification:* also referred to as "the imitator." Unconsciously, people use it in an attempt to identify with the personality and traits of another. Such behavior preserves one's ego or self, the organized conscious mediator between person and reality.

5. *Compensation:* the act of making up for a real or imagined inability or deficiency with a specific behavior to maintain self-respect or self-esteem. The person overcomes an inability by becoming proficient in another area. For example, a short girl may become the manager of a basketball team because she is not tall enough to qualify for the team. An unattractive man selects expensive, stylish clothes to draw attention to himself. This may occur at the conscious or unconscious level.

6. *Reaction-formation:* also referred to as overcompensation. The person exaggerates or overdevelops certain actions by displaying exactly the opposite behavior, attitude, or feeling from what he or she normally would show in a given situation. This mechanism is considered a protective drive by which the person prevents painful, undesirable, or unacceptable attitudes toward others from emerging. For example, a man who dislikes his mother-in-law may act very politely and courteously toward her. A woman who dislikes children may talk very lovingly to a friend's young son (although privately she considers him a brat). The conscious intent is often altruistic.

7. *Substitution:* the unconscious act of replacing a goal when it is blocked. Also defined as the replacement of consciously unacceptable emotions, drives, attitudes, or needs by those that are more acceptable. A student nurse in a baccalaureate program who feels unable to master the clinical competencies and elects to become a respiratory technician is using the mechanism of substitution. This mechanism is used to reduce frustration and promote feelings of satisfaction or success.

8. *Displacement:* a mechanism that serves to transfer feelings such as frustration, hostility, or anxiety from one idea, person, or object to another. The substitute target is less threatening and allows the person to release emotional reac-

tions. Have you ever slammed a door when you were angry or yelled at one person when you were angry at another? If so, you displaced your feelings toward the original person to an object or another person. Parents often displace feelings of anger or frustration toward their children because they are more tolerant recipients of such displacement than other adults.

9. *Restitution or undoing:* the negation of a previous consciously intolerable action or experience to reduce or alleviate feelings of guilt. For example, a man sends flowers to his fiancée after he embarrassed her at a cocktail party. A mother, who sent her son to his room because he broke a dish, decides to let him stay up an hour later to watch television.

10. *Projection:* often termed the "scapegoat" defense mechanism. The person rejects unwanted characteristics of self and assigns them to others. The person may blame others for faults, feelings, or shortcomings that are unacceptable to self. A man who is late for work states, "My wife forgot to set the alarm last night so I overslept." After spilling a glass of milk while playing cards with a friend, a 10-year-old tells his mother, "Johnny made me spill the milk. He told me to hurry up and play." A common retort is "You made me do it!" or "See what you made me do!"

11. *Symbolization:* an object, idea, or act represents another through some common aspect and carries the emotional feeling associated with the other. External objects may become outward representations of internal ideas, attitudes, or feelings. The engagement ring symbolizes love and a commitment to another person. Symbolization allows emotional self-expression.

12. *Regression:* retreating to past levels of behavior that reduce anxiety, allow one to feel more comfortable, and permit dependency. A 27-year-old woman acts like a 17-year-old on her first date with a fellow employee. A five-year-old boy who is toilet trained becomes incontinent during his father's hospitalization. Both people have regressed to earlier developmental levels to reduce feelings of anxiety.

13. *Sublimation:* the rechanneling of consciously intolerable or socially unacceptable impulses or behaviors into activities that are personally or socially acceptable. For example, a college student who has hostile feelings rechannels them by joining the debate team. An aggressive person volunteers to head the United Fund drive in the community.

14. *Denial:* the unconscious refusal to face thoughts, feelings, wishes, needs, or reality factors that are intolerable. Denial is also defined as blocking the awareness of reality by refusing to acknowledge its existence. A man who is told he has terminal cancer denies the diagnosis by telling his family he had a little tumor on his lung and his doctor "removed all of it." A woman denies that her marriage is failing by telling her estranged husband that all couples go through marital slumps and "things will be better tomorrow."

15. *Introjection:* attributing to oneself the good qualities of another; symbolically taking on the character trait of another person by "ingesting" the philosophy, ideas, knowledge, customs, mores, or attitudes of that person. Psychiatric patients have claimed to be Mary Magdalene, Jesus Christ, Moses, and other biblical or well known people. They have been observed dressing and acting like the personage they profess to be. One patient who claimed to be Moses grew a beard and long hair, wore a blanket and sandals, and read his Bible daily. He refused to participate in activities unless he was called Moses.

16. *Conversion:* the transferring of a mental conflict into a physical symptom to release tension or anxiety. For example, a woman experiences sudden blindness after witnessing a robbery. A man develops paralysis of his lower extremities after he learns that his wife has terminal cancer.

17. *Fantasy:* imagined events or mental images (*e.g.,* daydreaming) to express unconscious conflicts, gratify unconscious wishes, or prepare for anticipated future events. Individuals who play the lottery often fantasize what they would do if they won the jackpot. One state has named the lottery "Fantasy 5."

18. *Isolation:* the process of separating an unacceptable feeling, idea, or impulse from one's thoughts (also referred to as emotional isolation). For example, an oncologist is able to care for a terminally ill cancer patient by separating or isolating feelings or emotional reactions to the patient's inevitable death. The oncologist focuses on the treatment, not the prognosis.

19. *Dissociation:* the act of separating and *detaching* a strong, emotionally charged conflict from one's consciousness. This detached information is blocked from conscious awareness, which allows the person to defer or postpone experiencing an emotional impact or painful feelings. A woman who was raped was found wandering a busy highway in torn, disheveled clothing. When examined by the emergency room physician, the woman was exhibiting symptoms of traumatic amnesia. She separated and detached her emotional reaction to the rape from her consciousness.

20. *Intellectualization:* the act of transferring emotional concerns into the intellectual sphere. The person uses reasoning as a means of avoiding confrontation with unconscious conflicts and their stressful emotions. A man shows no emotional response to the "Dear John" letter he received from his fiancée; instead, he tells his roommate he is trying to figure out why she changed her mind about the upcoming wedding. The man is using intellectualization as a method of avoiding confrontation with his fiancée.

Defense mechanisms are categorized in various ways: healthy to unhealthy; sophisticated to primitive; most frequently to least frequently used. Such lists of defense mechanisms have been developed after extensive research of several psychological, sociologic, and psychiatric nursing texts and are based on the degree of personality disintegration and reality distortion that can occur when the mechanisms are used frequently. Although denial is listed as unhealthy, it can be a healthy mechanism if used for a short period during the grieving process. A woman who has just been informed of her husband's death may use denial as a temporary protective measure, postponing a confrontation with reality. If she is able to work through the denial stage and progress to the other stages of the grieving process, denial has not caused her personality to disintegrate. A middle-aged man who is told he has cirrhosis of the liver because of alcoholism ignores his doctor's recommendations and continues to drink. A few weeks later he is admitted to the hospital for portal hypertension and hemorrhaging esophageal varices. The use of denial has been detrimental to his health physically and emotionally and has distorted the reality of his prognosis, making it an unhealthy mechanism.

Significant Others or Support People

Although mental health can be maintained by means of positive interpersonal communication, facing one's emotions, and using ego defense mechanisms, people may reach out to other individuals or groups for support during periods of increased stress or anxiety. Such people are referred to as *significant others* or *support people*. For instance, labor and delivery is generally considered to be a normal, healthy biologic process; however, many women desire the presence or encouragement of a support person, one who assists the woman in coping with the stress and anxiety that may occur during the labor and delivery process as well as during the postpartum recovery period.

Support people or significant others can be anyone that the person feels comfortable with, trusts, and respects. A support person can act as a sounding board, simply listening while one vents various feelings or emotions, or he or she may interact as the need arises. People who enjoy coffee breaks with coworkers may look on these coworkers as people to whom they can relate their troubled feelings. Nurses need to help people to identify support people as well as to suggest people who might be supportive. A cancer patient who has just been told he has six months to live needs someone to help him work through the grieving process. A young mother hospitalized for emergency surgery would certainly benefit from the support of a significant other as she makes arrangements for the care of her children at home and prepares for surgery. A teenager whose parents are contemplating a divorce may need to explore feelings of guilt, anger, or resentment. A paraplegic just starting a new job may need a supportive person available 24 hours a day. These people could develop symptoms of mental illness if they are unable to cope with the various stressors they encounter. Crisis intervention, which generally occurs when someone is *unable to take action on his or her own* to solve a problem, is discussed in a separate chapter.

Summary

Various definitions of mental health and mental illness have been presented, as well as the factors that influence the development of mental health: (1) inherited characteristics; (2) nurturing during childhood; and (3) life circumstances. Agreed-on characteristics of mental health were summarized. A comparison of mental health and mental illness was explored. Misconceptions about mental illness were summarized. Methods of maintaining mental health, such as effective interpersonal communication, dealing directly with one's emotions, and using ego defense mechanisms were discussed. Five levels of communication were described to demonstrate one's willingness to communicate verbally with others. They include (1) cliché conversations; (2) reporting facts; (3) revealing ideas and judgments; (4) spontaneous, here-and-now emotions; and (5) open, honest communication. Healthy and unhealthy ways of dealing with one's emotions were compared, with focus on (1) awareness of one's emotional responses; (2) capability of experiencing negative emotions; (3) ability to examine the intensity of such emotions and sharing these emotional responses with others; and (4) ability to think through emotional reactions rather than letting the emotion rule one's actions. The dynamics of 20 defense mechanisms were discussed, including purpose, definitions, and examples. The importance of the presence of significant others or support people was explained.

Learning Activities

I. Clinical Activities
   A. Evaluate your nurse–patient interactions:
      1. What communication level did you use during these interactions?
      2. Identify defense mechanisms used by the patient and yourself. What purpose do you feel each served?
   B. Evaluate the reports you received on each assigned patient:
      1. Identify the communication level used during this report.
      2. Discuss your emotional reactions to the report.
      3. State how you handled these emotional reactions.
   C. Identify the support people or significant others available to each assigned patient. If none is available, what would you do?
II. Independent Activities
   A. Identify the following examples of defense mechanisms:
      1. Mary Jones has just been told her husband has cancer. She asks the doctor to repeat some laboratory work because she feels certain that the technician made a mistake.

2. When asked if she would care to talk about her husband's condition, Mary Jones says, "I'd rather not talk about it right now."

3. Mr. Jones died after a brief illness. When asked about the funeral, Mrs. Jones says, "I can't recall or remember anything about it except that there were a lot of people there."

4. Bill Smith imitates the characteristics and actions of one of the actors on his favorite television show.

5. Jane, a rather unattractive woman, dresses like a fashion plate to attract attention.

6. A person who has a strong desire to drink alcohol condemns the use of alcohol by others.

7. A person who has just been admitted to a mental institution states, "I'm really not sick. I'm just in here to get a rest."

8. Charlet Green always wanted to be a registered nurse. When she realized that her grades were not good enough to stay in the nursing program, she decided to become a medical receptionist.

9. Jim Williams, an executive whose day did not go smoothly, immediately criticizes his wife when he arrives home for dinner.

10. Ted Rule, who has difficulty playing basketball, was cut from the basketball team during tryouts. He states, "I got cut because the coach doesn't like me."

11. Carl White witnessed an accident while en route to work. He describes the accident to his secretary, who comments, "You're as cool as a cucumber. Didn't the accident upset you?"

12. A young prizefighter becomes very upset with his father and attempts to throw a right punch. His right arm becomes paralyzed as he tries to move it.

13. A person rechannels hostile impulses into debating, sports, or business activities.

14. Kevin Martin, age 22, sulks and pouts after his fiancée refuses to go to a boxing bout with him.

15. A shy 15-year-old girl daydreams about being glamorous, beautiful, and rich.

B. Read one of the following for personal growth:

1. E. Berne: *What Do You Say After You Say Hello?*
2. M. Edelson: *The Idea of a Mental Illness.*
3. M. James and D. Jongeward: *Born to Win.*
4. S. Jourard: *The Transparent Self: Self-Disclosure and Well-Being.*
5. J. Powell: *Happiness Is an Inside Job.*
6. R. Schuller: *Power Thoughts.*
7. L. Madow: *Anger: How to Recognize and Cope with It.*
8. V. Satir: *Self Esteem.*

Critical Thinking Questions

1. Select and describe examples of your own healthy behavior to illustrate three of Maslow's Characteristics of Mental Health. Pick one characteristic that you need to work on and create a care plan for yourself that will help you grow in this area.
2. You have been asked to make a presentation to a local ladies club whose members are especially interested in maintaining their mental health as they age. Outline a 20-minute presentation that includes basic information on mental health, misconceptions of mental illness, and maintenance of mental health.
3. The physician has just explained to your patient test results that indicate a need for additional medication. The physician hurries out and you observe that the patient is confused and upset. Identify on which of the five levels of communication the physician and patient are functioning. How might you use level 1 communication to gain the patient's trust? Describe the verbal and nonverbal components of your message.

Self-Test

1. List the factors that influence the development of mental health or mental illness.
2. Name a positive state in which a person is responsible, self-directive, and displays self-awareness.
3. Maternal deprevation and parental rejection are examples of:
4. List the characteristics of mental health as described by Maslow.
5. State at least five comparisons of mental health and mental illness.
6. Explain the five levels of communication as discussed in this chapter.
7. List ways to handle one's emotions in a positive manner while interacting with others.
8. Explain how defense mechanisms promote or help one to maintain mental health.
9. Match the following:

   1. Rationalization   a. "I'd rather not discuss my problems with you."
   2. Repression   b. "Sorry I'm late. My car kept stalling."
   3. Compensation   c. A laboratory technician is unhappy with the work and elects to become a medical secretary.
   4. Undoing   d. An accountant is unable to recall the reason for an argument with the boss.

5. Suppression	e. A paraplegic becomes a competitive arm wrestler.
6. Displacement	f. One yells at the dog after an argument with one's spouse.
7. Substitution	g. A doctor compliments the head nurse after criticizing the nurse earlier.
8. Symbolization	h. A 41-year-old dresses like a teenager.
9. Regression	i. A hostile, aggressive young man becomes a boxer.
10. Denial	j. One recites the Pledge of Allegiance or salutes the flag.
11. Conversion	k. A person living on the slope below a glacier disregards the danger it presents.
12. Sublimation	l. A young woman suddenly experiences chest pain after arguing with her husband.

10. Why are denial, projection, and introjection considered to be *unhealthy* ego defense mechanisms?

11. Explain the importance of a support person or significant other.

SELECTED REFERENCES

Altrocchi, J. (1980). *Abnormal behavior*. New York: Harcourt Brace Jovanovich.

American Psychiatric Association. (1980). *A psychiatric glossary* (5th ed.). Washington, DC: American Psychiatric Press.

Barry, P. D. (1994). *Mental health and mental illness* (5th ed.). Philadelphia: J. B. Lippincott.

Ebersole, P., & Hess, P. (1985). *Toward healthy aging: Human needs and human response*. St. Louis: C. V. Mosby.

Freud, A. (1946). *The ego and the mechanisms of defense*. New York: International Universities Press.

Johnson, B. S. (1997). *Adaptation and growth: Psychiatric–mental health nursing* (4th ed.). Philadelphia: Lippincott–Raven Publishers.

Maslow, A. (1954). *Motivation and personality*. New York: Harper & Row.

Powell, J. (1969). *Why am I afraid to tell you who I am?* Allen, TX: Argus Communications.

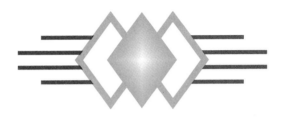

CHAPTER 2

HISTORY AND TRENDS IN PSYCHIATRIC NURSING

T he twenty years in this era (1915–1935) brought an awakening of interest in raising standards of care in psychiatric work, a growing realization of the role of nurses and the nursing profession in the needed improvements, and gradual inclusion in basic nursing curricula of the dominant psychiatric concepts available at this time.

Hildegard E. Peplau, 1956, in Smoyak & Rouslin, Classics (1982)

1 Define psychiatric nursing.

2 Discuss the treatment of mentally ill people during the Middle Ages.

3 Describe how the following people contributed to the history and trends in psychiatric nursing:

> Philippe Pinel
>
> Benjamin Rush
>
> Dorothea Dix
>
> Clifford Beers
>
> Linda Richards

4 State the educational objectives of psychiatric nursing during the early twentieth century as described by the National League for Nursing (NLN).

5 State the purpose of the "Standards of Psychiatric Mental Health Clinical Nursing Practice."

6 Describe the progress of psychiatric nursing during the twentieth century.

 Introduction

Psychiatric–mental health nursing is the diagnosis and treatment of human responses to actual or potential mental health problems. It is a specialized area of nursing practice that uses theories of human behavior as its scientific framework and requires the purposeful use of self as its art of expression. It is concerned with the promotion of optimum health for society. Comprehensive services focus on prevention of mental illness, health maintenance, management of or referral of mental and physical health problems, diagnosis and treatment of mental disorders and their sequelae, and rehabilitation (Haber & Billings, 1993).

According to the *Statement on Psychiatric–Mental Health Clinical Nursing Practice* (American Nurses' Association, 1994), psychiatric nurses must be able to make rapid comprehensive assessments; use effective problem-solving skills in making complex clinical decisions; act autonomously as well as collaboratively with other professionals; be sensitive to issues such as ethical dilemmas, cultural diversity, and access to mental health care for underserved populations; be comfortable working in decentralized settings; and be sophisticated about the costs and benefits of providing care within fiscal constraints (p. 7).

Early Civilization

Psychiatric nursing came into being between 1770 and 1880 during a series of reform movements concerning the treatment of persons with mental illness. Before that time, during the era of organic explanations, spirits were thought to possess the body and had to be driven away to effect a cure. The ancient Greeks, Romans, and Arabs believed emotional disorders were an organic dysfunction of the brain. They used a variety of treatment approaches such as sedation, good nutrition, good physical hygiene, music, and recreational activities.

During the fifth century B.C., Hippocrates described a variety of personalities or temperaments and proposed that mental illness was a disturbance of four body fluids or "humors," resulting alternately from heat, cold, dryness, and moisture. Aristotle concluded that the mind was associated with the heart, and a Greek physician, Galen, stated that the emotional or mental disorders were associated with the brain. The Greeks used temples as hospitals and provided an environment of fresh air, sunshine, and pure water to promote healing for the mentally ill. Riding, walking, and listening to the sounds of a waterfall were examples of therapeutic care.

 Middle Ages

During the Middle Ages, an era of alienation, social exclusion, and confinement, the humane treatment of mental illness suffered a setback while various theories pertaining to demonic possession became evident. Persons who displayed abnormal behavior were considered to be lunatics, witches, or demons possessed by evil spirits. Superstition, mysticism, magic, and witchcraft prevailed as patients were locked in asylums, flogged, starved, tortured, or subjected to the procedure of bloodletting. Beheading, hanging, and burning at the stake were common occurrences. Exorcism was practiced in some monasteries. People who were considered to be mad were isolated by confinement to large houses and institutions for social order. They were beaten for disobedience, chained, and placed in cages or closets. Patients suffering from a mental illness were subjected to cruel forms of torture. Physicians described symptoms of (1) depression, (2) paranoia, (3) delusions, (4) hysteria, and (5) nightmares. Persons displaying such symptoms were thought to be incompetent and potentially dangerous. The first mental hospital, Bethlehem Royal Hospital, was opened in England. Pronounced "Bedlam," the name came to symbolize the inhumane treatment of patients who were exhibited for twopence a look. Harmless inmates sought charity on the streets.

During the eighteenth century, an era of reason and observation, Philippe Pinel, a French physician, was placed in charge of La Bicêtre, a hospital for mentally ill persons in Paris. He began more humane treatment of patients with a mental illness by removing chains and advocating humane treatment instead. Pinel classified the patients according to observable behaviors, developed a case history on each, and kept records of their conversations with him.

Weyer, a German physician, is considered to be the first psychiatrist because of his descriptions of several diagnostic categories.

Eighteenth and Nineteenth Centuries

Benjamin Rush, often called "the father of American psychiatry," wrote the first American textbook on psychiatry and encouraged more humane treatment of persons with mental illness. In 1783, during an era of moral treatment, he joined the staff of Pennsylvania Hospital and insisted that intelligent, kind attendants be hired to read to the patients, talk to them, and share in their activities.

In 1843, Thomas Kirkbridge attempted to establish a training school for attendants at Pennsylvania Hospital to assist physicians in the care of mentally ill patients.

By 1872, New England Hospital for Women and Children and Women's Hospital of Philadelphia had established schools of nursing, but no psychiatric services were available. During this period, Dorothea Lynde Dix, a Boston teacher, spent much of her time working for improved conditions for mentally ill persons. She devoted her life to the cause of building state mental hospitals to meet the needs of patients suffering from mental disorders. The nurse's role was to oversee the care given and to ensure the smooth operation of the ward. Housekeeping duties, dietary management, and laundry care were considered nursing responsibilities.

As hospitals were established by the middle of the nineteenth century to provide long-term custodial care for mentally ill persons, humane treatment became more prevalent. In 1882, the first psychiatric training school was established at McLean Hospital in Belmont, Massachusetts. It was considered to be the first formally organized school for nurses in a hospital for mentally ill patients.

In 1890, trained nurses were employed on nursing staffs of state mental hospitals. These nurses were relieved of menial tasks and were able to develop their skills to provide therapeutic nursing care. By the end of the nineteenth century there was a growing appreciation of the therapeutic role of the psychiatric nurse. Duties included (1) assisting the physician; (2) administering sedative drugs; and (3) providing hydrotherapeutic measures (*e.g.*, hot and cold douches, continuous baths, and wet-sheet packs).

Twentieth Century

During the twentieth century, the mental health movement was strongly influenced by the publication of a book written by Clifford Beers, titled *A Mind That Found Itself* (1908). He spent approximately three years as a patient in mental institutions and described his observations and experiences. Beers used his influence to organize the National Society for Mental Hygiene in 1909, now known as the National Association for Mental Health. As a result of public awareness, large state mental hospitals were built in rural areas, where the patients could receive the benefits of fresh air, sunshine, and a rural environment.

In 1915, Linda Richards, the first graduate nurse in the United States and often referred to as "the first American psychiatric nurse," suggested that mentally ill patients receive the same quality care as physically ill patients. She stated that caring for the mentally ill required a degree of patience and tact that the average student did not possess. Clinical experience in state mental hospitals provided students with a chance to cultivate these qualities. Several advancements occurred as the National Committee on Mental Hygiene and the American Nurses' Association promoted study of mentally ill persons by publishing journal articles. Textbooks focusing on psychiatric nursing practice were written, and the National League for Nursing conventions discussed undergraduate psychiatric nursing education (1915–1935). These educational objectives included

1. Teaching the student nurse the relationship between physical and mental illness and the application of nursing principles to mental health nursing
2. Teaching the student nurse the causes of mental disease or illness and modern methods of treatment
3. Teaching the student nurse how to assess behaviors of patients who are mentally ill, so that they may recognize early signs or symptoms
4. Teaching the student nurse the relationship of environmental conditions and mental disorders
5. Teaching the student nurse to be resourceful, versatile, and adaptable while giving individualized care (Smoyak, 1982)

Clinical experiences in psychiatric hospitals were considered an essential part of the student nurses' basic experience and were standardized in 1937. Students were given the opportunity to care for patients with varying degrees of mental disorders, including organic diseases. Experiences focused on hydrotherapy; physical, occupational, recreational, and diversional therapy; and patient education. Nursing interventions included emphasizing cleanliness, proper elimination, and adequate nutrition, as well as supervising continuous baths to promote relaxation.

By 1939, approximately one half of all nursing schools provided psychiatric nursing courses for students, but participation in such courses did not become a requirement for nursing licensure until 1955.

Phenothiazines and other major tranquilizers were developed in the treatment of major symptoms of psychoses, enabling patients to be more responsive to therapeutic care. Open-door policies were implemented in large mental institutions, allowing patients to leave the units or wards under supervision.

In 1963, the Community Mental Health Act authorized funding for the establishment of community health centers to provide the following services to the public: (1) emergency mental health care, such as crisis centers and telephone hot lines; (2) inpatient care or hospitalization; (3) partial hospitalization such as daycare centers and therapeutic communities; (4) after-care, including halfway houses and foster homes; and (5) consultation services, as provided in counseling centers. The deinstitutionalization of patients from state mental hospitals to community living was considered a positive move; however, lack of federal funding resulted in an increase of the number of those who were homeless. The Community Mental Health Act played an important part in the specialization of psychiatric nursing services.

During the present century, psychiatric nursing also began to evolve as a clinical specialty. Nurses were previously involved as managers and coordinators of activities as they provided therapeutic care based on the medical model. By advanced study and clinical practice experienced in a master's program in psychiatric nursing, clinical specialists and nurse practitioners are able to gain expert knowledge in the care and prevention of psychiatric disorders.

Box 2-1 summarizes other events influencing psychiatric nursing. Box 2-2 (on p. 30) provides research examples of the biologic aspects of mental illness.

 ## Standards of Psychiatric–Mental Health Clinical Nursing Practice

In 1967, the *Statement on Psychiatric Nursing Practice* was published by the American Nurses' Association (ANA). A revision followed in 1976. Belief that scope of practice is linked to practice standards resulted in the publication of *Standards of Psychiatric–Mental Health Nursing Practice* in 1982. Broader general standards of nursing practice are delineated in the *Standards of Clinical Nursing Practice* (ANA, 1991b).

Standards are authoritative statements used by the nursing profession to describe the responsibilities for which nurses are accountable. They provide

BOX 2-1 Other Events Influencing Psychiatric Nursing

The following is a chronologic listing of other important events influencing psychiatric nursing:

1856 to 1929 Emil Kraepelin differentiated manic–depression psychosis from schizophrenia and stated that schizophrenia was incurable.

1856 to 1939 Sigmund Freud introduced psychoanalytic theory and therapy. He explained human behavior in psychological terms and proved that behavior can be changed in certain situations.

1857 to 1939 Eugene Bleuler described the psychotic disorder of schizophrenia (formerly referred to as *dementia praecox*).

1870 to 1937 Alfred Adler focused on the area of psychosomatic medicine, referring to organ inferiority as the causative factor.

1875 to 1961 Carl Jung described the human psyche as consisting of a social mask (persona), hidden personal characteristics (shadow), feminine identification in men (anima), masculine identification in women (animus), and the innermost center of the personality (self).

1920 Harriet Bailey wrote first textbook on psychiatric nursing, Nursing Mental Diseases.

1930s Insulin shock therapy, pentylenetetrazol (Metrazol) therapy, electroconvulsive therapy, and prefrontal lobotomy were introduced to treat mentally ill patients with psychotic disorders.
International Committee for Mental Hygiene was established.
The Hill-Burton Act funded the building of psychiatric units.

1940s The Mental Health Act of 1946 set up funding of graduate nursing programs to prepare clinical specialists.

1946 to 1971 Care of mentally ill persons was brought into the mainstream of health care.
National Mental Health Act provided funds for professional training programs.
World Federation for Mental Health provided funds for research and education.

(continued)

BOX 2-1 Other Events Influencing Psychiatric Nursing (Continued)

1947	Helen Render wrote *Nurse–Patient Relationships in Psychiatry*.

1947   Helen Render wrote *Nurse–Patient Relationships in Psychiatry*.

1949   The National Institute of Mental Health was established to (1) provide grants-in-aid; (2) fund training programs and demonstration projects; and (3) provide support for research.

1952   Hildegard E. Peplau wrote *Interpersonal Relations in Nursing*, a text that provided the basis for the development of therapeutic roles in nurse–patient relationships. This book was of paramount importance in the development of psychiatric nursing as a profession.

1955   Joint Commission on Mental Illness and Health was developed to study and evaluate needs and resources.

1961   World Psychiatric Association examined the social consequences of mental illness.

1963 to 1979   Economic Opportunity Act stressed improvement of social environments to prevent the development of mental illness.

The Mental Retardation Facilities and Community Mental Health Centers Construction Act provided federal funds to help state and local agencies decentralize mental health care; provided community services and facilities to treat substance abusers; and proposed that community mental health programs include special programs to treat children and the elderly.

Fifty graduate psychiatric nursing programs were established in the United States.

Private psychiatric hospitals and psychiatric units were established in general hospitals.

Insurance companies provided coverage for psychiatric care.

Deinstitutionalization and community living for mental patients was emphasized, focusing on teaching them activities of daily living (ADLs) and self-care.

Canadian and American nurses laid groundwork for formation of North American Nursing Diagnosis Association.

BOX 2-1 Other Events Influencing Psychiatric Nursing (Continued)

1980s Mental Health Systems Act (1980), designed to strengthen existing community efforts and to develop new initiatives, was never implemented due to 1981 legislation.
Omnibus Budget Reconciliation Act (1981) drastically curtailed federal funding for health care services.
Emphasis placed on American Nurses' Association (ANA) specialty certification exam.

1990s Insurance companies made drastic cuts in coverage for psychiatric care.
Formation of National Alliance for the Mentally Ill (NAMI).
Greater emphasis placed on the biologic aspects of mental illness and on advances in neuropharmacology (Box 2-2).

direction for professional nursing practice and a framework for the evaluation of practice. They also define the nursing profession's accountability to the public and the client outcomes for which nurses are responsible.

Standards of Psychiatric–Mental Health Clinical Nursing Practice (ANA, 1994) is divided into two sections, *Standards of Care* and *Standards of Professional Performance*.

Standards of Care

Standard I. Assessment The psychiatric–mental health nurse collects client health data.

Standard II. Diagnosis The psychiatric–mental health nurse analyzes the assessment data in determining diagnoses.

Standard III. Outcome Identification The psychiatric–mental health nurse identifies expected outcomes individualized to the client.

Standard IV. Planning The psychiatric–mental health nurse develops a plan of care that prescribes interventions to attain expected outcomes.

Standard V. Implementation The psychiatric–mental health nurse implements the interventions identified in the plan of care.

BOX 2-2 Examples of Research on Biologic Aspects of Mental Illness

Examples of research presented at the 17th Collegium Internationale Psychopharmacologicum Congress included the following findings:

- Schizophrenia may be caused by a virus, autoimmune phenomena, or frontal lobe dysfunction.
- Chronic alcoholics (approximately 60%) may experience cerebral atrophy, cortical shrinkage, and ventricular dilatation in the frontal lobe. Electroencephalograms are poorly synchronized.
- Increased episodes of depression and mania cause changes in brain structure and function, which lead to treatment-resistant depression.
- Alcoholics can be delineated as type A or B subgroups based on the disease's etiologic elements, onset and course, presenting symptoms, and drinking pattern.
- A combination of electroconvulsive therapy and lithium may achieve rapid control of an acute manic episode.
- Prozac may significantly improve the clinical symptoms of bulimia.
- Endozepine-4, a newly described brain chemical, is likened to endogenous diazepam (Valium).
- Untreated hypothyroidism may play an unheralded role in treatment resistance and the development of rapid cycling in bipolar patients.
- Clozaril has proven to be a safe, effective drug for psychotic patients with a history of neuroleptic malignant syndrome.
- Desyrel and Eldepryl have proved effective in the management of behavioral symptoms of Alzheimer's disease.
- Serotonin reuptake inhibitors such as Prozac augment previously ineffective tricyclic therapy in the treatment of depression.

(Other examples are included within the text.)

Standard Va. Counseling The psychiatric–mental health nurse uses counseling interventions to assist clients in improving or regaining their previous coping abilities, fostering mental health, and preventing mental illness and disability.

Standard Vb. Milieu Therapy The psychiatric–mental health nurse provides, structures, and maintains a therapeutic environment in collaboration with the client and other health care providers.

Standard Vc. Self-Care Activities The psychiatric–mental health nurse structures interventions around the client's activities of daily living to foster self-care and mental and physical well-being.

Standard Vd. Psychobiological Interventions The psychiatric–mental health nurse uses knowledge of psychobiologic interventions and applies clinical skills to restore the client's health and prevent future disability.

Standard Ve. Health Teaching The psychiatric–mental health nurse, through health teaching, assists clients in achieving satisfying, productive, and healthy patterns of living.

Standard Vf. Case Management The psychiatric–mental health nurse provides case management to coordinate comprehensive health services and ensure continuity of care.

Standard Vg. Health Promotion and Health Maintenance The psychiatric–mental health nurse employs strategies and interventions to promote and maintain mental health and prevent mental illness.

The following interventions (Vh–Vj) may be performed only by the certified specialist in psychiatric–mental health nursing.

Standard Vh. Psychotherapy The certified specialist in psychiatric–mental health nursing uses individual, group, and family psychotherapy, child psychotherapy, and other therapeutic treatments to assist clients in fostering mental health, preventing mental illness and disability, and improving or regaining previous health status and functional abilities.

Standard Vi. Prescription of Pharmacologic Agents The certified specialist uses prescription of pharmacologic agents in accordance with the state nursing practice act, to treat symptoms of psychiatric illness and improve functional health status.

Standard Vj. Consultation The certified specialist provides consultation to health care providers and others to influence the plans of care for clients, and to enhance the abilities of others to provide psychiatric and mental health care and effect change in systems.

Standard VI. Evaluation The psychiatric–mental health nurse evaluates the client's progress in attaining expected outcomes.

Standards of Professional Performance

Standard I. Quality of Care The psychiatric–mental health nurse systematically evaluates the quality of care and effectiveness of psychiatric–mental health nursing practice.

Standard II. Performance Appraisal The psychiatric–mental health nurse evaluates her or his own psychiatric–mental health nursing practice in relation to professional practice standards and relevant statutes and regulations.

Standard III. Education The psychiatric–mental health nurse acquires and maintains current knowledge in nursing practice.

Standard IV. Collegiality The psychiatric–mental health nurse contributes to the professional development of peers, colleagues, and others.

Standard V. Ethics The psychiatric–mental health nurse's decisions and actions on behalf of clients are determined in an ethical manner.

Standard VI. Collaboration The psychiatric–mental health nurse collaborates with the client, significant others, and health care providers in giving care.

Standard VII. Research The psychiatric–mental health nurse contributes to nursing and mental health through the use of research.

Standard VIII. Resource Utilization The psychiatric–mental health nurse considers factors related to safety, effectiveness, and cost in planning and delivering client care.

Psychiatric Nursing in the Twentieth Century

Schools of nursing offer a variety of programs in psychiatric nursing. Licensed practical nursing schools generally address the topics of human behavior or mental health and mental illness, and may integrate mental health concepts into various courses such as pediatrics, obstetrics, and the aging process. Psychiatric nursing clinical experience usually is not offered in such one-year programs, although state board examinations do include questions pertaining to basic mental health concepts. If a licensed practical nurse elects to continue training to become a registered nurse, psychiatric nursing experience needs to be obtained in a ladder program.

Associate degree programs may offer a 5- to 10-week course in psychiatric nursing with or without clinical rotation and psychiatric or mental health settings. Some schools integrate psychiatric nursing concepts throughout the two-year program, after core courses in developmental or abnormal psychology. Psychiatric nursing experience may occur in a medical–psychiatric unit, private psychiatric hospital, state psychiatric facility, or community mental health setting. Emphasis is on nursing intervention under the direction of a more experienced registered nurse.

Baccalaureate schools usually provide more time for psychiatric nursing and clinical experiences, and place a greater emphasis on theoretical foundations, the assessment process, statistics, group dynamics, patient and family education, and the nurse's role in preventive care.

Graduate schools offering a master's degree in psychiatric or mental health nursing usually require 48 to 50 hours of core courses, clinical experience, research, electives, and a practicum. Available courses may focus on leadership, life cycle, conceptual bases, physiologic bases, and client assessment. The graduate student may elect to become a clinical nurse specialist or a nurse practitioner, depending on the courses available.

Currently, the field of psychiatric nursing offers a variety of opportunities for specialization. Examples include nurse liaison in the general hospital, therapist in private practice, consultant, educator, expert witness in legal issues, employee assistance counselor, mental health provider in long-term care facilities, and association with a mobile psychiatric triage unit.

Psychiatric nursing experience as a student provides a valuable foundation for a variety of career opportunities after graduation. The following lists such positions and gives examples of how psychiatric nursing experience can be an asset.

Career Opportunities	Examples
Obstetric nursing	Helping the mother in labor and/or support person cope with anxiety or stress during labor and delivery
	Providing support to bereaved parents in the event of fetal demise, inevitable abortion, or the birth of an infant with congenital anomalies
	Providing support to an unwed mother who must decide whether to keep her child or give the child up for adoption

(continued)

Career Opportunities	Examples
Oncologic nursing	Helping cancer patients or other terminally ill individuals on oncology units to work through the grieving process
	Providing support groups for families of terminally ill patients
Industrial (occupational health) nursing	Implementing or participating in industrial substance abuse programs for employees and/or their families
	Providing crisis intervention during an industrial accident or the acute onset of a physical or mental illness (e.g., heart attack or anxiety attack)
	Teaching stress management
Public health nursing	Assessing the person both physically and psychologically (e.g., the newly diagnosed diabetic may develop a low self-concept, or the recovering stroke patient may exhibit symptoms of depression due to a slow recovery)
Office nursing	Assisting the patient in explaining somatic or emotional concerns during the assessment process
	Providing support with the problem-solving process when people call the office and the physician is unavailable
	Acting as a community resource person
Emergency room nursing	Providing crisis intervention as the need arises (e.g., during natural disasters, accidents, or unexpected illnesses causing increased anxiety, stress, or immobilization)

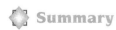 Summary

Psychiatric nursing began to emerge as a nursing subspecialty around 1880 with the establishment of schools of nursing specializing in psychiatric training. This chapter focused on the history of and trends in psychiatry and psychiatric nursing by discussing the treatment of mentally ill persons during the periods of early civilization, the Middle Ages, and the eighteenth, nineteenth, and twentieth centuries, mentioning the contributions of Hippocrates, Aristotle, Galen, Pinel, Weyer, Rush, Kirkbridge, Dix, Beers, and Richards. The *Standards of Psychiatric–Mental Health Clinical Nursing Practice* were included, as well as a chronologic listing of important acts and events influencing psychiatric nursing. An overview of student psychiatric nursing experiences for licensed practical nurses, associate degree nurses, baccalaureate nurses, and graduate students was presented. Examples of how a psychiatric nursing experience can be an asset for graduate nurses working in obstetric, oncologic, industrial, public health, office, and emergency room settings were given.

Critical Thinking Questions

1. During the Middle Ages, persons who displayed abnormal behavior were often treated inhumanely. Today, many mentally ill persons end up on the streets of our large cities. Analyze how society today handles persons with mental illness and compare the social, political, and economic issues that affect care for this segment of the population.
2. The American Nurses' Association issued *Standards of Psychiatric–Mental Health Nursing Practice* in 1982. Why are standards of practice necessary and what is the nurse's responsibility regarding standards?
3. The 1981 Omnibus Budget Reconciliation Act curtailed the funding of the Mental Health Systems Act of the previous year. This loss of funding prevented the implementation and strengthening of community efforts for mental health programs. How might nurses become aware of political, social, and economic events that could affect this patient population? How might nurses advocate for patients who have been lost from programs because of lack of funding?

Self-Test

1. Define psychiatric nursing.
2. State how the following pertain to the history of psychiatric nursing:
   a. Era of organic explanations
   b. Era of alienation, social exclusion, and confinement
3. Match the following:

1. Hippocrates	a.	Devoted time to the cause of building state mental hospitals
2. Philippe Pinel	b.	Removed chains from mentally ill patients and advocated the use of kindness
3. Benjamin Rush	c.	First graduate nurse and first American psychiatric nurse
4. Dorothea Dix	d.	Wrote the first American textbook on psychiatry
5. Linda Richards	e.	Proposed that mental illness was a disturbance of four fluids or "humors"

4. State the origin of the word "Bedlam."
5. Compare psychiatric nursing duties during the time Dorothea Dix worked for improved conditions for mentally ill persons and 1890, when trained nurses were employed in state mental institutions.
6. Discuss how Clifford Beers influenced psychiatry and psychiatric nursing.
7. List the educational objectives of psychiatric nursing as stated by the National League for Nursing conventions (1915–1935).
8. Discuss the function of the Community Mental Health Act of 1963.
9. Review the "Standards of Psychiatric–Mental Health Clinical Nursing Practice" and summarize the role of the psychiatric nurse.
10. State the contributions of the following people to psychiatric nursing:
    a. Harriet Bailey
    b. Helen Render
    c. Hildegard E. Peplau
11. Discuss the application of psychiatric nursing concepts in other fields of nursing, such as
    a. Emergency room nursing
    b. Public health nursing
    c. Oncologic nursing
    d. Obstetric nursing

SELECTED REFERENCES

American Nurses' Association. (1982). *Standards of psychiatric and mental health nursing practice*. Kansas City: Author.

American Nurses' Association. (1991b). *Standards of clinical nursing practice*. Kansas City: Author.

American Nurses' Association. (1992). *Working definition: Nurses in advanced clinical practice*. Washington, DC: Author.

American Nurses' Association. (1994). *A statement on psychiatric–mental health clinical nursing practice and standards of psychiatric–mental health clinical nursing practice*. Washington, DC: American Nurses Publishing.

Banes, J. S. (1983, March). An ex-patient's perspective of psychiatric treatment. *Journal of Psychosocial Nursing and Mental Health Services*.

Gaines, J. E. (1995, Spring/Summer). Who's on first? *Advanced Practice Nurse*.

Haber, J., & Billings, C. (1993, February). Primary mental health care: A vision for the future of psychiatric-mental health nursing. ANA Council Perspectives.

Hahn, M. S. (1995, July). Turning back time. *Advance for Nurse Practitioners*.

Ray, G. L., & Hardin, S. (1995, September). Advanced practice nursing: Playing a vital role. *Advanced Practice Nurse Sourcebook*.

Robinette, A. L. (1996, July). PCLNs: Who are they: How can they help you? *American Journal of Nursing*.

Smoyak, S., & Rouslin, S. (Eds.). (1982). *A collection of classics in psychiatric nursing literature*. Thorofare, NJ: Charles B. Slack.

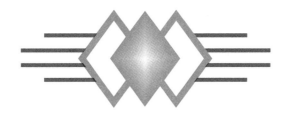

CHAPTER 3

COMMUNITY MENTAL HEALTH

C ommunity mental health describes a change in the focus of psychiatric–mental health care from the individual to the individual in interaction with his environment. It also describes a place where comprehensive care is delivered.

Bloom, 1977

1 Define community mental health.

2 Discuss the significant events in the history of community mental health.

3 Identify the major concepts of community mental health.

4 Compare the different types of community support services.

5 Explain the programs of the community mental health center.

6 Describe the varied roles of the community mental health nurse.

Introduction

During the 7th Annual U.S. Psychiatric and Mental Health Congress, November 17 through November 20, 1994 in Washington, DC, the topic of mental health financing and health care reform was addressed. S. Sharfstein, MD noted that care and treatment of mental illness and substance abuse is being transformed by the economics of health care. The managed care "revolution" is a result of cost-containment pressures and a pervasive sense of insecurity on the part of Americans who worry about being able to afford needed medical as well as psychiatric care. This "revolution," the formation of Health Maintenance Organizations (HMOs), Preferred Provider Organizations (PPOs), and a reduction in government funding of mental health services through Medicare and Medicaid, will have a direct bearing on the degree of quality and innovation preserved in the community mental health environment.

Community mental health can best be described as "a movement, an ideology or a perspective that promotes early, comprehensive treatment in the community, accessible to all, and that derives its values, beliefs, knowledge and practices from the behavioral and social sciences" (Panzetta, 1985). The type of mental health services that are provided in the community may include emergency psychiatric care/crisis intervention; partial hospitalization and day treatment programs; case management; community-based residential treatment programs; aftercare and rehabilitation; consultation and support; and psychiatric home care. The primary goal of community mental health is to deliver comprehensive care by a professional multidisciplinary team using innovative treatment approaches. Miller (1981) describes five major ideological beliefs influencing community mental health: (1) involvement and concern with the total community population; (2) emphasis on primary prevention; (3) orientation toward social treatment goals; (4) comprehensive continuity of care; and (5) belief that community mental health should involve total citizen participation in need determination, policy establishment, service delivery, and evaluation of programs.

 ## History of Community Mental Health

The community mental health movement, often considered to be the third revolution in psychiatry, gained a prominent position in the early 1960s. Before this time, psychiatric treatment had occurred primarily in institutions or hospitals. Examples of the few very early community programs included a farm program established in New Hampshire in 1855; a cottage plan in Illinois in 1877; and in 1885 community boarding homes for patients who were discharged from the state hospitals in Massachusetts. Although successful, these initial efforts were limited until after World War II, when the social, economic, and political factors were favorable to stimulate the community mental health movement.

In 1946, the National Mental Health Act provided funding for the states to develop mental health programs outside of the state hospitals, and for the establishment of the National Institute of Mental Health (NIMH) in 1949. Early in 1952, an international committee from the World Health Organization (WHO) defined the components of community mental health as out-patient treatment, rehabilitation, and partial hospitalization. Later in that decade, state and federally funded programs mandated the broadening of services to include 24-hour emergency walk-in services, community clinics for state hospital patients, traveling mental health clinics, community vocational rehabilitation programs, halfway houses, and night and weekend hospitals. In October of 1963, president John F. Kennedy, who supported the improvement of mental health care, approved major legislation significantly strengthening community mental health. This legislation, the Community Mental Health Centers Act, authorized the nationwide development of community-based mental health centers (CMHCs). It was believed that these centers would provide more effective and comprehensive mental health treatment than the often remote state-run institutions that previously served as the primary place of care for the psychiatric patient.

In conjunction with these congressional mandates, states began the massive process of "deinstitutionalization," moving chronically mentally ill patients from the state hospitals back to their community homes or to community-supervised facilities. This movement, a controversial and much-debated social policy, occurred within the framework of the major and comprehensive social reforms of the 1960s. The federally funded CMHCs were also mandated to provide all of the comprehensive services for this new population, some of whom had been in institutions for as many as 20 to 25 years. Throughout the 1970s and 1980s, the CMHCs and the services they provided expanded; today their primary focus is the treatment of the chronic psychiatric client.

The positive and negative effects of deinstitutionalization continue significantly to influence the field of community mental health. Unfortunately, the federal government has not provided a financial budget necessary to meet the needs of seriously ill mental health patients.

Concepts of Community Mental Health

Panzetta (1985) has documented eight fundamental concepts of mental health that he and others believe are the foundation for community mental health:

1. The use of a multidisciplinary team, with its members consisting of psychiatrist, psychologist, social workers, nurses, and mental health counselors
2. The prevention of mental illness
3. Early detection and treatment
4. A comprehensive, multifaceted treatment program
5. Continuity of care
6. Group and family therapy
7. Environmental and social support and intervention
8. Community participation, support, and control

In their well documented description of overall community health services, Solomon and Davis (1985) discuss the belief that community mental health is based on identified needs of the specific population. The results of their comprehensive survey indicate that over 85% of the community population identified had a need for community mental health services. Crosby (1987) wrote that community-focused mental health services were based on the premise that confined institutional living did not assist the resident with a psychiatric illness to acquire the needed skills to reintegrate into community life. He claimed that community treatment could provide the wide range of needed services, would ensure more support from family and friends, and could strengthen the psychiatric client's need for independence and self-care. Crosby further promoted the theory that all community mental health should be based on the concepts of structure, support, and conceptual awareness for adaptation to societal norms and expectations.

Types of Community Mental Health Services

Psychiatric Emergency Care: Psychiatric Triage

The Community Mental Health Act of 1963 mandated that the community make the necessary provisions for psychiatric emergency care. It was believed that accessible emergency services were needed to provide crisis intervention, to prevent unnecessary hospitalizations, and to attempt to decrease chronicity and dependence on institutional care. At that time, providing these critical support services placed additional pressure on communities because of the increased population of chronically mentally ill patients residing outside of institutions. Jails were often inappropriate, psychiatrists were either over-burdened or uncooperative, and mental health centers operated only during regular business hours. Community mental health administrators and clinicians responded either by establishing an emergency clinic at the local community mental health center or by contracting with a general hospital in the same catchment area to provide the emergency care on a 24-hour-a-day basis. Because of the psychiatric client's increasing reliance on these emergency services within the past decade, hospitals have assumed a key role in the provision and management of crisis intervention and psychiatric emergency care. Nurius (1983–1984) notes that they often function as the "revolving door" between patients and the mental health services network and are oriented toward providing crisis stabilization services. The research that Nurius and others have conducted indicates that the people who most use the community-based emergency services tend to be young, unemployed veterans of the mental health system, and either chronically mentally ill or chronic substance abusers.

The psychiatric emergency room is often located in a separate room or a specially allocated section of the hospital emergency room. The triage staff members may include a variety of psychiatric disciplines: psychiatric nurses, social workers, mental health counselors, and marriage and family therapists. The primary focus is on crisis stabilization through employment of the therapeutic interview, and immediate mobilization of available community- and client-centered resources and support systems. An advanced registered nurse practitioner or clinical nurse specialist may supervise the triage area. The nurse may have a collaborative agreement with a consulting psychiatrist to prescribe necessary psychotropic medication or to support admission to a psychiatric inpatient unit. The staff who provide these critical services must be knowledgeable and skillful in the areas of (1) psychiatric assessment, including the administration of a complete mental status exam; (2) application of crisis intervention theories; (3) individual and family counseling; and (4) resources in the specific community that can provide emergency housing, financial aid, and medical and psychiatric hospitalization.

Many small community hospitals do not have in-house psychiatric services. Clinical nurse specialists or advanced registered nurse practitioners may serve as psychiatric nurse liaisons in the general hospital setting. They may be employed by the hospital or have a contractual agreement to provide psychiatric services as needed. This nurse liaison may assist with discharge planning and provide follow-up care when indicated.

Day Treatment/Partial Hospitalization

The first day-treatment program (also known as day hospital or partial hospitalization) in North America was established in Montreal, Canada, shortly after the end of World War II. Day-treatment programs are usually located either in or near the community mental health center or in an inpatient treatment facility (*i.e.*, psychiatric hospital). The partial hospitalization program, or day-treatment program, is usually a 30- to 90-day treatment program that operates for 6 to 8 hours per day, 5 days a week. Most of these programs are able to accommodate up to 25 persons who are not dysfunctional enough to require hospitalization but who need more structured and intensive treatment than traditional outpatient services alone can provide.

These community partial hospitalization programs are usually supervised by a psychiatrist and are staffed by psychologists, social workers, psychiatric nurses, family therapists, activities therapists, and mental health counselors. Multidisciplinary assessments usually include a physical exam; a complete psychiatric evaluation; psychological, educational, and nursing assessments; a substance abuse assessment; and a psychosocial history. A treatment plan, which is usually formulated within 10 days of admission to the program, is reviewed weekly by the multidisciplinary treatment team.

Each day-treatment program offers a variety of treatment methods that may include

1. Individual therapy
2. Group therapy
3. Therapeutic education or vocational training
4. Drug and alcohol education
5. Recreational therapy
6. Expressive therapies (art, movement, psychodrama)
7. Family therapy/multifamily groups
8. Client and family education

Research has shown that, as these day-treatment/partial hospitalization programs have increased in communities, they have been very successful. Such programs have resulted in fewer hospitalizations, a decrease in psychiatric symptoms, more successful work experiences, and better overall social functioning in the community. In addition, with the current climate of containment for health care costs and with the utilization of limited health care resources coming under increasing scrutiny, there is an increased awareness that the partial hospitalization programs will assume a major role within community mental health systems.

Psychiatric Services in Long-term Care

The long-term care environment is rapidly changing as a result of the development of subacute units and transitional care and rehabilitation services. The prevalence of psychiatric disorders has increased. Delivery of services is shaped by federal legislation and evolving regulations. The Nursing Home Reform Act of the Omnibus Budget Reconciliation Act of 1987 sets forth guidelines regarding the admission of persons with psychiatric disorders. In response to these guidelines, psychiatric and psychological services are now provided in most facilities. Advanced registered nurse practitioners working in collaboration with physicians or psychiatrists are reimbursed for services including consultation or diagnostic interview, follow-up visits to monitor response to medication, brief individual psychotherapy, full individual psychotherapy, group psychotherapy, family psychotherapy, and consultation with family/medical staff. The patients most in need of nursing home admission are those who also have the greatest need for psychiatric services.

Residential Programs

In many communities, residential placements are a key element in the services provided by community mental health boards. They have become one of the leading areas of program expansion in the care of the psychiatric client. Numerous patients now are able to leave a long-term hospital or institutional care for another structured living situation. Historically, the first community program of this type, called Tueritian House, was established in New York City shortly after World War II. Today, there are thousands of innovative residential treatment programs throughout the United States. In 1982, the American Psychiatric Association issued a typology of these community care residential facilities:

1. *Group homes:* halfway houses, therapeutic community homes, group foster homes
2. *Personal care homes:* boarding homes, congregate care facilities, social rehabilitation residential programs

3. *Foster homes:* domiciliary care, group foster homes, transitional care facilities
4. *Satellite housing:* apartment clusters, transitional residences, independent living with aftercare support
5. *Independent living:* lodgings, single-room occupancy with therapeutic support

Each type of residential program offers different support services and is staffed in a variety of ways. The services provided include shelter, food, house-keeping, personal care and supervision, health care, individual or group counseling, vocational training or employment, and leisure and socialization opportunities. The staffing for these residential programs also varies considerably, ranging from professional psychiatric staff being present at all times in the facility to provide support and supervision, to staff being only on call for crisis intervention and stabilization. Continued research into these programs has led many community mental health experts to conclude that they are a successful means of therapeutic support and intervention, and are particularly effective with the chronically mentally ill client (Talbott, 1985).

Psychiatric Home Care

In the 1960s, in conjunction with the increasing emphasis on community mental health, programs were established to treat the psychiatric client at home with visiting nurse home care. One of these early projects, in Louisville, Kentucky, had clients with acute schizophrenia living at home with their families. These clients were visited at least weekly by a public health nurse or a nurse from the local Visiting Nurses Association. The nurse's role was to conduct a psychiatric assessment, dispense medication, and provide individual and family counseling. In addition, home clients consulted with a psychiatrist every few months for evaluation. During the 1970s, these types of community programs declined as the focus increasingly centered on residential and day-treatment programs; however, in the latter part of the 1980s, the concept of psychiatric home care was revitalized as community resources became scarcer. Pelletier (1988) writes that "psychiatric home care can fill the gap in the mental health continuum of care by providing nursing resources as adjunctive to outpatient treatment." Research further supports the concept that home care is an extremely valuable service and economically feasible; it also presents a significant opportunity for psychiatric–mental health nursing.

Independent psychiatric–mental health nurse practitioners who have acquired contracts with various insurance companies or who are providers for Medicare and Medicaid are able to provide psychiatric services in the home environment. Provisions have been made by Medicare and Medicaid to use a billing code that indicates a "house call" was made. Individuals who have had a chronic psychiatric illness for at least two years may apply for Medicare or Medicaid health care coverage. Therefore, patients may be children, adolescents, adults, or elderly persons. Mobile crisis center units, home health care agencies, and the Visiting Nurses Association all provide psychiatric care in private homes, assisted living units, and group homes.

The Health Care Financing Administration (HCFA) has established criteria for the provision of psychiatric home care services:

1. A psychiatrist must certify that the client is homebound.
2. The client must have a DSM-IV psychiatric diagnosis that is acute or an acute exacerbation of a chronic illness.
3. The client must require the specialized knowledge, skills, and abilities of a psychiatric registered nurse.

Richie and Lusky (1987) have identified three major client populations that use this community service. The first group is the elderly who do not have histories of chronic mental illness but who are experiencing acute psychological and developmental problems. A common client in this group is an elderly person who lives alone and is exhibiting increasing physical limitations that cause severe isolation and major depression. The second population is the chronically mentally ill client who requires long-term medication and ongoing supportive counseling. Such a client is often diagnosed with schizophrenia, bipolar illness, depression, or schizoaffective disorders. The third population is made up of clients in need of crisis intervention and short-term psychotherapy. Richie and Lusky define the major functions of psychiatric home care as the provision of comprehensive care, ongoing interdisciplinary collaboration, and accountability to client and community.

Role of Community Mental Health Center in Aftercare and Rehabilitation

The CMHC also provides support and rehabilitation for the client who has been recently discharged from a psychiatric hospital. Many of these clients require a minimum of support with weekly or biweekly individual or family therapy and medication evaluation. Most of these psychiatric clients, however, represent the chronically mentally ill population. They experience repeat hospitalizations and require a diversity of support functions from the treatment team at the CMHC. Therapeutic services that most CMHCs provide include

1. *Medication.* The use of psychotropic medication is generally regarded as essential in the treatment of chronically ill clients. The individual often continues this medication regime after the acute symptoms have subsided and he or she returns to the community. It is the responsibility of the CMHC psychiatrist or advanced registered nurse practitioner to conduct a full medication assessment and to supervise a safe and strategic medication care plan.
2. *Individual and family therapy.* Throughout the past several years, there have been many significant developments in the field of community-based family therapy with the psychiatric client. Family interventions focus on altering the emotional climate within the family and reducing stress. Significant emphasis is placed on educating the family about the client's illness and teaching more effective communication and problem-solving skills.
3. *Crisis intervention.* The psychiatric client in the community is vulnerable to stress and often lacks the self-care skills to cope with unexpected stressful situations. The CMHCs usually assume responsibility for 24-hour crisis intervention by contracting with hospital emergency rooms or by establishing their own hot line or psychiatric emergency room.
4. *Social skills training.* Many of the CMHC clients lack social skills and experience much difficulty in maintaining good interpersonal relationships. In response to this need, many centers have established social skills training programs that use treatment methods such as role playing and individual and group therapy to teach new interpersonal skills.
5. *Medical care.* It is estimated that between 30% and 60% of psychiatric clients recently discharged from a psychiatric hospital suffer from a significant physical illness. Poor physical health is also one of the most important factors that affects the recovery of psychiatric clients in the community. A comprehensive treatment program at a CMHC should include a means of obtaining medical services for clients through contracting or referral. Laboratory service is also provided to monitor drug levels, liver profiles, electrolytes, and so forth.
6. *Vocational training.* Many community clients also experience difficulty in finding a suitable job. Unemployment statistics in the United States for recently discharged psychiatric patients have been estimated as high as 70%. Many CMHCs offer programs that focus on job skills, interviewing techniques, writing resumes, filling out applications, and job searching. To be fully effective, these vocational rehabilitative programs should continue once the CMHC client obtains a job, because she or he will need continued skills training, support, and stress management.

Managed Care

The current trend of managed care focuses on short-term, inpatient crisis stabilization in the event that the patient does not respond to outpatient case management. Insurance companies or managed care providers are insisting on precertification for inpatient care. Once the individual is admitted to a psychiatric facility, continued stay certification is usually limited to four or five days of care. The individual's discharge plan dictates the type of follow-up care that will be provided. The freedom to select a psychiatrist or therapist is limited by managed care contracts to preferred providers who have established working relationships with select hospitals.

 Problems Related to Community Mental Health Care

According to 1985 statistics provided by the NIMH, there were approximately 2.8 million chronically mentally ill persons living in residential sites such as nursing homes, households, long-term psychiatric facilities, and group homes. The homeless made up approximately 200,000 of the chronically mentally ill. Included in the 2.8 million were approximately 100,000 individuals who experienced the "revolving-door syndrome" (*i.e.*, repeated, short-term admissions to psychiatric facilities).

Limited funding has created fragmented services provided by community mental health staff. Centers located in various catchment areas (specific geographic areas) may not be readily accessible to special populations such as children, the elderly, the homeless, minority groups, or individuals living in rural communities. Furthermore, services in some remote areas may be limited because of a shortage of mental health professionals.

Overcrowding of CMHCs can result as hospitals precipitously discharge some clients to provide room for more acutely disturbed individuals.

 Role of the Community Mental Health Nurse

Nurses have a major role in the provision of quality services for the psychiatric client in the community. Psychiatric nurses were initially included with other health care professionals in the movement of the 1960s to deinstitutionalize and move significant numbers of hospitalized patients back to the community. Nurses assumed positions in the newly established CMHCs and provided the necessary aftercare services. These early community projects encouraging the use of nurses were based on the belief that psychiatric nurses would provide optimal transition from the hospital to the community. In the 1970s and

1980s, the role of the community health nurse continued to expand as nurses assumed key leadership positions in all types of community programs, including day treatment, residential homes, community mental health prevention programs, and psychiatric home-care programs. The psychiatric nurse practicing in the community today provides counseling, support, and coordination of care and health teaching. The role is comprehensive and challenging, requiring adaptability and flexibility. A nurse clinician with an advanced degree may function as a nurse therapist using individual, group, and family therapy. Prescriptive privileges are endorsed by the department of professional regulation in various states. Many insurance companies, as well as government-funded Medicare and Medicaid programs, approve reimbursement for services provided in the home, in long-term care facilities, or in community-based mental health settings.

Dr. Jeanne Miller (1981), in emphasizing the need for a clear theoretical framework for the practice of community mental health nursing, describes two areas of concern to community mental health nurses. The first area is the attempt by nurses to improve the quality of direct care of clients through such means as primary nursing, psychiatric home care, and case management. At the same time, community mental health nurses are becoming more concerned about societal and community conditions that may contribute to health problems and to the needs of persons with mental illness. Miller further states that community mental health nurses must continue to broaden their role to include a more holistic approach in the assessment, planning, and implementation of community services. In the 1990s and beyond, the community nurse will need to respond to the increasingly complex challenge of providing optimal mental health care by going beyond the traditional roles of psychiatric nursing. Miller and others encourage these specialized nurses to go beyond providing therapy and education to include interventions that reduce vulnerability to mental illness and enhance strengths in the individual and the community.

Summary

Several definitions of community mental health were presented. A history of community mental health was briefly discussed along with the Community Mental Health Acts of the 1960s. A description of the major concepts supporting the foundation of community mental health was explored. The community-based programs that were described in detail included psychiatric emergency care or triage, day treatment or partial hospitalization, residential programs, and psychiatric home care. The role of the advanced registered nurse practitioner in the long-term care setting was explained. The mainstay of most community mental health programs, the community mental health center, was presented along with an outline of the therapeutic services that most community mental health centers provide. Managed care was addressed. Problems related to community mental health care were identified. The chapter concluded with a discussion of the role of the community mental health nurse and the importance of establishing a clear theoretical framework for the practice of community mental health nursing.

Learning Activities

I. Clinical Activities
   A. If possible, spend a few days in your community-based agencies: a community mental health center, a psychiatric emergency room, and a day-treatment program.
   B. Describe the types of services available in these community mental health agencies.
   C. Establish a therapeutic relationship with a client, using community mental health resources.
   D. Spend time with several different community mental health nurses and differentiate among their varying roles and responsibilities.
II. Independent Activities
   A. Obtain a list of the mental health resources in your community.
   B. Visit several of these agencies to obtain information on the services that they provide.
   C. Read J. Miller's "Theoretical Basis for the Practice of Community Mental Health Nursing," in *Issues in Mental Health Nursing, 3*, 1981.

Critical Thinking Questions

1. Interview a local community mental health nurse about the system in which she or he works. How does that system match up to Panzetta's eight fundamental concepts for community mental health?
2. Visit a group home or halfway house in a local community. What type of support services, staffing, and therapeutic interventions are available? What are the strengths and weaknesses of this type of program? After assimilating this information, discuss how a group home might be accepted into the neighborhood where you live.
3. How do current social, economic, and political factors help or hinder those homeless persons who need community mental health services? What is nursing's role with this population?

Self-Test

1. State the five beliefs that influence community mental health.
2. Describe the Community Mental Health Centers Act of 1963.
3. List five of the eight fundamental concepts that are the basis for community mental health.
4. Explain the concept of psychiatric emergency care and the services provided by the psychiatric emergency room.
5. Identify three types of community care residential facilities.
6. Differentiate the treatment methods that may be included in a day-treatment or partial hospitalization program.
7. Describe the nursing interventions for a community mental health nurse.

SELECTED REFERENCES

Baker, F. M. (1995, December). Misdiagnosis among older psychiatric patients. *Journal of the National Medical Association.*

Connolly, P. M. (1991, January). Services for the underserved: A nurse-managed center for the chronically mentally ill. *Journal of Psychosocial Nursing and Mental Health Services.*

Crosby, R. (1987, January). Community care of the chronically mentally ill. *Journal of Psychosocial Nursing and Mental Health Services.*

Dittenbrenner, H. (1993, June). Psychiatric home care: An overview. *Caring.*

Foley, M. E., Fahs, M. C., Eisenhandler, J., & Hyer, K. (1995, September/October). Satisfaction with home healthcare services for clients with HIV: Preliminary findings. *Journal of the Association of Nurses in AIDS Care.*

Grossman, D. (1996, July). Cultural dimensions in home health nursing. *American Journal of Nursing.*

Hellwig, K. (1993, December). Psychiatric home care nursing: Managing patients in the community setting. *Journal of Psychosocial Nursing and Mental Health Services.*

Hochberger, J. M., & Fisher-James, L. (1992, April). Discharge group for chronically mentally ill. *Journal of Psychosocial Nursing and Mental Health Services.*

Joyce, B., Staley, D., & Hughes, L. (1990, June). Staying well: Factors contributing to successful community adaptation. *Journal of Psychosocial Nursing and Mental Health Services.*

Maurin, J. T. (1990, July). Case management: Caring for psychiatric clients. *Journal of Psychosocial Nursing and Mental Health Services.*

Miller, J. (1981, March). Theoretical basis for the practice of community mental health nursing. *Issues in Mental Health Nursing.*

Nurius, P. (1983–1984). Emergency psychiatric services: A study of changing utilization patterns and issues. *International Journal of Psychiatry in Medicine, 13.*

Panzetta, A. (1985, November). Whatever happened to community mental health? Portents for corporate medicine. *Hospital and Community Psychiatry.*

Pelletier, L. (1988, March). Psychiatric home care. *Journal of Psychosocial Nursing and Mental Health Services.*

Pittman, D. C., Parsons, R., & Peterson, W. (1990, November). Easing the way: A multifaceted approach to day treatment. *Journal of Psychosocial Nursing and Mental Health Services.*

Ricci, M. S. (1990, August). The new after-care clinic: Treating individuals rather than masses. *Journal of Psychosocial Nursing and Mental Health Services.*

Richie, F., & Lusky, K. (1987, Fall). Psychiatric home health nursing: A new role in community mental health. *Community Mental Health Journal.*

Robinson, G. M., & Pinkney, A. A. (1992, May). Transition from the hospital to the community: Small group program. *Journal of Psychosocial Nursing and Mental Health Services.*

Rosenzweig, L. (1992, June). Psychiatric triage: A cost-effective approach to quality management in mental health. *Journal of Psychosocial Nursing and Mental Health Services.*

Solomon, P., & Davis, J. (1985, Spring). Meeting community service needs of discharged psychiatric patients. *Psychiatric Quarterly.*

Strumpf, N. E. (1994, December). Innovative gerontological practices as models for health care delivery. *Nursing and Health Care.*

Talbott, J. (1985, September). Community care for the chronically mentally ill. *Psychiatric Clinics of North America.*

Wilkinson, L. (1991, December). A collaborative model: Ambulatory pharmacotherapy for chronic psychiatric patients. *Journal of Psychosocial Nursing and Mental Health Services.*

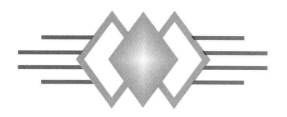

CHAPTER 4

LEGAL ISSUES

The field of psychiatric nursing is especially affected by the law . . . the nurse must be acutely aware of not only her patients' rights but her own potential liabilities.

Zeuli, 1991

1 State the purpose of the Nurse Practice Act.

2 Describe the various forms of nursing malpractice.

3 Compare criteria for voluntary and involuntary admission to a psychiatric facility.

4 Discuss the concept of competency and the role of an appointed guardian.

5 Discuss the impact of the Omnibus Reconciliation Act (OBRA) on placement of patients with psychiatric disorders in long-term care facilities.

6 Compare the legal rights of adults and minors admitted to psychiatric facilities.

7 Explain forensic psychiatry and the role of the psychiatric nurse.

Introduction

Nursing as a profession is influenced in each state by legislative acts referred to as the Nurse Practice Act. The practice of psychiatric nursing demands a knowledge of the law, particularly the rights of patients and the quality of their care. Historically, the care of those deemed mentally ill included questionable practices such as the loss of individual rights.

In the early 1900s, all states had accepted the doctrine of charitable immunity or Good Samaritan Act. By the mid-1970s, most states had revoked the doctrine, and "the malpractice crisis" occurred. Health care risk management developed, preventive law in medicine was addressed, and the American Nurses' Association developed standards of psychiatric–mental health clinical nursing practice. Currently, a nurse practicing in the psychiatric–mental health clinical setting is responsible for providing care consistent with the American Nurses' Association code of ethics (Box 4-1).

Nursing Malpractice

The nursing malpractice law is generally based on fault. It must be shown that the nurse's conduct fell below a level that society considers acceptable before the nurse can be held legally liable.

BOX 4-1 American Nurses' Association Code of Ethics

1. The nurse provides services with respect for human dignity and the uniqueness of the client, unrestricted by considerations of social or economic status, personal attributes, or the nature of health problems.
2. The nurse safeguards the client's right to privacy by judiciously protecting information of a confidential nature.
3. The nurse acts to safeguard the client and the public when health care and safety are affected by the incompetent, unethical, or illegal practice of any person.
4. The nurse assumes responsibility and accountability for individual nursing judgments and actions.
5. The nurse maintains competence in nursing.
6. The nurse exercises informed judgment and uses individual competence and qualifications as criteria in seeking consultation, accepting responsibilities, and delegating nursing activities to others.
7. The nurse participates in activities that contribute to the ongoing development of the profession's body of knowledge.
8. The nurse participates in the profession's efforts to implement and improve standards of nursing.
9. The nurse participates in the profession's efforts to establish and maintain conditions of employment conducive to high-quality nursing care.
10. The nurse participates in the profession's effort to protect the public from misinformation and misrepresentation and to maintain the integrity of nursing.
11. The nurse collaborates with members of the health professions and other citizens in promoting community and national efforts to meet the health needs of the public.

From American Nurses' Association (1985). *Code for Nurses (With Interpretive Statements)*. Kansas City, MO: Author. Reprinted with permission from the American Nurses' Association.

Conduct that falls below the standard of care established by law for the protection of others and involves an unreasonable risk of harm to a patient is negligence. The following four elements must be present to constitute negligence (Calloway, 1986):

1. Failure to act in an acceptable way
2. Failure to conform to the required standard of care

3. Approximate cause, which requires that there be a reasonably close connection between the defendant's conduct and the resultant injury (*i.e.*, the performance by the health care provider caused the injury)
4. Actual damage has occurred

Other forms of malpractice include intentional torts, assault and battery, defamation, invasion of privacy, and false imprisonment by the inappropriate use of restraints. Intentional torts refer to willful or wanton conduct with disregard of the interests of others. Assault is an act that puts another person in apprehension of being touched or of bodily harm without consent. Battery is unlawful touching of another without consent. Defamation refers to injury to a person's reputation or character through oral or written communications to a third party. Unwarranted exploitation of one's personality or private affairs is an invasion of privacy. Last, false imprisonment is the intentional and unjustifiable detention of a person against his or her will. Detention can occur by use of physical restraint, barriers, or threats of harm (Calloway, 1986).

In the psychiatric clinical setting, knowledge of the law and the bill of rights for mental health patients, plus quality patient care greatly reduce the risk of malpractice litigation. Legal issues could arise in various practice settings involving situations such as child abuse, breach of confidentiality, failure to provide for informed consent, family violence, mental retardation, prenatal substance abuse, rape, sexual assault, spouse abuse, and suicide. For example, if a patient is admitted to a psychiatric facility involuntarily (has not signed the voluntary admission form or consent for treatment), emergency orders are necessary to provide any type of nursing interventions. Touching the patient, giving medication, or completing a physical examination could result in a malpractice suit based on a complaint of assault and battery.

Admission Criteria Based on Competency

Hospitalization can be traumatic or supportive, depending on the situation, attitude of family and friends, response of staff, and type of admission. Admissions to a psychiatric facility can occur as an emergency or scheduled admission. Both types of admission may occur on a voluntary or involuntary basis. Voluntary patients have the right to refuse any type of treatment prescribed and may initiate their own discharge at any time. The attending physician may write the order as a routine discharge or AMA (against medical advice) if the physician feels the patient should remain in the facility but does not wish to invoke the involuntary admission procedure.

If patients are a threat to themselves or others, they may be admitted and detained for at least 72 hours by an involuntary admission. For example, in most states a physician, licensed clinical psychologist, master's prepared psychiatric nurse, or master's prepared licensed clinical social worker may initiate involuntary admission. The form for involuntary admission usually states that the following conditions exist:

1. There is reason to believe said person is mentally ill and
   a. has refused voluntary examination after conscientious explanation and disclosure of the purpose of the examination; or
   b. is unable to determine for herself or himself where examination is necessary; and
2. Either
   a. without care or treatment said person is likely to suffer from neglect or refuse to care for self; or
   b. there is substantial likelihood that in the near future said person will inflict serious bodily harm on self or another person

If within 72 hours the patient's condition does not improve and the patient does not sign the voluntary admission forms authorizing treatment and continued stay in the facility, first and second opinions by two psychiatrists are completed and a court hearing is set. As a result of information presented at the hearing, the patient may be court-ordered to remain in the facility for a specified period of time (involuntary commitment) or the patient may be released from the facility.

Individuals may decide to elope from a facility. If they were admitted under a voluntary status, they can be brought back to the facility only if they again voluntarily agree. If they refuse to return, the physician must discharge them or initiate involuntary commitment procedures.

If individuals admitted to a psychiatric facility are not competent to make decisions (*e.g.*, incapable of giving informed consent), a guardian will be appointed by the court to make decisions for them. Guardianship may continue after they are released from the facility or transferred to a long-term care psychiatric institution.

Psychiatric Patients in Long-term Care Facilities

As of August 1, 1988, new regulations regarding the admission of patients with psychiatric disorders to long-term care facilities (nursing homes) have been established. These regulations, based on the Omnibus Reconciliation Act of 1987 (OBRA), state that a long-term care facility must not admit, on or after January 1, 1989, any new resident needing active treatment for mental illness or mental retardation. A screening document called the Preadmission

Screening and Annual Resident Review (PSARR) is supposed to determine whether the patient needs active psychiatric treatment. If a patient resides in a long-term care facility and requires psychiatric treatment, the proper course of action may be unclear. Should the patient be discharged, transferred to a psychiatric facility, or treated in the facility? This confusion also impedes discharge planning for patients admitted to psychiatric treatment facilities. Some long-term care facilities are willing to admit psychiatric patients if they are stabilized and followed by a psychiatrist or psychiatric nurse practitioner.

 Bill of Rights for Mental Health Patients

Psychiatric patients who voluntarily seek help retain civil rights during hospitalization. Involuntarily committed patients lose the right to liberty. The following is a summary of patient or client rights as stated by the Protection and Advocacy Bill for Mentally Ill Individuals Act of 1986 and the Joint Commission on Accreditation of Hospitals (JCAH). They include the rights to

1. Receive treatment, including (a) a humane psychological and physical environment; (b) adequate treatment in a least restrictive environment; (c) a current, written, individualized treatment plan; and (d) informed consent concerning one's condition, progress, explanations of procedures, risks involved, alternative treatments, consequences of alternative treatments, and any other information that may help the patient to make an intelligent, informed choice
2. Refuse treatment, unless such action endangers others, or withdraw from treatment if risks outweigh benefits
3. A probable cause hearing within 3 court days of admission to secure a speedy recovery from involuntary detention if found sane in a court of law (writ of *habeas corpus*)
4. Privacy and confidentiality: Information, records, and correspondence may be disclosed only with the patient's written consent. The exception occurs when the public becomes endangered; the patient is transferred to another facility; the patient's attorney, law enforcement officers, or a court requests information; the patient participates in research; or insurance companies require information to complete insurance claims.
5. Communicate freely with others by letter, telephone, or visits, unless such activities are specifically restricted in one's treatment plan
6. Personal privileges: (a) wearing one's own clothing; (b) maintaining personal appearance to individual taste; and (c) receiving the basic necessities of life
7. Maintain one's civil rights, including the right to (a) be legally represented; (b) be employed; (c) hold public office; (d) vote; (e) execute a will; (f) drive; (g) marry; (h) divorce; or (i) enter into a contract

8. Religious freedom and education
9. Maintain respect, dignity, and personal identity
10. Maintain personal safety and assert grievances
11. Transfer and continuity of care
12. Access to own records
13. Explanation of cost of services
14. Aftercare: Individuals discharged from mental health facilities have the right to adequate housing and aftercare planned by professional staff.

 ## Legal Rights of Minors

State laws vary regarding the age and legal rights of minors such as the right to purchase cigarettes or alcoholic beverages, obtain an abortion, or obtain medical treatment without consent. In the past, parents or guardians made decisions regarding admissions to psychiatric facilities and commitment for treatment. In most states, a minor who has not been court-ordered to receive treatment is privileged to a voluntariness hearing at the time of admission to a facility. An objective professional such as the registered nurse asks the minor in a private interview if he or she has voluntarily agreed to obtain psychiatric care or if coercion has occurred. The U.S. Supreme Court has stated that such a neutral fact finder has the authority to refuse admission of a minor if a parent has erred in the decision to have the minor institutionalized or to seek treatment for mental health care.

 ## Forensic Psychiatry

The evaluation of competency of an individual to stand trial and the person's mental condition at the time of an alleged crime constitute the specialized area of mental health care referred to as forensic psychiatry. If the defendant meets legally prescribed criteria, an insanity plea may be entered by the defense. The defendant is then involuntarily committed to a forensic unit for a period of approximately 30 to 90 days to be evaluated by mental health professionals. At the completion of the evaluation, which includes a variety of tests to determine if an insanity defense exists, the court is informed of the recommendations and a hearing may be scheduled to determine the court's order for release or continuation of mandatory treatment.

 ## Summary

This chapter focuses on legal issues specific to psychiatric–mental health nursing. The topic of nursing malpractice was addressed by describing negligence, intentional torts, assault and battery, invasion of privacy, and false imprisonment by the use of restraints. The common types of admissions based on competency were described, including the initiation of an involuntary commitment and guardianship appointment. Regulations regarding admission of psychiatric patients to long-term care facilities were explained. The bill of rights for mental health patients was summarized. The legal rights of minors were stated, and a brief description of forensic psychiatry was given.

Learning Activities

I. Clinical Activities
   A. Examine patient charts in the clinical setting to determine each patient's admission status. Discuss findings during clinical conference.
   B. Obtain a copy of your state's involuntary commitment forms to review and discuss in clinical conference.
   C. If possible, attend an involuntary commitment hearing and discuss the process with the assigned social worker or case manager.
   D. Assess the understanding of legal rights by a patient who is a minor.
II. Independent Activities
   A. Visit a local mental health center to assess the type of milieu provided. What type of individuals utilize the center? What is their legal status?
   B. Obtain and review a copy of your state's Nurse Practice Act.
   C. Investigate the availability and cost of malpractice insurance for psychiatric nurses.

Critical Thinking Questions

1. You are working on the evening shift of a psychiatric facility when you are asked to admit a new patient. As you begin your assessment, the patient informs you he has been brought there against his will and he does not intend to stay. You notice that neither the voluntary admission form nor the consent for treatment has been signed. You excuse yourself and inform the charge nurse of your findings. She brushes you off, saying, "Don't worry, get him admitted and then I'll talk to him." What do you do?

2. While working in a long-term care facility, you begin to admit a new patient. She informs you that she is under the care of a psychiatrist, but "Don't worry, my hallucinations are mostly controlled." Keeping in mind the Omnibus Reconciliation Act of 1987, what actions must you take?

3. For several days you have been caring for a 15-year-old woman who was admitted for episodes described by her parents as "outbursts of rage." She confides in you that her parents forced her to come to the hospital and she feels like a prisoner. What do you need to consider before taking action?

Self-Test

1. Differentiate voluntary from involuntary admission.
2. Define competency, informed consent, and guardianship.
3. State the purpose of the Nurse Practice Act.
4. Describe the four elements that constitute negligence.
5. Cite examples of intentional tort, assault and battery, defamation, invasion of privacy, and false imprisonmentx by the inappropriate use of restraints.
6. Explain the impact of OBRA on nursing home residents with psychiatric disorders.
7. List five rights of patients with psychiatric disorders.
8. Explain the purpose of forensic psychiatry.

SELECTED REFERENCES

American Hospital Association. (1974). *A patient's bill of rights.* Chicago: Author.

American Nurses' Association. (1994). *Standards of psychiatric–mental health clinical nursing practice.* Washington, DC: Author.

Barry, P. D. (1994). *Mental health and mental illness* (5th ed.). Philadelphia: J. B. Lippincott.

Birkett, D. P. (1991). *Psychiatry in the nursing home: Assessment, evaluation and intervention.* New York: The Haworth Press.

Calloway, S. D. (1986). *Nursing and the law.* Eau Claire, WI: Professional Education Systems, Inc.

Calloway, S. D. (1986). *Statutes affecting nursing practice.* Eau Claire, WI: Professional Education Systems, Inc.

Haddad, A. (1994, March). Acute care decisions: Ethics in action. *RN.*

Hahn, M. S. (1995, February). The political process of changing the nurse practice act. *Advance for Nurse Practitioners.*

Johnson, B. S. (1997). *Adaptation and growth: Psychiatric–mental health nursing.* (4th ed.). Philadelphia: Lippincott–Raven Publishers.

Sadoff, R. L. (1992). *Psychiatric malpractice: Cases and comments for clinicians.* Washington, DC: American Psychiatric Press.

Sullivan, G. H. (1994, May). Home care: More autonomy, more legal risks. *RN.*

Weiss, E. S. (1990, August). The right to refuse: Informed consent and the psychosocial nurse. *Journal of Psychosocial Nursing and Mental Health Services.*

Zeuli, L. B. (1991). Legal considerations in mental health nursing practice. In Gary, F., & Kavanagh, C. K., *Psychiatric Mental Health Nursing.* Philadelphia: J. B. Lippincott.

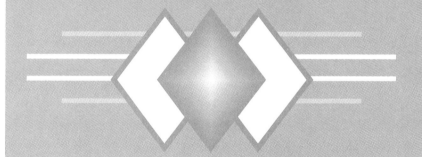

UNIT II

Components of Psychiatric–Mental Health Nursing

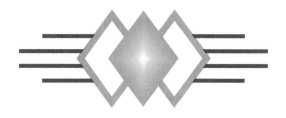

CHAPTER 5

THE NURSING PROCESS: ASSESSMENT OF PSYCHIATRIC PATIENTS

> **K**nowledge of psychosocial assessment theory is mandatory if we are to support our patients' adaptation. Knowledge of theory is the first essential, since we must know what we are looking for. The second part, equally essential, is to know how to intervene when a problem is spotted.
>
> *Barry, 1996*

1 State the purpose of a psychiatric assessment.

2 Discuss the significance of cultural diversity in psychiatric–mental health nursing.

3 List three factors that constitute a comprehensive psychiatric assessment.

4 Define the following terminology:

Blocking

Circumstantiality

Flight of ideas

Perseveration

Verbigeration

Neologism

Mutism

Inappropriate affect

5 Differentiate delusions of reference, grandeur, self-deprecation, alien control, nihilism, and somatic concerns.

6 Describe auditory, visual, olfactory, gustatory, and tactile hallucinations.

7 Differentiate between obsessions and compulsions.

8 State how information obtained during the assessment process is transmitted to members of the health care team.

9 List the criteria for charting psychiatric nurses' progress notes.

Introduction

The nursing process is a six-step problem-solving approach that serves as an organizational framework for the practice of nursing. It sets the practice of nursing in motion and serves as a monitor of quality nursing care. This chapter focuses on the first step, which is the assessment of patients with psychiatric disorders.

Assessment

The assessment phase of the nursing process includes the collection of data about a person, family, or group by the methods of observation, examination, and interviewing. Two types of data are collected: objective and subjective.

Objective data include information obtained verbally from the patient, as well as the results of inspection, palpation, percussion, and auscultation during an examination. Subjective data are obtained as the patient, family members, or significant others provide information spontaneously, during direct questioning, or during the health history.

The psychiatric–mental health nurse uses a nursing assessment tool to obtain factual information, observe appearance and behavior, and evaluate the patient's mental or cognitive status. A sample nursing assessment form for an adult or adolescent is reproduced in Appendix A. The Folstein Mini-Mental State Exam, used to determine the presence or absence of dementia, is shown in Box 5-1 (on p. 70). Examples of other assessment tools used to diagnose the presence of specific psychiatric disorders include the Hamilton Anxiety Rating Scale, Hamilton Rating Scale for Depression, Beck Depression Inventory, Geriatric Depression Scale, Yale–Brown Obsessive Compulsive Rating Scale, Global Deterioration Scale, Brief Cognitive Rating Scale, and screening tests to determine the presence of alcoholism, referred to as MAST and CAGE. The assessment process enables the psychiatric–mental health nurse to make sound clinical judgments and plan appropriate interventions.

During hospitalization or outpatient treatment such as partial hospitalization, a psychosocial history is obtained by the social worker and a psychiatric evaluation is completed by the attending physician. Other assessments utilized in the psychiatric setting are psychological testing and the neurological examination. A physical examination is performed to rule out any physiologic causes of disorders such as anxiety, depression, or dementia. Many facilities require medical clearance before or within 24 hours of admission to avoid medical emergencies in the psychiatric setting.

Transcultural Perspectives

The "browning of America" refers to changes in the U.S. population and to the belief that by the middle of the twenty-first century, the average resident will trace his or her ancestry to non-European parts of the world such as Africa, Asia, Mexico, or Puerto Rico. The psychiatric nurse must possess sensitivity, knowledge, and skills to provide care to such culturally diverse groups of clients to avoid labeling persons as noncompliant, resistant to care, or abnormal. For example, the act of suicide is accepted in some cultures as a means to escape identifiable stressors such as terminal illness, criticism from others, or spinsterhood (Kavanaugh in Andrews & Boyle, 1995).

Individuals may require the assistance of an interpreter to overcome language barriers. Cultural beliefs and practices of clients may differ from those of the nurse conducting the assessment. Environmental conditions may not be

BOX 5-1 The Folstein Mini–Mental State Exam

Instructions: Ask all questions in the order listed and score immediately. Record total number of points.

	Maximum Score	Score	Question
Orientation	5	( )	1. Ask the patient to name the year, season, date, day, and month. (1 *point each*)
	5	( )	2. Ask the patient to give his/her whereabouts: state, county, town, street, floor. (1 *point each*)
Registration	3	( )	3. Ask the patient to repeat three unrelated objects that you name. Repeat them and continue to repeat them until all three are learned. (1 *point each*)
Attention and Calculation	5	( )	4. Ask the patient to subtract 7 from 100, stopping after five subtractions, or to spell the word "world" backwards. (1 *point for each correct calculation or letter*)
Recall	3	( )	5. Ask the patient to repeat the three objects previously named. (1 *point each*)
Language	2	( )	6. Display a wrist watch and ask the patient to name it. Repeat this for a pencil. (1 *point each*)
	1	( )	7. Ask the patient to repeat this phrase: "No ifs, ands, or buts!" (1 *point*)
	3	( )	8. Have the patient follow a three-point command such as, "Take a paper in your right hand, fold it in half, and put it on the floor." (1 *point each*)
	1	( )	9. On a blank piece of paper write, "Close your eyes!" Ask the patient to read it and do what it says. (1 *point*)

BOX 5-1 **The Folstein Mini–Mental State Exam** (Continued)

	Maximum Score	Score	Question
Language	1	( )	10. Ask the patient to write a sentence on a blank piece of paper. It must be written spontaneously. Score correctly if it contains a subject and a verb and is sensible (correct grammar and punctuation are not necessary). (1 *point*)
	1	( )	11. Ask the patient to copy a design you have drawn on a piece of paper (two intersecting pentagons with sides about one inch). (1 *point*)

TOTAL SCORE: (Maximum score = 30)

SCORING: Score of 23 or less: high likelihood of dementia
         Score of 25–30: normal aging or borderline

Adapted from Folstein, J. F., Folstein, S. E., & McHugh, P. R. (1975). *Mini–mental state: A practical method for grading the cognitive state of patients for the clinician.* Oxford: Pergamon Press.

revealed by individuals seeking treatment to avoid the possibility of prejudgment by the health care provider.

Talking openly and communicating with the patient can provide valuable information about compliance and behavior. The most important thing the psychiatric nurse can do is to acknowledge that a difference does exist (Hahn, November 1995).

 Appearance

General appearance includes physical characteristics, apparent age, peculiarity of dress, cleanliness, and use of cosmetics. A person's general appearance, including facial expressions, is a manner of nonverbal communication in which emotions, feelings, and moods are related. For example, depressed people often neglect their personal appearance, appear disheveled, and wear drab-looking clothes that are generally dark in color, reflecting a depressed mood. The facial expression may appear sad, worried, tense, frightened, or distraught. Manic patients may dress in bizarre or overly colorful outfits, wear heavy layers of cosmetics, and don several pieces of jewelry.

Behavior, Attitude, and Normal Coping Patterns

The interviewer assesses patients' actions or behavior by considering the following factors:

1. Do they exhibit strange, threatening, or violent behavior? Are they making an effort to control their emotions?
2. Is there evidence of any unusual mannerisms or motor activity, such as grimacing, tremors, tics, impaired gait, psychomotor retardation, or agitation? Do they pace excessively?
3. Do they appear friendly, embarrassed, evasive, fearful, resentful, angry, negativistic, or impulsive? Their attitude toward the interviewer or helping persons can facilitate or impair the assessment process.
4. Is behavior overactive or underactive? Is it purposeful, disorganized, or stereotyped? Are reactions fairly consistent?

Patients should be asked how they normally cope with a serious problem or with high levels of stress if they are in contact with reality and able to respond to such a question. Responses to this question enable the interviewer to assess patients' present ability to cope as well as their judgment. Have they lost this ability? Do they need to develop new coping measures? Their behavior may be the result of inadequate coping patterns.

Paranoid or suspicious persons may isolate themselves, appear evasive during a conversation, and demonstrate a negativistic attitude toward the nursing staff. Such activity is an attempt to protect oneself by maintaining control of a stressful environment.

Personality Style and Communication Ability

"The manner in which the patient talks enables us to appreciate difficulties with his thought processes. It is desirable to obtain a verbatim sample of the stream of speech to illustrate psychopathologic disturbances" (Small, 1980, p. 8).

Factors to be considered while assessing patients' ability to communicate and interact socially include the following:

1. Do they speak coherently? Does the flow of speech seem natural or logical, or is it illogical, vague, and loosely organized? Do they enunciate clearly?
2. Is the rate of speech slow, retarded, or rapid? Do they fail to speak at all or respond only when questioned?
3. Do patients whisper or speak softly, or do they speak loudly or shout?
4. Is there a delay in answers or responses, or do patients break off their conversation in the middle of a sentence and refuse to talk further?
5. Do they repeat certain words and phrases over and over?
6. Do they make up new words that have no meaning to others?
7. Is their language obscene?
8. Does their conversation jump from one topic to another?
9. Do they stutter, lisp, or regress in their speech?
10. Do they exhibit any unusual personality traits or characteristics that may interfere with their ability to socialize with others or adapt to hospitalization? For example, do they associate freely with others or do they consider themselves "loners?" Do they appear aggressive or domineering during the interview? Do they feel that people like them or reject them? How do they spend their personal time?
11. Are they members of a minority or culturally diverse group?

The following terminology usually is used to describe impaired communication observed during the assessment process: (1) blocking, (2) circumstantiality, (3) flight of ideas, (4) perseveration, (5) verbigeration, (6) neologisms, and (7) mutism. These terms are defined as follows by the American Psychiatric Association (1980) and Rowe (1989):

Blocking

This impairment is a sudden stoppage in the spontaneous flow or stream of thinking or speaking for no apparent external or environmental reason. Blocking may be due to preoccupation, delusional thoughts, or hallucinations; for example, while talking to the nurse, a patient stated, "My favorite restaurant is Chi-Chi's. I like it because the atmosphere is so nice and the food is . . ." Most often found in schizophrenics during audio hallucinations.

Circumstantiality

In this pattern of speech the person gives much unnecessary detail that delays meeting a goal or stating a point. For example, when asked to state his occupation, a patient gave a very detailed description of the type of work he did. Commonly found in manic disorder and some organic mental disorders.

Flight of Ideas

This impairment is characterized by overproductivity of talk and verbal skipping from one idea to another. The ideas are fragmentary, although talk is continuous. Connections between the parts of speech often are determined by chance of associations; for example: "I like the color blue. Do you ever feel blue? Feelings can change from day to day. The days are getting longer." Most commonly observed in manic disorders.

Perseveration

Perseveration is the persistent, repetitive expression of a single idea in response to various questions. Found in some organic mental disorders and catatonia.

Verbigeration

This term describes meaningless repetition of incoherent words or sentences. Observed in certain psychotic reactions and organic mental disorders.

Neologism

A neologism is a new word or combination of several words coined or self-invented by a person and not readily understood by others; for example: "His *phenologs* are in the dryer." Found in certain schizophrenic disorders.

Mutism

This impairment is refusal to speak even though the person may give indications of being aware of the environment. Mutism may occur from conscious or unconscious reasons. Observed in catatonic schizophrenic disorders, profound depressive disorders, and stupors of organic or psychogenic origin.

Other terminology, such as loose association, echolalia, and clang association, is described in the chapter discussing schizophrenic disorders.

Emotional State or Affect

Affect is defined as "the outward manifestation of a person's feelings, tone, or mood. Affect and emotion are commonly used interchangeably" (American Psychiatric Association, 1980, p. 3). "The relationship between mood and the content of thought is of particular significance. There may be a wide divergence between what the patient says or does on the one hand and his emotional state as expressed objectively in his face or attitudes" (Small, 1980, p. 10).

A lead question such as "What are you feeling?" may elicit such responses as "nervous," "angry," "frustrated," "depressed," or "confused." The person should be asked to describe the nervousness, anger, frustration, or confusion. Is the person's emotional response constant or does it fluctuate during the assessment? The interviewer should record a verbatim reply to questions concerning the patient's mood and note whether an intense emotional response accompanies the discussion of specific topics. Affective responses may be appropriate, inappropriate, flat, or blunted. An emotional response out of proportion to a situation is considered inappropriate.

Under ordinary circumstances, a person's affect varies according to the situation or subject under discussion. The person with emotional conflict may have a persistent emotional reaction based on this conflict. It is imperative that the examiner or observer identify the abnormal emotional reaction and explore its depth, intensity, and persistence. Such an inquiry could prevent a depressed person from attempting suicide.

Content of Thought

The American Psychiatric Association defines thought disorder as "a disturbance of speech, communication, or content of thought, such as delusions, ideas of reference. . . . A thought disorder can be caused by a functional emotional disorder or an organic condition" (1980, p. 131). Small (1980) and Rowe (1989) describe those thought contents more commonly exhibited during a psychiatric examination: (1) delusions, (2) hallucinations, (3) depersonalization, (4) obsessions, and (5) compulsions.

Delusions

A delusion is a fixed false belief not true to fact and not ordinarily accepted by other members of the person's culture. It cannot be corrected by an appeal to the reason of the person experiencing it. Delusions occur in various types of psychotic disorders, such as organic mental disorder and schizophrenic disorder, and in some affective disorders. Box 5-2 (on p.76) describes various types of delusions.

Hallucinations

Hallucinations are sensory perceptions that occur in the absence of an actual external stimulus. They may be auditory, visual, olfactory, gustatory, or tactile in nature. Hallucinations occur in substance-use disorders, schizophrenia, and manic disorders. Examples of the types of hallucinations are presented in Box 5-3 (on p.77).

Depersonalization

Depersonalization is described as a feeling of unreality or strangeness concerning self, the environment, or both; for example, patients have described out-of-body sensations in which they view themselves from a few feet overhead. These peo-

BOX 5-2 Types of Delusions

Type	Description
Delusions of reference or persecution	The person believes that he or she is the object of environmental attention or is being singled out for harassment. "The police are watching my every move. They're out to get me."
Delusions of alien control	The person believes his or her feelings, thoughts, impulses, or actions are controlled by an external source. "A spaceman sends me messages by TV and tells me what to do."
Nihilistic delusions	The person denies reality or existence of self, part of self, or some external object. "I have no head."
Delusions of self-deprecation	The individual feels unworthy, ugly, or sinful. "I don't deserve to live. I'm so unworthy of your love."
Delusions of grandeur	A person experiences exaggerated ideas of her or his importance or identity. "I am Napoleon!"
Somatic delusions	The person entertains false beliefs pertaining to body image or body function. The person actually believes that she or he has cancer, leprosy, or some other terminal illness.

ple may feel they are "going crazy." Causes of depersonalization include prolonged stress and psychological fatigue, as well as substance abuse. This feeling has been described in schizophrenia, bipolar disorders, and depersonalization disorders.

Obsessions

"Obsessions are insistent thoughts, recognized as arising from the self, usually regarded by the patient as absurd and relatively meaningless, yet they persist despite his endeavors to rid himself of them" (Small, 1980, p. 13). Persons who experience obsessions generally describe their thoughts as "thoughts I can't get rid of" or "I can't stop thinking of things . . . they keep going on in my mind over and over again." Obsessions are typically seen in obsessive–compulsive disorders.

BOX 5-3 Types of Hallucinations

Type	Example
Auditory hallucination	AS tells you that he hears voices frequently while he sits quietly in his lounge chair. He states, "The voices tell me when to eat, dress, and go to bed each night!"
Visual hallucination	Ninety-year-old EK describes seeing spiders and snakes on the ceiling of his room late one evening as you make rounds.
Olfactory hallucination	AJ, a 65-year-old psychotic patient, states that she smells "rotten garbage" in her bedroom, although there is no evidence of any foul-smelling material.
Gustatory (taste) hallucination	MY, a young patient with organic brain syndrome, complains of a constant metallic taste in her mouth.
Tactile hallucination	NX, a middle-aged woman undergoing symptoms of alcohol withdrawal and delirium tremens, complains of feeling "worms crawling all over (her) body."

Compulsions

A compulsion is "an insistent, repetitive, intrusive and unwanted urge to perform an act contrary to one's ordinary wishes or standards" (American Psychiatric Association, 1980, p. 21). If the person does not engage in the repetitive act due to an inner need or drive, he or she usually experiences feelings of tension and anxiety. Compulsions are frequently seen in obsessive–compulsive disorders.

Orientation

During the assessment, patients are asked questions regarding their ability to grasp the significance of their environment, an existing situation, or the clearness of conscious processes. In other words, are they oriented to person, place, and time? Do they know who they are, where they are, or what the date is? Levels of orientation and consciousness are subdivided as follows: confusion, clouding of consciousness, stupor, delirium, dream state, and coma. A brief description of each is presented in Box 5-4.

BOX 5-4 Levels of Orientation and Consciousness

Level	Description
Confusion	Disorientation to person, place, or time, characterized by bewilderment and complexity
Clouding of consciousness	Disturbance in perception or thought that is slight to moderate in degree, usually owing to physical or chemical factors producing functional impairment of the cerebrum
Stupor	A state in which the person does not react to or is unaware of the surroundings. The person may be motionless and mute but conscious
Delirium, or acute brain syndrome	Confusion accompanied by altered or fluctuating consciousness. Disturbance in emotion, thought, and perception is moderate to severe. Usually associated with infections, toxic states, head trauma, and so forth
Dream state	Disturbed, clouded, or confused consciousness in which the person may not be aware of surroundings. Visual or auditory hallucinations may occur. May last several minutes to a few days
Coma	Loss of consciousness

 Memory

Memory, or the ability to recall past experiences, is divided into recent and long term. Recent memory is the ability to recall events in the immediate past and up to two weeks previously. Long-term memory is the ability to recall remote past experiences such as the date and place of birth, names of schools attended, occupational history, and chronologic data relating to previous illnesses. Small (1980) states that memory defects may result from lack of attention, difficulty with retention, difficulty with recall, or any combination of these factors. Loss of recent memory may be seen in patients with chronic organic brain syndrome, acute organic brain syndrome, or depression. Long-term memory loss usually is due to a physiologic disorder resulting in brain dysfunction. Three disorders of memory are (1) hypermnesia or an abnormally pronounced memory, (2) amnesia or loss of memory, and (3) paramnesia or falsification of memory.

 Intellectual Ability

The person's ability to use facts comprehensively is an indication of intellectual ability. During the assessment the person may be asked general information such as (1) to name the last three presidents, (2) to calculate simple arithmetical problems, and (3) "to correctly estimate and form opinions concerning objective matters" (Small, 1980, p. 16). The person may be asked a question such as "What would you do if you found a wallet in front of your house?" The examiner is able to evaluate reasoning ability and judgment by the response given. Abstract and concrete thinking abilities are evaluated by responses to proverbs such as "an eye for an eye and a tooth for a tooth."

 Insight Regarding Illness or Condition

Does the person consider himself or herself ill? Does the patient understand what is happening? Is the illness threatening to the patient? Insight is defined as self-understanding, or the extent of one's understanding of the origin, nature, and mechanisms of one's attitudes and behavior. Patients' insights into their illness or condition range from poor to good, depending on the degree of psychopathology present.

 Neurovegetative Changes

Does the patient exhibit changes in psychophysiologic functions such as sleep patterns, eating patterns, energy levels, sexual functioning, or bowel functioning? Depressed persons usually complain of insomnia or hypersomnia, loss of appetite or increased appetite, loss of energy, decreased libido, and constipation, which are all signs of neurovegetative changes. Persons who are diagnosed as psychotic may neglect their nutritional intake, appear fatigued, sleep excessively, and ignore elimination habits (sometimes to the point of developing a fecal impaction).

 Recording of Assessments

Information obtained during the assessment process is relayed to the members of the health care team in the form of a summary of the history and physical examination, a summary of the social history, a summary of the psychological testing, and multidisciplinary progress notes. Nurses can provide invaluable pertinent information if they follow the criteria of good recording. Such information is significant to the members of the interdisciplinary team, who use these notes as an aid in planning treatment and disposition of patients. Thorough charting shows progress, lack of progress, or regression on the part of the patient. The details of the patient's conduct, appearance, and attitude are significant. Increased skill in observation and recording result in more concise charting. Charting is also important in research because it is an accurate record of the symptoms, behavior, treatment, and reactions of the patient. Charting is recognized by legal authorities, who frequently use the notes for testimony in court.

The basic criteria for charting psychiatric nursing progress notes are listed here. The notes should be

1. Objective: The nurse records what the patient says and does by stating facts and quoting the patient's conversation.
2. Descriptive: The nurse describes the patient's appearance, behavior, and conversation as seen and heard.
3. Complete: A record of examinations, treatments, medications, therapies, nursing interventions, and the patient's reaction to each should be made on the patient's chart. Samples of the patient's writing or drawing should be preserved.
4. Legible: Psychiatric nursing notes should be written legibly, with the use of acceptable abbreviations only, and no erasures. Correct grammar and spelling are important, and complete sentences should be used.
5. Dated: It is very important to note the time of entry. For example, MS has been quiet and withdrawn all day; however, later in the evening she becomes agitated. The nurse needs to state the time at which MS's behavior changed, as well as describe any pertinent situations that might be identified as the cause of her behavioral change.
6. Logical: Presented in logical sequence
7. Signed: By the person making the entry

 Example of Nursing Progress Notes

Various forms of documentation are used to record nursing progress notes, including SOAP (subjective data, objective data, assessment, and plan of care) and DAP (objective and subjective data, assessment, and plan of care). Progress notes should reflect the effectiveness of treatment plans. Multidisciplinary progress notes have become more prevalent as they depict a chronologic picture of the patient's response to various therapeutic interventions.

An example of DAP nursing notes using the multidisciplinary progress note format is presented in Box 5-5. Problems identified in the nursing care plan and addressed in documentation are entered in the column labeled "Problem Number." Both objective and subjective data are included under "data" (D). Subjective data include what the patient states about thoughts, feelings, behaviors, or problems, whereas objective data refers to the nursing observations or measurements related to vital signs, appearance, and behavior.

BOX 5-5 Example of DAP Nursing Progress Notes

Date and Time	Problem Number	Name and Title	Multidisciplinary Progress Notes
2/7/92 9:00 A.M.	#1	ARNP	D: RK was eating breakfast at 8:00 A.M. when she began to perspire profusely and stated, "I don't know what's wrong with me, but I feel jittery inside. I feel like something terrible is going to happen." When asked to describe her feelings, RK replied, "I can't. I just have an awful feeling inside." Affect blunted. Pallor noted. Tearful during interaction. Minimal eye contact. Voice tremulous. P = 120, R = 28, BP = 130/80. No signs of acute physical distress noted at this time. A: Expressing fear of the unknown and inability to maintain control of her emotions. Recognizes she is experiencing symptoms of anxiety but is unable to use effective coping skills. P: Encourage verbalization of feelings when able to interact/communicate needs Explore presence of positive coping skills Administer prescribed antianxiety agent Monitor response to medication

Note. Problem #1 refers to *Ineffective Individual Coping.
*NANDA-approved nursing diagnosis.

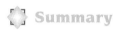 **Summary**

Assessment of the psychiatric patient includes a mental status examination, the psychological counterpart of a physical examination. Transcultural perspectives were discussed. Data obtained during this assessment were discussed in depth, including appearance; behavior, attitude, and normal coping patterns; personality style and communication ability; emotional state or affect; content of thought; orientation; memory; intellectual ability; insight regarding illness or condition; and neurovegetative changes. Several purposes of assessment were stated. Criteria for charting psychiatric nursing progress notes were listed. An example of DAP nursing progress notes was given.

Learning Activities

I. Clinical Activities
  A. Assess the following areas of your assigned patient:
    1. Appearance
    2. Behavior
    3. Attitude
    4. Ability to communicate
    5. Emotional state or affect
    6. Content of thought
    7. Orientation
    8. Memory
    9. Intellectual ability
    10. Insight regarding illness
  B. Summarize the data obtained to give an informative report about the patient's mental health status.
  C. Chart pertinent information using descriptive, noninterpretive data.
II. Independent Activities
  A. Use the following nonverbal behavior assessment guide while communicating with fellow students or friends:
    1. State any significant nonverbal behavior, such as finger tapping, tics, or poor eye contact.
    2. State the possible reason for or meaning of the behavior, such as fear, anxiety, boredom, or impatience.
  B. List nursing interventions for the identified behavior.
III. Case Study Behavioral Assessment
  A. WJ, a 45-year-old patient admitted for emergency surgery for a bleeding ulcer, is referred to the psychiatric unit for a consultation because of

symptoms of depression and anxiety. This married man has four children, two of whom are still living at home while attending college. He runs his own business and often works 10 to 12 hours each day. He had one previous hospitalization 2 years ago, when he had surgery for cancer of the colon.

WJ is alert and oriented in ICU but gets little sleep at night. While awake, he watches the nurses carefully and is very pleasant when he converses with them. When he calls for a nurse and one does not respond immediately, WJ begins to shout until someone arrives. His requests are often minor and could have waited.

The staff isn't certain how much WJ knows about his latest surgery, but his response is "I'm glad it wasn't cancer. Maybe this happened to slow me down." He usually terminates such discussions by stating that he has to rest and suggests that the attending staff care for other patients "who are sicker" than he is.

B. From the information given:

1. List the possible stressors before and during hospitalization.
2. Describe WJ's present coping mechanisms.
3. While providing nursing care for WJ, identify stressors that the staff may experience.
4. Write informative nursing progress notes regarding WJ's behavior.

Critical Thinking Questions

1. Spend several hours in the cafeteria or library observing the general appearance (physical characteristics, facial expressions, apparent age, dress, hygiene, and use of cosmetics) of those who enter. Do these aspects of general appearance blend appropriately in the persons you observe? What have you learned? How might you continue to hone your observation skills?

2. As you assess Mr. Chan, you notice that he stops his answers in mid-sentence and also uses words that are unfamiliar to you. How would you continue your assessment to determine if he is blocking and using neologisms, or if there is a cultural or language barrier?

3. To assess how a patient normally copes with a problem, it can be helpful to provide a scenario, ask the patient to identify and talk through the problem, and then listen to the patient's problem-solving methods. (Such scenarios must be applicable to the individual patient.) What kind of scenario might you provide to a 16-year-old male, a 45-year-old laid-off worker, and a 76-year-old widow?

Self-Test

1. State the purpose of a psychiatric assessment or determination of a person's mental health status.
2. List data obtained during a psychiatric assessment.
3. Explain why cultural diversity must be addressed during the assessment process.
4. What term describes overproductivity of talk characterized by verbal skipping from one idea to another?
5. Giving much unnecessary detail while speaking is referred to as what trait?
6. State the term that describes emitting the same verbal or motor response repeatedly to verbal stimuli.
7. What is the term for a sudden stoppage in the spontaneous flow of thought or speech for no apparent external or environmental reason?
8. Differentiate among the following thought processes:
   Delusion of grandeur
   Nihilistic delusion
   Hallucination
   Depersonalization
   Obsession
9. Describe the following six levels of orientation and consciousness:
   Confusion
   Clouding of consciousness
   Stupor
   Delirium
   Dream state
   Coma
10. Explain the phrase *neurovegetative changes.*
11. State the purposes of assessment besides the evaluation of mental status.
12. State the criteria for charting psychiatric nurses' progress notes.

SELECTED REFERENCES

American Psychiatric Association. (1980). *A psychiatric glossary* (5th ed.). Washington, DC: American Psychiatric Press.

Andrews, M. M., & Boyle, J. S. (1995). *Transcultural concepts in nursing care* (2nd ed.). Philadelphia: J. B. Lippincott.

Barry, P. D. (1994). *Mental health and mental illness* (5th ed.). Philadelphia: J. B. Lippincott.

Barry, P. D. (1996). *Psychosocial nursing assessment and intervention* (3rd ed.). Philadelphia: Lippincott–Raven Publishers.

Carpenito, L. J. (1995). *Nursing diagnoses: Application to clinical practice* (6th ed.). Philadelphia: J. B. Lippincott.

Folstein, J. F., Folstein, S. E., & McHugh, P. R. (1975). *Mini-mental state: A practical method for grading the cognitive state of patients for the clinician.* Oxford: Pergamon Press.

Grossman, D. (1996, July). Cultural dimensions in home health nursing. *American Journal of Nursing.*

Hahn, M. S. (1995, September). Minority nurse practitioners: What are the issues? *Advance for Nurse Practitioners.*

Hahn, M. S. (1995, November). Providing health care in a culturally complex world. *Advance for Nurse Practitioners.*

Johnson, B. S. (1996). *Adaptation and growth: Psychiatric–mental health nursing* (4th ed.). Philadelphia: Lippincott–Raven Publishers.

Jost, K. E. (1995, July). Psychosocial care: Document it. *American Journal of Nursing.*

Rowe, C. J. (1989). *An outline of psychiatry* (9th ed.). Dubuque, IA: Brown Publishing.

Simms, C. (1995, April). How to unmask the angry patient. *American Journal of Nursing.*

Small, S. M. (1980). *Outline for psychiatric examination.* East Hanover, NJ: Sandoz Pharmaceuticals.

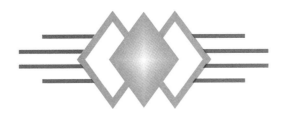

CHAPTER 6

THE NURSING PROCESS: NURSING DIAGNOSIS AND INTERVENTION

The nursing diagnosis is a statement that describes the human response (health state or actual/potential altered interaction pattern) of an individual or group which the nurse can legally identify and for which the nurse can order the definitive interventions to maintain the health state or to reduce, eliminate, or prevent alterations.

Carpenito, 1995

1 State the purpose of using the nursing diagnosis in a psychiatric setting.

2 Discuss the three types of nursing diagnoses identified by Carpenito (1991).

3 Describe the rationale for using outcome identification as part of the nursing process.

4 Explain the development of a nursing care plan in the psychiatric setting.

5 Discuss the nurse's role during the implementation of nursing interventions.

6 State the rationale for the evaluation phase of the nursing process.

Introduction

As stated in Chapter 5, the nursing process consists of six steps and uses a problem-solving approach. This chapter focuses on the remaining five steps: statement of a nursing diagnosis; outcome identification; formulation of a plan of nursing care; implementation of nursing actions or interventions; and evaluation of the patient's response to interventions. The nursing process has been referred to as an ongoing, systematic series of actions, interactions, and transactions.

Nursing Diagnosis and Outcome Identification

The nursing diagnosis is a statement of an existing problem or of a potential health problem that a nurse is both licensed and competent to treat. In 1990, the North American Nursing Diagnosis Association (NANDA) defined nursing diagnosis as "a clinical judgment about individual, family, or community responses to actual or potential health problems/life processes."

The psychiatric–mental health nurse analyzes the assessment data before determining a nursing diagnosis. The diagnosis provides the basis for selection of nursing interventions to achieve expected outcomes and improve the individual's health status.

Expected outcomes are measurable goals that are realistic in relation to the individual's present and potential capabilities. The outcomes are formulated by the nurse, patient, significant others, and interdisciplinary team members when possible. Expected outcomes serve as a record of change in the patient's health status (American Nurses' Association, 1994).

Carpenito (1995) classifies nursing diagnoses as actual, risk or high risk, possible, wellness, and syndrome. An actual nursing diagnosis is based on validated data; a risk or high-risk nursing diagnosis is based on the patient's degree of vulnerability to development of a specific problem; a possible nursing diagnosis describes a suspected problem requiring additional data to confirm or rule out its presence; a wellness nursing diagnosis focuses on clinical judgment about an individual, group, or community transitioning from a specific level to a higher level of wellness; and a syndrome nursing diagnosis refers to a cluster of actual or high-risk diagnoses that are predicted to be present because of a certain event or situation (Table 6-1).

Carpenito (1995) also states that nursing diagnoses should not be written in terms of cues, inferences, goals, patient needs, or nursing needs. Caution is advised regarding making legally inadvisable or judgmental statements as part of the nursing diagnosis. Last, nursing diagnostic statements should not be stated or written to encourage negative responses by health care providers, the patient, or the family.

The nursing diagnoses, as developed by NANDA, are incomplete for psychiatric–mental health nursing practice. Therefore, the development of a list of over 50 nursing diagnostic categories was supported by the Executive Committee of the Division of Psychiatric and Mental Health Nursing Practice of the American Nurses' Association in 1984. The diagnostic categories are included in Box 6-1. The asterisk (*) denotes NANDA-approved nursing diagnoses. The entire list of NANDA-approved nursing diagnoses appears in Appendix C. The American Nurses' Association task force continues to work on the development of a single classification system that will incorporate psychiatric nursing diagnoses.

TABLE 6-1 NURSING DIAGNOSIS TERMS: EXAMPLES AND DEFINITIONS

Type	Diagnosis
Actual	*Ineffective Individual Coping related to forced relocation as evidenced by clinical symptoms of depression (*e.g.,* insomnia, lack of appetite, apathy, low self-esteem)
High Risk	*High Risk for Violence (self-harm) as evidenced by presence of suicidal ideation
Possible (Potential for)	*Noncompliance related to inability to follow directions (*e.g.,* how to take medication) secondary to impaired hearing and poor memory
Wellness	*Potential for Enhanced Family Processes
Syndrome	*Rape-Trauma Syndrome

*NANDA-approved nursing diagnosis.

BOX 6-1 **Nursing Diagnoses in Psychiatric–Mental Health Nursing**

Aggression (mild, moderate, severe, extreme/violent)
Agitation
Anger
*Anxiety (mild, moderate, severe, extreme/panic)
Bizarre Behavior
Boredom
*Communication, Impaired Verbal
*Coping, Family, Potential for Growth
*Coping, Ineffective Individual
Crisis, Maturational or Situational
*Decisional Conflict (Specify)
*Defensive Coping
Depression
*Diversional Activity Deficit
Elopement, Risk for
Emotional Lability
*Family Processes, Altered
*Fear
*Grieving, Anticipatory or Dysfunctional
*Growth and Development, Altered
Guilt
*Health Maintenance, Altered
*Hopelessness
Impulse Control, Altered
*Injury, Risk for
*Knowledge Deficit (Specify)
*Loneliness, Risk for
Manipulation
*Noncompliance (Specify)
*Nutrition, Altered: Less Than Body Requirements
*Parenting, Altered (actual, risk for)
Perception/Cognition, Altered
Post-Overdose Syndrome
*Post-Trauma Response
*Powerlessness
*Rape-Trauma Syndrome
Regressed Behavior
Resource Management, Impaired (Specify)

BOX 6-1 Nursing Diagnoses in Psychiatric–Mental Health Nursing (Continued)

Ritualistic Behavior
*Self-Care Deficit
Self-Concept Disturbance (identity, self-esteem, body image, or role performance)
*Sexual Dysfunction
*Sleep Pattern Disturbance
*Social Interaction, Impaired
Somatization
*Spiritual Distress
Substance Abuse (alcohol)
Substance Abuse (drugs)
Suicide, Risk for
Suspiciousness
Wellness-Seeking Behavior

*NANDA-approved nursing diagnoses.

 Examples of Nursing Diagnoses

The following are examples of nursing diagnoses identified by student nurses who assessed patients in the medical–psychiatric setting.

1. Fifty-two-year-old man with congestive heart failure and metabolic acidosis. This man's chief complaint was shortness of breath. History revealed two heart attacks, chronic constipation, and kyphosis. The student nurse noted the following nursing diagnoses pertaining to psychological needs:
Moderate *Anxiety related to physical condition and hospitalization as evidenced by voice tremors, increased verbalization, increased muscle tension, and diaphoresis
*Ineffective Individual Coping related to loss of independence secondary to relocation and change in physical status
*Sleep Pattern Disturbance related to anxiety secondary to physical illness
Potential for *Sexual Dysfunction related to fear and anxiety secondary to physical illness

2. Forty-five-year-old woman with chronic congestive heart failure and lymphoma, admitted for chemotherapy. Chief complaints included shortness of breath, rapid weight loss, and fatigue. The following nursing diagnoses were made pertaining to the patient's psychological needs:

   *Anticipatory Grieving related to terminal condition as exhibited by denial, anger, and statement "I don't have long to live"

   Self-Concept Disturbance due to alterations in body image as evidenced by negative statements about self

   *Ineffective Individual Coping demonstrated by the increased use of suppression, projection, dissociation, and denial

   Acute *Anxiety related to illness, hospitalization, and separation from spouse as evidenced by increased restlessness, rapid pulse, and increased questioning about illness

Formulation of Plan of Nursing Care

The next phase of the nursing process is the development of a plan of care to guide therapeutic intervention and achieve expected outcomes. The plan of care is individualized, identifies priorities of care, identifies effective interventions, and includes patient education to achieve the stated outcomes. The responsibilities of the psychiatric–mental health nurse, client, and interdisciplinary team members are indicated. Documentation of the plan of care should allow access to it by team members and modification of the plan as necessary (American Nurses' Association, 1994).

Priority setting considers the urgency or seriousness of the problem or need and its impact on the person. Is there a threat to the person's life, dignity, or integrity? Are there problems or needs that negatively affect the patient? Do problems exist that affect normal growth and development? Maslow's hierarchy of needs usually is used as a guide for problem solving during the formulation of a plan of care. These needs include physical needs, safety, love and belonging, self-esteem, and self-actualization.

Ideally, goal setting occurs as the nurse and patient mutually discuss and state expected outcomes. If the patient is actively psychotic and unable to participate in the development of the care plan, the mental health team formulates a plan of care for the patient. Goals can be short term as well as long term to evaluate the patient's progress. Short-term goals are also referred to as objectives for care that may be achieved as stepping stones to reach a long-term goal. Long-term goals are expected to be achieved over a period of weeks or months. Goals should be realistic and achievable; measurable, observable, and behavioral; patient centered; and time designated.

General principles to be considered in writing care plans include the following:

1. Individualize or personalize the plan of care according to the nursing diagnoses or problem list. Ask yourself, "If a person who knew nothing about the patient read the care plan, what would be learned about the patient's needs?"
2. Use simple, understandable language to communicate information about the patient's care.
3. Be specific when stating nursing actions.
4. Prioritize nursing care (*e.g.*, list nursing actions for effective airway clearance before those for impaired physical mobility or sexual dysfunction).
5. State short- and long-term goals.
6. Indicate the responsible party for each nursing intervention.

During licensure surveys by Medicare, Joint Commission, or Veterans Administration, surveyors expect to see the name and title of the individual responsible for specific nursing interventions.

 ## Implementation of Nursing Actions/Interventions

During this phase of the nursing process, the nurse uses various skills to perform or assist the patient in performing specific activities; promote independence and self-care whenever possible; engage in patient education; counsel new patients as the need arises; and implement nursing orders (*e.g.*, measure abdominal girth, monitor intake and output, or spend 30 minutes every shift talking with the patient).

 ## Evaluation

The evaluation phase of the nursing process focuses on the patient's status, progress toward goal achievement, and ongoing reevaluation of the care plan. Four possible outcomes may occur: (1) the patient may respond favorably or as expected to nursing interventions; (2) short-term goals may be met but long-term goals may remain unmet; (3) the patient may be unable to meet or achieve any goals; and (4) new problems or needs may be identified. All members of the multidisciplinary treatment team, as well as the patient, should be encouraged to provide feedback regarding the effectiveness of the plan of care. As a result of the evaluation process, the care plan is maintained, modified, or totally revised. A brief sample care plan for the patient with the DSM-IV diagnosis of depression is shown in Nursing Care Plan 6-1.

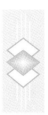

NURSING CARE PLAN 6-1
The Patient with Depression

Nursing Diagnosis: *Ineffective Individual Coping related to depression in response to death of spouse

Goal: Before discharge the patient will demonstrate a beginning adaptation to the loss.

Nursing Interventions	Outcome Criteria
	Within 48 to 72 hours, the patient will do the following:
Encourage verbalization of feelings.	Begin to verbalize feelings to staff
Identify past coping skills.	Identify one or two effective coping skills
Explore current support systems.	Identify one or two available support systems
Educate about grief process.	Identify present stage of grief process
Administer antidepressant medication; instruct patient about medication and its common side effects.	Demonstrate an understanding of the purpose of the specific antidepressant medication and its common side effects

*NANDA-approved nursing diagnosis.

 Summary

The previous chapter focused on assessment, the first step of the nursing process. This chapter focused on the remaining five steps: statement of a nursing diagnosis, outcome identification, formulation of a plan of nursing care, implementation of nursing actions or interventions, and evaluation of the patient's response to interventions. A definition of nursing diagnosis was cited. Psychiatric nursing diagnoses, denoting those approved by NANDA, were listed. Principles to be considered in writing a care plan were given. The rationale for the evaluation process, including four possible outcomes or responses to care, was discussed. A brief sample care plan for a patient with the nursing diagnosis of Ineffective Individual Coping related to depression was given.

Learning Activities

I. Clinical Activities
   A. Using the steps of the nursing process, develop a care plan for an assigned patient in the psychiatric setting, focusing on psychological or emotional needs. List responsible persons for each nursing intervention.

B. Evaluate the care plan daily and modify or revise it when necessary.
II. Independent Activities
   A. Read the following articles listed in the references:
      1. Catherman, A. (1990, June). Biopsychosocial nursing assessment: A way to enhance care plans. *Journal of Psychosocial Nursing and Mental Health Services.*
      2. Jost, K. E. (1995, July). Psychosocial care: Document it. *American Journal of Nursing.*
   B. Develop a care plan for the patient described in the following paragraph. Focus on emotional or psychological needs.

     A 50-year-old man complains of chronic low back pain from degenerative disk disease and other somatic symptoms. He alleges that he is disabled and cannot work or pursue his hobbies owing to his back pain. This person was divorced approximately 6 years ago at age 44 and described the divorce in great detail during his initial assessment. He refers to himself as a failure, stating, "I never could do anything well enough to please my father and then my marriage ended in divorce. Things never did go right for me. I don't have any friends." He alleges that he has difficulty falling asleep at night, has lost 18 pounds the past year, and "does not feel like" eating. He has no social or civic involvements and alleges financial problems because he is receiving only social security disability benefits of $637.00 per month. During the interview his voice became tremulous as he discussed his divorce. He rubbed the arm of the chair incessantly, chain-smoked four cigarettes, and complained of headaches, dizziness, restlessness in his legs, and back pain.

Critical Thinking Questions

1. Identify your own level of attainment according to Maslow's hierarchy of needs. Develop a care plan for yourself, being sure to include short- and long-term goals to promote your growth and development.
2. Every time you take report from Susan Fowler, RN, you find that her care plans are incomplete and the nursing actions don't seem appropriate for the patients as you assess them. What actions can you take to help the patients, Susan, and yourself?
3. Using a clinical case with which you are familiar, prepare a 10-minute presentation that will help the members of a multidisciplinary treatment team see the nursing process in action.

Self-Test

1. Name the six steps of the nursing process.
2. Benefits of using a nursing diagnosis include:
3. Which step of the nursing process includes setting priorities and goals?
4. Three purposes of a nursing care plan are:
5. Principles to consider when writing a care plan include:
6. State several activities that occur during the implementation of nursing intervention.
7. Describe the evaluation step of the nursing process.

SELECTED REFERENCES

Alfaro, R. (1990). *Applying nursing diagnoses and nursing process: A step-by-step guide* (2nd ed). Philadelphia: J. B. Lippincott.

American Nurses' Association. (1994). *Standards of psychiatric–mental health clinical nursing practice*. Washington, DC: Author.

Barry, P. D. (1994). *Mental health and mental illness* (5th ed.). Philadelphia: J. B. Lippincott.

Carpenito, L. J. (1991). *Handbook of nursing diagnoses* (4th ed.). Philadelphia: J. B. Lippincott.

Carpenito, L. J. (1995). *Nursing diagnosis: Application to clinical practice* (6th ed.). Philadelphia: J. B. Lippincott.

Catherman, A. (1990, June). Biopsychosocial nursing assessment: A way to enhance care plans. *Journal of Psychosocial Nursing and Mental Health Services*.

Johnson, B. S. (1997). *Adaptation and growth: Psychiatric–mental health nursing* (4th ed.). Philadelphia: Lippincott–Raven Publishers.

Jost, K. E. (1995, July). Psychosocial care: Document it. *American Journal of Nursing*.

McFarland, G. K., Wasli, E. L., & Gerety, E. K. (1997). *Nursing diagnoses and process in psychiatric mental health nursing* (3rd ed.). Philadelphia: Lippincott–Raven Publishers.

North American Nursing Diagnosis Association. (1992). Taxonomy II. St. Louis: Author.

North American Nursing Diagnosis Association. (1993). *Classification of nursing diagnoses: Proceedings of the Tenth Conference*. Philadelphia: J. B. Lippincott.

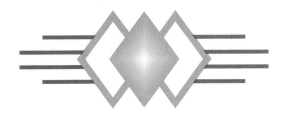

CHAPTER 7

THERAPEUTIC INTERACTIONS

Listen

When I ask you to listen to me and you start giving advice
you have not done what I asked.

When I ask you to listen to me and you begin to tell me why I
shouldn't feel that way, you are trampling on my *feelings*.

When I ask you to listen to me and you feel you have to *do*
something to solve my problem, you have failed me,
strange as that may seem.

Listen! All I asked, was that you listen, not talk or do—
just hear me.

Advice is cheap: 10 cents will get you both Dear Abby and
Billy Graham in the same newspaper.

And I can do for myself; I'm not helpless. Maybe discouraged
and faltering, but not helpless.

When you do something for me *that I can and need to do for myself*,
you contribute to my fear and weakness.

But, when you accept as a simple fact that I do feel what I
feel, no matter how irrational, then I can quit trying to
convince you and can get about the business of
understanding what's behind this irrational feeling.

And when that's clear, the answers are obvious and I don't
need advice.
Irrational feelings make sense when we understand what's
behind them.
Perhaps that's why prayer works, sometimes, for some people
because God is mute, and he doesn't give advice or try to
fix things. "They" just listen and let you work it out for
yourself.
So, please listen and just hear me. And, if you want to talk,
wait a minute for your turn; and I'll listen to you.

Anonymous

LEARNING OBJECTIVES

1 Describe a therapeutic interaction.
2 Define the process of communication.
3 State the factors that influence communication.
4 Explain how one may develop good communication skills.
5 Discuss how communication blocks can occur.
6 Compare social and therapeutic interactions.
7 List essential conditions for a therapeutic relationship to occur as
described by Carl Rogers.
8 Describe the elements of nonverbal communication.
9 Explain the phases of a therapeutic relationship.
10 Cite examples of interpersonal therapeutic techniques.
11 Discuss the interaction or process recording.

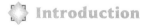 Introduction

According to Webster's, an *interaction* is a mutual or reciprocal action that can
occur between or among people. Interaction that facilitates growth, development, maturity, improved functioning, and improved coping is considered therapeutic (Rogers, 1961).

Therapeutic communication, relationship, intervention, environment, and milieu all are terms that refer to nurse–patient interactions. The focus of this chapter is to discuss the nurse's ability to establish a therapeutic relationship through communication and interaction.

Communication

The process of communication includes three elements: the sender, the message, and the receiver. Communication is the giving and receiving of information. The sender prepares or creates a message when a need occurs and sends the message to a receiver or listener, who then decodes it. The receiver may then return a message or feedback to the initiator of the message. Communication is a learned process influenced by a person's attitudes, sociocultural or ethnic background, past experiences, knowledge of subject matter, and ability to relate to others. Interpersonal perceptions also affect our ability to communicate because they influence the initiation and response of communication. Such perception occurs through the senses of sight, sound, touch, and smell. Environmental factors that influence communication include time, place, and the presence of one or more persons.

The factors influencing communication follow:

1. *Attitude.* Attitudes are developed in various ways and may be the result of interaction with the environment, assimilation of others' attitudes, life experiences, intellectual processes, or a traumatic experience. Descriptive terms include accepting, caring, prejudiced, judgmental, and open or closed minded.
2. *Sociocultural or ethnic background.* People of French or Italian heritage often are referred to as gregarious and talkative, willing to share thoughts and feelings. People from Southeast Asian countries such as Thailand or Laos, who often are referred to as quiet and reserved, may appear stoic and reluctant to discuss personal feelings with persons outside their families.
3. *Past experiences.* Previous positive or negative experiences influence one's ability to communicate. For example, children who have been told continually to be quiet, or to speak only when spoken to, may become withdrawn and noncommunicative. Teenagers who have been "put down" by parents or teachers whenever attempting to express any feelings may develop a poor self-image and feel their opinions are not worthwhile. As a result, they avoid interacting with others.
4. *Knowledge of subject matter.* A person who is well educated or knowledgeable about certain topics may feel more secure when discussing these topics with others. A word of caution: knowledgeable people need to communicate with

others at the level of understanding of others. The receiver of the message may neglect to ask questions, not wanting to appear ignorant, and as a result, may not receive the correct information.

5. *Ability to relate to others.* Some people are "natural-born talkers" who claim to have "never met a stranger." Others may possess an intuitive trait that enables them to say the right thing at the right time and relate well to people. "I feel so comfortable talking with her," "She's so easy to relate to," and "I could talk to him for hours" are just a few comments made about people who have the ability to relate to others. Such an ability can also be a learned process, the result of practicing communicative skills over a period of time.

6. *Interpersonal perceptions.* Satir (1976) warns the reader to beware of looking without seeing, listening without hearing, touching without feeling, moving without awareness, and speaking without meaning. The following passage reinforces the importance of perception: "I know that you believe you understand what you think I said, but I'm not sure you realize that what you heard is not what I said" (Lore, 1981, p. 63).

7. *Environmental factors such as time, place, and the presence of people.* Timing is quite important during a conversation. Consider the child who has misbehaved and is told by his mother, "Just wait till your father gets home." By the time father does arrive home, the child may not be able to relate to him regarding the incident that occurred earlier. Some people prefer to "buy time" to handle a situation involving a personal confrontation. They want time to think things over or "a cooling-off period." The place in which communication occurs, as well as the number of people present, has a definite influence on interactions. A subway, crowded restaurant, or grocery store would not be a desirable place to conduct a disclosing, serious, or philosophic conversation.

🞧 Nonverbal Communication

As mentioned earlier, communication can be verbal, written, or nonverbal. The last is considered a more accurate description of true feelings because people have less control over nonverbal reactions. Nonverbal communication includes position or posture, gestures, touch, physical appearance, facial expressions, vocal cues, and distance or spatial territory.

1. *Position or posture.* The position one assumes can designate authority, cowardice, boredom, or indifference. For example, a nurse standing at the foot of a patient's bed with arms folded across chest gives the impression that the nurse is in charge of any interaction that may occur. A student nurse slumped in a chair, doodling on a pad, gives the appearance of boredom.

2. *Gestures.* Pointing, finger tapping, winking, hand clapping, eyebrow raising, palm rubbing, hand wringing, and beard stroking are examples of nonverbal gestures that communicate various thoughts and feelings. Reflect on these gestures and your reactions to them. What gestures are common in your nonverbal communication? Do they betray feelings of insecurity, anxiety, or apprehension, or do they express feelings of power, enthusiasm, eagerness, or genuine interest?

3. *Touch.* Hand shaking, hugging, holding hands, and kissing all denote positive feelings for another person. Reactions to touch depend on age, sex, cultural background, interpretation of the gesture, and appropriateness of the touch. The nurse should exercise caution when touching people. The depressed or grieving patient may respond to touch as a gesture of concern, whereas the sexually promiscuous person may consider touching an invitation to sexual advances. An abused child may recoil from the nurse's attempt to comfort, whereas the dying patient may be comforted by the presence of a nurse sitting by the bedside silently holding the patient's hand.

4. *Physical appearance.* People who are depressed may pay little attention to their appearance. They may appear unkempt and unconsciously don dark-colored clothing, reflecting their depressed feelings. Confused or disoriented persons may forget to put on items of clothing, put them on inside out, or dress inappropriately. Weight gain or weight loss also may be a form of nonverbal communication. People who exhibit either may be experiencing a low self-concept or feelings of anxiety, depression, or loneliness. The manic patient may dress in brightly colored clothes with several items of jewelry and excessive make-up. People with a positive self-concept may communicate such feelings by appearing neat, clean, and well dressed.

5. *Facial expressions.* A blank stare, startled expression, sneer, grimace, and broad smile are examples of facial expressions denoting one's innermost feelings. Clowns use facial expressions to convey feelings of sadness, happiness, surprise, and disgust, as well as other emotional reactions. Commercials on television and billboard advertisements make use of facial expressions to sell various products.

6. *Vocal cues.* Pausing or hesitating while conversing, talking in a tense or flat tone, or speaking tremulously are vocal cues that can agree with or contradict one's verbalization. Speaking softly may indicate a concern for another, whereas speaking loudly may be the result of feelings of anger or hostility. For example, a person who is admitted to the hospital for emergency surgery may speak softly but tremulously, stating, "I'm okay. I just want to get better and go home as soon as possible." The nonverbal cues should indicate to the nurse that the patient is not okay and the patient's feelings should be explored.

7. *Distance or spatial territory.* Hall (1966) describes four zones of distance awareness used by adult, middle-class Americans. They include the intimate, personal, social, and public zones. Actions that involve touching another body, such as love-making and wrestling, occur in the intimate distance zone. The personal zone refers to an arm's length distance of approximately one and one-half feet to four feet. Physical contact, such as hand holding, still can occur. This is the zone in which therapeutic communication occurs. The social zone, in which formal business and social discourse occurs, occupies a space of 4 feet to 12 feet. The public zone, in which no physical contact and little eye contact occurs, ranges from 12 feet to 25 feet. People who maintain communication in this zone remain strangers.

Communication Skills

The following suggestions are given to enable the nurse to develop good communication skills for effective therapeutic interactions.

1. *Know yourself:* What motivates your interest in helping others? Identify your emotional needs so that they don't interfere with the ability to relate to others. Be aware of any mood swings that you may exhibit. Patients are very sensitive to the emotions and reactions of helping persons. One student stated at the beginning of a therapeutic interaction, "Mr. Williams asked me what was wrong today. I tried not to show that I had a headache. He said I wasn't my usual cheery self. I'm surprised he realized I wasn't feeling up to par."

2. *Be honest with your feelings:* Don't wear a mask to protect yourself or avoid contact with others. Your body language, gestures, and tone of voice can reveal your true feelings or reactions to patient behavior. Your nonverbal communication may contradict your spoken word if you are not honest with the patient. Nurses who work with cancer patients often find it hard to relate to terminally ill persons. They may avoid contact as much as possible, so that their emotions are not revealed to the patients when they are asked questions such as, "Will I be getting better?", "Is it cancer?", or "Am I going to die?" It is okay to cry with a terminally ill patient who is emotionally upset or depressed.

3. *Be secure in your ability to relate to people:* Don't allow the behavior of others to threaten or intimidate you. Remember that all behavior has meaning. Ask yourself, "What is the patient trying to communicate?"

4. *Be sensitive to the needs of others:* Listen attentively by using eye-to-eye contact, focusing your attention on the speaker, and assuming a personal

distance of one and one-half feet to four feet. Use tact and diplomacy while conversing with others.

5. *Be consistent:* Consistency in what you say and do encourages the development of trust.

6. *Recognize symptoms of anxiety:* Knowing anxiety when it appears in yourself and those you relate to is important. Anxiety impairs communication if the person is unable to concentrate or express feelings.

7. *Watch your nonverbal reactions:* Be aware of your body language because it punctuates and modifies verbal messages. Use gestures cautiously to emphasize meanings, reactions, or emotions.

8. *Use words carefully:* When relating to others, these words should be used cautiously: I, you, they, it, but, yes, no, always, never, should, and ought. Satir (1976) refers to these words as "powerful words" that may be used thoughtlessly, appear to be accusations, be easily misunderstood, cause confusion or ambivalence, or imply stupidity.

9. *Recognize differences:* The fact that people may have cultural, personality, or age differences, or may have conflicting loyalties, can impair communication.

10. *Recognize and evaluate your own actions and responses:* Are you open or closed minded, cooperative or uncooperative, and supportive or nonsupportive, when you converse with someone? Are you available when needed or do you tend to put someone on hold if you are busy? Never cut a conversation short in the middle of a self-disclosing interaction. Refer the person to someone whom you feel can be supportive regarding the issues at hand.

✦ Ineffective Communication

Stalls can occur during the process of communication. The nurse needs to be aware of the various reasons for ineffective communication. These reasons include

1. Ineffective communication skills used by the helping person. The nurse may not send the message intended. A list of effective interpersonal communication skills and examples of each are presented later in this chapter.

2. Failure to listen on the part of the helping person. Some individuals are doers rather than listeners. They focus on task-oriented nursing instead of therapeutic communication. The patient also may not hear the message sent because of a variety of reasons, such as stress, anxiety, fear, denial, or anger.

3. Conflicting verbal and nonverbal messages. Ambivalence on the part of the sender may confuse the receiver, who senses conflicting signals and doubts the helping person's interest in him or her.

4. A judgmental attitude. Someone who displays prejudice or a judgmental attitude when relating to others may never really get to know the person.

A sensitive person may pick up on judgmental attitudes and refuse to relate to others, thinking that all people are judgmental. A student nurse in post-clinical conference shared that her assigned patient was quite defensive as she attempted to relate to him. She later learned that he was labeled a juvenile delinquent because he had lived in a low socioeconomic part of town. His parents were migrant workers and left the children to care for each other while they worked in the fields. The patient related experiences that he had had with teachers as he attended various schools. He was shunned by the middle-class students and stereotyped as a member of the street gangs.

5. Misunderstanding because of multiple meanings of English words. Consider the word *cup*. It may mean a drinking receptacle, a hole on a golf green, or a winner's cup (trophy). The sender should select words that are not confusing in meaning.

6. False reassurance. Cliches such as "Everything will be okay" or "Don't worry, the doctor will make you well" are considered examples of false reassurance. No one can always predict or guarantee the outcome of a situation. There are too many variables, such as a person who desires to maintain a sick role, nonsupportive families, or an illness that is irreversible (*e.g.*, cancer or multiple sclerosis). Patients who receive false reassurance quickly learn not to trust people if they do not respond to treatment as predicted.

7. Giving advice rather than encouraging the person to make decisions, however small they may be. Giving advice may facilitate dependency and may also cause the patient to feel inadequate because she or he is not given the opportunity to make choices pertaining to personal care. The patient will accept advice only when wanted. Feelings of dependency and inadequacy may occur and impair therapeutic communication if the patient receives no positive feedback during nurse–patient interactions. It is much more constructive to encourage problem solving by the patient.

8. Disagreeing with or criticizing a person who is seeking support. Belittling a person may result in the development of a low self-concept and inability to cope with stressors. Thoughts and feelings are not important, or so the patient thinks.

9. The inability to receive information because of a preoccupied or impaired thought process. The receiver may be prepared to hear a different message from the one sent. Someone who is preoccupied with thoughts is not as receptive to messages as a person with a clear mind. Impaired thought processes, such as delusions or hallucinations, also interfere with communication. A person who hears voices saying she or he is being poisoned is not receptive to a nurse's request to take medication.

10. Changing the subject if one becomes uncomfortable with the topic being discussed.

Interactions

Two types of interactions—social and therapeutic—may occur when the nurse is working with patients or families who seek help for physical or emotional needs. Social interactions occur daily as the nurse greets the patient and passes the time of day, so to speak, with what is referred to as small talk. Comments such as "Good morning. It's a beautiful day out," "How are your children?", and "Have you heard any good jokes lately?" are examples of socializing. During a therapeutic interaction the nurse helps or encourages the patient to communicate feelings of perceptions, fears, anxieties, frustrations, expectations, and increased dependency needs. "You look upset. Would you like to share your feelings with someone?", "I'll sit with you until the pain medication takes effect," and "No, it's true that I don't know what it is like to lose a husband, but I would think it would be one of the most painful experiences one might have," are just a few examples of therapeutic communication.

A comparison of social interactions and therapeutic interactions as discussed by Purtilo (1978) appears in Box 7-1 (on p.106). Purtilo also recommends the following approaches when communicating in a therapeutic manner:

1. Translate any technical information into layperson's terms.
2. Clarify and restate any instructions or information given. Patients usually do not ask doctors or nurses to repeat themselves.
3. Display a caring attitude.
4. Exercise effective listening.
5. Do not overload the listener with information.

Rogers (1961) lists eight conditions essential for a therapeutic relationship to occur. They include

1. *Empathy*. The helper is able to zero in on the feelings of another person. To "walk in another's shoes" describes empathetic understanding because such action enables one to experience the feelings of another and respond to them. A person seeking help feels understood and accepted. The person is then able to relate to another, to explore feelings, and to try new behaviors.
2. *Respect*. The helper considers the person to be deserving of high regard and cares deeply for the person as a human being. Consistency on the part of the helper conveys respect.
3. *Genuineness*. The helper is sincere, honest, and authentic in responses. The helper becomes a role model as she or he meets the patient's needs rather than wants.

BOX 7-1 Social Versus Therapeutic Interactions

Social Interactions	Therapeutic Interactions
Social interaction may be referred to as doing a favor for another person, such as lending someone money, taking food to a housebound elderly couple, or giving advice to a young girl who has just broken her engagement.	Therapeutic interaction promotes the functional use of one's latent inner resources. Encouraging verbalization of feelings after the death of one's child or exploring ways to cope with increased stress are examples of therapeutic helping.
A personal or intimate relationship occurs.	A personal, but not intimate, relationship occurs.
The identification of needs may not occur.	Needs are identified by the person with the help of the nurse if necessary.
Personal goals may or may not be discussed.	Personal goals are set by the patient.
Constructive or destructive dependency may occur.	Constructive dependency, interdependency, and independency are promoted.
A variety of resources may be used during socialization.	Specialized professional skills are used while employing nursing interventions.

4. *Self-disclosure.* Exposing a view of one's attitudes, feelings, and beliefs is self-disclosure. It can occur on the part of the helper as well as the patient. Appropriate self-disclosure by the helper provides a role for the other person to model, allowing the person to become more open, reveal more about self, and feel more secure.

5. *Concreteness and specificity.* The ability to identify feelings by skillful listening requires the helper to be realistic, not theoretical, while assisting the person in expressing specific feelings. The helper should not expect a patient to be a textbook picture of an illness and stereotype or label symptoms.

6. *Confrontation.* Discussing discrepancies in the person's behavior must be done in an accepting manner after the helper has established a good rapport with the person. Those with emotional problems may perceive themselves

differently than they think others regard them. Such feelings may result in anxiety and inappropriate behavior in an attempt to reconcile these perceived discrepancies.

7. *Immediacy of relationship.* Recognizing one's own feelings and sharing them with the patient is essential to a therapeutic relationship. The helper needs to be able to share spontaneous feelings, but not necessarily all of them. The sharing of too many negative expressions can be detrimental during the beginning of a relationship. Once a relationship exists, the helper shares spontaneous feelings when the helper feels the patient will profit from such a discussion.

8. *Self-exploration.* If the patient is to make progress, he or she needs to engage in self-exploration. Feelings of discomfort or fear may initially emerge; however, the more the patient investigates feelings, the more he or she learns to cope and adapt.

Confidentiality

Confidentiality is important during a nurse–patient interaction. The patient has a right to privacy. All information concerning the patient is considered personal property and is not to be discussed with other patients or outside the hospital setting. When discussing a patient, as in preclinical or postclinical conference, the patient's name and descriptive information that might identify the patient should not be mentioned. It may be necessary for a student nurse to reassure a patient that confidentiality will be maintained except when (1) the information may be harmful to the patient or others; (2) the patient does not intend to comply with the treatment plan; and (3) the patient threatens self-harm. One way to convey this is simply to state, "Only information that will be helpful in assisting you toward recovery will be provided to others on the staff." The student nurse has an obligation to share such information with the nursing staff or with the patient's doctor. Family members should be told that permission must be obtained from patients 18 years of age and older before the attending physician, social worker, or other members of the health care team can discuss the patient's progress with them.

Therapeutic Relationships: Establishing Roles

Peplau (1952) describes six subroles of the psychiatric nurse during a therapeutic relationship. They are teacher, mother surrogate, technical nurse, manager, socializing agent, and counselor or nurse-therapist. For example, the nurse-manager is responsible for creating a therapeutic environment in which the patients feel safe and accepted. The subrole of teacher enables the nurse to educate patients about specific illnesses and medication prescribed to promote stabilization of their condition. Social skills such as participating in groups are promoted by the nurse who acts as a socializing agent. The nurturing needs of patients who are unable to carry out simple tasks are met by the subrole of mother surrogate. Vital signs checks, medical or surgical treatment procedures, administration of medication, and physical assessment are usually completed by the technical nurse. Finally, the nurse-therapist or counselor uses therapeutic skills to help patients identify and deal with various stressors or problems that have resulted in dysfunctional coping. Each of these roles can be effective during the various phases of the therapeutic relationship.

During the therapeutic relationship, patients may distort their perceptions of others. Therefore, they may relate to the nurse not on the basis of the nurse's realistic attributes, but wholly or chiefly on the basis of interpersonal relationships existing in their environment. This behavior is referred to as transference or paratoxic distortion (Yalom, 1985). Countertransference occurs when the nurse responds unrealistically to the patient's behavior or interaction. Negative transference can interfere with the development of a therapeutic relationship.

The One-to-One Nurse–Patient Relationship

Peplau (1952) discusses the phases of one-to-one nurse–patient relationships established in psychiatric–mental health nursing. Such relationships can be divided into three phases: initiating or orienting, working, and terminating. The phases are effective in both inpatient and outpatient settings. Following is a summary of each of the phases, including therapeutic tasks or goals to be accomplished.

Initiating or Orienting Phase

The first step of the therapeutic relationship is called the initiating or orienting phase. During this phase, the nurse sets the stage for a one-to-one relationship by becoming acquainted with the patient. Both the nurse and the patient may experience anxiety when they first meet. A comment such as "Sometimes it's hard to talk to a stranger" is a good way to begin a discussion on initiating a relationship. Assessment of the patient occurs as the nurse and patient agree on the time, place, and duration of each meeting. Communication styles of the nurse and patient are explored to facilitate rapport and open communication as the patient begins to share innermost feelings and conflicts. The patient must feel accepted as she or he develops a feeling of trust toward the nurse. Allow the patient to set the pace of the relationship. The patient is a unique person who is ill and may be experiencing feelings of loneliness, fear, anger, disgust, despair, or rejection. As a patient, the person seeks comfort and help in handling various stressors. In doing so, the patient accepts another's assistance in problem solving or goal setting. The following tasks are to be accomplished during the initiating phase:

1. Building trust and rapport by demonstrating acceptance
2. Establishing a therapeutic environment
3. Establishing a mode of communication acceptable to both the patient and nurse
4. Initiating a therapeutic contract by establishing a time, place, and duration for each meeting, as well as the length of time the relationship will be in effect
5. Assessing the patient's strengths and weaknesses

Working Phase

The second phase of the therapeutic relationship is known as the working or middle phase. The patient begins to relax, trusts the nurse, and is able to discuss mutually agreed-upon goals with the nurse as the assessment process continues and a plan of care develops. Perceptions of reality, coping mechanisms, and support systems are identified at this time. Alternative behaviors and techniques are explored to replace those that are maladaptive. The nurse and patient discuss the meaning behind such behavior, as well as any reactions by the nurse such as fear, intimidation, embarrassment, or anger. During the working phase, the patient is able to focus on unpleasant, painful aspects of life with the nurse's supportive help. Therapeutic tasks accomplished during the working phase include

1. Exploring perception of reality
2. Developing positive coping behaviors
3. Identifying available support systems
4. Promoting a positive self-concept
5. Encouraging verbalization of feelings
6. Developing a plan of action with realistic goals
7. Implementing the plan of action
8. Evaluating the results of the plan of action
9. Promoting independence

Terminating Phase

The final step of the therapeutic relationship is the terminating phase. The nurse terminates the relationship when the mutually agreed-upon goals are reached, the patient is transferred or discharged, or the nurse has finished the clinical rotation. As separation occurs it is not uncommon for the patient to exhibit regressive behavior, demonstrate hostility, or experience sadness. The patient may attempt to prolong the relationship as clinical symptoms of separation anxiety are experienced.

Termination needs to occur if a therapeutic relationship is to be a complete process. Preparation for termination begins during the initiating phase.

Some mutually accepted goals resulting in the termination of a therapeutic relationship include the ability to

1. Provide self-care and maintain one's environment
2. Demonstrate independence and work interdependently with others
3. Recognize signs of increased stress or anxiety
4. Cope positively when experiencing feelings of anxiety, anger, or hostility
5. Demonstrate emotional stability

 Interpersonal Techniques

Box 7-2 lists therapeutic interpersonal communication techniques and examples of each.

BOX 7-2 Examples of Therapeutic Communication Techniques

Techniques	Examples
Using silence	
Accepting	Yes. That must have been difficult for you.
Giving recognition or acknowledging	I noticed that you've made your bed.
Offering self	I'll walk with you.
Giving broad openings or asking open-ended questions	Is there something you'd like to do?
Offering general leads or door-openers	Go on. You were saying . . .
Placing the event in time or in sequence	When did your nervousness begin?
Making observations	I notice that you're trembling. You appear to be angry.
Encouraging description of perceptions	What does the voice seem to be saying? How do you feel when you take your medication?
Encouraging comparison	Has this ever happened before? What does this resemble?
Restating	*Patient:* I can't sleep. I stay awake all night. *Nurse:* You can't sleep at night.

BOX 7-2 Examples of Therapeutic Communication Techniques (Continued)

Techniques	Examples
Reflecting	*Patient*: I think I should take my medication. *Nurse*: You think you should take your medication?
Focusing on specifics	This topic seems worth discussing in more depth. Give me an example of what you mean.
Exploring	Tell me more about your job. Would you describe your responsibilities?
Giving information or informing	His name is . . . I'm going with you to the beauty shop.
Seeking clarification or clarifying	I'm not sure that I understand what you are trying to say. Please give me more information.
Presenting reality or confronting	I see no elephant in the room. This is a hospital, not a hotel.
Voicing doubt	I find that hard to believe. Did it happen just as you said?
Encouraging evaluation or evaluating	Describe how you feel about taking your medication. Does participating in group therapy enable you to discuss your feelings?
Attempting to translate into feelings or verbalizing the implied	*Patient*: I'm empty. *Nurse*: Are you suggesting that you feel useless?
Suggesting collaboration	Perhaps you and your doctor can discuss your home visits and discover what produces your anxiety.
Summarizing	During the past hour we talked about your plans for the future. They include . . .
Encouraging formulation of a plan of action	If this situation occurs again, what options would you have?
Asking direct questions	How does your wife feel about your hospitalization?

Interaction or Process Recording

Interaction (or process) recording is a tool used to analyze nurse–patient inter-actions and is seen in various formats. It is used to teach communication skills to student nurses in the clinical setting, focusing on verbal and nonverbal com-munication. The following format has been used successfully in an associate degree program:

> Patient's initials:
> Age:
> Diagnosis:
> Goal of interaction: State your goal.
> Description of environment: Give a visual description of the setting in which the conversation took place, including noise level and odors, as well as the patient's physical appearance.
> Verbal communication: State the communication verbatim, including what the patient states and your responses. List in sequential order and identify therapeutic and nontherapeutic techniques used during the conversation. Identify any defense mechanisms used by the patient.
> Nonverbal communication: Include your thoughts and feelings, as well as any facial expressions, gestures, position changes, or changes in eye con-tact, voice quality, and voice tone by the patient or yourself.
> Evaluation of this interaction: Discuss whether the goal was met. What changes would you make, if any, after evaluating this interaction?

Excerpts of an interaction recording by a second-year associate degree stu-dent during her clinical rotation on a medical floor in a general hospital are given. Although the patient was diagnosed as having acute low back pain, the staff had observed symptoms of anxiety and suggested that the student and patient would both benefit from the assignment.

 ## Example of Process Recording

> Patient's initials: JW
> Age: 33
> Diagnosis: Acute low back pain
> Goal of interaction: To identify the cause of his low back pain and explore methods of alleviating pain

Description of environment: A private room at the end of the corridor with no offensive odors or disturbing noises. The room is rather bare, with no evidence of get-well cards, pictures, or plants.

The patient was dressed in a hospital gown and was found lying with his back to the door as I entered the room. The lights were turned off and the curtains were drawn.

Description of interaction:

Student	Patient

1. "Good morning. My name is . . . I will be your nurse for this morning." (Smiling; speaking softly; gazing directly at JW while walking to the side of the bed.)
  a. Giving recognition
  b. Giving information
  c. Offering self
	1. "Oh, How long will you be here?" (Turns over in bed and briefly gazes at me with a blank facial expression; speaks in a low voice.)

2. "I'll be here until 1:30. I understand you are having back pain. Could you describe the pain to me?"
  a. Giving information
  b. Encouraging description of perceptions
	2. "It started when I was moving a chair in my living room after my son spilled some spaghetti on the rug." (Maintains eye contact and grimaces as he sits up in bed.)

3. "Tell me about the pain." (Maintaining eye contact while sitting in the chair beside his bed.) a. Exploring	3. "It's a sharp, stabbing pain that occurs whenever I move from side to side or try to get up and walk."

The patient confided in the student that he had experienced episodes of low back pain since he was 25 years old. He stated that although he had no history of injury to his back, the pain occurred whenever he was working and either had an argument with his boss or worried about financial problems at home. This was his third hospitalization within 1 year, and the family doctor suggested that he talk with a counselor because the results of his physical examination were negative. The interaction resumed as follows:

Student	Patient
4. "How do you feel about your doctor's recommendation?" (Maintaining eye contact; sitting) a. Encouraging description of perceptions	4. "I guess he knows what he is doing." (Serious expression; breaks eye contact; fingers sheets nervously.)
5. "Perhaps you and the counselor can discover the cause of your back pain? Then you'll be able to prevent future hospitalizations." a. Suggesting collaboration	5. "I hope so. I can't afford to miss any more work."

Evaluation of interaction: JW was quite receptive to any questions or comments I made and readily discussed his hospitalization for lower back pain. He is willing to undergo counseling at the suggestion of his family doctor to identify the cause of his recurrent pain. I feel this interaction was effective because it showed JW I cared about him as a person and showed an active interest in his physical condition.

⚙ Summary

The process of communication and the three elements necessary to interact with another person—sender, message, and receiver—were discussed. Influencing factors that determine the outcome of communication include attitudes, socioeconomic or ethnic background, past experiences, knowledge of subject matter, the ability to relate to others, interpersonal perceptions, and environmental factors. The effects of nonverbal communication behaviors or reactions such as the posture or position one assumes, gestures, touch, physical appearance, facial expressions, vocal clues, and distance or spacial territory were explored. Ten suggestions for developing good communication skills were listed, focusing on honesty, consistency, sensitivity, security, and careful selection of words relating to others. Ten communication blocks or stalls such as a judgmental attitude, ambivalence, false reassurance, failure to listen, giving advice, disagreeing with or criticizing the patient, the inability to receive information, and the use of ineffective communication skills were discussed. Two types of interactions, social and therapeutic, were compared. Rogers' eight essential conditions for a therapeutic relationship were summarized: empathy, respect, genuineness, self-disclosure, concreteness or specificity, confrontation, immediacy of relationship, and self-exploration. Confidentiality was explained, with focus on the nurse's responsibility to the patient. Six subroles of the psychiatric nurse were described. Three phases of the therapeutic relationship were discussed—orienting or initiating phase, working phase, and terminating phase. Therapeutic tasks of each phase were stated. A list of therapeutic interpersonal communication techniques and examples of each were included for reference. An example of the interaction or process recording was given, with an explanation of its purpose.

Learning Activities

I. Clinical Activities
   A. Establish a therapeutic relationship with a patient. Identify therapeutic and nontherapeutic techniques during your interactions.
   B. Observe various nonverbal gestures and facial expressions of patients and personnel in the clinical setting. List those nonverbal reactions used most frequently. Discuss your reactions to each individual observed.
II. Independent Activities
   A. The following instructions pertain to therapeutic interactions. Share your responses in postclinical conference.
      1. Explain why a nurse's personality is considered by some to be the most effective tool in establishing a therapeutic interaction.
      2. State how one's personality could be detrimental to a therapeutic relationship.
      3. Describe how you would handle feelings of anger or annoyance generated by a patient's behavior.
   B. Role-play the following:
      1. A social interaction with a 19-year-old, newly admitted male patient
      2. The orienting phase of a therapeutic interaction with a 23-year-old female patient exhibiting symptoms of depression
      3. The terminating phase of a therapeutic relationship with a 33-year-old man with the diagnosis of alcoholism
   C. Describe possible reactions or behaviors of patients during the following phases of the nurse–patient relationship:
      1. Initial or orienting phase
      2. Working phase
      3. Terminating phase

D. After reviewing the list of therapeutic communication techniques listed in the chapter, state those techniques you commonly use and explain why.

Critical Thinking Questions

1. You enter Ms. Martin's room and find her crying quietly. She looks up and tells you that her doctor has just told her she needs surgery. Encourage her to explore her fears, anxieties, and feelings with you, using Purtilo's and Rogers' essentials of therapeutic communication.
2. Discuss the three phases of the one-to-one nurse–patient relationship described by Peplau with another nurse. Share experiences with patients where you have and have not been able to accomplish the appropriate goals of each phase. Collaborate with your mentor to analyze your therapeutic interactions and develop strategies for improving them.
3. After studying your own use of therapeutic techniques, you realize that you are reluctant to give information and ask direct questions. What do you need to do to improve your use of these techniques?

Self-Test

1. Describe the purpose of each phase of the therapeutic relationship.
2. Explain the communication process.
3. List the factors influencing communication.
4. Explain a stall or communication block and why it may occur.
5. Explain the importance of honesty, sensitivity, and consistency when developing communication skills.
6. Differentiate between social and therapeutic communication.
7. Explain the difference between sympathy and empathy.
8. What purpose does confrontation serve in a therapeutic interaction?
9. Why is confidentiality important in nursing?
10. Explain the statement, "Don't invade his spatial territory."
11. State the purpose of a process or interaction recording.

SELECTED REFERENCES

Carpenito, L. J. (1995). *Nursing diagnosis: Application to clinical practice* (6th ed.). Philadelphia: J. B. Lippincott.

Emrich, K. (1989, December). Helping or hurting? Interacting in the psychiatric milieu. *Journal of Psychosocial Nursing and Mental Health Services.*

Hall, E. (1966). *The hidden dimension.* New York: Doubleday.

Havens, L. (1986). *Making contact: Use of language in psychotherapy.* Cambridge, MA: Harvard University Press.

Lore, A. (1981). *Effective therapeutic communication.* Bowie: Robert J. Brady.

Peplau, H. (1952). *Interpersonal relations in nursing.* New York: Putnam.

Purtilo, R. (1978). *Health professionals/patient interaction* (2nd ed.). Philadelphia: W. B. Saunders.

Rogers, C. (1961). *On becoming a person.* Boston: Houghton Mifflin.

Rosenberg, L. (1990, November). The use of therapeutic correspondence: Creative approaches in psychotherapy. *Journal of Psychosocial Nursing and Mental Health Services.*

Satir, V. (1976). *Making contact.* Berkeley, CA: Celestial Arts.

Simms, C. (1995, April). How to unmask the angry patient. *American Journal of Nursing.*

Yalom, I. D. (1985). *The theory and practice of group psychotherapy.* New York: Basic Books.

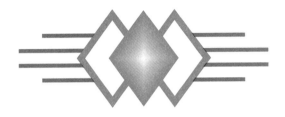

CHAPTER 8
THE THERAPEUTIC MILIEU

M ilieu therapy embraces the idea that a client's difficulties in relating to others often contribute to the development of problems in responding and adapting to the environment.

Baskerville in Psychiatric Mental Health Nursing
by McFarland and Thomas, 1991

1 Differentiate between therapeutic milieu and therapeutic community.

2 List criteria for a therapeutic milieu.

3 Define psychiatric–mental health team.

4 List the disciplines that participate in the promotion of a therapeutic milieu.

5 Differentiate the nurse's role in the following conceptual models of patient care:

    Biological

    Psychological

    Behavioral

    Interpersonal

    Existential

    Nursing

6 State the goals of psychotherapy.

7 Differentiate between operant conditioning and systematic desensitization.

8 Discuss nursing interventions during electroconvulsive therapy.

9 Explain the importance of assessing a patient's spiritual needs.

 ## Introduction

Milieu therapy and therapeutic milieu are terms used interchangeably to describe an environment that is organized to assist patients to control problematic behavior and to use various adaptive psychosocial skills in coping with self, others, and the environment. The focus is on social relationships as well as occupational and recreational activities. Deinstitutionalization, the use of psychotropic agents, respect for patient rights, creation of the multidisciplinary treatment team, and use of therapeutic groups are changes that have contributed to the development of a therapeutic milieu.

 ## Developing the Therapeutic Milieu

The Joint Commission on Accreditation of Hospitals (JCAH) has set forth a comprehensive list of standards to serve as a guide in the development of a therapeutic milieu. These standards serve as criteria for JCAH accreditation surveys.

Therapeutic milieus can exist in a variety of settings, such as the hospital, community, home, or private practice of a counselor or therapist. Regardless of the setting, certain criteria must be met to help patients to develop a sense of self-esteem and personal worth, to feel secure, to establish trust, to improve their ability to relate to others, and to return to the community. The milieu should

1. Be purposeful and planned to provide safety from physical danger and emotional trauma. It should have furniture to facilitate a homelike atmosphere with privacy and provisions for physical needs, as well as promote opportunities for interaction and communication among patients and personnel.
2. Provide a testing ground for new patterns of behavior while patients take responsibility for their actions. Behavioral expectations should be explained to patients, including the existing rules, regulations, and policies.
3. Be consistent when setting limits. This criterion reflects aspects of a democratic society. All patients are treated as equally as possible with respect to restrictions, rules, and policies.
4. Encourage participation in group activities and free-flowing communication in which patients have the freedom to express themselves in a socially acceptable manner.
5. Provide respect and dignity to patients. Adult–adult interactions should prevail, when appropriate, promoting equal status of interactors and exchange of interpersonal information, and avoiding any "power plays." Patients should be encouraged to use personal resources to resolve problems or conflicts.
6. Convey an attitude of overall acceptance and optimism. Conflict between staff members must be handled and resolved in some manner to maintain a therapeutic environment. Patients are perceptive of such reactions and may feel that they are the cause of conflicts among personnel.
7. Continually assess and evaluate patients' progress, modifying treatment and nursing interventions as needed.

The Ward Atmosphere Scale (WAS) is an instrument used to evaluate the effectiveness of a therapeutic milieu (Moos, 1974). Ten subscales are rated by staff and patients to provide information regarding what actually exists and what should exist. Subscale items focus on

1. Staff control of rules, schedules, and patient behavior
2. Program clarity of day-to-day routine
3. Measurement of patient involvement in social functioning, attitudes, and general enthusiasm
4. Practical preparation of the patient for discharge and transition into the community

5. Supportive atmosphere of staff, doctors, and peers toward patients
6. Degree of spontaneity the environment allows the patient to express feelings freely
7. Promotion of responsibility, self-direction, and independence as well as staff response to patient suggestions or criticisms
8. Order and organization of the unit, including staff and patient responses
9. Encouragement of verbalization of personal problems by patients
10. Encouragement of verbalization of feelings such as anger and the channeling of feelings into appropriate behavior.

This instrument is appropriate to evaluate inpatient settings, partial hospitalization programs, day treatment centers, and community-based mental health programs.

Mental Health Team

Members of several disciplines participate in the promotion of a therapeutic milieu. Referred to as the psychiatric–mental health team, members include psychiatric nurses; psychiatric nurse assistants, or technicians; psychiatrists; clinical psychologists; psychiatric social workers; occupational, educational, art, musical, psychodrama, recreational, play, and speech therapists; chaplains; dietitians; and auxiliary personnel. A summarized description of these disciplines follows:

Discipline	Description
Psychiatric nurse	A registered nurse who specializes in mental health nursing by employing theories of human behavior and the therapeutic use of self. Gives holistic nursing care by assessing the patient's mental, psychological, and social status. Provides a safe environment, works with patients dealing with everyday problems, provides leadership, and assumes the role of patient advocate.
	Nurses with a master's degree, clinical specialty, or certification in psychiatric–mental health nursing conduct individual, family, or group therapy. In certain states, the nurse practitioner is granted prescriptive privileges.
Psychiatric technician or nurse assistant	High school graduate who receives in-service education pertaining to the job description. Assists the mental health team in maintaining a therapeu-

(text continues on page 126)

Discipline	Description
	tic environment, providing care, and supervising patient activities.
Psychiatrist	Licensed physician with at least three years of residency training in psychiatry, including two years of clinical psychiatric practice.
	Specializes in the diagnosis, treatment, and prevention of mental and emotional disorders.
	Conducts therapy sessions and serves as leader of the mental health team. Prescribes medication and somatic treatment.
Clinical psychologist	Has a doctoral degree in clinical psychology, is licensed by state law, and has completed a psychology internship (supervised work experience).
	Provides a wide range of services, from diagnostic testing, interpretation, evaluation, and consultation to research. May treat patients individually or in a group therapy setting.
Psychiatric social worker	Possesses a baccalaureate, master's, or doctoral degree. Uses community resources and adaptive capacities of individuals and groups to facilitate positive interactions with the environment. Conducts the intake interview; family assessment; individual, family, and group therapy; discharge planning; and community referrals.
Occupational therapist	Possesses a baccalaureate or master's degree in occupational therapy. Uses creative techniques and purposeful activities, as well as therapeutic relationship, to alter the course of an illness. Assists with discharge planning and rehabilitation, focusing on vocational skills and activities of daily living (ADL) to raise self-esteem and promote independence.
Educational therapist	College graduate who specializes in the field of educational therapy. Determines effective instructional methods, assessing the person's capabilities and selecting specialized programs to promote these capabilities. May include remedial classes, special education for "maladjusted" children, or continuing education for hospitalized students with emotional or behavioral problems (*e.g.*, anorexia nervosa, depression, or substance abuse).
Art therapist	College graduate with a master's degree and specialized training in art therapy. Encourages spontaneous

(continued)

Discipline	Description
	creative art work to express feelings of emotional conflicts. Assists the patient in analyzing expressive work. Uses basic child psychiatry to diagnose and treat emotional or behavioral problems. Attention is paid to the use of colors as well as symbolic or real-life figures and settings. (For example, one dying child drew a series of sailboats on the ocean, beginning with colorful sails and ending with drab gray just before his death. He had interpreted the sailboats as his body sailing the sea of life and death.)
Musical therapist	College graduate with a master's degree and training in music therapy. Focuses on the expression of self through music such as singing, dancing, playing an instrument, or composing songs and writing lyrics. Deanna Edwards, a musical therapist who originally worked with Kübler-Ross, uses music to relate to the elderly, dying, and emotionally disturbed. (She has written such songs as "Teach Me to Die," "Put My Memory in Your Pocket," and "Catch a Little Sunshine.") Music therapy promotes improvement in memory, attention span, and concentration and provides an opportunity for one to take pride in one's achievement.
Psychodrama therapist	College graduate with advanced degree and training in group therapy. This therapy is also referred to as role-playing therapy. People are encouraged to act out their emotional problems through dramatization and role playing. This type of therapy is excellent for children, adolescents, and people with marital or family problems. The therapist helps the people to explore past, present, and potential experiences through role play and assists group members in developing spontaneity and successful interactional tools. The audience may participate by making comments about and interpretations of the people acting.
Recreational or activity therapist	College graduate with a baccalaureate or master's degree and training in recreational or activity therapy. Focuses on remotivation of patients by directing their attention outside themselves to relieve preoccupation with personal thoughts, feelings, and attitudes. Patients learn to cope with stress through activity. Activities are planned to meet specific needs and encourage the development of leisure-time activities or hobbies. Recreational

Discipline	Description

therapy is especially useful with those people who have difficulty relating to others (*e.g.*, the regressed, withdrawn, or immobilized person). Examples of recreational activity include group bowling, picnics, sing-alongs, and bingo. One group of student nurses presented a puppet show during a sing-along for patients with organic brain syndrome. The people related well to the puppets, who visited them individually, because they encouraged singing. The students also dressed like clowns as they recruited sedentary patients to participate in activities. The clowns tossed balloons at stroke patients who responded by hitting the balloons with their affected limbs (exercise that is considered active range-of-motion activity) and tossing beanbags into baskets. A volunteer, under the direction of the recreational therapist, visited the patients daily with her pet poodle as she delivered mail. The patients responded positively to the poodle.

Play therapist — A psychiatrist, licensed psychologist, psychiatric nurse, psychiatric social worker, or other person trained in counseling. A play therapist observes the behavior, affect, and conversation of a child who plays in a protected environment with minimal distractions, using games or toys provided by the therapist. The therapist tries to gain insight into the child's thoughts, feelings, or fantasies and helps the child to understand and work through emotional conflicts. One child was observed hitting the boy doll and calling him stupid. The therapist explored the child's behavior and discovered that he was a victim of child abuse.

Speech therapist — College graduate with a master's degree and training in speech therapy. Speech therapists assess and treat disturbed children or people who have developmental language disorders involving nonverbal comprehension, verbal comprehension, and verbal expression. Failure to develop language may occur as a result of deafness, severe mental disability, gross sensory deprivation, institutionalization (*e.g.*, an orphanage) or an abnormality of the central nervous system. The speech therapist may work with a neurologist or otologist in such cases.

(continued)

Discipline	Description
Chaplain	College graduate with theological or seminary education. Identifies the spiritual needs of the patient and support persons and provides spiritual comfort as needed. If appropriately trained, a chaplain may act as a counselor. The chaplain may attend the intake interview and staff meetings to provide input about the patient as well as to plan holistic health care.
Dietitian or clinical nutritionist	Person with graduate level education in the field of nutrition. The dietitian serves as a resource person to the psychiatric–mental health team as well as a nutritional counselor for clients with eating disorders, such as anorexia nervosa, bulimia, pica, and rumination.
Auxiliary personnel	Refers to volunteers, housekeepers, or clerical help who come in contact with patients. Such persons receive inservice training on how to deal with psychiatric emergencies as well as how to interact therapeutically with patients.

Mental health teams consist of people from a variety of disciplines, depending on the needs of the patients and the therapeutic milieu. Because of budgetary constraints, it is not uncommon for the occupational or activity therapist to serve as the recreational, occupational, music, and art therapist, especially in smaller, privately owned, or community-based hospitals.

 Conceptual Models or Frameworks of Patient Care

Various models or frameworks of care exist within the therapeutic milieu. Each model considers aspects of human behavior, methods of assessment and treatment, and implications for nursing interventions. This section focuses on the original models of care as well as nursing theories used in psychiatric–mental health nursing.

Biological Model (Kraepelin)

The biological or medical model states that mental illness is a disease that is the result of a specific etiology affecting the brain and emphasizes physical, chemical, genetic, environmental, and neurologic causes. As a result, signs and symptoms or syndromes provide the basis for a differential diagnosis, which then determines the treatment. The psychiatrist or attending physician may prescribe antipsychotic or antidepressant drugs, while at the same time using interpersonal treatment approaches that vary from intensive to brief, superficial therapy sessions. The physician avoids placing the blame for deviant behavior on the patient. The nurse who functions under the biological model deals with the patient's somatic complaints as well as responses to psychopharmacology, electroconvulsive therapy, psychosurgery, and hydrotherapy. This model is considered particularly useful in treating acute schizophrenic and depressed patients. It is used frequently in modern psychiatric care and encourages research pertaining to the causes of mental illness. *The Diagnostic and Statistical Manual of Mental Disorders* (DSM-IV) is used to evaluate clinical syndromes, personality disorders, and physical disorders.

Psychological Model (Freud, Sullivan, Erikson)

The psychological or psychoanalytic model states that the personality is pathologic or defective owing to developmental conflicts such as childhood deprivation, confused communication between parent and child, or poor family relationships. Negative experiences due to the inability to cope can result in adult neurosis as well as other pathologic disorders. This model uses psychotherapy or psychoanalysis to bring the person's unconscious problems to the awareness level. Free association (the verbalization of thoughts as they occur without censorship) and the interpretation of dreams are techniques used to help the patient recognize intrapsychic conflict. Emphasis is placed on revealing unconscious conflicts. Nurses who work in an environment that uses the psychological model help the patient to handle here-and-now problems by developing more positive coping skills. A surrogate parent role may be necessary temporarily while the nurse encourages the patient to explore and interpret feelings and behavior.

Behavioral Model (Pavlov, Watson, Skinner)

Proponents of the behavioral model believe that learned abnormal behavior is used to avoid uncomfortable experiences or to seek positive reinforcement. Such behavior becomes habitual and needs to be modified or unlearned through treatment approaches such as desensitization, aversive control, extinction, shaping, assertiveness training, relaxation therapy, or operant conditioning. The patient is not encouraged to explore the past or underlying conflicts. Behavioral approaches are useful for some personality disturbances, adjustment disorders, and behavioral disorders, and are considered complete when the symptoms disappear. The nurse participates in the treatment regimen by setting limits, teaching the patient relaxation techniques, promoting assertiveness, and focusing on the characteristics of mental health. The nurse also works closely with the clinician and patient, for example, during the desensitization process of anxiety disorders such as agoraphobia.

Interpersonal Model (Horney, Fromm, Reich, Sullivan)

The interpersonal model stresses that behavior is the result of interpersonal relationships and early life experiences including infancy. Anxiety can occur during a disturbed mother–child relationship and is a major factor in personality development as well as the development of all emotional illnesses and psychopathology. Intrapsychic conflicts or conflicts within one's personality are derived from interpersonal conflicts. Treatment approaches focus on exploration of patients' progress through the stages of personality development and ability to relate to others. As patients communicate with the clinician or nurse, they experience a closeness that enables them to develop trust, enhance self-esteem, and demonstrate healthy behavior. The nurse functions in various roles: (1) resource person, (2) teacher, (3) leader, (4) surrogate, and (5) counselor. Therapy terminates when the patient is able to establish satisfying interpersonal relationships.

Existential Model (Sartre, Heidegger, Kierkegaard)

The existential approach stresses the here-and-now in the evaluation of a personality disorder by focusing on three aspects of the person's ability to relate: the person and self, the person and others, and the person and the world in which he or she lives. The person develops deviant behavior when out of touch with self or environment. Such behavior is the result of inhibitions or restrictions that are self-imposed and prevent the person from choosing possible alternative behaviors. The person feels helpless, sad, and lonely, and is unable to engage in rewarding interpersonal relationships. Such people tend to allow tradition and the demands of others to dominate behavior or reactions. Encounter approaches (meeting of two or more persons who appreciate each other's existence) include confrontation about one's behavior and responsibility for it, searching for the meaning of one's life, exploring one's life goals and intent to accomplish them, and enhancing one's self-awareness (Stuart and Sundeen, 1995).

Nursing Model: Interpersonal Theory (Peplau)

In the past, psychiatric–mental health nursing followed the medical model. Nurses were taught and supervised by psychiatrists. Peplau was responsible in part for the emergence of theory-based mental health nursing practice. Peplau believed the nurse served as therapist, counselor, socializing agent, manager, technical nurse, mother surrogate, and teacher. Her interpersonal theory focuses primarily on the nurse–client relationship in which problem-solving skills are developed. Four phases occur during the interactive process: orientation, identification, exploitation, and resolution (Meleis, 1997).

Analysis of this theory (Johnson, 1997) reveals its limitations when used in short-term, acute care nursing settings, where hospitalizations last for only a few hours or a few days. It is also ineffective if the client is considered to be a group of individuals, a family, or a community. Peplau's theory is effective in long-term care settings, home health, and inpatient psychiatric–mental health settings where time allows for the development of a nurse–client relationship and, it is hoped, a resolution to promote health.

Nursing Model: Behavioral Nursing Theory (Orem)

Orem's theory focuses on self-care deficit and proposes that the recipients of nursing care are persons who are incapable of continuous self-care or independent care because of health-related or health-derived limitations (Johnson, 1997; McFarland & Thomas, 1997). Human beings are described as integrated wholes who function biologically, symbolically, and socially. Because of their self-care deficits, a nurse, family member, or friend may educate or consult with the individual to improve the deficit. This theory is used in the psychiatric–mental health setting, where individuals may neglect self-care needs such as eating, drinking, rest, personal hygiene, and safety.

Nursing Model: Theory of Adaptation (Roy)

Roy's theory of adaptation was modeled from a behavioral theory and states that human beings use coping mechanisms to adapt to both internal or external stimuli. Two major internal coping mechanisms are the regulator and cognator. The regulator mechanism refers to the individual's physiologic response to stress. The cognator mechanism pertains to perceptual, social, and information-processing functions. Coping behavior occurs in four adaptive modes: physiologic, self-concept, role function, and interdependence. Individuals sustain health through the integration of the four modes of adaptation. This theory is used in the psychiatric–mental health setting as the nurse develops a plan of care to assist the patient in adapting to changes in physiologic needs, self-concepts, role functions, and interdependent relationships during health and illness (Johnson, 1997; McFarland & Thomas, 1997).

Nursing Model: Systems-oriented Nursing Theory (Rogers)

Rogers' theory focuses on the outcome of nursing. It defines nursing as a humanistic science for maintaining and promoting health, preventing illness, and caring for and rehabilitating the sick and disabled. This theory is based on four major premises. In summary, they are that the human organism is in continuous interaction with the environment; the human organism has an energy field that is in constant interaction with energy fields of the environment and other organisms; energy fields appear as organized patterns and designs; and human beings have the capacity to transcend concepts of time–space interaction (Johnson, 1997; Meleis, 1997). This nursing model is used in the psychiatric–mental health setting to promote symphonic interaction and harmony between humans and the environment by repatterning human environmental fields or providing assistance in mobilizing inner resources or energy fields (Meleis, 1997). Therapeutic touch, guided imagery, humor, and meditation are used by nurses to promote symphonic interaction and harmony or well-being (McFarland & Thomas, 1997).

Eclectic Approach

The eclectic approach is an individualized style that incorporates the patient's own resources as a unique person with the most suitable theoretical model. Therapists may specialize in one particular conceptual model or combine aspects of different ones. The therapist realizes there is no one way to deal with all of life's stresses or problems of living and is open to new ideas and approaches as the need arises.

 ## Treatment Modalities in the Therapeutic Milieu

There are as many treatment modalities as there are books written about the care of psychiatric patients. Chapters include information on relationship therapies, alternative therapies, somatic therapies, psychosocial intervention, intervention modes, helping relationships, and crisis intervention.

Some of the more common categories of treatment modalities that are discussed in this chapter include psychotherapy, behavior therapy, management therapy, and somatic therapy. Crisis intervention, group therapy, and family therapy are discussed in separate chapters. Virtual reality is now being used to treat individuals with phobic disorders; however, research findings are limited at this time.

Psychotherapy

Psychotherapy has been referred to as a process in which a person attempts to relieve symptoms, resolve problems, or seek personal growth by entering into an implicit or explicit contract with a psychotherapist.

The goals of psychotherapy include reducing patient discomfort or pain, improving the patient's social functioning, and improving the patient's ability to perform or act appropriately. These goals are achieved by

1. Establishing a therapeutic therapist–patient relationship
2. Providing an opportunity for the patient to release tension as problems are discussed
3. Assisting the patient in gaining insight about the problem

4. Providing the opportunity to practice new skills
5. Reinforcing appropriate behavior as it occurs
6. Providing consistent emotional support

Types of individual psychotherapy include psychoanalysis, uncovering therapy, hypnotherapy, reality therapy, and supportive therapy. Following is a summary of each type.

Psychoanalysis   The term *psychoanalysis*, introduced by Freud, is used to describe a lengthy method of psychotherapy in which the patient talks in an uncontrolled, spontaneous manner termed "free association." The therapist assists the patient in exploring repressed anxieties, fears, and images of childhood by interpreting dreams, emotions, and behaviors. A reliving experience is encouraged by the therapist to enable the patient to deal with once harmful emotions. Sessions last approximately 45 minutes, 4 to 5 days a week for approximately 3 to 5 years. It is an expensive form of therapy.

Uncovering Therapy   Uncovering therapy, also referred to as intensive, insight, or investigate psychotherapy, assists the person in gaining insight by uncovering conflicts, mainly unconscious, so that they can be treated openly and effectively. The patient then "works through" the conflict through repeated exploration of the newly gained insight.

Hypnotherapy   Hypnotherapy is an adjunct to psychotherapy used to help people learn to relax, effect behavioral change, control attitudes, and uncover repressed feelings and thoughts. The therapist places the person in a trance and encourages discussion of emotional conflicts. A person who undergoes hypnosis usually is submissive, abandons control, and responds with a high degree of mental and physical suggestibility. Hypnosis is considered effective in the treatment of overeating, smoking, and other addictive disorders. A hypnotized person cannot be forced to perform actions that conflict with the person's values and beliefs.

Reality Therapy   Reality therapy is based on the premise that persons who are mentally unhealthy are irresponsible. They cannot meet all of their basic needs, and they refuse to face reality. Responsibility either was never learned or was abandoned at some point in life. The therapist helps the person to overcome denial of the real world and meet needs by assuming responsibility for actions. This is done as the therapist becomes involved in an active relationship with the patient, rejects unrealistic behavior displayed by the patient, and teaches the patient better ways to meet needs in the real world. Reality therapy stresses the present because the past cannot be changed. It also forces the patient to make value judgments by facing issues of right and wrong, and by assuming responsibility for actions.

Supportive Therapy Supportive psychotherapy is used to handle conscious conflicts or current problems. The therapist uses techniques such as reassurance, unburdening, environmental modification, persuasion, and clarification. Reassurance helps the patient to regain self-confidence and decrease feelings of fear and anxiety. Psychological reassurance occurs, for example, when parents are told it is normal to experience occasional feelings of hostility and aggression toward one's children.

Ventilating one's feelings through conscious, free expression is referred to as unburdening. Two purposes are served by unburdening: (1) sharing one's feelings, which makes them appear less intense; and (2) revealing oneself, resulting in a form of self-punishment. A middle-aged man placed an apology in a local newspaper to a childhood classmate he had accused of stealing a sandwich. The article stated that he had felt guilty for several years and had to unburden himself even if the classmate did not see the apology.

Environmental modification or manipulation is done to relieve a patient's symptoms and distress. Advising a young mother to hire a babysitter so that she can have time to herself, placing a child in a foster home because of a poor interpersonal relationship with the parents, who are undergoing a divorce, or suggesting that a middle-aged man take a vacation to overcome feelings of prolonged or unresolved grief are examples of environmental modification or manipulation.

Persuasion is used to give direct suggestions to influence behavior and may include an element of environmental modification. For example, a teenager who smokes and drinks excessively when feeling stressed is told to try jogging, swimming, or other physical exercise to release tension, anxiety, or frustration.

Clarification is a process by which the therapist helps the patient to gain a clearer picture of reality by understanding feelings and behavior. Explaining to a man with alcoholism that his illness is a result of a poor self-image or to a woman that she needs to be hospitalized because of self-destructive behavior are both examples of clarification of reality.

Behavior Therapy

Behavior therapy is "a mode of treatment that focuses on modifying observable and, at least in principle, quantifiable behavior by means of systematic manipulation of the environment and behavioral variables thought to be functionally related to the behavior" (American Psychiatric Association, 1980, p. 13). It aims to eliminate symptoms such as temper tantrums or bed-wetting or to develop desirable behavior. Behaviorists believe that problem behaviors are learned and therefore can be eliminated or replaced by desirable behaviors through new learning experiences.

Rowe (1989) lists the following general principles of behavior therapy:

1. Faulty learning can result in psychiatric disorders.
2. Behavior is modified through the application of principles of learning.
3. Maladaptive behavior is considered to be excessive or deficient; thus, behavior therapy seeks to promote appropriate behavior and decrease or eliminate the frequency, duration, or place of occurrence of inappropriate behavior.
4. One's social environment is a source of stimuli that support symptoms; therefore, it also can support changes in behavior through appropriate treatment measures.

Behavior techniques include behavior modification, systematic desensitization, aversion therapy, cognitive behavior therapy, assertiveness training, implosive therapy, and limit setting. A discussion of each follows.

Behavior Modification and Systematic Desensitization Two models of learning theory are used in behavior modification: Pavlov's theory of conditioning, which states that a stimulus elicits a response (a Red Delicious apple stimulates one's salivary glands); and Skinner's operant conditioning theory, which states that the results of a person's behavior determine whether the behavior will recur in the future (a child is given a spanking when he breaks a dish while playing with it). In operant conditioning, good behavior is rewarded with physical reinforcers (food) or social reinforcers (approval, tokens of exchange), and these reinforcers are withheld if maladaptive behavior occurs. Such rewards generally encourage positive or good behavior, bringing about a change in attitudes and feelings. Operant conditioning has been successful in teaching language to autistic children, teaching ADLs and social skills to cognitively disabled children and adults, and teaching social skills to regressed psychotic patients.

Systematic desensitization is useful with Pavlov's theory of conditioning. This behavior therapy eliminates patients' fears or anxieties by stressing relaxation techniques that inhibit anxious responses. Patients are taught various ways to relax as they vividly imagine a fear. For example, a mail carrier is intensely afraid of dogs because he was bitten by one. He is taught relaxation techniques and then is asked to visualize a dog several yards away. He is instructed to imagine himself walking toward the dog, and whenever he becomes anxious he is instructed to divert his attention by using a relaxation technique. This imagined role-playing situation continues until the man no longer experiences anxiety. The next step would be to approach a live dog slowly while using relaxation techniques to decrease anxiety. Therapy is successful if the patient loses his intense fear of dogs.

Aversion Therapy This type of therapy uses unpleasant or noxious stimuli to change inappropriate behavior. The stimulus may be a chemical, such as Antabuse or apomorphine, used to treat alcoholics; electrical, such as a pad and buzzer apparatus, used to treat children who have urinary incontinence while sleeping; or visual, such as the films of an auto accident shown to drivers who are arrested for speeding or for driving while under the influence of alcohol or drugs. Aversion therapy has been used in the treatment of alcoholism and compulsive unacceptable or criminal social behavior.

Cognitive Behavior Therapy This behavioral approach uses confrontation as a means of helping patients restructure irrational beliefs and behavior. In other words, the therapist confronts the patient with a specific irrational thought process and helps to rearrange maladaptive thinking, perceptions, or attitudes. Thus, by changing thoughts, a person can change feelings and behavior. Cognitive behavior therapy is considered a choice of treatment for depression and adjustment difficulties. Rational emotive therapy is a type of cognitive therapy that is effective with groups whose members have similar problems.

Assertiveness Training During assertiveness training, patients are taught how to relate appropriately to others using frank, honest, and direct expressions, whether these are positive or negative in nature. In other words, one voices opinions openly and honestly without feeling guilty. One is encouraged not to be afraid to show an appropriate response, negative or positive, to an idea or suggestion. Many people are unable to say how they feel and hold back their feelings. Others may show inconsiderate aggression and disrespect for the rights of others. Assertiveness training teaches one to ask for what is wanted, take a position on various issues, and initiate specific action to obtain what one wants while respecting the rights of others. Such training is beneficial to mentally ill as well as mentally healthy persons.

Implosive Therapy or Flooding Implosive therapy is the opposite of systematic desensitization. Persons are exposed to intense forms of anxiety producers, either in imagination or in real life. Such flooding is continued until the stimuli no longer produce disabling anxiety. It is used in the treatment of phobias and other problems causing maladaptive anxiety.

Limit Setting Limit setting is an important aspect of the therapeutic milieu. Limits reduce anxiety, minimize manipulation, provide a framework for the patient to function, and enable a patient to learn to make requests. Eventually the patient learns to control her or his own behavior. The first step in limit setting is to give advanced warning of the limit and the consequences that will follow if the patient does not adhere to the limits. Choices should be provided whenever possible. This allows the patient a chance to participate in the limit setting. For example, a 17-year-old substance abuse patient is informed that he is to keep his room orderly, practice good personal hygiene, and attend therapy sessions twice a week. If he does not follow these rules or regulations, he is to forfeit one or more of his privileges. He will be allowed to state his feelings about the limits and to decide which of his privileges will be discontinued temporarily.

The consequence of limit setting should neither provide a secondary gain (*e.g.*, individual attention) nor lower self-esteem. The consequence should occur immediately after the patient has exceeded the limit. Consistency must occur with all personnel on all shifts acting to contribute to a person's security and to convey to the patient that someone cares.

Management Therapy

Occupational, educational, art, music, and recreational activities all have psychotherapeutic values and are called management therapy.

Occupational therapy uses purposeful activities as a way of meeting a person's needs and provides for personal change and growth. Creative media such as clay, woodburning, or painting are used to express creative needs or feelings and conflicts that a person is unable to express verbally. Activities such as rug weaving or sanding provide outlets for the release of anger, hostility, and frustration. The therapist also may focus on activities that improve living skills, such as grocery shopping, cooking, and self-care.

Somatic Therapy

The biologic treatment of mental disorders is referred to as somatic therapy. It includes clinical psychopharmacology (use of psychotropic drugs), electroconvulsive therapy (ECT), psychosurgery, and physiotherapy. Such approaches are used to treat the patient by improving physical and psychological well-being. A discussion of each follows.

Clinical Psychopharmacology   Also referred to as pharmacotherapy, chemotherapy, psychotropic drug therapy, psychoactive drug therapy, and the use of psychotherapeutic drugs, this somatic regimen has changed psychiatric treatment more than any other single development. Modern psychopharmacology played an important role in the deinstitutionalization of patients who were mentally ill and the success of community-based treatment centers. For the most part, acute psychotic patients, who were once on locked wards and restrained, are able to function with moderate to minimal supervision without restraints, hydrotherapy, or ECT. Hyperactive and depressed patients can be

medicated so that they do not harm themselves or others while receiving psychiatric treatment. (Antipsychotic drugs, antidepressant drugs, lithium, antianxiety agents, sedative-hypnotics, and anti-parkinson agents are discussed in the chapter on Psychopharmacology.)

Electroconvulsive Therapy Introduced by Cerletti and Bini in 1937, ECT (or electroshock) uses electric current to induce convulsive seizures. Electronarcosis is a type of ECT that produces a sleeplike state; electrostimulation avoids producing convulsions by using anesthetics and muscle relaxants. ECT is indicated in the treatment of severe depressions, psychosis, catatonia, or mania; in situations in which the patient shows no response to drug therapy; or when rapid results are necessary.

The following is a step-by-step description of the ECT procedure:

1. A thorough physical including heart, lung, and bone examination should precede any treatment.
2. The patient should not eat or drink at least 4 hours before treatment.
3. Vital signs are taken 30 minutes before treatment.
4. Instruct the patient to empty the bladder just before or after vital signs are taken.
5. Remove dentures, contact lenses, metal hair accessories, or any prosthesis that may conduct electricity or injure the patient during treatment.
6. A sedative may be given to decrease anxiety.
7. An atropine-like drug, Robinul, is given to dry up body secretions and prevent aspiration.
8. The patient is given a quick-acting anesthetic such as Brevital after being placed on a padded mat or table.
9. Medication such as Anectine is given to produce muscle paralysis or relaxation and prevent severe muscle contractions.
10. Oxygen may be administered by way of an Ambu bag if spontaneous respirations are decreased.
11. A plastic airway is usually in place to prevent biting of the tongue or obstruction of the airway.
12. Two electrodes are applied to the temples to deliver electrical shock.
13. The limbs may be restrained gently to prevent fractures during a severe clonic seizure. Usually the seizure is barely noticeable; slight toe twitching, finger twitching, or goose bumps may occur.
14. The patient awakens approximately 20 to 30 minutes after treatment and appears groggy and confused.
15. Vital signs are taken during the recovery stage. The nurse stays with the patient until the patient is oriented and able to care for self.

Six to twelve treatments (one treatment two to three times a week) are generally required to be effective. During ECT, memory gradually returns over a period of two to three weeks, although the patient may not recall events immediately surrounding treatment.

Cardiac patients are considered poor risks, as are patients with brain tumors or aneurysms. Side effects include memory disturbances and rare skeletal complications such as vertebral compressions or fractures.

Psychosurgery (Lobotomy)

Originating in 1936, psychosurgery is a surgical intervention to sever fibers connecting one part of the brain with another or to remove or destroy brain tissue. It is designed to affect the patient's psychological state, including modification of disturbed behavior, thought content, or mood. Prefrontal lobotomy and transorbital lobotomy are the two types of psychosurgery still used in research and treatment centers for chronic patients and for those who have not responded to other recommended approaches.

Physiotherapy

Hydrotherapy and massages are used for their relaxing effects in the treatment of psychiatric patients. The effects are short-lasting and the treatments produce few side effects, if any. In the past, hydrotherapy was used to treat agitated and depressed patients by the application of wet packs and cold sheets. Tubs also were used to contain restrained patients in hot or cold water for a period of time. Present-day hydrotherapy includes hot baths, whirlpool baths, showers, and swimming pools.

Spiritual Care of the Psychiatric Patient

When a person enters a hospital, he brings along his spiritual beliefs—possibly intensified by his illness. These beliefs can effect both his recovery rate and his attitude toward treatment.

Pumphrey, 1977, p. 64

Respecting the faith is but one small aspect of our total concern for clients, and is, perhaps, also a much overlooked aspect of tender loving care.

Peck, 1981, p. 158

The first statement was made by a chaplain; the second by a nurse. Both are attuned to the spiritual needs of hospitalized patients, whether they have physical or emotional problems. If the nurse is to establish a therapeutic relationship with a patient, she first needs to establish trust, which is in turn built on faith.

The initial interview should include a cultural assessment, focusing on the patient's existing support system. Who are trusted persons? What religious practices are part of the cultural background? Does the patient exhibit any spiritual needs? Does he or she indicate a belief in home remedies or cultural practices as part of treatment?

Some religious groups condemn modern scientific practice, whereas others support medicine in general. The nurse needs to be familiar with the attitudes and requirements of various religious groups to be effective while giving care.

Once the nurse has established a therapeutic relationship with a patient, the nurse should inform the mental health care team of the patient's spiritual needs. As a care plan is developed, the help of the chaplain or other personnel the patient feels should be involved with the treatment may be elicited. This should be done in conjunction with the members of the mental health team, who must consider the patient's spiritual as well as physical and psychological needs.

Protective Care of the Psychiatric Patient

Protective care of the psychiatric patient focuses on providing observation and care so that the patient does not injure self, injure others, or become injured when around other patients. The patient must be supervised so as not to use poor judgment, lose self-respect, destroy property, embarrass others, or leave the hospital without permission. Specific nursing interventions are given in various chapters focusing on suicide, disorientation, confusion, and so on.

Summary

The terms *therapeutic milieu* and *community* are defined in this chapter. A therapeutic milieu (1) is purposeful and planned; (2) provides a testing ground; (3) reflects a democratic atmosphere; (4) encourages social interaction; (5) respects the individual; (6) conveys an attitude of acceptance and optimism; and (7) continually assesses and evaluates the patient's progress, modifying treatment and nursing interventions as the need arises. A summarized description of each of the following members of the mental health team was given: psychiatric nurse, nurse assistant or technician, psychiatrist, clinical psychologist, psychiatric social worker, various therapists (including occupational, educational, art, music, psychodrama, recreational, play, and speech therapists), chaplain, and dietitian. The following conceptual models of patient care, including the role of the psychiatric nurse, were discussed: biological, psychological, behavioral, interpersonal, and existential.

Nursing theories by Peplau, Orem, Roy, and Rogers were described. The term *eclectic approach* was explained. Treatment modalities in the therapeutic milieu were presented according to the following categories: psychotherapy, behavior therapy, management therapy, and somatic therapy. The following behavior techniques were presented: (1) behavior modification, (2) systematic desensitization, (3) aversion therapy, (4) cognitive behavior therapy, (5) assertiveness training, (6) implosive therapy, and (7) limit setting. Somatic therapy, the biologic treatment of mental disorders, focused on clinical psychopharmacology, ECT, psychosurgery, and physiotherapy. A step-by-step description of ECT, and nursing intervention, was discussed. Spiritual care and protective care of the psychiatric patient were also discussed.

Learning Activities

 I. Clinical Activities
   A. Evaluate the psychiatric setting in which you receive your clinical experience. Does it meet the criteria of a therapeutic milieu? If not, list changes necessary to establish a therapeutic milieu.
   B. List the members of the mental health team.
   C. Identify conceptual models of patient care being used.
   D. Are the following identifiable as part of the therapeutic milieu?
     1. Limit setting
     2. Protective care
     3. Management therapy
 II. Independent Activities
   A. Interview a member of the mental health team. Ask the following questions:
     1. How do you view your role as a member of the psychiatric–mental health team?
     2. What are your goals for the unit?
     3. What are your goals for a specific patient? On which model of therapeutic intervention are these goals based?
   B. Read one or more of the references on
     1. Musical therapy
     2. Spiritual needs of hospitalized patients
   C. Develop a nursing care plan for a patient receiving ECT.

Critical Thinking Questions

 1. Using the Ward Atmosphere Scale (WAS), assess the unit where you have your clinical experience. How many of the 10 subscales are met on this unit? What are your recommendations for improvement? How might you go about implementing these recommendations?
 2. Mr. Clayton is a 56-year-old veteran with a history of depression and alcoholism who has been admitted for the third time this year. What questions

would you focus on if you were operating under the biological model? the psychological model? the behavioral model? and the social model? How might the answers to those questions be merged to implement a plan of care?

3. Although Assertiveness Training is listed as a treatment modality under Behavior Therapy, it is a useful method of communication for nurses. Explore Assertive Communication—assess your communication skills and identify strategies for improving your own assertiveness. Discuss how assertive behavior can assist the nursing profession to come into its own.

Self-Test

1. State three purposes of a therapeutic milieu.
2. Explain the rationale for protective care of the psychiatric patient.
3. Describe the purpose of limit setting.
4. List functions of each of the following in the mental health setting:
   Psychiatrist
   Clinical psychologist
   Psychiatric social worker
   Psychiatric nurse
   Chaplain
5. State the purpose of psychodrama.
6. Match the following models of care and their descriptions.

1. Psychological	a. Mental illness is the result of a specific factor affecting the brain.
2. Biological	b. Focuses on recreational, occupational, and social competencies of the patient.
3. Existential	c. The personality is defective owing to a developmental conflict.
4. Behavioral	d. Learned abnormal behavior needs to be modified or unlearned.
	e. Stresses the present in evaluating a personality disorder.

7. Explain the difference between the theories of Peplau, Orem, Roy, and Rogers as they apply to the psychiatric–mental health setting.
8. Complete the following:
   1. The adjunctive therapy used to help people uncover repressed feelings or thoughts or to effect behavioral change (*e.g.*, to stop smoking) is:
   2. Intensive insight therapy is also referred to as:

3. Psychological reassurance, unburdening, and clarification are examples of:
4. The elimination or replacement of desirable behaviors by means of new learning experiences is known as:
5. Token economy or rewarding a person for good behavior is called:
6. The use of noxious stimuli to change inappropriate behavior is called:
7. Contraindications for ECT include:
8. Side effects of ECT are:

SELECTED REFERENCES

American Psychiatric Association. (1980). *A psychiatric glossary* (5th ed.). Washington, DC: American Psychiatric Press.

Berne, E. (1964). *Games people play*. New York: Grove Press.

Bowers, J. J. (1992, June). Therapy through art: Facilitating treatment of sexual abuse. *Journal of Psychosocial Nursing and Mental Health Services*.

Buxman, K. (1991, December). Humor in therapy for the mentally ill. *Journal of Psychosocial Nursing and Mental Health Services*.

Glaister, J. A., & McGuinness, T. M. (1992, May). The art of therapeutic drawing: Helping chronic trauma survivors. *Journal of Psychosocial Nursing and Mental Health Services*.

Johnson, B. S. (1997). *Adaptation and growth: Psychiatric–mental health nursing* (4th ed.). Philadelphia: Lippincott–Raven Publishers.

Johnston, N. J., & Baumann, A. (1992, April). A process-oriented approach: Selecting a nursing model for psychiatric nursing. *Journal of Psychosocial Nursing and Mental Health Services*.

Mackey, R. B. (1995, April). CE credit: Discover the healing power of therapeutic touch. *American Journal of Nursing*.

McFarland, G. K., & Thomas, M. D. (1991). *Psychiatric–mental health nursing: Application of the nursing process*. Philadelphia: Lippincott–Raven Publishers.

Meleis, A. I. (1997). *Theoretical nursing: Development and progress* (3rd ed.). Philadelphia: Lippincott–Raven Publishers.

Moos, R. H. (1974). *Evaluating treatment environments: A social–ecological approach*. London: Wiley.

Peck, M. L. (1981, February). The therapeutic effect of faith. *Nursing Forum*.

Pumphrey, J. (1977, December). Recognizing your patient's spiritual needs. *Nursing 77*.

Rowe, C. (1989). *An outline of psychiatry* (9th ed.). Dubuque, IA: William C. Brown.

Stepnick, A., & Perry, T. (1992, January). Preventing spiritual distress in the dying patient. *Journal of Psychosocial Nursing and Mental Health Services*.

Stuart, G., & Sundeen, S. (1995). *Principles and practice of psychiatric nursing* (5th ed.). St. Louis: C. V. Mosby.

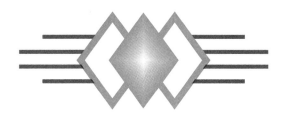

CHAPTER 9

CRISIS INTERVENTION

C risis is a danger because it threatens to overwhelm the individual or his family and it may result in suicide or a psychotic break. It is also an opportunity because during times of crisis individuals are more receptive to therapeutic influence.

Aguilera & Messick, 1986

1 Define the term *crisis.*

2 List the characteristics of a crisis.

3 Describe the phases of a crisis.

4 Differentiate the six classifications of a crisis according to severity.

5 Discuss how the following balancing factors can influence the development of a crisis:

    Realistic perception of the event

    Adequate situational support

    Adequate coping mechanisms

6 Define crisis intervention.

7 State the goals of crisis intervention.

8 Describe the steps of crisis intervention.

9 Discuss the importance of legal immunity for the crisis worker.

 ## Introduction

Most people exist in a state of equilibrium; that is, their everyday lives contain some degree of harmony in their thoughts, wishes, feelings, and physical needs. Such an existence generally remains intact unless there is a serious interruption or disturbance of one's biologic, psychological, or social integrity. As undue stress occurs, one's equilibrium can be affected and one may lose control of feelings and thoughts, thus experiencing an extreme state of emotional turmoil. When this occurs, one may be experiencing a crisis.

A crisis may be maturational or situational. A maturational crisis is an experience such as puberty, adolescence, young adulthood, marriage, or the aging process, in which one's life-style is continually subject to change. These are the normal processes of growth and development that evolve over an extended period and require the person to make some type of change. An example of a maturational crisis is retirement, in which a person faces the loss of a peer group as well as a status identity. A situational crisis refers to an extraordinarily stressful event that could affect an individual or family regardless of age group, or socioeconomic or sociocultural status. Examples include economic difficulty, illness, accident, divorce, or death.

Characteristics of a Crisis

A crisis usually occurs suddenly, when a person, family, or group of individuals is inadequately prepared to handle the event or situation. Normal coping methods fail, tension rises, and feelings of anxiety, fear, guilt, anger, shame, and helplessness may occur. Most crises are generally short in duration, lasting 24 to 36 hours; rarely do they last longer than four to six weeks. They can cause increased psychological vulnerability, resulting in potentially dangerous, self-destructive, or socially unacceptable behavior, or they can provide an opportunity for personal growth. The outcome of a crisis depends on the availability of appropriate help (Mitchell & Resnik, 1981).

 ## Phases of a Crisis

Eric Lindemann (1965) is considered by most to be the father of crisis theory. His theory evolved from the study of grief responses in families of victims of the Coconut Grove fire in Boston in 1943. Gerald Caplan (1964) contributed to the concept of crisis theory after World War II while working with immigrant mothers and children. Each described stages or phases of a crisis. Following is a summary of the various phases generally described by theorists: (1) precrisis; (2) impact; (3) crisis; (4) resolution; and (5) postcrisis. The general state of equilibrium in which a person is able to cope with everyday stress is called the *precrisis phase*. When a stressful event occurs, the person is said to be experiencing the *impact phase*. For example, a young couple is told by their pediatrician that their five-year-old son has inoperable cancer. Once the shock is over, the young parents become acutely aware of their son's critical illness and poor prognosis. This is an extraordinarily stressful event and a threat to their child's life as well as to their integrity as a family. They are in the *crisis phase* and may experience much confusion, anxiety, and disorganization because they feel helpless and are unable to cope with the son's physical condition. When the young parents are able, with or without intervention of others, to regain control of their emotions, handle the situation, and work toward a solution concerning their son's illness, they are in the *resolution phase* of a crisis. If they are able to resume normal activities while living through their son's hospitalization and illness, they are in the *postcrisis phase*. Such an experience may produce permanent emotional injury or may make the young parents feel a stronger bond with each other and their son, depending on their ability to cope. These phases are described in Box 9-1.

BOX 9-1 Phases of a Crisis

Phases	Description
Precrisis	State of equilibrium or well-being
Initial impact or shock	High level of stress
	Inability to reason logically
	Inability to apply problem-solving behavior
	Inability to function socially
	Helplessness
	Anxiety
	Confusion
	Chaos
	Disorganization
	Possible panic
	May last a few hours to a few days
Crisis or defensive retreat	Inability to cope results in attempts to redefine the problem, avoid the problem, or withdraw from reality.
	Ineffective, disorganized behavior interferes with daily living.
	Denial of problem
	Rationalization about cause of the situation
	Projection of feelings of inadequacy onto others
	May last a brief or prolonged period of time
Recoil, acknowledgment, or beginning of resolution	Acknowledges reality of the situation
	Attempts to use problem-solving approach by trial and error
	Tension and anxiety resurface as reality is faced.
	Feelings of depression, self-hate, and low self-esteem may occur.
Resolution, adaptation, and change	Occurs when the person perceives the crisis situation in a positive way
	Successful problem solving occurs.
	Anxiety lessens.

Phases	Description
	Self-esteem rises.
	Social role is resumed.
Postcrisis	May be at a higher level of maturity and adaptation owing to acquisition of new positive coping skills, or may function at a restricted level in one or all spheres of the personality due to denial, repression, or ineffective mastery of coping and problem-solving skills
	Persons who cope ineffectively may express open hostility, exhibit signs of depression, or abuse alcohol, drugs, or food.
	Symptoms of neurosis, psychosis, chronic physical disability, or socially maladjusted behavior may occur.

BOX 9-1 Phases of a Crisis (Continued)

Classification of Crises According to Severity

A classification system developed by Burgess and Baldwin (1981) systematically describes six types of crises based on the severity of the situation. A brief summary of each classification follows:

Class 1: Dispositional crisis in which a problem is presented with a need for immediate action, such as finding housing for the homeless during subzero temperatures.

Class 2: Life transitional crisis that occurs during normal growth and development, such as going away to college or experiencing a planned pregnancy.

Class 3: Crisis due to a sudden, unexpected, traumatic external stress such as the loss of a home during a hurricane or earthquake.

Class 4: Maturational or developmental crisis, in which the stress is internal and involves psychosocial issues such as questioning one's sexual identity or lacking the ability to achieve emotional independence.

Class 5: Crisis due to a preexisting psychopathology such as depression or anxiety that interferes with activities of daily living (ADL) or various areas of functioning.

Class 6: Psychiatric emergencies such as attempted suicide, drug overdose, or extreme agitation resulting in unpredictable behavior or the onset of an acute psychotic disorder.

Paradigm of Balancing Factors

Aguilera and Messick (1986) illustrate a paradigm of balancing factors that determine whether a crisis occurs as the result of a stressful event. These factors, which can effect a return to equilibrium, are (1) realistic perception of an event; (2) adequate situational support; and (3) adequate coping mechanisms to help resolve a problem.

A realistic perception occurs when a person is able to distinguish the relationship between an event and feelings of stress. For example, a 45-year-old executive recognizes the fact that his company is on the verge of bankruptcy because of inefficient projected financial planning by the board of trustees. He does not place the blame on himself and view himself as a failure, although he realizes the seriousness of the situation and feels stressed. His *perception* rather than the actual event will determine his reaction to the situation.

The executive may discuss the situation with a financial consultant, a lawyer, or the firm's accountant. Such persons available in the environment are considered to be situational supports because they reflect appraisals of one's intrinsic and extrinsic values. Support by these people may prevent a state of disequilibrium and crisis from occurring. The less readily available emotional or environmental support systems (*i.e.*, family or friends) are, the more overwhelming or hazardous will the person define the event, thus increasing vulnerability to crisis.

Coping mechanisms are those methods usually used to deal with anxiety or stress and reduce tension in difficult situations. They may be conscious or unconscious, revealing themselves in behavioral responses such as denial, intellectualization, productive worrying, grieving, crying, aggression, regression, withdrawal, or repression. The executive may cope by burying himself in his work, calling an emergency meeting of the board of trustees to discuss the situation, or withdrawing from the situation. Coping mechanisms are used during early developmental stages and, if found effective in maintaining emotional stability, will become a part of a person's life-style in dealing with daily stress. The person who has met developmental tasks and achieved a level of personal maturity usually adapts more readily in a crisis. Additional factors that may influence the development of a crisis include the physical and emotional status of a person, previous experience with similar situations, and cultural influences.

Using the crisis theory paradigm (Aguilera & Messick, 1986), a comparison of what could happen in the presence or absence of adequate balancing factors during a stressful situation, that of the young parents whose son has cancer, is presented (Table 9-1).

Description of Crisis

Stressful Event A young couple is told that their son has inoperable cancer.

State of Disequilibrium Occurs The impact of their son's illness results in feelings of increased anxiety, tension, and helplessness. They experience a threatened loss: their son's life.

TABLE 9-1 BALANCING FACTORS

Realistic Perception of the Event: Prognosis of illness is poor because the cancer is inoperable.	**Distorted Perception**: Question seriousness of illness
Adequate Situational Support: Receive support of pastor, parents, and close friends	**Inadequate Situational Support**: No religious affiliation; decline help from the hospital chaplain; poor interpersonal relationship with both sets of parents; no close friends to turn to for help
Adequate Coping Skills: Able to discuss their feelings and thoughts with each other, family members, and friends	**Inadequate Coping Skills**: Unable to communicate openly with each other; each blames the other for not recognizing signs of their son's illness earlier.

Resolution of Problem: Able to apply problem-solving process
 	
Decide to
  Stay with their son and make the most of their time together as a family.
  Provide the best medical care possible to keep their son comfortable.
Anxiety lessens after the problem-solving process applied.
Able to carry on with routine daily activities while son is hospitalized.
	Problem Unresolved: Uncertain what to do about son's illness; confusion, anxiety, and feelings of helplessness persist. Usual coping mechanisms do not alleviate the fear of a threatened loss. They avoid reality with overactivity.

Crisis Resolving: Achieving equilibrium	**Crisis Not Resolving**: Experiencing severe or extraordinary stress that is precipitated by the son's illness

Need to Restore Equilibrium Parents recognize the need to decrease feelings of anxiety, tension, and helplessness so that they can handle their own feelings and their son's illness.

 Definition and Goals of Crisis Intervention

"Crisis intervention is an active but temporary entry into the life situation of an individual, a family, or a group during a period of stress" (Mitchell & Resnik, 1981, p. 11). It is an attempt to resolve an immediate crisis when a person's life goals are obstructed and usual problem-solving methods fail. The patient or client is called on to be active in all steps of the crisis intervention process, including clarifying the problem, verbalizing feelings, identifying goals and options for reaching goals, and deciding on a plan.

Crisis intervention can occur in a variety of settings—for example, the home, community, emergency room, industrial dispensary, classroom, surgical intensive care unit, or psychiatric unit. The generic approach focuses on a particular kind of crisis with direct encouragement of adaptive behavior, general support, environmental manipulation, and anticipatory guidance. The individual approach stresses the present, shows little or no concern for the developmental past, and places an emphasis on the immediate causes of disequilibrium. It can be used as secondary or tertiary prevention and can be effective in preventing future crises.

The goals of crisis intervention are

1. To decrease emotional stress and protect the crisis victim from additional stress.
2. To assist the victim in organizing and mobilizing resources or support systems to meet unique needs and reach a solution for the particular situation or circumstances that precipitated the crisis. It is hoped that this action will enable the individual to understand the relationship of past life experiences to current stress, prevent hospitalization, reduce the risk of chronic maladaptation, and promote adaptive family dynamics.
3. To return the crisis victim to a precrisis or higher level of functioning.

 Steps in Crisis Intervention

Aguilera and Messick (1986) list four steps in the process of crisis intervention. They are (1) assessment; (2) planning therapeutic intervention; (3) implementing techniques of intervention; and (4) resolution of the crisis and anticipatory planning (evaluation).

When working with a developmental crisis (also referred to as maturational or internal crisis) or a situational crisis (also referred to as accidental or external crisis), the crisis worker should be aware of the following usual occurrences (Lego, 1984):

1. Most crises occur suddenly, without warning, therefore, there is inadequate prior preparation to handle such a situation.
2. The person in crisis perceives it to be life threatening.
3. There is a decrease or loss of communication with significant others.
4. Some displacement from familiar surroundings or significant others occurs.
5. All crises have an aspect of an actual or perceived loss involving a person, object, idea, or hope.

Assessment

The first step in the assessment process is to identify the degree of disruption the individual is experiencing. Is the individual anxious, depressed, fearful, confused, disoriented, suicidal, or homicidal? The second step is to assess the individual's perception of the event. Is it realistic or distorted? Does she or he perceive the situation as a threat to self-esteem or well-being? Some individuals are unaware of the significance of the event in their lives. Attention is also given to present coping skills and the availability of support systems on whom the individual can rely for continued support.

Formulation of nursing diagnoses is the next step. Examples include *anxiety, *fear, *ineffective individual coping, *impaired verbal communication, high risk for injury, or *altered family processes.

Planning Therapeutic Intervention

With information gained through the assessment process, and the formulation of one or more nursing diagnoses, several specific interventions are proposed. Johnson (1997) states that individuals must learn to ask for help and realize the potential for growth during a crisis. They should be involved in the choice of alternative coping methods and encouraged to make as many arrangements as possible by themselves. If significant others are involved, their needs and reactions must also be considered. Strengths and resources of all persons providing support should be identified.

*NANDA-approved nursing diagnosis.

Implementing Therapeutic Intervention

Therapeutic intervention depends on preexisting skills, the creativity and flexibility of the crisis worker, and the rapidity of the person's response. The crisis worker helps the person to establish an intellectual understanding of the crisis by noting the relationship between the precipitating factor and the crisis. She or he also helps the crisis victim to explore coping mechanisms, remember or recreate successful coping devices used in the past, or devise new coping skills. Reducing immobility caused by anxiety and encouraging verbalization of feelings is an immediate goal of the crisis worker. An attempt also is made to establish new supportive and meaningful relationships and experiences, reopening the person's social world.

The following therapeutic techniques are used while performing crisis intervention:

1. Display acceptance and concern, and attempt to establish a positive relationship.
2. Encourage the person to discuss present feelings, such as denial, guilt, grief, or anger.
3. Help the person to confront the reality of the crisis by gaining an intellectual as well as an emotional understanding of the situation. Do not encourage the person to focus on *all* the implications of the crisis at once.
4. Explain that the person's emotions are a normal reaction to the crisis.
5. Avoid giving false reassurance.
6. Clarify fantasies, contrasting them with facts.
7. Do not encourage the person to place the blame for the crisis on others because such encouragement prevents the person from facing the truth, reduces the person's motivation to take responsibility for behavior, and impedes or discourages adaptation during the crisis.
8. Set limits on destructive behavior.
9. Emphasize the person's responsibility for behavior and decisions.
10. Assist the person in seeking help with ADL until resolution occurs.
11. Evaluate and modify nursing intervention as necessary.

Resolution and Anticipatory Planning

During the evaluation phase or step of crisis intervention, reassessment must occur to ascertain that the intervention is reducing tension and anxiety successfully rather than producing negative effects. Reinforcement is provided whenever necessary while the crisis work is reviewed and accomplishments of the crisis victim are emphasized. Assistance is given to formulate realistic plans for the future, and the person is given the opportunity to discuss how present experiences may help in coping with future crises.

Crisis Intervention Modes

The steps in crisis intervention just presented usually are evident during individual crisis counseling. Persons may elect to participate in a crisis group that resolves various crises through use of the group process (seen in self-awareness groups, personal growth groups, or short-term group therapy). Such groups generally meet for four to six sessions. They provide support and encouragement to persons who depend on others for much of their sense of personal fulfillment and achievement.

Family crisis counseling includes the entire family during sessions lasting approximately six weeks. This type of counseling is considered the preferred method of crisis intervention for children and adolescents.

Telephone hot lines such as CONTACT and ADAPT are provided by suicide prevention and crisis intervention counseling centers on a 24-hour basis. They are usually staffed by volunteers who have had intensive training in telephone interviewing and counseling and can give the person in crisis immediate help.

Mental health crisis intervention services are often hospital based or tied to community mental health centers. Mobile crisis units are now used especially to provide services to the homebound, geriatric patients, or individuals who live in rural areas. Outreach programs in rural communities have been known to reduce psychiatric hospitalizations by approximately 60%.

 ## Legal Aspects of Crisis Intervention*

Since 1980, the National Crisis Prevention Institute (CPI) has trained over 100,000 human service providers in the technique of nonviolent crisis intervention. Participants are trained to recognize an individual in crisis and prevent an emotionally or physically threatening situation from escalating out of control. Crisis intervention training helps eliminate staff confusion, develops self-confidence among staff, and promotes teamwork.

Most people are not required by law to help a person in crisis; however, there are some exceptions such as police officers, firefighters, and emergency medical personnel. In certain states, doctors and nurses also are expected to provide help during an emergency or crisis situation. They generally have legal immunity while providing reasonable and prudent care according to a set of previously established criteria and should not hesitate to aid people who need their help.

The criteria or standards of care for a person providing crisis intervention state that the person who begins to intervene in a crisis is obligated to continue the intervention unless a more qualified person relieves him or her. Discon-

*The following information is a summary of simple, broad statements regarding the legal aspects of crisis intervention and in no way is intended to provide legal counsel. The intent of the author is to inform the crisis worker of the potential for legal liabilities.

tinuing care constitutes abandonment, and the care-giver is liable for any damages suffered as a result of the abandonment. Unauthorized or unnecessary discussion of the crisis incident is considered a breach of confidentiality. Touching a crisis victim without the victim's permission could result in a charge of battery. Permission can be obtained verbally or by non-verbal actions that express a desire for help. Implied consent is permission to care for an unconscious crisis victim to preserve life or prevent further injury. "Failure to act in a crisis carries a greater legal liability than acting in favor of the treatment" (Mitchell & Resnik, 1981, p. 34). Negligence may be charged if a person is injured by the actions of a crisis worker; however, the victim must prove that the worker acted with a blatant disregard for standard care. Usually the charge is dropped if the care-giver can prove he or she acted in a prudent and reasonable manner.

Summary

This chapter focused on the theory of crisis intervention by defining a crisis, listing the characteristics of a crisis, and describing the phases or stages of a crisis. The six classifications of a crisis were described according to severity and an example of each was cited. The paradigm of balancing factors used to determine whether a crisis occurs during an exceptionally stressful situation was presented. A definition and the goals of crisis intervention were stated. The four steps of crisis intervention were summarized, including (1) assessment, (2) planning therapeutic intervention, (3) implementing therapeutic intervention, and (4) resolution and anticipatory planning (evaluation). Crisis intervention modes of group process, family crisis counseling, telephone counseling, and mobile crisis visits were discussed. Basic legal aspects of crisis intervention were presented to inform the crisis worker of the potential for legal liabilities.

Learning Activities

I. Clinical Activities
   A. Identify the crisis event that contributed to the hospitalization of your patient.
   B. Discuss the circumstances of the crisis in an effort to evaluate the patient's understanding of the situation.
   C. Identify coping mechanisms used by your patient in his or her effort to establish equilibrium.
   D. Identify the support systems of your patient.
   E. List the therapeutic interventive measures used by health care personnel.
   F. Evaluate effectiveness of interventive measures.
II. Independent Activities
   A. Read Aguilera, D., & Messick, J. (1986). *Crisis intervention: Theory and methodology.* St. Louis: C. V. Mosby.

B. Review Swanson, A. Crisis intervention (1984). In S. Lego (Ed.). *The American handbook of psychiatric nursing.* Philadelphia: J. B. Lippincott. Complete the following:
   1. State the basic concepts of crisis intervention.
   2. Describe the characteristics of crisis intervention.
   3. Compare developmental and situational crises.
   4. State general and specific guidelines during crisis intervention as described by Swanson.
C. Using crisis intervention theory, develop a nursing care plan for a 73-year-old, widowed white woman who, living alone in an apartment, just attempted suicide by inflicting superficial lacerations on her left wrist.
D. Explore the legal aspects of crisis intervention in your state.

Critical Thinking Questions

1. You have just completed the toughest exam of your nursing education. A classmate has been struggling with her grades and is sure she has been unsuccessful. As you listen to her, you realize her perception is distorted and she is exhibiting inadequate coping skills. How might you help her use balancing factors to prevent her from having a crisis?
2. Interview a family member about a family crisis (*e.g.*, a death, illness, injury, or divorce). Analyze how the family went through the phases of crisis. Did some family members come to resolution and others remain in crisis longer? What is the difference in the coping abilities of those different family members? What does this tell you about your family's ability to handle crises?
3. Create a fact sheet about the legal aspects of crisis intervention in your state. Prepare a 15-minute inservice and share the information you researched with your classmates.

Self-Test

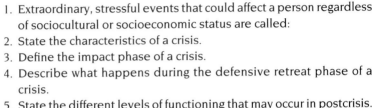

1. Extraordinary, stressful events that could affect a person regardless of sociocultural or socioeconomic status are called:
2. State the characteristics of a crisis.
3. Define the impact phase of a crisis.
4. Describe what happens during the defensive retreat phase of a crisis.
5. State the different levels of functioning that may occur in postcrisis.
6. Give examples of situational supports in your life.
7. List coping mechanisms that you think you would use if you were told you failed a final examination in psychiatric nursing.
8. State the purpose of crisis intervention.

9. Describe common causes of developmental and situational crises.
10. List examples of nursing diagnoses that may be formulated during the assessment process of crisis intervention.
11. Cite several therapeutic techniques the nurse can use during crisis intervention.
12. Explain the rationale for the following crisis intervention modes:
    Family crisis counseling
    Telephone hot lines or counseling centers
    Mobile crisis units
13. Discuss the legal aspects of crisis intervention.

SELECTED REFERENCES

Aguilera, D., & Messick, J. (1986). *Crisis intervention: Theory and methodology* (5th ed.). St. Louis: C. V. Mosby.

Anderson, D. B. (1991, March). Never too late: Resolving the grief of suicide. *Journal of Psychosocial Nursing and Mental Health Services.*

Austin, L. S. (1992). *Responding to disaster: A guide to mental health professionals.* Washington, DC: American Psychiatric Press.

Blair, D. T., & New, S. A. (1991, November). Assaultive behavior: Know the risks. *Journal of Psychosocial Nursing and Mental Health Services.*

Burgess, A. W., & Baldwin, B. A. (1981). *Crisis intervention: Theory and practice.* Englewood Cliffs, NJ: Prentice Hall.

Caplan, G. (1964). *Principles of preventive psychiatry.* New York: Basic Books.

Carpenito, L. J. (1995). *Nursing diagnosis: Application to clinical practice* (6th ed.). Philadelphia: J. B. Lippincott.

Hradek, E. A. (1988, May). Crisis intervention and suicide. *Journal of Psychosocial Nursing and Mental Health Services.*

Johnson, B. S. (1997). *Psychiatric–mental health nursing: Adaptation and growth* (4th ed.). Philadelphia: Lippincott–Raven Publishers.

Lego, S. (Ed.). (1984). *The American handbook of psychiatric nursing.* Philadelphia: J. B. Lippincott.

Lindemann, E. (1965). Symptomatology and management of acute grief. In H. J. Pared (Ed.). *Crisis intervention: Selected readings.* New York: Family Service Association of America.

Mitchell, J., & Resnik, H. L. P. (1981). *Emergency response to crisis.* Bowie, MD: Robert J. Brady.

Servellen, G. V., Nyamathi, A. M., & Mannion, W. (1989, December). Coping with a crisis: Evaluating psychological risks of patients with AIDS. *Journal of Psychosocial Nursing and Mental Health Services.*

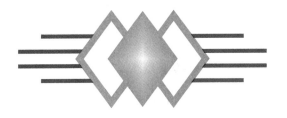

CHAPTER 10

GROUP THERAPY

G roups are a crucial part of life experience for people. . . . They constitute a potent force for prevention and remediation of personal and social problems.

Brill, 1978

1 State the purpose of group therapy.

2 Identify at least six primary factors considered to be essential components of group therapy.

3 Define the terms *open* and *closed groups*.

4 Explain the stages of group development.

5 Describe the qualifications of the nurse–therapist.

6 Differentiate between group task functions and maintenance functions.

 ## Introduction

The use of group therapy as a treatment method has long been effective in resolving many mental health problems. Many people are members within a number of groups, for inherent in human nature is the desire and drive to join others in similar activities and pursuits. Baker (1985) lists the following reasons for the efficacy of groups: collective management of behavior, stimulation of personal growth and satisfaction, improved sociability, decreased social isolation, and improved psychological well-being. The advantages of group therapy include decreased isolation, opportunities for helping others, interpersonal learning and development of coping skills, decreased dependence, and transference to the therapist while developing the ability to listen to other group members. The use of group therapy on an inpatient unit can help integrate patients into the overall treatment program, develop cohesion and support among the patients, and provide an opportunity for patients to be more assertive while decreasing their fears of exploring personal issues and feelings. Nudelman (1986) writes that groups can be a valuable treatment element, encouraging members to use one another's assets to foster their own growth. She further hypothesizes that growth occurs because each member obtains benefits in (1) becoming more aware of self, (2) learning what behaviors are more acceptable, (3) developing therapeutic and supportive relationships, and (4) improving communication.

 ## Definition of Group Therapy

Nudelman (1986) defines *group therapy* as "an identifiable system comprised of at least three people who share a common goal." She proposes that group therapy helps members be knowledgeable about their goals and work toward their achievement. Psychological forces are operative in group therapy, and each member is affected by the unique behaviors, personality traits, and emotional energy of the others in the group. Sadock (1985) suggests that in group therapy members gain personal insights, improve their interpersonal relationships, change destructive behaviors, and make necessary alterations in their personality. Gardner and LaSalle (1987) define group therapy as the treatment of emotional stress and disorder through the means of group method and process. Within their proposed framework, group processes are planned, goal-oriented, systematic, and based on sound theoretical theories. Yalom (1985), considered to be one of the leading practitioners in the field of group therapy, believes that therapy groups are composed of many forms, with the major emphasis on the importance of the "here-and-now" experience.

Therapeutic groups focus on the stress and emotional problems that can arise in relation to a physical illness, a developmental crisis, or a lack of social adjustment. These functional groups assume the complex task of attempting to prevent further emotional distress and disturbance. Therapeutic groups usually center on a specific theme and are educational in nature. The leaders of these groups hope to teach members to cope better with the emotional stress they are experiencing and, if possible, to eliminate the sources of stress. Gardner and LaSalle (1987) identify the following goals:

1. Decrease sense of isolation
2. Promote readjustment to former community involvement and relationships
3. Enhance the skills of problem solving

Some examples of therapeutic groups are groups of persons with a terminal illness, growth groups for the elderly, groups for mothers who are expecting their first child, or groups for families who have a child with spina bifida or other birth defects.

Adjunctive groups make use of specialized activities such as sensory and perceptual stimulation, socialization, and reality orientation. One example of this type of group would be a daily orientation group for chronically ill psychotic patients on a short-term hospital inpatient unit.

 Historical Overview

The use of groups as a therapeutic method has been in effect since the early 1900s. Dr. Joseph Pratt, a physician practicing in Massachusetts, initially treated tuberculosis patients individually. Gradually he began to meet with them weekly in a small group to educate them about their chronic disease, to help alleviate feelings of depression and hopelessness, and to provide support and encouragement for participants to follow through with their treatment regime. In 1919 Dr. Cody Marsh, a psychiatrist and ordained minister, became the first practitioner to apply Dr. Pratt's theories to the treatment of institutionalized psychiatric patients. Shortly thereafter, Dr. Jacob Mareno, a Viennese psychiatrist, was credited with first defining the term *group psychotherapy*.

In 1921, Freud wrote his classic *Group Psychology and Analysis of the Ego*. He described the many differences between groups with leaders and those without, emphasizing the need to have a qualified group leader to reduce members' anxiety. During the 1930s, many more psychologists and psychiatrists became interested in this new method of treatment and began to explore the use of various kinds of groups in their practice. In support of these endeavors, Dr. Slanson founded the first professional group therapy organization, the American Group Psychotherapy Association. During World War II, group therapy experienced significant growth when this method provided optimal treatment for both military and civilian populations. Because there were a limited number of qualified, trained professionals at that time, group therapy allowed a therapist to treat more people in a timely and effective manner.

After the war, in the 1950s and 1960s, therapists expanded the traditional psychoanalytic approach and became more creative in employing various types of groups such as encounter groups, sensitivity training groups, and self-growth and development groups. Later, a variety of social workers, family counselors, nurses, and other professionals began the practice of group therapy. Members from several of the mental health disciplines participate as cotherapists.

Characteristics of Group Therapy

Many essential elements are common to all types of group therapy. Group therapy differs most significantly from individual therapy in that it is more effective in treating problems with interpersonal relationships; it creates a heightened sense of risk and vulnerability; and it allows psychiatric clients a greater opportunity for reality testing and experiencing mutual concern and support. On the other hand, members of groups may feel more vulnerable, frightened, and at risk, and the transference process may be diluted.

Yalom (1985) has identified 11 primary factors as essential components of group therapy:

1. *Instillation of hope* is the first and often most important factor. White (1987) describes people participating in the group experience as initially feeling demoralized and helpless, and points out that providing them with hope is therefore a most worthwhile achievement. Clients should be encouraged to believe that they can find help and support within the group and that it is realistic to expect that problems will eventually be resolved.

2. *Universality* can be defined as the sense of realizing that one is not completely alone in any situation. Group members often identify this factor as a major reason for their seeking group therapy. During the sessions, members are encouraged to express complex and often very negative feelings in the hope that they will experience understanding and support from others with similar thoughts and feelings.

3. *The imparting of information* includes both didactic instruction and direct advice, and refers to the imparting of specific educational information plus the sharing of advice and guidance among members. The transmission of this information also indicates to each member the others' concern and trust.

4. *Altruism* in therapy groups benefits members through the act of giving to others. Clients have the experience of learning to help others, and in the process they begin to feel better about themselves. Both the group therapist and the members can offer invaluable support, insight, and reassurance while allowing themselves to gain self-knowledge and growth.

5. *The corrective recapitulation of the primary family group* allows members within the group to correct some of the perceptions and feelings associated with unsatisfactory experiences they have had with their family. The participants receive feedback as they discuss and relive early familial conflicts and experience corrective responses. Family roles are explored, and members are encouraged to resolve unfinished family business.

6. *The development of socializing techniques* is essential within the group as members are given the opportunity to learn and test new social skills. Persons also receive information about maladaptive social behaviors.

7. *Imitative behavior* refers to the process in which members observe and model their behaviors after one another. Imitation is an acknowledged therapeutic force; a healthy group environment provides valuable opportunities for experimenting with desired changes and behaviors.

8. *Interpersonal learning* includes the gaining of insight, the development of the transference relationships, the experience of correcting emotional thoughts and behaviors, and the importance of learning about oneself in relation to others.

9. *Group cohesiveness* is the development of a strong sense of group membership and alliance. Ideally, each member should feel acceptance and approval from all others within the group. The concept of cohesiveness refers to the degree to which a group functions as a supportive problem-solving unit. This factor is essential in ensuring optimal individual and group growth.

10. *Catharsis*, similar to group cohesiveness, involves members relating to one another through the verbal expression of positive and negative feelings.

11. *Existential factors* that are constantly operating within the group make up Yalom's final factor. These intangible issues encourage each group member

to accept the motivating idea that he or she is ultimately responsible for his or her own life choices and actions.

Taylor (1982) expands Yalom's theory and states that members of group therapy reflect persons in the larger society, and that group conditions replicate reality. Within this structure, group participants present their concerns and problems and in return receive direct feedback and resolutions. Sadock's (1985) view is that the key elements of group therapy involve the expression of feelings, the group atmosphere, the various types of member participation, and the skill and expertise of the group leader.

Types of Therapy Groups

There are a wide variety of therapy groups that make use of the major theoretical frameworks. Lego (1982) classifies all group therapy as either open or closed. *Open groups* do not have established boundaries; members may join and leave the group at different times. Group cohesion and leadership stability are identified as major elements. *Closed groups* may have either a set membership, a specific time frame, or both of these components. Specific membership may address the needs of a particular kind of client, such as a group of female college students who are bulimic or an aftercare group for previously hospitalized patients. Most closed groups require members to start the group at the same time and then terminate the group after a predetermined length of time. Both open and closed therapy groups are used extensively in inpatient and outpatient treatment settings.

Marram (1978) describes five models of group therapy that on a continuum range from supportive to psychoanalytic group therapy. His five groups are as follows:

1. *Support groups* focus on increasing the members' adaptation, self-esteem, and sense of emotional well-being.
2. *Reeducation and remotivation groups*, often very beneficial for psychiatric clients who are withdrawn or socially isolated, attempt to increase communication and interaction among members to foster more acceptable and appropriate behaviors.
3. *Problem-solving therapy groups* focus on the resolution of specific problems that patients have identified.
4. *Insight without reconstruction groups* have group leaders who place their major emphasis on interpersonal communication and work on effecting change by increasing the members' cognitive and emotional understanding of their problems.

5. *Personality reconstruction groups* make use of psychoanalytic theory and encourage the members to explore former relationships and problems and their impact on the present.

 Establishing a Group

Personal treatment philosophies as well as individual patient needs determine the selection of group therapy participants. Consideration is given to the desired size of the group (usually no larger than 10 members), diagnosis of participants, age, sex, intellectual level, verbal or communication skills, motivation, and social skills. During the selection process, a decision is made as to whether the group will be homogenous or heterogenous in nature. For example, a group focusing on women's issues such as single parenting may not be therapeutic for adolescents, women in their 70s, or male patients. Conversely, a group focusing on loss and grief could be suitable for various age groups, either sex, and persons married, widowed, single, or divorced.

Examples of groups conducted in a 40-bed adult unit include task-oriented, co-dependency, loss and grief, medication, spiritual quest, women's issues, men's issues, eating disorders, substance abuse, cognitive skills, and discharge planning groups.

Attention is also paid to the environmental setting. Room temperature, lighting, sound, furnishings, privacy, location, and seating arrangements are important factors that contribute to an atmosphere conducive to therapeutic group process.

 Stages of Group Development

All therapy groups have three major phases: a beginning or orientation phase, a middle or working phase, and an ending or termination phase. During each of these three stages, significant issues concerning group growth and development arise and are dealt with by the group. The key issues involve dependency and interdependency. Tuckman (1965) identified the primary focus as the completion of a specific task, viewing all interactions among members as related to that task. Tuckman, as an acknowledged expert, proposed that the phases of group development were

1. *Forming:* Group members are concerned with orientation.
2. *Storming:* Group members are resistant to task and group influence.
3. *Norming:* The resistance to the group is overcome by the members.
4. *Performing:* The group enters the problem-solving stage, and creative solutions emerge.

Regardless of the name, the initial phase of any group therapy is often one of much stress and anxiety for group members. Each is concerned with how she or he will fit into the group as the group norms and acceptable behaviors are identified. During this stage there may be frequent testing, minimal disclosure, and periods of awkwardness and uncomfortable silence. The major task is for the group to resolve these initial feelings and to achieve a sense of group identification and definition of purpose. The tasks of the leader are to create a supportive and accepting environment, to promote unification, and to encourage verbalization of feelings.

During the middle phase, the working phase, the group becomes more cohesive and members explore relationships and conflicts. The group begins to express all kind of feelings, both positive and negative, and unhealthy behaviors are openly confronted. Throughout this stage there may still be evidence of continued resistance as increased pressure is placed on members to participate in risk taking. The major tasks for members during the working phase are to develop a sense of reliance on each other, to assume a heightened sense of responsibility for the group direction, and to maintain trust and openness within the group relationships. The therapist's role is to encourage members to explore their conflicts and goals, to identify repetitive behaviors, and continually to clarify the group goals and tasks.

During the final stage of group therapy, termination may occur in several different ways, depending on whether the group is open or closed. As the members prepare to leave, they reflect on the insights and growth that they have made within the group. They share feedback with one another as they experience ambivalence about leaving the group. Most members feel both sadness and optimism as they anticipate the future. They may feel a sense of loss and rejection by the group, and feelings of anger, envy, and hostility may surface. The group therapist assumes a less active role during the termination phase as he or she helps the members to integrate the changes and to say goodbye. Nudelman (1986) recommends that the therapist conduct an exit interview with each group member to review the individual's progress and to make an accurate evaluation of the group experience. The therapist hopes, as members leave the group, that they are more realistic in their perception of themselves, have an increased sense of self-esteem, are more resourceful in resolving problems, and are better able to assume responsibility for all facets of their lives.

❀ Role of the Nurse

With all of these groups there are numerous opportunities for nurses to assume the role of group leader, group therapist, or co-therapist. Three major qualifications that a nurse should meet to be an effective leader of group therapy include

1. Theoretical preparation through lectures, reading, formal course work, seminars, and workshops
2. Supervised practice in the role of co-leader and leader
3. Personal experience as a group therapy member

Most mental health professionals agree that the minimal degree for a group therapist is a master's degree. Most master's programs for nurses are now offering this necessary preparation. On the baccalaureate and associate levels, nurses need to have an understanding of group therapy and process, and may be actively involved in leading therapeutic and adjunctive groups.

In a therapy group, the nurse therapist has both task and maintenance role functions. Group task functions are concerned with the more practical issues of leading a group, whereas group maintenance functions focus on less tangible group process (Box 10-1). It is important for nurses to know about these role functions and to become skillful in their administration.

Three basic styles of group leadership are described as autocratic, democratic, or laissez-faire. An autocratic leader generally does not encourage active participation or interaction among group members. Such leaders maintain authority and control over group members. Democratic leaders encourage active participation,

---

BOX 10-1 Nurse–Therapist Task and Maintenance Role Functions in Group Therapy

Task Role Functions	Maintenance Role Functions
1. Identify the goals and plans for the group.	1. Orient group members to purpose and goals.
2. Select an appropriate time and place for the group.	2. Observe and comment on group process.
3. Seek necessary administrative permission.	3. Propose questions and interventions based on theoretical framework.
4. Select appropriate members for the group.	4. Facilitate creative problem solving.
5. Decide on a cotherapist.	5. Maintain group's direction in pursuit of task.
6. Decide whether the group will be open or closed.	6. Act as a support and resource person.
7. Decide frequency and length of group sessions.	7. Promote termination.

value the input and feedback of group members, and promote cohesiveness among the group members as they develop problem-solving and decision-making skills. Leaders who use the laissez-faire style allow much freedom within the group setting. If the group members are not highly motivated, task oriented, or knowledgeable, group tasks or goals may not be met (Johnson, 1997).

 ## Summary

The effective use of group therapy as a treatment modality was initially discussed. Definitions of group treatment were proposed, differentiating between therapy groups, therapeutic groups, and adjunctive groups. A brief historical overview of groups as a therapeutic method was presented. The characteristics of group therapy included a discussion of Yalom's (1985) 11 primary factors. The wide variety of therapy groups was identified and several examples were given. The three stages of group development were reviewed. The chapter concluded with a discussion of the role of the nurse as a group leader or group therapist, including leadership styles.

Learning Activities

I. Clinical Activities
 A. Design and implement a small, short-term therapeutic group that meets weekly, assuming the role of group leader or co-leader.
 B. Observe and keep a record of your observations on group process; share these with your co-leader and instructor.
 C. Identify what the group is experiencing.
 D. Observe several different therapeutic groups and differentiate between their goals and purposes.
II. Independent Activities
 A. Obtain a comprehensive list of self-help groups in the community.
 B. Visit several of these self-help groups to obtain information about each group.
 C. Read one or more of the references on group therapy.

Critical Thinking Questions

1. Familiarize yourself with community support groups. Visit an open group and a closed group several times. Which of Yalom's 11 essential components of groups did you see in action? Was there a difference between the open and closed groups?

2. In what stages of group development were the groups? How did the group leaders handle those stages?
3. What task role functions and maintenance role functions did you see each group leader use? Were they effective?

Self-Test

1. Identify 3 of Yalom's 11 therapeutic factors that influence all groups.
2. Describe the differences between an open group and a closed group.
3. Define therapy groups, therapeutic groups, and adjunctive groups.
4. List five types of therapy groups.
5. Describe the three stages of group development.
6. Briefly explain the history of group therapy.
7. Discuss the role of the nurse–therapist or group leader.

SELECTED REFERENCES

Baker, N. (1985, November). Reminiscing in group therapy for self worth. *Journal of Gerontological Nursing*.

Barry, P. D. (1994). *Mental health and mental illness* (5th ed.). Philadelphia: J. B. Lippincott.

Brill, N. I. (1978). *Working with people: The helping process* (2nd ed.). Philadelphia: J. B. Lippincott.

Gardner, K., & LaSalle, P. (1987). Small groups and their therapeutic forces. In G. Stuart & S. Sundeen (Eds.). *Principles and practice of psychiatric nursing*. St. Louis: C. V. Mosby.

Johnson, B. S. (1997). *Adaptation and growth: Psychiatric–mental health nursing* (4th. ed.). Philadelphia: Lippincott–Raven Publishers.

Lego, S. (1982). Group psychotherapy. In J. Haber, A. M. Leach, S. Schudy, et al. (Eds.). *Comprehensive psychiatric nursing* (2nd ed.). New York: McGraw-Hill.

Marram, G. (1978). *The group approach in nursing practice* (2nd ed.). St. Louis: C. V. Mosby.

Nudelman, E. (1986, September). Group psychotherapy. *Nursing Clinics of North America*.

Pollack, L. E. (1990, May). Improving relationships: Groups for inpatients with bipolar disorder. *Journal of Psychosocial Nursing and Mental Health Services*.

Sadock, B. J. (1985). Group psychotherapy, combined psychotherapy and psychodrama. In H. L. Kaplan & B. J. Sadock (Eds.). *Comprehensive textbook of psychiatry* (6th ed.). Baltimore: Williams & Wilkins.

Staples, N. R., & Schwartz, M. (1990, February). Anorexia nervosa support group: Providing transitional support. *Journal of Psychosocial Nursing and Mental Health Services*.

Taylor, C. M. (1982). Interventions with groups. In C. M. Taylor (Ed.). *Essentials of psychiatric nursing* (4th ed.). St. Louis: C. V. Mosby.

Teets, J. M. (1990, December). What women talk about: Sexuality issues of chemically dependent women. *Journal of Psychosocial Nursing and Mental Health Services.*

Tuckman, B. (1965). Developmental sequence in small groups. *Psychological Bulletin, 63.*

White, E. (1987, February 18). Well supported. *Nursing Times.*

Yalom, I. D. (1985). *The theory and practice of group psychotherapy* (3rd ed.). New York: Basic Books.

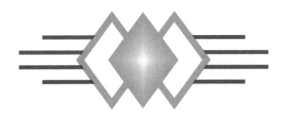

CHAPTER 11

FAMILY THERAPY

I nterest in the family *of* the psychiatric patient has blended over the years to interest in the family *as* the psychiatric patient. This conceptual focus on the family as a whole instead of one individual member is the key element of the family therapy approach.

Jones, 1980

Introduction

Families are an integral part of society. They consist of two or more persons and may include children. All family members influence one another as they interact and support one another in performing basic functions necessary for the family's well-being. In the family setting, members learn how to relate to and communicate with others. The family also influences personal development. If the family has a positive influence on its members, they will have a sense of self-worth and positive self-esteem, and will become productive members of society.

Duvall's Theory of the Family Life Cycle

The family is a developing system that must progress in the right way for the child's development to be healthy. According to Duvall's (1977) theory, there are predictable successive stages of growth and development within the life cycle of every family. Family developmental tasks refer to growth responsibilities achieved by a family unit as well as individual developmental requisites. The interfacing of individual developmental needs and family tasks is not always possible and may lead to conflict, resulting in poor interpersonal relationships, the development of individual emotional problems, or a family crisis. An understanding of the eight stages of the family life cycle gives the nurse guidelines for analyzing family growth and health promotion needs as well as the ability to provide therapeutic intervention when conflict arises. Box 11-1 summarizes each of

BOX 11-1 Duvall's Eight Stages of the Family Life Cycle

Stage	Description of Family Tasks
I. Beginning families (no children; commitment to each other)	Establishing a mutually satisfying marriage by learning to live together and provide for each other's personality needs Relating harmoniously to three families: each respective family and the one being created by marriage Family planning: whether to have children and when Developing a satisfactory sexual and marital role adjustment
II. Early childbearing (begins with birth of first child and continues until infant is 30 months)	Developing a stable family unit with new parent roles Reconciling conflicting developmental tasks of various family members Jointly facilitating developmental needs of family members to strengthen each other and the family unit Accepting the new child's personality
III. Families with preschool children (first-born child 2½ years old; continues until age 5)	Exploration of environment by children Establishment of privacy, housing, and adequate space Husband-father becomes more involved in household responsibilities Preschooler develops a more mature role and assumes responsibilities for self-care

(continued)

BOX 11-1 **Duvall's Eight Stages of the Family Life Cycle (Continued)**

Stage	Description of Family Tasks
	Socialization of children such as attending school, church, sports
	Integration of new family members (second or third child)
	Separation from children as they enter school
IV. Families with school-aged children (firstborn child ages 6 to 13)	Promoting school achievement of children
	Maintaining a satisfying marital relationship because this is a period when it diminishes
	Promoting open communication within the family
	Accepting adolescence
V. Families with teenagers	Maintaining a satisfying marital relationship while handling parental responsibilities
	Maintaining open communication between generations
	Maintaining family ethical and moral standards by the parents while the teenagers search for their own beliefs and values
	Allowing children to experiment with independence
VI. Launching-center families (covers the first child through last child leaving home)	Expanding the family circle to include new members by marriage
	Accepting the new couple's own life-style and values
	Devoting time to other activities and relationships by the parents

BOX 11-1 Duvall's Eight Stages of the Family Life Cycle (Continued)	
Stage	**Description of Family Tasks**
VII. Families of middle years ("empty nest" period through retirement)	Reestablishing the wife and husband roles as the children achieve independent roles
	Assisting aging and ill parents of the husband and wife
	Maintaining a sense of well-being psychologically and physiologically by living in a healthy environment
	Attaining and enjoying a career or other creative accomplishments by cultivating leisure-time activities and interests
	Sustaining satisfying and meaningful relationships with aging parents and children
	Strengthening the marital relationship
VIII. Families in retirement and old age (begins with retirement of one or both spouses, continues through the loss of one spouse, and terminates with the death of the other spouse)	Maintaining satisfying living arrangements
	Maintaining marital relationships
	Adjusting to a reduced-income
	Adjusting to the loss of a spouse

Duvall's eight stages, including the age and school placement of the oldest child, which affects the responsibilities of the family members.

 Emerging Changes in Families

Families in the United States have undergone several changes in the last 50 years. A variety of living styles and arrangements have emerged. Alternatives to the traditional nuclear family (father, mother, and children) include single-parent households, blended families, communes, and cohabitation between unmarried persons. As women join the work force in greater numbers, changes occur in child care, child-rearing practices, and role sharing. Dual-career families in which both the husband and wife are working mean that husbands must assume some roles that mothers and wives traditionally performed. These changes in the traditional nuclear family have made it necessary for parents to teach their children new skills to help them cope in today's society.

Healthy Functioning Families

It is difficult to find much research on the so-called normal family, although there is much literature published about dysfunctional or pathogenic families. However, healthy families demonstrate specific characteristics: (1) the ability to communicate thoughts and feelings, and (2) parental guidance in determining the functioning level of the total family. In addition, the healthy family expects interactions among its members to be unreserved, honest, attentive, and protective; whereas interactions in the unhealthy family tend to be reserved, guarded, or antagonistic (Goldenberg & Goldenberg, 1980).

In the healthy functioning family, no single member dominates or controls another. Instead, there is a respect for the individuation of other family members and their points of view and opinions, even if the differences lead to confrontation or altercation. Such family members participate in activities together, whereas members of dysfunctional families tend to be isolated from one another and may try to control others in the family. Although power is found in healthy families in the parent coalition (union or alliance), it is not used in an authoritarian manner. Children are allowed to express opinions, negotiations are worked out, and power struggles do not ensue. Good communication patterns are paramount (Goldenberg & Goldenberg, 1980).

A healthy and well-functioning family encourages personal autonomy and independence among its members, but individuality is not obscured. Family members are able to adapt to the changes that occur with normal growth and development and to cope with separation and loss.

Each family should progress through certain specific stages of development, which include bonding, independence, separation, and individuation. Ego boundaries should be clearly developed. By the time members reach adolescence, they begin to function more independently. Increased independence requires an adjustment in the relationship of all family members. However, family members should not function so independently of each other that the family system is impaired or the rights of individual family members are violated, because this can lead to distress in the family. Other problems that may cause distress include marital disharmony, differing child-rearing techniques, the acute physical illness of a member, or a member who is emotionally ill.

Dysfunctional Families

The characteristics of dysfunctional families are the antithesis of healthy functioning families. Issues of power persist and are not resolved. No identified leader or parent helps take control and establish some sense of order. Instead, the family experiences chaos, which results from leadership that may be changing from one member to another over short periods of time. Control or power is attempted through intimidation instead of open communication and negotiation. The lack of leadership sometimes makes it difficult to determine who fulfills the parental role and who fulfills the child's. This confusion encourages dependency, not autonomy, and individuation is not enhanced. When all family members have similar thoughts and feelings, it is viewed as family closeness and not as a loss of autonomy (Goldenberg & Goldenberg, 1980).

In dysfunctional families, communication is not open, direct, or honest; usually it is confusing to other family members. Little warmth is demonstrated. All these experiences tend to undermine each member's individual thoughts, feelings, needs, and emotions so that they are regarded as unimportant or unacceptable. Also, in dysfunctional families, children and adults may be performing roles that are inappropriate to their age, sex, or personality characteristics. For example, a mother of a seven-year-old daughter and a three-year-old son may expect the daughter to take care of the son and help prepare meals. This expectation can create distress in the daughter because of the amount of responsibility that is being placed on her, and because she is being forced to fulfill the role of a mother. If such expectations persist, it could result in a dysfunctional family system.

 Culturally Diverse Families

Andrews and Boyle (1995) discuss transcultural nursing as it applies to families and the community. The ability to communicate through the use of the same language is necessary if one is to understand cultural diversity. Duvall's stages of the family life cycle do not apply to all cultures because of differences in family and kinship systems, social life, political systems, language and traditions, religion, health beliefs and practices, and cultural norms. It is imperative that the nurse–therapist consider these differences when assessing family members for therapy to avoid labeling a family as dysfunctional because of cultural differences.

 History of Family Therapy

In the 1950s, psychotherapists began looking not only at individuals with problems but at the pattern of relationships that corresponded with family problems. These psychotherapists included Murray Bowen, Nathan Ackerman, Salvador

Minuchin, Jay Haley, and Virginia Satir. They began changing their approach from treating only the individual to including the family to help increase therapeutic effectiveness. This change in therapeutic approach was based on the belief that until the family pattern was changed, the individual's behavior would remain fixed.

This approach corresponds with another method: viewing the family as a system of relationships, such as between parent and child, brother and sister, mother and daughter. Each member of the family must be able to communicate in a productive and healthy way with other members within the system. If there is a breakdown in the system, all members are affected. Thus, a change or disruption in one family member affects the family system and all its members.

Family Therapy

Family therapy is a technique that uses a psychotherapeutic approach in helping family members gain insight into their problems and change behavior and emotions from dysfunctional to healthy. Using this method, the family can perform the basic functions necessary for the well-being of all its members. Therapy is indicated when the family does not perform its basic functions adequately. The therapist views the family as the patient and looks at the family members in relationship to the individual patient. Therapists also encourage family involvement in the treatment of individual family members.

Family therapy differs from individual therapy, however. In the former it is assumed that outside or external influences play a major role in personality development and the regulation of members' lives. In individual therapy, however, it is believed that internal or intrapsychic thoughts, feelings, and conflicts are the major components of personality development (Goldenberg & Goldenberg, 1980).

Traditionally, the person who seeks treatment is considered the patient. If the problem is within the individual and he or she is not affected by outside influences or family members, individual treatment can be helpful and can bring about improvement in the individual's behavior. If the patient's behavior is due to a dysfunctional family system, however, improvement will not be as significant or last as long. Some therapists believe that if an individual's behavior can be changed, it will eventually have an impact on that person's family and positive changes will thus occur. Others believe that the person who is ill and improves will regress to old patterns of behavior or to other types of dysfunctional behavior when placed back in the family.

Changes in families occur during family therapy because of the individual's desire to conform to the group of family. As problems are worked through by the family, the individual members become cognizant of their mutual problems, of specific areas that are distorted, and of the family members' needs. Each individual member's role(s) should become clear. Sometimes scapegoating occurs: the family needs to maintain a "sick" person in the family or a scapegoat to aid the denial of family pathology. Once the family is able to perceive this scapegoating, family therapy focuses on family problems instead of on the individual who was the scapegoat (Cohen & Lipkin, 1979).

If one person in a family becomes dysfunctional, interaction often occurs between a "normal" family and the dysfunctional member. The relationship may become entwined, causing the "normal" member to become unhealthy if the dysfunctional member's behavior and ability to function improve.

Different Therapies

Because family therapy is a relatively new therapeutic method of helping individuals, there are a number of different approaches. Jones (1980) describes seven orientations to family therapy, which are briefly discussed in the following paragraphs.

Integrative Approach

Nathan Ackerman, considered by some to be the grandfather of family therapy, used the integrative approach. To varying degrees, he rejected the view of the family as a system (a view nearly all other therapists hold). His focus was on family values. Ackerman believed in interlocking pathology, which occurs when an individual's problems are locked into a neurotic interaction.

Therapists using the integrative approach consider the interactions between the person and her or his social environment. The family needs to share concern for each member's welfare. A problem arises if there is too much fluidity or rigidity of family-role relationships. These relationships are analyzed so that therapy focuses on the family dynamics of illness.

Psychoanalytic Approach

Therapists using the psychoanalytic approach base many of their views on Freud's work, believing that family members are affected by each member's psychological makeup. Individual behaviors are regulated by the family's feedback system. Problems arise from this feedback system when there is an internalization process or introjection of parental figures. This occurs from an unconscious incorporation of another's personality into one's own.

Psychoanalytic therapy is intensive over a long period of time and focuses on cognitive, affective, and behavioral components of family interaction. A goal is to guide the family members who exhibit pathology into a restructuring change in their personality.

Bowen Approach

Murray Bowen's approach to family therapy viewed the family as consisting of emotional and relationship systems. He believed an individual's behavior is a response to the behavior of another person. The intellect is not autonomous but is responsive to the other's feelings, and logical reasoning is impaired. Bowen's therapy is similar to the psychoanalytic approach. Problems arise if there is internalization or introjection of parental figures. Pathology develops if a family member is dominated by the feelings of those around him or her, and boundaries of self are not clearly differentiated from the family system. Thus, relationships with others can cause emotional disturbance in the individual.

Therapy is based on therapeutic strategies that are teachable, and is geared toward helping the person differentiate between feeling and thinking. Bowen believed that appropriate responses could be taught. A goal is to help each member not to be dominated by the feelings of others but to achieve a better differentiation of self.

Structural Approach

Structuralists, like the well known Salvador Minuchin, view the family as a system of individuals. The family develops a set of invisible rules and laws that evolve over a period of time and are understood by all family members. A hierarchical system or structure develops within the family. Problems arise if family boundaries become enmeshed (tangled with no clear individual roles) or disengaged (individual detaches self from the family). Problems also arise when a family cannot cope with change.

The structural therapist observes the activities and functions of family members. Therapy is short-term and action-oriented. It is geared toward changing the family organization and its social context. A holistic view of the family is developed, focusing on influences that family members have on one another. Guidance is given toward developing clear boundaries for individual members and toward changing the family's structural pattern.

Interactional or Strategic Approach

The interactional or strategic approach uses communication theory and was pioneered by Virginia Satir and Jay Haley. The therapist studies the interactions between and among family members, recognizing that change in one family member occurs in relation to change in another family member. Family members develop a calibration and feedback system so that homeostasis may be maintained. Interactionists agree with structuralists that a set of invisible laws emerges in the family relationship and problems arise if these family rules are ambiguous. When power struggles develop within a family, strategies employed to control the situation may provoke symptoms. These symptoms are interpersonal, with at least one family member contributing to the dysfunction of another.

Therapy is based on the concept of homeostasis. According to this concept, as one member gains insight and becomes better, another family member may become worse. Communication is considered the basis for all behavior. Therapy deals with the interpersonal relationships among all family members and focuses on why the family is in therapy and what changes each member expects. The family thus helps set goals for the treatment approach.

Social Network or Systemic Approach

Some therapists believe that the family operates as a social network. They believe that healing comes from social relationships. Problems ensue if the family social network loses its ability to recover quickly from illness or change. A systems approach is utilized but is not clearly defined. The growth model is used to understand emotional difficulties that arise during different stages of development.

Therapy emphasizes the natural healing powers of the family. It involves bringing several people together as a social network. For the first few meetings, this may encompass people who are outside of the family but have similar ideals and goals. Family members are helped to set goals for optimal outcomes or solving of problems.

Behaviorist Approach

Behaviorists believe that the family is a system of interlocking behaviors, that one type of behavior causes another. They deny internal motivating forces, but believe individuals react to external factors and influences. The individual learns that he or she obtains satisfaction or rewards from certain responses to other individuals. Behavior is thus learned. Problems arise when maladaptive behavior is learned and reinforced by family members, who respond either positively or negatively. Sometimes a particular behavior is exhibited to gain attention.

Therapy includes interpreting family members' behavior but not necessarily changing it, although change may be brought about by restructuring interpersonal environments. Therapy is thus based on an awareness process as well as on behavioral change. Therapeutic approaches using principles of learning theory are taught. In an effort to bring about change, positive reinforcement is given for desired behavior. Approaches are direct and clearly stated. The family is involved in goal setting for desired outcomes, and a contract may be established for this purpose.

Goals of Family Therapy

When meeting with a family or identified patient in a family, it is important for the therapist to assess the family's problems. Goals may need to be modified according to the family's value system. The therapist needs to have insight into her or his own value system so as not to influence the direction of treatment.

What the family identifies as problems may not be what the therapist identifies as problems owing to differences in values, culture, and socioeconomic class. The therapist needs to remember to work on the problems the family identifies or to explain to the dysfunctional family why the therapist sees the problems differently. The family, not the therapist, should provide the information for and determine the direction of change when goals are being set. Each family member should state her or his goals and the outcomes expected from the therapy. If the therapist and family are from similar backgrounds, the problems identified and the methods of resolving them tend to be more similar.

A major goal of family therapy is to facilitate positive changes in the family. Other goals include fostering open communication of thoughts and feelings and promoting optimal functioning in interdependent roles. The therapist needs to assess the various roles each family member fulfills and determine if these roles are rigid or inflexible. In addition, the therapist needs to function as a role model and demonstrate how to deal with conflicts. Developing contracts for the family members may be useful in goal setting (*e.g.*, keeping a room clean, having fewer quarrels, paying more attention to the needs of other family members).

Initially, the therapist determines which family members need to participate or continue in family therapy and how the problems of the identified patient(s) interlock with the relationships of other family members. This interlocking relationship may need to be modified. Finally, the therapist helps family members take a realistic view of their relationships with one another and the overall effect of their behavior on each other.

Stages of Family Therapy

The three main stages of family therapy are the initial interview, the intervention or working phase, and the termination phase.

The Initial Interview

Usually a family therapist is contacted by telephone by the identified patient or by another family member regarding the identified patient. The caller expresses concern regarding the problem or symptom(s), and the family therapist sets up an appointment for an initial interview with the family. Most therapists ask all family members to be present at that time. Later, the therapist may decide that not all members need to be present at the family sessions (for example, very young children may be excluded). The information gleaned from all family members at the initial interview can be invaluable during later sessions. During the initial interview, some therapists gather data regarding family history; other therapists focus on the present functioning of the family (Goldenberg & Goldenberg, 1980).

If a certain family member is reluctant to come in for the initial interview, it may be helpful if the therapist states the rationale for seeing all family members at that time. For example, the therapist could state that the problem affects all members of the family and that it is important to attend. The therapist can explain that therapy will not be effective without that member's attendance and input.

An outline of a family assessment guide used to obtain information during the initial interview is shown in Box 11-2.

Haley (1977) identified specific stages during an initial interview in which the therapist facilitates the process of determining which problems the family has identified as needing attention. These stages include

1. *Engagement stage:* The family is met and put at ease.
2. *Assessment stage:* Problem(s) that concern the family are identified.
3. *Exploration stage:* The therapist and family explore additional problems that may have a bearing on present family concerns.
4. *Goal-setting stage:* The therapist synthesizes all the information, and the family members state what they would like to see changed.
5. *Termination stage:* The initial interview ends, an appointment is set for the next session, and it is determined which family members need to attend.

During the initial interview, the therapist must be able to assess and synthesize all the information the family has given and formulate ideas or interventions for bringing about positive changes to resolve the identified problems.

BOX 11-2 Family Assessment Guide

I. Construction of a family genogram

II. Description of the family in relation to the community, focusing on ethnicity, socioeconomic class, educational level, and religion

III. Description of presenting problems, focusing on each family member's perception of the identified problems

IV. Identification of communication patterns focusing on who speaks to whom, tone of voice, emotional climate, and manner by which emotions are expressed

V. Identification of roles of family members as supportive, antagonistic, critical, scapegoat, rescuer, or victim. Are there family coalitions, pairings, triangles, or splits?

VI. Developmental history of the family in general and of the presenting problems

VII. Family's expectations of therapy

The Intervention or Working Phase

The goal of the working phase is to help the family accept and adjust to change (Goldenberg & Goldenberg, 1980). During this phase, the therapist needs to identify the strengths and problems of the family. Otto (1963) has identified 12 family strengths. The therapist should determine which of these strengths are present in the family seeking help. Identified strengths are useful in helping the family remain stable when other relationships seem threatened by change. According to Otto, these strengths are

1. The ability to provide for the physical, emotional, and spiritual needs of each family member
2. The ability to be sensitive to the needs of family members
3. The ability to communicate feelings, emotions, beliefs, and values effectively
4. The ability to provide support, security, and encouragement to enhance creativity and independence
5. The ability to initiate and maintain growth-producing relationships within and without the family system
6. The capacity to maintain and create constructive and responsible community relationships in the neighborhood, school, town, and local and state governments
7. The ability to grow with and through children
8. The ability for self-help and the ability to accept help when appropriate
9. The ability to perform family roles flexibly
10. The ability to show mutual respect for the individuation and independence of each family member
11. The ability to use a crisis as a means of growth
12. The ability to have a concern for family unity and loyalty, and for cooperation among family members

During this second phase families do a lot of working, and the therapist participates in the therapeutic process. Usually family sessions occur once a week for approximately one hour. Some family members may be motivated to participate in order to help the identified patient. Other members may be reluctant to participate owing to fears of having family secrets revealed. It would be unusual if all family members were willing and eager to participate in family therapy sessions. The therapist can ask all members their view of the problem, what they would like to see changed, and their thoughts and feelings about other members of the family. Through this technique, the therapist can learn a great deal about the problems and conflicts that are occurring in the family system (Goldenberg & Goldenberg, 1980).

Soon the family members will be able to recognize that the therapist's role is to clarify and interpret communication as well as to offer suggestions and guidance. The therapist does not assume the role of a parent, child, or arbitrator. The therapist facilitates open, honest communication among family members. Learning appropriate methods of expressing themselves may cause some stress in family members, especially if there has been hostility, angry outbursts, or little communication. Also, some sessions—particularly those dealing with conflicts and altercations—may make family members feel uncomfortable. As therapy continues, family members will begin to realize that relationships can change. They will recognize that roles do not have to be fixed and rigid; they may change as personal growth occurs within the family. Family members will become more autonomous. If the sessions are helpful and changes occur in the family, alterations in behavior rather than increased family understanding and insight may be the cause. Increased understanding, however, does occur to a certain degree over a period of time.

Termination Phase

Sometimes families want to terminate the sessions prematurely. This desire may be indicated by behavior. Family members begin to be late or do not show up for scheduled appointments, or not all members continue to participate, as agreed on the initial interview. Such behavior may occur if the family perceives that a certain type of change is threatening to the family's present functioning. At this point, it is important for the therapist to review the identified problems with the family and renegotiate the contract and number of family sessions. This review is helpful in recognizing which problems remain and which goals have been met.

If the family has achieved the goals and the identified specific problems have been resolved, then it is time to initiate the termination phase. However, the therapist should remember that no family terminates therapy without experiencing some problems. Also, some family members may be somewhat reluctant to terminate the sessions. Nevertheless, termination should take place. By now, the family has learned how to solve its own problems in a healthy manner, has developed its own internal support system, and has learned to communicate in an open, honest, and direct manner. Power has been appropriately assigned and redistributed, and family members are able to work out and resolve problems at home without the therapist's help or interventions. The original problems or symptoms have been alleviated, and it is time for termination of family therapy sessions (Goldenberg & Goldenberg, 1980). Referral may be made to family support groups such as Parents Anonymous, Toughlove, or Families Anonymous.

Nurse's Role in Family Therapy

The clinical nurse specialist or nurse practitioner with a graduate degree in psychiatric nursing has received supervised clinical experience and has extensive knowledge and skills in psychiatric and mental health nursing. Specialists can function in a variety of highly skilled roles, one of which is serving as a family therapist (Cain, 1986).

Involving the family when one of the family members becomes ill is not new to nursing. During the initial assessment, whether for medical or emotional illnesses, nurses obtain information about the patient's family members, including grandparents, aunts, and uncles. Nurses include family members in health education and teaching. However, viewing the family as a specialty, in and of itself, is relatively new for psychiatric nurses. Nurses functioning in this role conduct family assessments, participate in family teaching and education, and also provide family therapy (Cain, 1986). The nurse family therapist obtains a detailed family history for at least three generations to gain information as to how the family has functioned in the past and how it is currently functioning.

One assessment tool that nurses can use in determining the family's constellation of members is a genogram, a diagram of family member relationships, usually over three generations. The genogram is simple to use and can convey a great deal of information about the family.

In a genogram, the names of family members are placed on horizontal lines to indicate separate generations. Any children are denoted by vertical lines. The children are ranked from oldest to youngest, going from left to right. The symbols used to depict each individual family member are usually squares for males and circles for females. Inside the square or circle is the family member's name and age. Outside of the symbols pertinent information can be written, such as *cancer, stroke, depressed, workaholic,* and so on. Other symbols can be used to denote marriage, death, adoption, divorce, separation, miscarriage, abortion, or twins. A basic genogram is depicted in Figure 11-1 (Wright & Leahey, 1984).

It can readily be seen how this simple tool can provide a lot of information in one perusal. A family is often interested in doing a genogram because it gives them a diagram of family relationships, including significant information. The genogram is useful in teaching the family members about family systems. It is important for family members to begin to understand the roles they fill and how their roles influence the family system. Once they realize that roles are learned and that they have the choice of altering their roles, change can occur. At that point the family can begin to work on its problems (Cain, 1986).

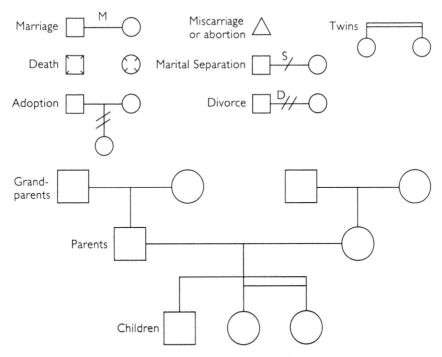

FIGURE 11-1 Simple Genogram with Common Symbols

🌼 Common Nursing Diagnoses

Nursing diagnoses are used to identify functional characteristics of families. Carpenito (1995) describes the following nursing diagnoses specific to families:

> *Family Coping, Compromised, Ineffective
> *Family Coping: Disabling, Ineffective
> *Family Coping: Potential for Growth
> *Family Processes, Altered
> *Family Processes, Altered: Alcoholism
> *Parental Role Conflict
> *Parenting, Altered

A definition, defining characteristics, and related factors are described. Outcome criteria are listed. Nursing interventions are provided to assist the nurse, and references are included for additional information.

*NANDA-approved nursing diagnosis

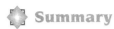 **Summary**

Family therapy, which began in the 1950s, is a psychotherapeutic approach to helping family members achieve an optimal level of functioning. When problems are not resolved, the family is in a state of dysfunction. A healthy functioning family interacts in an open, attentive, and caring manner with its various members. Communication is straightforward and helpful. A dysfunctioning family exhibits hostility, resentment, and a lack of positive communication between its members.

This chapter discussed Duvall's theory of the family life cycle and compared healthy functioning families to dysfunctional families. Reference was made to the assessment of culturally diverse families. The purpose of family therapy was explained and various orientations to family therapy were briefly discussed. Goals of family therapy were stated and the three stages were described. An outline of a family assessment guide was given. The nurse's role as a therapist was explained. Common nursing diagnoses used to identify functional characteristics of families were included.

Learning Activities

I. Clinical Activities
   A. Care for a patient and his or her family, which exhibits dysfunctional patterns in the family system.
   B. Identify the dysfunctional characteristics of the family.
   C. Identify the strengths of the family.
   D. Determine if the family members exhibit any insight into their problems.
   E. Identify the various roles of each member.
   F. Determine if family members express a desire to be helped and involved with family therapy.

II. Independent Activities
   A. Read one of the following to increase your knowledge base of family therapy:
      Barker, *Basic Family Therapy*
      Friedman, *Family Nursing: Theory and Assessment*
      Hoffman, *Foundation of Family Therapy*
      Minuchin and Fishman, *Family Therapy Techniques*
   B. Using Otto's list of family strengths, determine which strengths are present in a family that is seeking help.
   C. Assess your family's cultural background and value system. Is your cultural background and value system the same as or different from the family that is seeking help?
   D. Complete a genogram of the family seeking help.

Critical Thinking Questions

1. Interview three members of your family, preferably of different gender and age, using Otto's 12 family strengths. How does each member perceive the family? What differences in perception occur with gender and age? How do their perceptions match your own? Does this information provide a picture of strength or dysfunction?
2. Identify three different types of families (*e.g.*, nuclear, blended, homosexual). Assess each family for its ability to handle crises. What similarities and differences did you ascertain?
3. Create a genogram of your family going back as far as possible. What patterns of disease, marriage, and so forth can you assess? What did you learn about roles in your family and what might you do with that information?

Self-Test

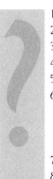

1. Define family therapy.
2. List the characteristics of a healthy functioning family.
3. List the characteristics of a dysfunctional family.
4. Explain why Duvall's theory does not apply to all families.
5. Cite several approaches to family therapy.
6. Describe the following stages of family therapy:
   Initial interview
   Intervention or working phase
   Termination phase
7. Describe how family therapy differs from individual therapy.
8. Discuss the goals of family therapy.
9. Explain how a genogram is helpful in family therapy.

SELECTED REFERENCES

Andrews, M. M., & Boyle, J. S. (1995). *Transcultural concepts in nursing care* (2nd ed.). Philadelphia: J. B. Lippincott.

Barry, P. D. (1994). *Mental health and mental illness* (5th ed.). Philadelphia: J. B. Lippincott.

Bowen, M. (1978). *Family therapy in clinical practice.* New York: Jason Aronson.

Cain, A. (1986, September). Family therapy: One role of the clinical specialist in psychiatric nursing. *Nursing Clinics of North America.*

Carpenito, L. J. (1995). *Nursing diagnoses: Application to clinical practice* (6th ed.). Philadelphia: J. B. Lippincott.

Cohen, R., & Lipkin, G. (1979). *Therapeutic group work for health care professionals.* New York: Springer.

Duvall, E. (1977). *Marriage and family development* (5th ed.). Philadelphia: J. B. Lippincott.

Goldenberg, I., & Goldenberg, H. (1980). *Family therapy: An overview*. Monterey, CA: Brooks/Cole.

Haley, J. (1977). *Problem solving therapy*. San Francisco: Jossey-Bass.

Johnson, B. S. (1997). *Adaptation and growth: Psychiatric–mental health nursing* (4th ed.). Philadelphia: Lippincott–Raven Publishers.

Jones, S. (1980). *Family therapy: A comparison of approaches*. Bowie, MD: Robert J. Brady.

McFarland, G. K., & Thomas, M. D. (1991). *Psychiatric mental health nursing: Application of the nursing process*. Philadelphia: J. B. Lippincott.

Minuchin, S. (1974). *Families and family therapy*. Cambridge: Harvard University Press.

Minuchin, S., & Fishman, H. C. (1981). *Family therapy techniques*. Cambridge: Harvard University Press.

Otto, H. (1963, February). Criteria for assessing family strength. *Family Process*.

Satir, V. (1967). *Conjoint family therapy* (3rd ed.). Palo Alto, CA: Science and Behavior Books.

Whitfield, C. L. (1989). *Healing the child within: Discovery and recovery for adult children of dysfunctional families*. Deerfield Beach, FL: Health Communications.

Wright, L., & Leahey, M. (1984). *Nurses and families: A guide to family assessment and intervention*. Philadelphia: F. A. Davis.

Wright, L. M. (1990, February). Trends in nursing of families. *Journal of Advanced Nursing*.

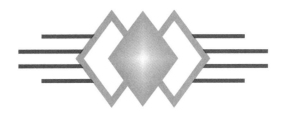

CHAPTER 12

PSYCHOPHARMACOLOGY

Medications function best to alleviate specific symptoms (*e.g.*, delusions, panic attacks). Psychotherapy, in contrast, functions best to resolve specific issues (*e.g.*, marital fights). . . . To compare the two is akin to asking whether the length or width of the football field determines its size.

Maxmen, 1991

1 Define the term *psychopharmacology*.

2 State the rationale for the administration of the following types of psychotropic medication:

   Antipsychotic drugs

   Antianxiety agents and sedative-hypnotics

   Antidepressants

   Antimanic agents

   Anticonvulsants

   Anticholinergic/antiparkinson agents

3 Define the following terminology:

   Extrapyramidal side effects

   Parkinsonism

   Akathisia

   Acute dystonic reactions

   Akinesia

   Tardive dyskinesia

   Neuroleptic malignant syndrome

4 Explain the role of the nurse in psychopharmacology, including guidelines to be considered when administering psychotropic medication.

Introduction

Psychotropic or psychoactive drugs are chemicals that affect the brain and nervous system; alter feelings, emotions, and consciousness in various ways; and frequently are used therapeutically in the practice of psychiatry to treat a broad range of mental and emotional illnesses. "In the mid-1950s . . . 500,000 patients were hospitalized in the United States for mental illness. By 1973, the number of hospitalized mental patients had fallen to 250,000, largely due to the use of psychoactive drugs" (Walker, 1982, p. 209). Psychopharmacology changed the role of the nurse by making effective treatment accessible to mentally ill persons.

Categories of psychotropic drugs include (1) antipsychotic drugs, (2) antianxiety agents, (3) sedative-hypnotics, (4) antidepressants, (5) antimanic agents, and (6) anticonvulsants. Anticholinergic or antiparkinson drugs are utilized to alleviate extrapyramidal symptoms or side effects. Each category is discussed with the focus on principles or rationale for therapy; contraindications, precautions, and side effects; implications for nursing actions; and patient and family education when applicable. Med Alerts are included, focusing on drug–drug interactions and unusual side effects.

Daily dosage ranges for each classification of drugs, listed by both generic and trade name, are given. The reference source is *Psychotropic Drugs Fast Facts* (Maxmen, 1991) and the *Guide to Psychotropic Agents* (Bristol-Myers Squibb Co., 1996).

Medicating the Psychiatric Patient

Bernstein (1988, p. 25) cites several guidelines to be considered when medicating the patient with a psychiatric disorder. They are included in Box 12-1 (on p. 192)

Antipsychotic Agents or Neuroleptics

The major clinical use of antipsychotic agents or neuroleptics is in the treatment of psychoses such as schizophrenia, mania, paranoid disorders, organic dementia, psychotic depression, and organic brain syndrome. Symptoms include impaired communication or the inability to relate to others, delusions, hallucinations, lack of responsiveness to the external environment, and the inability to identify reality. Antipsychotic agents provide symptomatic control of the patient by blocking the activity of dopamine, a chemical normally occurring in the brain and having the potential to produce psychotic thinking. Too much dopamine causes nerve impulses in the brain stem to be transmitted faster than normal, resulting in strange thoughts, hallucinations, and bizarre behavior. Blocking this activity of dopamine lessens or prohibits the development of such thoughts and behavior. Antipsychotic agents also have antiemetic properties; they have been used to treat intractable hiccoughs and have been used in combination with other drugs for pain control. However, "Antipsychotic medication does not cure social withdrawal, apathy, and interpersonal difficulties that are found in schizophrenics and other psychotic individuals. Psychotherapy is needed to help with these problems" (Walker, 1982, p. 213).

Commonly used antipsychotic agents include phenothiazines (*e.g.*, Thorazine, Mellaril, Prolixin, Trilafon, Serentil, Stelazine, and Vesprin) and nonphenothiazines (*e.g.*, Clorazil, Navane, Haldol, Loxitane, and Moban). Clozaril and Loxitane are recommended for use in the treatment of schizophrenia. A new drug, Risperdal, has been used to treat both the positive and negative symptoms of schizophrenia. It is classified as a benzisoxazole derivative that produces

BOX 12-1 Psychopharmacologic Guidelines

1. Rational pharmacotherapy requires decisions as to when and when not to medicate.
2. Emotional responses to ordinary life situations should generally not be medicated.
3. Psychiatric illnesses such as depression and psychosis generally require pharmacotherapy.
4. Failure to medicate properly may prolong the patient's illness and suffering.
5. Irrational use of medications may lead to simultaneous adverse reactions to multiple drugs.
6. Detailed medical and psychiatric history as well patient attitudes toward medication are needed.
7. Appropriate medication must be carefully chosen.
8. The dose should be titrated according to response and adverse effects; the "standard dose" seldom is optimal.
9. All medications should be temporarily withheld if unexplained adverse response occurs.
10. It is generally advisable to start only one medication at a time, and to observe the patient before others are added.
11. Lack of desired response may indicate that the patient is not taking medication as directed.
12. The physician must be aware of the possible lack of bioequivalence among generic drug preparations.
13. The addicting potential of sedatives such as benzodiazepines should be kept in mind.
14. Interactions between various psychotropic drugs and between psychotropic and nonpsychotropic drugs, as well as potential interactions between alcoholic beverages and various medications, must be considered in prescribing medication.
15. Physicians must be aware of increased sensitivity and persistence of various drugs in elderly patients, and the interactions between underlying medical conditions and psychotropic drugs.
16. Before prescribing medication, the potential risks and benefits of treatment must be discussed with patient.

minimal extrapyramidal side effects, and is used in treating psychotic symptoms in adult and geriatric patients. Efficacy has not been established in the treatment of children or adolescents.

Contraindications and Side Effects

Contraindications of the use of neuroleptics include a history of drug hypersensitivity, severe depression, bone marrow depression or blood dyscrasias, and brain damage.

Patients with a history of impaired liver function, cardiovascular disease, hypertension, glaucoma, diabetes, Parkinson's disease, peptic ulcer disease, epilepsy, or pregnancy should be observed closely when they are taking neuroleptics.

Side effects of antipsychotic drugs include the following:

1. Drowsiness, lethargy and inactivity. Persons exhibiting these symptoms should avoid driving or operating hazardous machinery.
2. Dry mouth, nasal congestion, and blurred vision
3. Skin reactions such as urticaria and dermatitis
4. Pigmentation of the skin and eyes and photosensitivity or phototoxicity
5. Constipation or urinary retention
6. General orthostatic hypotension during the first two weeks of treatment
7. Alteration in sexual functioning owing to a diminished sex drive
8. Seizures due to a lowering of the seizure threshold
9. Agranulocytosis (generally within first eight weeks of treatment)
10. Hyperglycemia
11. Mild ECG changes
12. Gastrointestinal distress such as nausea or heartburn
13. Weight gain
14. Edema

Although the list of side effects is lengthy, they usually are mild. They can be annoying, however, and should be treated as soon as they are recognized.

Extrapyramidal Side Effects

Extrapyramidal side effects or adverse neurologic effects may occur during the early phase of drug therapy. They are classified as parkinsonism, akathisia, and acute dystonic reactions. Tardive dyskinesia may occur after short-term use of moderate doses, although it generally occurs after long-term use and high-dose therapy. A summary of these neurologic effects and their treatment is presented in Box 12-2. Clozapine (Clozaril) differs from other neuroleptics or antipsychotic

(*text continues on page 196*)

BOX 12-2 Extrapyramidal Side Effects and Neuroleptic Malignant Syndrome as Possible Result of Treatment with Antipsychotic Agents

Side Effect	Definition/Symptoms	Onset	Treatment
Extrapyramidal side effects			
Parkinsonism	Motor retardation or akinesia, characterized by masklike appearance, rigidity, tremors, "pill rolling," salivation	Generally occurs after first week of treatment or before second month	Administer anticholinergic agent such as Cogentin or Artane
Akathisia (motor restlessness)	Constant state of movement, characterized by restlessness, difficulty sitting still, or strong urge to move about	Generally occurs two weeks after treatment begins	Rule out anxiety or agitation before administration of an anticholinergic agent
Acute dystonic reactions	Irregular, involuntary spastic muscle movement, wryneck or torticollis, facial grimacing, abnormal eye movements, backward rolling of eyes in the sockets (oculogyric crisis)	May occur anytime from a few minutes to several hours after first dose of antipsychotic drug	Administer anticholinergic agent; have respiratory support equipment available

Tardive dyskinesia (abnormal movements)	Most frequent serious side effect resulting from termination of the drug, during reduction in dosage, or after long-term, high-dose therapy. Characterized by involuntary rhythmic, stereotyped movements, tongue protrusion, cheek puffing, involuntary movements of extremities and trunk	Occurs in approximately 20% to 25% of patients taking antipsychotics for over two years	No treatment except discontinuation of antipsychotic agent; irreversible
Neuroleptic malignant syndrome (NMS)	Idiosyncratic, rare syndrome characterized by hyperpyrexia, severe muscle rigidity, altered consciousness, alterations in blood pressure, elevated creatinine phosphokinase, elevated white blood cell count.	May develop within hours after first dose or after years of continued drug exposure; more common in persons under 20 and over 60 years of age	Discontinue antipsychotic agent; have cardiopulmonary and renal support available; administer skeletal muscle relaxant (*e.g.*, dantrolene) or centrally acting dopamine receptor agonist (*e.g.*, bromocriptine)

agents because it does not cause extrapyramidal symptoms, including tardive dyskinesia. There is a relatively high risk of agranulocytosis; therefore, weekly white blood cell counts are recommended.

Implications for Nursing Actions

Patients receiving antipsychotic drug therapy should have an evaluation of blood pressure, complete blood count, liver function tests, and vision tests before therapy and at periodic intervals thereafter.

Nurses who administer antipsychotic drugs should be aware of the following precautions (Abrams, 1995; Karch, 1997):

1. If a single daily dose is ordered, give oral neuroleptics within one or two hours of bedtime whenever possible to aid sleep. Minor side effects are less bothersome at this time.
2. Avoid contact with concentrated solutions while preparing them because they are irritating to the skin and may cause contact dermatitis.
3. Liquid concentrates should be mixed with at least 60 ml of fruit juice or water just before administration to mask the taste of the concentrate and to avoid irritation of oral mucosa.
4. Do not give antipsychotic drugs subcutaneously unless specifically ordered because they may cause tissue irritation. They should be given as deep intramuscular injections. The Z-track method is used when giving decanoate injections (Haldol Decanoate, Prolixin Decanoate).

Persons receiving neuroleptic medication should be observed for the following:

1. Therapeutic effects of the drugs, such as decreased agitation, decreased hallucinations, and increased socialization. Intramuscular injections of Prolixin and Haldol are used when patients are noncompliant.
2. A decrease in nausea and vomiting if the drug is given as an antiemetic
3. Drug-induced extrapyramidal side effects, early signs of tardive dyskinesia, and neuroleptic malignant syndrome
4. Anticholinergic side effects, respiratory depression, and hypersensitivity
5. Signs of agranulocytosis (e.g., sore throat, fever, and discomfort)
6. Drug-induced, endocrine-related changes: menstrual irregularities, breast enlargement, lactation, and changes in libido
7. Signs of jaundice, high fever, upper abdominal pain, nausea, diarrhea, and skin rash
8. See Med Alert in Box 12-3 regarding drug–drug interactions.

BOX 12-3 Med Alert (Psychotropic Medication)

Dosages of neuroleptics or antipsychotic drugs are reduced when given to children, adolescents, or the elderly. Nevertheless, drug interactions can occur. Following is a summary of drug–drug interactions to be considered when providing care to patients receiving neuroleptic drugs:

1. Neuroleptics can potentiate the effects of CNS depressants, antidepressants, anticholinergic agents, phenytoin, beta blockers, antibiotics such as tetracycline, thiazide diuretics, antihypertensives, surgical muscle relaxants, and quinidine.
2. Neuroleptics can reduce the effects of lithium, anticonvulsants, antibiotics, postganglionic blocking agents, antiparkinson agents, methyldopa, and hypoglycemic agents.
3. The effects of neuroleptics can be increased by the concomitant use of antidepressants, beta blockers, barbiturates, and methyldopa.
4. The effects of neuroleptics can be reduced by the concomitant use of lithium, cimetidine, antidiarrheal drugs, antacids, and anticholinergic agents.

The Abnormal Involuntary Movement Scale is used to assess individuals for extrapyramidal side effects. The rating scale code is 0 (no side effects) to 4 (severe effects). Areas assessed include facial and oral movements, extremity movements, trunk movements, global movements, and denture status. The total score may range from 0 to 42.

An Antipsychotic Drug Use Assessment Form is used in long-term care to monitor appropriate use of psychotropic drugs for geropsychiatric patients. The intent is to limit the use of these drugs to appropriate diagnoses or specific behavior (e.g., dementia with agitation); evaluate efficacy of the drug; monitor for side effects; attempt gradual dose reduction unless medical contraindication is documented by the physician; and provide therapeutic alternatives such as behavioral intervention, environmental modification, and modification of staff approach.

Patient Education

Patients need to be informed about the planned drug therapy, length of time it takes to achieve therapeutic results, and possible side effects of drug therapy. They should be instructed to report any physical illnesses or unusual side effects and to avoid taking over-the-counter drugs or any medications prescribed by another physician. Table 12-1 lists daily dosages of common antipsychotic agents. The following is a list of instructions for patients and family members regarding antipsychotic drug therapy:

1. Alcohol and sleeping pills cause drowsiness and decrease one's awareness of environmental hazards. Sleeping pills, alcohol, and other medication should be avoided during drug therapy. Driving or operating hazardous machinery also should be avoided while taking antipsychotic drugs.
2. Patients should avoid being in direct sunlight for an extended time to prevent sunburn or pigmentation of the skin.
3. Individuals should be instructed not to increase, decrease, or cease taking drugs without discussing this step with the physician. The drug should be withdrawn slowly to avoid nausea or seizures.
4. The patient should be told that antacids may decrease the absorption of antipsychotic drugs from the intestinal tract, thus altering the effects.
5. To avoid falls or other injuries, the patient should be made aware of the possibility of dizziness and syncope from postural hypotension for about an hour after receiving medication or following the injection.

TABLE 12-1 DAILY DOSAGE OF COMMONLY USED ANTIPSYCHOTIC AGENTS

Generic Name	Trade Name	Dosage Range (mg/day)
chlorpromazine	Thorazine	25 mg–2000 mg
clozapine	Clozaril	75 mg–700 mg
fluphenazine	Prolixin	1 mg–30 mg
fluphenazine decanoate	Prolixin Decanoate	12.5 mg–100 mg
haloperidol	Haldol	1 mg–100 mg
haloperidol decanoate	Haldol Decanoate	12.5 mg–100 mg
mesoridazine	Serentil	30 mg–400 mg
molindone	Moban	15 mg–200 mg
olanzepine	Zyprexa	5 mg–10 mg
perphenazine	Trilafon	4 mg–64 mg
risperidone	Risperdal	0.5 mg–16 mg
thioridazine	Mellaril	40 mg–800 mg
thiothixene	Navane	1 mg–60 mg
trifluoperazine	Stelazine	2 mg–80 mg

6. Good oral hygiene should be practiced to avoid mouth infections, dental caries, and ill-fitting dentures. An annual dental examination should be performed.
7. If children are in the home, tablets or capsules should be kept in a safe place to avoid their being mistaken for candy.
8. Injectable drugs such as Prolixin Decanoate or Haldol Decanoate are usually given every two to four weeks to patients who are noncompliant regarding use of prescribed medication.
9. Antipsychotic agents may provoke seizures in patients with seizure disorders.

Antianxiety Agents and Hypnotics

Antianxiety agents (*i.e.*, sedatives) and hypnotics share many characteristics and are referred to collectively as hypnosedatives, although antianxiety agents are primarily used to treat daytime tension and hypnotics to relieve insomnia. Antianxiety agents, also referred to as anxiolytics, may be used to manage withdrawal symptoms associated with chronic alcoholism, to control convulsions, and to produce skeletal muscle relaxation.

The four basic classes of anxiolytics include benzodiazepines, antihistamines, beta blockers, and buspirone. Fluvoxamine maleate (Luvox) is classified as a selective serotonin reuptake inhibitor (SSRI) and is used to treat obsessive–compulsive disorder (OCD). Clomipramine hydrochloride (Anafranil) is a tricyclic drug used to control OCD or in those patients with concomitant depression.

Commonly used benzodiazepines include chlordiazepoxide (Librium), clonazepam (Klonopin), diazepam (Valium), oxazepam (Serax), clorazepate (Tranxene), lorazepam (Ativan), prazepam (Centrax), and alprazolam (Xanax). They should be used for a short time, one or two weeks, because of their potential for abuse, toxicity, and lethal overdose. These nonbarbiturate benzodiazepines work selectively on the limbic system of the brain, which is responsible for emotions such as rage and anxiety. They produce tranquilizing effects without much sedation and may numb emotions, taking away one's enthusiasm and zest for life. Individuals who take 40 mg or more of diazepam daily for several months may experience seizures and die if they stop taking it abruptly. When used in combination with alcohol, these drugs can be lethal. Benzodiazepines interfere with normal coping mechanisms; increase irritability, aggressiveness, and hostility when taken over an extended time; and increase chances of depression.

Many antihistamines are available to treat a wide variety of medical problems such as allergic and dermatologic reactions, motion sickness, nausea and vomiting, and drug-induced extrapyramidal symptoms. The most commonly used antihistamines to treat anxiety are hydroxyzine hydrochloride (Atarax), hydroxyzine pamoate (Vistaril), and diphenhydramine hydrochloride (Benadryl).

Beta blockers are used to diminish tachycardia, benign essential tremors, impulsivity, and agitation associated with anxiety. The most commonly used beta blockers include propranolol (Inderal), atenolol (Tenormin), metapolol (Lopressor), and nadolol (Corgard).

Buspirone (Buspar) is an anxiolytic agent that has approximately one third the potential for abuse or physical dependence compared to benzodiazepines. It produces less sedation with fewer side effects that impair cognition and performance.

Hypnotics are used to induce a state of natural sleep, reduce periods of involuntary awakenings during the night, and increase total sleep time. There are three classifications of hypnotics. Benzodiazepines include estazolam (ProSom), flurazepam (Dalmane), quazepam (Doral), temazepam (Restoril), and triazolam (Halcion). Barbiturates include amobarbital (Amytal), butabarbital (Butisol), pentobarbital (Nembutal), phenobarbital (Luminal), and secobarbital (Seconal). Barbiturate-like compounds include chloral hydrate (Noctec), ethchlorvynol (Placidyl), methyprylon (Noludar), and zolpidem(Ambien). Tolerance can occur within 7 to 14 days, resulting in physical dependence after a month or more of use.

Contraindications and Side Effects

Persons diagnosed with porphyria should not be placed on antianxiety therapy because these agents aggravate the symptoms of acute intermittent porphyria. Caution should be used when prescribing these agents for patients with impairment of respiratory, liver, or kidney function, as well as for depressed persons with possible suicidal tendencies.

Physical dependence may occur if these drugs are taken in large quantities for prolonged periods, and on abrupt withdrawal, an abstinence syndrome can occur. Symptoms include nausea, vomiting, hypotension, fatigue, sleep disturbance, fever, delirium, and potentially fatal grand mal seizures within 12 hours to 2 weeks.

Implications for Nursing Actions

Before administering antianxiety agents or hypnotics, the nurse should assess the person's mental and physical status to avoid the risk of adverse side effects. Pregnant women or those breast-feeding should not be placed on antianxiety agents because of the risk of these side effects. If a patient complains of a sleep disturbance, the causative factor should be identified if possible. Appropriate nursing measures to promote relaxation, such as a warm drink or a backrub, should first be tried as alternatives to the administration of hypnotics.

When administering antianxiety or hypnotic drugs, the nurse should do the following (Abrams, 1995; Karch, 1997):

1. Give the daily dose at bedtime to promote sleep, minimize adverse reactions, and allow more normal daytime activities to occur.

2. Administer intramuscular dosages deeply and slowly into large muscle masses because they are irritating to tissues and can cause pain at the site of injection. The Z-track method is generally used to avoid irritation of tissue.
3. Observe for therapeutic effects.
4. Observe for adverse side effects such as oversedation, hypotension, pain at the injection site, skin rashes, and paradoxic excitement. Symptoms of paradoxic excitement include hostility, rage, confusion, depersonalization, or hyperactivity. Rare side effects include gastrointestinal discomfort, nausea, vomiting, menstrual irregularities, blood dyscrasias, photosensitivity, and nonthrombocytopenic purpura.
5. Lorazepam (Ativan) can be given sublingually for rapid absorption.
6. See Med Alert in Box 12-4 regarding drug–drug interactions.

BOX 12-4 Med Alert (Antianxiety Agents and Hypnotics)

Dosages of anxiolytics and hypnotics are reduced when given to children, adolescents, or the elderly. Following is a summary of drug–drug interactions and unusual side effects to be considered when providing care to patients receiving antianxiety or sedative-hypnotic agents:

1. Alcohol, narcotic analgesics, TCAs, and CNS depressants can cause an increase in CNS depression when used concurrently with this classification of psychotropic medication.
2. Displacement of digoxin from serum proteins can occur when taken concurrently with Buspar.
3. Hyertension can occur when Buspar and MAOIs are combined during therapy.
4. Prothrombin times may vary during anticoagulant therapy.
5. The use of Tagamet (cimetidine) reduces the clearance of Valium and Xanax.
6. Benzodiazepines may decrease the actions of Tegretol.
7. Erythromycin may inhibit the metabolism of Valium and Librium.
8. Beta blockers may decrease the effects of insulin and oral antidiabetic agents.
9. Beta blockers may increase the effects of thyroxine, phenytoin, clonidine, and phenothiazines.
10. Coadministration of Luvox with Seldane or Hismanol is contraindicated.
11. Avoid use of Xanax in patients who have severe pulmonary disorders.

Patient Education

Patients should be told the name of the drug, dose, and schedule of treatment, as well as the expected course of treatment. Tables 12-2 and 12-3 list daily dosages of common antianxiety agents and hypnotics. Patients should not alter the dose of medication nor should they drive or operate hazardous equipment. Instructions to patients and family members include the following:

1. Avoid mixing alcoholic beverages, antihistamines, or antipsychotic drugs with antianxiety agents because they can increase the depressant effects of those agents, possibly causing death.
2. Avoid ingesting large amounts of beverages containing caffeine, a stimulant, because it can decrease the effects of hypnotic agents.
3. Report symptoms of fever, malaise, sore throat, petechiae, easy bruising or bleeding, and skin rash.
4. Sudden cessation of these agents can cause rapid eye movement or rebound effects such as insomnia, dreams, nightmares, hyperexcitability, agitation, or convulsions.
5. Avoid excessive use of these drugs to prevent the onset of substance abuse or addiction.
6. Hypnotics are ineffective as analgesics.

TABLE 12-2 DAILY DOSAGE OF COMMONLY USED ANTIANXIETY AGENTS

Generic Name	Trade Name	Dosage Range (mg/day)
atenolol	Tenormin	50 mg–200 mg
alprazolam	Xanax	0.5 mg–8 mg
buspirone	BuSpar	15 mg–60 mg
chlordiazepoxide	Librium	10 mg–100 mg
clomipramine hydrochloride	Anafranil	25 mg–250 mg
clorazepate dipotassium	Tranxene	7.5 mg–90 mg
diazepam	Valium	2 mg–40 mg
diphenhydramine hydrochloride	Benadryl	25 mg–300 mg
fluvoxamine maleate	Luvox	50 mg–300 mg
lorazepam	Ativan	1.0 mg–10 mg
oxazepam	Serax	30 mg–120 mg
propranolol	Inderal	40 mg–120 mg

TABLE 12-3 DAILY DOSAGE OF COMMONLY USED HYPNOTICS

Generic Name	Trade Name	Dosage Range (mg/day)
estazolam	ProSom	1 mg–2 mg
flurazepam	Dalmane	15 mg–30 mg
pentobarbital	Nembutal	50 mg–200 mg
secobarbital	Seconal	100 mg–200 mg
temazepam	Restoril	15 mg–30 mg
zolpidem	Ambien	5 mg–10 mg

Antidepressants or Mood Elevators

Antidepressants are used to treat depressive disorders caused by emotional or environmental stressors, losses, drugs, disease states such as cerebral vascular accidents, or depression that cannot be related to an identifiable cause. These drugs are classified as tricyclic antidepressants (TCAs), monoamine oxidase inhibitors (MAOIs), SSRIs, and atypical antidepressants. Psychostimulants such as methylphenidate (Ritalin) and pemoline (Cylert) may be used concurrently in the presence of treatment-resistant depression.

Tricyclic antidepressants increase the level of the neurotransmitters, serotonin or norepinephrine, in the space between nerve endings. Neurotransmitters carry messages from one nerve cell to another and a deficiency in these transmitters is thought to cause depression. Choice of medication depends on which chemical is thought to be deficient in the nerve endings.

Monoamine oxidase inhibitors prevent the metabolism of neurotransmitters, but are used less frequently than the TCAs because they are less effective, must be given for longer periods of time before they are beneficial, are more toxic, have a longer duration of action, and may cause adverse reactions if taken with tyramine-rich foods.

Selective serotonin reuptake inhibitors represent the latest advancement in pharmacotherapy. They inhibit the 5-HT system uptake of indoleamine (serotonin). Abnormalities in the 5-HT function can result in disturbance of mood, anxiety, alteration of cognition, aggressive behavior, or alteration in sexual drive.

Atypical antidepressants commonly used to treat depression include bupropion (Wellbutrin), trazodone (Desyrel), maprotiline (Ludiomil), venlafaxine (Effexor) nefazodone hydrochloride (Serzone), and mirtazapine (Remeron).

Tricyclic Antidepressants

Tricyclic antidepressants generally are used to treat symptoms of depression, for example, insomnia, decreased appetite, decreased libido, excessive fatigue, indecisiveness, difficulty thinking and concentrating, somatic symptoms, irritability, and feelings of worthlessness. These agents are considered effective in 85% of those people who exhibit symptoms of depression. Those individuals receiving tricyclic agents usually show an increased mental alertness and physical activity with mood elevation within a few days after initial therapy is begun. People on antidepressant drug therapy continue on the medication for several months to allow neurotransmitters to return to normal levels and to achieve a reversal of the depressive episode. Other disorders that usually respond to TCAs include agoraphobia, borderline personality disorder, dysthymic disorder, OCD, panic disorder, and schizoaffective disorder (Maxmen, 1991). Examples of TCAs commonly used to treat depression include nortriptyline (Pamelor), imipramine (Tofranil), doxepin (Sinequan), and desipramine (Norpramin).

Contraindications and Side Effects Women who are pregnant or breast-feeding and persons recovering from a myocardial infarction or who have a severe liver or kidney disease should not be given TCAs. Caution should be used when administering these drugs to persons with asthma, urinary retention, hyperthyroidism, glaucoma, cardiovascular disorders, benign prostatic hypertrophy, alcoholism, epilepsy, and schizophrenia.

Common side effects of tricyclic drugs include dry mouth, blurred vision, tachycardia, urinary retention, and constipation. Less frequently encountered side effects include loss of appetite, insomnia, hypotension, anxiety, and increased intraocular pressure. Potentially dangerous side effects of tricyclic drug therapy include agranulocytosis, jaundice, increased seizure susceptibility in epileptic patients, and prolongation of atrioventricular conduction time. Acute toxicity due to overdose may occur.

Implications for Nursing Actions The nurse should (1) asses the patient's level or severity of depression, including the presence of suicidal ideation, (2) note any side effects, (3) monitor for drug interactions, and (4) observe for therapeutic effects of TCAs. Several drugs increase the effects of these agents. They include antihistamines, atropine, alcohol, narcotic analgesics, benzodiazepines, and urinary alkalizers, such as sodium bicarbonate. Barbiturates, nicotine, and chloral hydrate decrease the effects of TCAs (Abrams, 1995; Karch, 1997).

Within two or three weeks after the initial dose, tricyclic drugs should reach a serum plasma level at which optimal response occurs (therapeutic window); therefore, if no therapeutic response is observed within four to eight weeks, another drug usually is prescribed.

Because these agents may cause urinary retention and constipation, the patient should be observed for abdominal distention. Patients on high doses should be observed for signs of seizure activity. Orthostatic hypotension, tachycardia, or arrhythmias may occur; therefore, any significant changes should be reported and the medication adjusted accordingly.

Patient Education Patients undergoing antidepressant drug therapy should be instructed to

1. Take drugs as prescribed. No attempt should be made to alter the dosage. Table 12-4 provides daily dosages of commonly used tricyclic and atypical antidepressants. Therapeutic effects may not occur for two to three weeks after initial therapy. Plasma levels may be ordered to monitor dosage.
2. Avoid taking over-the-counter cold remedies or other drugs without the physician's knowledge.

TABLE 12-4 DAILY DOSAGE OF COMMONLY USED TRICYCLIC AND ATYPICAL ANTIDEPRESSANTS

Generic Name	Trade Name	Dosage Range (mg/day)
Tricyclic Antidepressants		
amitriptyline	Amitril, Elavil, Endep	50 mg–300 mg
amoxapine	Asendin	50 mg–400 mg
desipramine	Norpramin, Pertofrane	75 mg–300 mg
doxepin	Sinequan, Adapin	75 mg–300 mg
imipramine	Tofranil	75 mg–300 mg
clomipramine	Anafranil	25 mg–300 mg
nortriptyline	Aventyl, Pamelor	50 mg–150 mg
protriptyline	Vivactil	15 mg–60 mg
trimipramine	Surmontil	75 mg–300 mg
Atypical Antidepressants		
bupropion	Wellbutrin	200 mg–450 mg
maprotiline	Ludiomil	25 mg–225 mg
nefazodone hydrochloride	Serzone	100 mg–600 mg
trazodone	Desyrel	25 mg–600 mg
venlafaxine	Effexor	75 mg–375 mg

3. Inform other professionals who may treat the patient, such as a dentist or surgeon, of the drug therapy.
4. Report any side effects, such as fever, malaise, sore throat, sore mouth, urinary retention, fainting, irregular heartbeat, restlessness, mental confusion, or seizures.
5. Avoid excessive exercise and high temperatures because anticholinergic effects of these agents block perspiration.

Tricyclics are not addictive, but some patients may have a chronic deficiency in neurotransmitters, requiring them to take these agents over an extended period.

Monoamine Oxidase Inhibitors

As stated earlier, MAOIs are antidepressants that prevent the metabolism of neurotransmitters. They are generally effective when treating depression associated with acute anxiety attacks, phobic attacks, or many physical complaints; patients who fail to respond to tricyclic agents; and patients who are in the depressive phase of manic-depressive illnesses. MAOIs may be superior to TCAs in treating atypical depression (Maxmen, 1991).

Contraindications and Side Effects The list of conditions that prohibit the use of MAOIs is lengthy but is presented at this time to emphasize the caution that should be used when prescribing or administering these drugs.

1. Asthma
2. Cerebral vascular disease
3. Congestive heart failure
4. Hypertension
5. Hypernatremia
6. Impaired kidney function
7. Cardiac arrhythmias
8. Pheochromocytoma
9. Hyperthyroidism
10. Liver disease
11. Abnormal liver function tests
12. Severe headaches
13. Alcoholism
14. Glaucoma
15. Atonic colitis
16. Paranoid schizophrenia
17. Debilitated patients

18. Patients over age 60
19. Pregnancy
20. Children under age 16

Caution should be exercised when treating patients with a history of angina pectoris, pyloric stenosis, epilepsy, and diabetes mellitus.

Frequently seen side effects include abnormal heart rate, orthostatic hypotension, drowsiness or insomnia, headache, dizziness, blurred vision, vertigo, constipation, weakness, dry mouth, nausea, vomiting, and loss of appetite.

Hypertensive crisis may result if MAOIs are taken with tyramine-rich foods (e.g., aged cheese, avocados, guacamole dip, bananas, chicken livers, fava bean pods, canned figs, meat tenderizers, pickled herring, raisins, sour cream, soy sauce, and yogurt). Patients also should avoid drinking beer, Chianti and other red wines, and any caffeine-containing beverages. Meat tenderizers and yeast supplements should be restricted. Drugs that should be avoided include amphetamines, antiallergy and antihistaminic preparations, antihypertensive agents, levodopa, and meperidine. Toxic symptoms may not occur until 12 hours or later after drug ingestion.

Implications for Nursing Actions MAOIs are nonaddictive and are considered safe and effective if taken as directed. As with TCAs, observe the patient for signs of adverse effects, drug or food interactions, and therapeutic effects.

Drugs that increase the effects of MAOIs have been identified as anticholinergics, adrenergic agents, alcohol, levodopa, reserpine, meperidine, and guanethidine (Abrams, 1991).

To reach a maximum therapeutic effect, MAOIs may require two to six weeks of therapy. Beneficial response should be evident within three to four weeks.

Medication for overdose includes phentolamine (Regitine) for excessive pressor response and diazepam (Valium) for excessive agitation.

Patient Education Education regarding the use of MAOIs includes the following information:

1. Take the drugs as prescribed. Table 12-5 provides daily dosages of commonly used MAOIs. Avoid altering the dosage or discontinuing the use of the drug.
2. Avoid the ingestion of tyramine-containing foods, and caffeine-containing or certain alcoholic beverages.
3. Report any symptoms indicative of a hypertensive crisis, such as headache or heart palpitations.
4. Avoid overactivity because these agents may suppress anginal pain, a warning of myocardial ischemia.

TABLE 12-5 DAILY DOSAGE OF COMMONLY USED MAOIs		
Generic Name	Trade Name	Dosage Range (mg/day)
isocarboxazid	Marplan	10 mg–70 mg
phenelzine	Nardil	15 mg–90 mg
tranylcypromine	Parnate	20 mg–60 mg

5. Have vision checked periodically because optic toxicity may occur if therapy is given over an extended period.
6. Carry a Medic Alert card to inform emergency room staff about MAOIs.

Selective Serotonin Reuptake Inhibitors

This class of antidepressants has become popular because of its advantageous safety profile and its broad spectrum of potential indications. They are used in the treatment of depression alone or in the presence of concurrent disorders such as anxiety, panic attacks, eating disorders, sleep disorders, alcoholism or schizophrenia. Flexible dosing is another advantage because single doses may be given in the morning or at bedtime. Dosage titration usually occurs slowly to achieve a therapeutic level.

Contraindications and Side Effects If a patient has been managed on MAOIs, a 14-day drug clearance is required before initiating SSRI therapy. Caution should be used when SSRIs are prescribed concurrently with anticoagulants. Prothrombin times should be monitored closely. The dosages of theophylline and alprazolam are reduced to avoid excessive plasma concentrations of both drugs. Hismanal, Seldane, Valium, alcohol, and tryptophan are to be avoided.

Common side effects reported include nausea, diarrhea, constipation, tremor, insomnia, somnolence, dry mouth, headache, nervousness, anorexia, weight loss, sweating, and sexual dysfunction.

Implications for Nursing Actions Nursing interventions discussed previously under TCA and MAOI therapy are applicable. Special considerations include (1) advising patients to avoid use if pregnant or lactating, (2) administering the drug once a day, in the morning or evening, (3) arranging for lower doses in the elderly or in patients with hepatic or renal impairment, (4) increasing dosages at intervals of not less than once a week, (5) establishing suicide precautions for severely depressed patients, and (6) reporting any unusual side effects to the attending physician (Karch, 1997).

> **BOX 12-5 Med Alert (Antidepressants)**
>
> Dosages of antidepressants are reduced when given to children, adolescents, or the elderly. Pamelor, Prozac, and Sinequan are available in liquid form. Tofranil-PM and Elavil are available for intramuscular injection. Uncommon but potentially serious adverse effects that can occur during the administration of TCAs or atypical antidepressants include:
>
> 1. Heart block or arrhythmias
> 2. Onset of psychosis possibly secondary to anticholinergic effects as seen with the use of Elavil, Tofranil, Sinequan, or Surmontil
> 3. Mild confusional states due to sedating effects of Elavil, Sinequan, Ludiomil, or Surmontil
> 4. Seizures due to lowering of seizure threshhold, as with the use of Wellbutrin
> 5. Potential for withdrawal symptoms secondary to abrupt discontinuation of antidepressant drugs
>
> Specific drug–drug interactions have been listed in the discussion of each classification of antidepressant drugs. The U.S. Government Printing Office released a medical alert (February, 1995) stating severe CNS toxicity, hyperpyrexia, and death are recognized consequences when using Eldepryl concurrently with antidepressants (MAOIs, TCAs, and SSRIs).

Because certain drugs should not be given concurrently with SSRI therapy, the patient's chart and medication administration record should be marked clearly to avoid any adverse drug–drug interactions (Box 12-5).

Patient Education Patients undergoing SSRI drug therapy should be instructed to

1. Take the drugs as prescribed. Table 12-6 provides daily dosages for SSRI therapy. Avoid altering the dosage of the medication. Contact the physician before discontinuing the use of the drug.
2. Report any unusual symptoms such as tremors, nausea and vomiting, anorexia, weight loss, nervousness, or sexual dysfunction.
3. Avoid the use of Hismanal, Seldane, Valium, alcohol, and tryptophan.
4. Inform the physician if taking an anticoagulant or theophylline.
5. Avoid operating hazardous machinery, including an automobile, if drowsiness occurs.

TABLE 12-6 DAILY DOSAGE OF SELECTIVE SEROTONIN REUPTAKE INHIBITORS

Generic Name	Trade Name	Dosage Range (mg/day)
fluoxetine	Prozac	20 mg–50 mg
fluvoxamine	Luvox	50 mg–300 mg (utilized in depression associated with OCD)
paroxetine	Paxil	10 mg–50 mg
sertraline	Zoloft	25 mg–200 mg

6. Notify the physician if symptoms of depression worsen.
7. Keep the medication out of the reach of children.

Antimanic Agents (Lithium Salts)

Administration of lithium is considered the treatment of choice for the manic phase of the bipolar disorder formerly termed manic-depressive illness and for the long-term prophylaxis of this bipolar disorder. It has also been used in the treatment of depressive and schizoaffective disorders, aggression, and uncontrolled rage reaction.

Exactly how lithium produces therapeutic effects is unknown. It is not metabolized by the body; approximately 80% of a lithium dose is reabsorbed in the proximal renal tubules and excreted by the kidneys. It is believed to level out the activity of neurotransmitters in the area of the brain that controls emotions, thus preventing a decreased activity of nerve impulses, resulting in depression, or an increased activity, resulting in mania. Lithium also is thought to maintain a constant sodium concentration in the brain, regulating mood swings as well as impulses traveling along nerve cells.

Contraindications and Side Effects

Lithium should not be prescribed during pregnancy or in the presence of severely impaired kidney function. Caution should be used when prescribing lithium for patients who have heart disease; perspire profusely; are on a sodium-restricted diet; are hypotensive; have epilepsy, parkinsonism, or other central nervous system (CNS) disorders; or are dehydrated. Serum lithium concentrations may increase in the presence of extreme vomiting, diarrhea, or perspiration, resulting in lithium toxicity.

Common side effects include nausea, metallic taste, abdominal discomfort, polydipsia, polyuria, muscle weakness, fine hand tremors, fatigue, and mild diarrhea, as well as edema of the feet, hands, abdominal wall, or face. These effects may occur as early as two hours after the first dose is taken.

Lithium toxicity occurs when serum lithium levels exceed 1.5 to 2.0 mEq/liter and includes symptoms such as drowsiness, slurred speech, muscle spasms, blurred vision, diarrhea, dizziness, stupor, convulsions, coma, or death.

Implications for Nursing Actions

Patients undergoing lithium therapy should be given the drug during or after meals to decrease gastric irritation. Serum lithium levels should be taken at least twice a week during the initiation of therapy before stabilization of the manic episode. After stabilization, they should be taken at monthly intervals. Serum samples should be drawn 12 hours after a dose is administered; desired levels should reach 1.0 to 1.5 mEq/liter.

Patients should be observed for decreases in manic behavior and mood swings, adverse side effects, and drug interactions. Drugs that increase the effects of lithium include diuretics and anti-inflammatory agents such as Indocin. The effects of lithium are decreased by acetazolamide (Diamox), sodium bicarbonate, excessive amounts of sodium chloride, drugs with a high sodium content, and theophylline compounds. To avoid lithium toxicity, electrolytes, a thyroid profile, and a liver profile are routinely drawn.

Patient Education

Instructions should focus on the following information about lithium therapy during patient and family education:

1. Take the drug as directed. Table 12-7 provides the daily dosage of lithium salts. Do not alter the dosage or cease taking the prescribed drug. Lithium may require three to five weeks to be effective.
2. Do not decrease dietary salt intake unless instructed to do so by the physician because it increases the risk of adverse effects from lithium.
3. Maintain a high intake of fluids (three liters daily) unless contraindicated because of a physical disorder.
4. Avoid crash or fad diets.
5. Avoid excessive exercise in warm weather.
6. Regular blood lithium levels are necessary for safe, effective therapy. Blood samples should be taken 12 hours after the previous dose of lithium; therefore, do not take the morning dose until the serum sample has been taken. Other laboratory tests, including blood urea nitrogen, thyroid profile, electrolytes, and liver profile, are monitored to avoid adverse side effects.
7. Avoid taking other medications without the physician's knowledge because these may increase or decrease the effects of lithium.

TABLE 12-7 DAILY DOSAGE OF LITHIUM SALTS		
Generic Name	Trade Name	Dosage Range (mg/day)
lithium carbonate	Eskalith	900 mg–1800 mg in divided doses until serum levels reach 1.0–1.5 mEq/liter
	Lithane	
	Lithobid	
	Eskalith CR	
lithium citrate	Cibalith-s	Begin with 300 mg b.i.d. and gradually increase by 300-mg increments to achieve desired serum lithium level

8. Report any unusual symptoms, illness, or loss of appetite immediately to the physician.
9. Continue to take the drug despite an occasional relapse. Some patients respond slowly to lithium therapy.
10. Notify the doctor whenever a change in diet occurs because this may affect the lithium level.
11. Women should not breast-feed while taking lithium.
12. Schedule an annual physical examination.
13. Carry a Medic Alert card or wear a Medic Alert bracelet.

◈ Anticonvulsants

Anticonvulsant drugs are used to treat seizure disorders, which are not uncommon among individuals with psychiatric disorders. For example, individuals experiencing acute substance abuse withdrawal are given sedatives and anticonvulsant medications to prevent or treat seizures and delirium tremens. Other examples include individuals with organic mental disorders associated with Axis III physical disorders or conditions such as brain tumor, history of head injury, explosive personality, or epilepsy. Anticonvulsants may also be used to treat bipolar disorders, especially mania (Maxmen, 1991).

Commonly used anticonvulsants include valproic acid (Depakene), phenytoin (Dilantin), clonazepam (Klonopin), primidone (Mysoline), carbamazepine (Tegretol), and ethosuximide (Zarontin).

Contraindications and Side Effects

There are several chemical classifications of anticonvulsants: long-acting barbiturates, benzodiazepines, hydantoins, and succinimides. They may be used to control seizure activity such as petit mal (absence seizures), grand mal (tonic–clonic), psychomotor, akinetic and myoclonic, focal epileptic, or seizures associated with neurosurgery (Bristol-Meyers Squibb, 1996).

Anticonvulsants are contraindicated or must be used cautiously in patients with CNS depression. The presence of hepatic or renal damage, liver disease, or bone marrow depression prohibits the use of anticonvulsants. Increased incidence of birth defects may occur if used during pregnancy. Mothers who are breast-feeding should not take anticonvulsants.

Implications for Nursing Actions

Abrams (1995) and Karch (1997) cite the following nursing actions for anticonvulsant drug therapy:

1. Give on a regular schedule to maintain therapeutic blood levels.
2. Give oral anticonvulsant drugs with meals or fluid to reduce gastric irritation and decrease gastrointestinal side effects. Zantac (ranitidine) is often prescribed to eliminate gastric irritation.
3. Observe for therapeutic effects, which occur approximately 7 to 10 days after drug therapy is started.
4. Monitor for adverse side effects including CNS changes (*e.g.*, drowsiness, sedation, ataxia), gastrointestinal irritation, skin disorders, blood dyscrasias, respiratory depression, liver damage, gingival hyperplasia, hypocalcemia, and lymphadenopathy.
5. Observe for drug interactions.
6. Arrange for laboratory test to monitor liver function and serum drug levels.

Patient Education

Patients receiving anticonvulsant drug therapy should be instructed to

1. Inform the physician/psychiatrist of any known physical illnesses or pregnancy.
2. Inform the physician/psychiatrist of any medication or over-the-counter drugs he or she is presently taking.
3. Take medication with food or glass of fluid at the same time each day. Table 12-8 provides the daily dosage of commonly used anticonvulsants.
4. Ask for the same brand and form of drug when renewing prescriptions.
5. Follow directions when taking a liquid preparation of phenytoin (Dilantin).

TABLE 12-8 DAILY DOSAGE OF COMMONLY USED ANTICONVULSANTS

Generic Name	Trade Name	Dosage Range (mg/day)
carbamazepine	Tegretol	600 mg–1200 mg
clonazepam	Klonopin	1.5 mg–20 mg
ethosuximide	Zarontin	500 mg–1500 mg
phenytoin	Dilantin	300 mg–625 mg
primidone	Mysoline	500 mg–2000 mg
valproate	Depakote	60 mg/kg in divided doses
valproic acid	Depakene	1000 mg–3000 mg

6. Discuss monitoring blood levels of the prescribed drug to avoid reaching toxic levels.
7. Report any adverse side effects to physician/psychiatrist.

Anticholinergic/Antiparkinson Drugs

Anticholinergic/antiparkinson agents are the drugs of choice to treat extrapyramidal disorders, to treat idiopathic or postencephalitic Parkinson's disease, or to use as an adjunct to levodopa. Anticholinergic drugs are used to decrease salivation, spasticity, and tremors in people who have minimal symptoms or cannot tolerate levodopa. They may also be prescribed in combination with other antiparkinson drugs. Anticholinergic drugs are contraindicated in the presence of glaucoma, myasthenia gravis, gastrointestinal obstruction, prostatic hypertrophy, and urinary bladder neck obstruction. They must be used with caution in patients exhibiting symptoms related to cardiovascular disorders. Benztropine (Cogentin), biperiden (Akineton), trihexyphenidyl (Artane), and diphenhydramine (Benadryl) are examples of anticholinergic/antiparkinson drugs used to alleviate acute extrapyramidal symptoms.

Antiparkinson agents act to increase levels of dopamine or inhibit actions of acetylcholine in the brain to adjust levels of neurotransmitters. Antiparkinson agents are contraindicated in the presence of known hypersensitivity to specific drugs; in concomitant use with MAOIs, meperidine, and other opioids; and in the presence of uncontrolled hypertension, narrow-angle glaucoma, or breast-feeding. Examples include carbidopa and levodopa (Sinemet), bromocriptine (Parlodel), levodopa (Larodopa), and amantadine (Symmetrel).

Implications for Nursing Actions

Nursing actions for antiparkinson drug therapy cited by Abrams (1995) and Karch (1997) include the following:

1. Give antiparkinson agents with or immediately after food intake to prevent or reduce gastrointestinal distress.
2. Observe for therapeutic effects such as decreased salivation, tremor, and drooling (anticholinergic effects).
3. Observe for improvement in gait, balance, posture, speech, and self-care ability.
4. Monitor for adverse effects due to anticholinergic drugs (atropine-like effects) such as dry mouth, drowsiness, constipation, and urinary retention.
5. Monitor for adverse reactions to antiparkinson agents such as psychosis, depression, hallucinations, insomnia, and irritability.

Patient Education

As is true of other types of drug therapy, the patient receiving medication to lessen or reverse extrapyramidal side effects of psychotropic drugs should be instructed to follow the physician's instructions regarding dosage (Table 12-9). Other instructions for the patient and family members include the following:

1. Maintain an adequate amount of fluid intake (unless contraindicated) to prevent excessive dryness of the mouth. Taking the medication just before meals, chewing gum, or sucking on hard candies may alleviate this side effect.

TABLE 12-9 DAILY DOSAGE OF COMMONLY USED ANTICHOLINERGIC/ANTIPARKINSON AGENTS

Generic Name	Trade Name	Dosage Range (mg/day)
amantadine	Symmetrel	100 mg–300 mg
benztropine	Cogentin	0.5 mg–6 mg
biperiden	Akineton	2 mg–16 mg
bromocriptine	Parlodel	2.5 mg–100 mg
diphenhydramine	Benadryl	25 mg–200 mg
levodopa	Larodopa or Dopar	1,000 mg–8,000 mg
selegiline	Eldepryl	5 mg–10 mg
trihexyphenidyl	Artane	2 mg–15 mg

2. Avoid operating potentially hazardous machinery or driving an automobile if symptoms of blurred vision or drowsiness occur.
3. Report any side effects or unusual symptoms to the physician/psychiatrist.
4. Use caution when rising from a sitting or reclining position because of the possibility of postural hypotension and drowsiness.
5. Limit strenuous activities in hot weather because anticholinergic drugs may cause anhidrosis (the inability to sweat).
6. Have routine vision examinations to eliminate the possibility of the presence of glaucoma.
7. Limit use of alcohol, high-protein foods, and vitamin B_6 because they decrease therapeutic effects of levodopa.
8. Avoid taking MAOIs, TCAs, or SSRIs concurrently with Eldepryl.

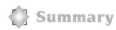 **Summary**

Psychotropic drugs are chemicals used therapeutically in the practice of psychiatry to treat a wide range of mental and emotional illness and are categorized as antipsychotic drugs, antianxiety agents, sedative-hypnotics, antidepressants, antimanic agents, and anticonvulsants. Antiparkinson agents also are used in the psychiatric setting. Each category was presented, focusing on the principle or rationale for therapy; contraindications, precautions, and side effects; and implications for nursing actions. Patient education was discussed, and examples of commonly used drugs and the daily dosage of each were given. Drug–drug interactions and unusual side effects were featured in Med Alerts.

Learning Activities

I. Clinical Activities
   A. Identify several psychotropic drugs prescribed in the clinical setting.
   B. State the rationale for the administration of each identified drug.
   C. Identify any side effects or drug–drug interactions.
   D. List nursing implications for each drug identified.

Critical Thinking Questions

1. Research and create a lesson plan to teach patients and families about antipsychotic agents. Collaborate with a pharmacy student and team teach this material to an appropriate group. How does the pharmacy student's focus differ from yours? What are the strengths you bring to this process and what are the pharmacy student's?

2. MAOIs present unique problems for the patients taking them. What member of the health care team would be of great assistance to you as you prepare patient education materials for this group of drugs?
3. We know that MAOIs alleviate symptoms and it is necessary for them to be taken to do so. Yet, in many of our large cities, homeless people with mental illnesses roam the streets with symptoms raging, medications forgotten. What might be done about this problem? What is nursing's role in this community mental health issue?

Self-Test

1. List five types of psychotropic drugs.
2. Explain the action of TCAs.
3. List the trade names of various TCAs.
4. Explain the action of MAOI antidepressants.
5. List the trade names of various MAOI medications.
6. List common side effects of antidepressant medications.
7. List conditions, other than depression, that appear to respond to antidepressant medications.
8. Explain why lithium is the drug of choice in the treatment of manic disorders.
9. State two reasons why lithium is considered a potentially dangerous drug.
10. List the disorders that appear to respond to lithium.
11. List side effects and toxicity levels of lithium.
12. List drug classifications that interact dangerously with lithium.
13. What are the absolute and relative contraindications in the use of lithium?
14. Compare the terms *neuroleptic* and *antipsychotic medication*.
15. List causes of those psychotic conditions that respond to the antipsychotic medications.
16. State symptoms that *do* and *do not* respond to the use of an antipsychotic medication.
17. List other disorders that respond to the use of an antipsychotic medication.
18. Explain the action of an antipsychotic medication.
19. Note drug interactions of various agents with antipsychotic medications.
20. List the trade names of various antipsychotic medications.
21. List the side effects of antipsychotic medications.
22. Define the term *extrapyramidal*.

23. Cite examples of extrapyramidal side effects.
24. List common anticholinergic/antiparkinson medications.
25. List common side effects of sedative-hypnotic medications.
26. State conditions that contraindicate the use of sedative-hypnotic medications.

SELECTED REFERENCES

Abrams, A. C. (1995). *Clinical drug therapy: Rationales for nursing practice* (4th ed.). Philadelphia: J. B. Lippincott.

American Psychiatric Association. (1990). *Benzodiazepine dependence, toxicity, and abuse.* Washington, DC: American Psychiatric Press.

Barrett, N., Ormiston, S., & Molyneux, V. (1990, February). Clozapine: A new drug for schizophrenia. *Journal of Psychosocial Nursing and Mental Health Services.*

Bernstein, J. G. (1988). *Handbook of drug therapy in psychiatry* (2nd ed.). Littleton, CO: PSG Publishing.

Blair, D. T., & Dauner, A. (1993, February). Neuroleptic malignant syndrome: Liability in nursing practice. *Journal of Psychosocial Nursing and Mental Health Services.*

Bostrom, A. C. (1988, June). Assessment scales for tardive dyskinesia. *Journal of Psychosocial Nursing and Mental Health Services.*

Bristol-Myers Squibb (1996). *Guide to psychotropic agents.* Secaucus, NJ: Pocket Prescribing, Inc.

Gerchufsky, M. (1996, March). The art and science of prescribing psychiatric medications: An outline for nurse practitioners. *Advance for Nurse Practitioners.*

Kane, J. M. (1992). *Tardive dyskinesia: A task force report of the American Psychiatric Association.* Washington, DC: American Psychiatric Press.

Karch, A. M. (1997). *Lippincott's nursing drug guide.* Philadelphia: Lippincott–Raven Publishers.

Lee, M. (1996, July). Drugs and the elderly: Do you know these risks? *American Journal of Nursing.*

Maxmen, J. S. (1991). *Psychotropic drugs fast facts.* New York: W. W. Norton.

New drug bulletin: Risperidone (Risperdal). (June, 1994). *RN.*

Norris, A. E., Eilsaver, S. C., & Del Medico, V. J. (1990, December). Carbamazepine treatment in psychosis: Implications for patient welfare and nursing practice. *Journal of Psychosocial Nursing and Mental Health Services.*

Popper, C. W., & Frazier, S. H. (Eds.). (1990, Spring). *Journal of Child and Adolescent Psychopharmacology.*

Schatzberg, A. F., & Nemeroff, C. B. (1995). *Textbook of psychopharmacology.* Washington, DC: American Psychiatric Press.

Shamoian, C. A. (Ed.). (1992). *Psychopharmacological treatment complications in the elderly.* Washington, DC: American Psychiatric Press.

Walker, J. (1982). *Everybody's guide to emotional well-being.* San Francisco: Harbor Publishing.

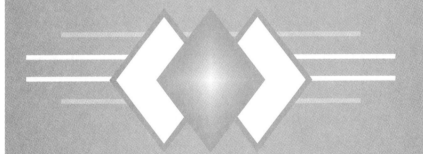

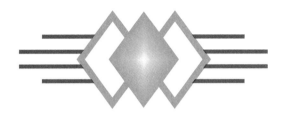

CHAPTER 13

THEORIES OF PERSONALITY DEVELOPMENT

P arents and their social groups teach children to recognize and express their emotions and to apply the correct emotion to the appropriate situation. They also legitimize the expression of some emotions and suppress the expressions of others. This depends on the stage of development of the child, the level of education of the family, and the cultural group to which the persons belong.

Boyle & Andrews, 1989

1   Define the term *personality*.

2   Summarize the concepts of the following theories:

   Freud's psychoanalytic theory

   Erikson's psychosocial theory

   Piaget's cognitive developmental theory

3   State the common feelings, behavior patterns, and social considerations to be assessed when one is working with minority groups.

4   Explain why the understanding of a person's cultural background (*e.g.*, Asian American) is crucial for appropriate nursing interventions.

5   Discuss the importance of a working knowledge of personality growth and development in the mental health setting.

6   Analyze the above-mentioned theories and their applicability to clinical practice.

Introduction

Personality is the total of a person's internal and external patterns of adjustment to life, determined in part by genetically transmitted organic endowment and by life experiences. Thus, the dynamics of personality development become increasingly complex throughout the life span as one continually interacts with the environment and experiences various stages of physical and psychological maturation. Factors influencing psychological maturation have been identified as genetic stressors, such as Down syndrome; environmental stressors, including parental relationships, peer relationships, and cultural and social experiences; individual accomplishments that are results of learning and adaptation; and one's mental health status at each developmental stage. Thus, a newborn infant reacts differently to a given environmental stimulus than does an adolescent, young adult, or elderly person.

Various theories of personality maturation are presented in developmental psychology classes as part of the curriculum in nursing programs. Generally, they are categorized as psychoanalytical, cognitive, behavioristic, and interpersonal. It is not the intent of this book to provide an in-depth chapter on these theories, but, rather, to present a summary of the more common theories such as those of Freud, Erikson, and Piaget.

Maslow's (1962, 1970) characteristics of mental health are described in Chapter 1. His hierarchy of human needs (*e.g.*, physiologic, safety, loving and belonging, esteem, and self-actualization) is discussed within the text. The relationship of developmental theories and conceptual models of nursing care is addressed in Chapter 8.

Freud's Psychoanalytic Theory

Freud's theory of personality development describes three major categories: the organization or structure of personality, the dynamics of personality, and the development of personality.

The organization or structure of the personality (Freud, 1960) consists of the *id*, which is an unconscious reservoir of primitive drives and instincts dominated by thinking and the pleasure principle; the *ego*, which meets and interacts with the outside world as an integrator or mediator and is the executive function of the personality that operates at all three levels of consciousness; and the *superego*, which acts as the censoring force or conscience of the personality and is composed of morals, mores, values, and ethics largely derived from one's parents. The superego operates at all three levels of consciousness also.

According to Freud's explanation of the dynamics of the personality, each person has a certain amount of psychic energy to cope with the problems of everyday living. The id's energy is used to reduce tension and may be exhibited, for example, by frequency of urination, daydreaming, or eating. The ego's energy controls the impulsive actions of the id and the moralistic and idealistic actions of the superego. One whose energy is controlled primarily by the superego generally behaves in an overly moralistic manner because the system monopolizing the psychic energy governs the person's behavior.

Freud explains the development of the personality by describing three levels of consciousness: the unconscious, preconscious (subconscious), and conscious. The unconscious level consists of drives, feelings, ideas, and urges outside of the person's awareness. This is the most significant level of consciousness because of the effect it has on behavior. A considerable amount of psychic energy is used to keep unpleasant memories stored in the unconscious level of the mind. The preconscious or subconscious level, midway between the conscious and unconscious levels, consists of feelings, ideals, drives, and ideas that are out of one's ongoing awareness but can be recalled readily. The conscious level of the personality is aware of the present and controls purposeful behavior.

Freud also describes five phases of psychobiologic process (psychosexual theory), which have a great impact on personality development: oral, anal, phallic or oedipal, latency, and genital. The oral phase (0–18 mos) is a period in which pleasure is derived mainly through the mouth by the actions of sucking or biting. During the anal phase (18 mos–3 yrs), attention focuses on the excretory function, and the foundation is laid for the development of the superego.

The phallic or oedipal stage (3–7 yrs) is a stage of growth and development in which the child identifies with the parent of the same sex, forms a deep attachment to the parent of the opposite sex, develops a sexual identity of male or female role, and begins to experience guilt. During the latency phase (7 yrs to adolescence), the person learns to recognize and handle reality, has a limited sexual image, develops an inner control over aggressive or destructive impulses, and experiences intellectual and social growth. The final stage of psychosexual development is the genital phase (puberty or adolescence into adult life), in which the individual develops the capacity for object love and mature sexuality. Identity and independence are established during this phase.

Erikson's Psychosocial Theory

Erikson (1968) emphasizes the concepts of identity or an inner sense of sameness that perseveres despite external changes, identity crisis, and identity confusion in the dynamics of personality development. He has identified eight psychosocial stages during one's life span: (1) sensory-oral (birth to 18 mos), characterized by the central task of trust versus mistrust; (2) muscular-anal (18 mos–3 yrs), characterized by autonomy versus shame and doubt; (3) locomotor-genital (3–5 yrs), characterized by initiative versus guilt; (4) latency (6–11 yrs), characterized by industry versus inferiority; (5) puberty and adolescence (12–18 yrs), involving identity versus role confusion; (6) young adulthood (19–40 yrs), characterized by intimacy versus isolation; (7) middle adulthood (41–64 yrs), characterized by generativity versus stagnation or self-absorption; and (8) late adulthood or maturity (65 yrs to death), characterized by ego integrity versus despair. These developmental stages are a series of normative conflicts that every person must handle. The two opposing energies (developmental crisis) must be synthesized in a constructive manner to produce positive expectations for new experiences. If the crisis is unresolved, the person does not develop attitudes that will be helpful in meeting future developmental tasks. Box 13-1 summarizes Erikson's psychosocial theory, focusing on the developmental stage, area of conflict and resolution, basic virtues or qualities acquired, and positive and negative behavior. Failure to resolve a challenge or conflict results in negative behavior or developmental problems. An opportunity to resolve such conflicts recurs later in one's life span.

Piaget's Cognitive Developmental Theory

Piaget's (1963) theory views intellectual development as a result of constant interaction between environmental influences and genetically determined attributes. Piaget's research focused on four stages of intellectual growth during

BOX 13-1 Summary of Erikson's Psychosocial Theory

Developmental Stage	Area of Conflict and Resolution	Basic Virtues or Qualities	Positive Behavior or Resolution of Conflict	Negative Behavior
Sensory-oral or early infancy (birth to 18 mos)	Trust vs mistrust	Drive and hope	Displays affection, confidence, gratification, recognition, and the ability to trust others	Suspicious of others, fears affection, projection
Muscular-anal or later infancy (18 mos–3 yrs)	Autonomy vs shame and doubt	Self-control and willpower	Cooperative, expresses oneself, displays self-control, views self apart from parents	Self-doubt, denial, dependency and co-dependency, low self-esteem, loss of self-control
Locomotor-genital or early child-hood (3–5 yrs)	Initiative vs guilt	Direction and purpose	Tests reality. Shows imagination, displays some ability to evaluate own behavior, exerts positive controls over self	Excessive guilt, feels victimized, passive, apathetic
Latency or middle childhood (6–11 yrs)	Industry vs inferiority	Method and competence	Develops a sense of duty, and scholastic and social competencies. Displays perseverance and interacts with peers in a less infantile manner	Feels inferior, lacks motivation, uncooperative, incompetent, unreliable
Puberty and adolescence (12–18 yrs)	Identity vs role confusion	Devotion and fidelity	Displays self-certainty, experiments with role, expresses ideologic commitments, chooses a career or vocation, and develops inter-	Self-doubt, dysfunctional relationships, rebellion, substance abuse

(continued)

BOX 13-1 Summary of Erikson's Psychosocial Theory (Continued)

Developmental Stage	Area of Conflict and Resolution	Basic Virtues or Qualities	Positive Behavior or Resolution of Conflict	Negative Behavior
Young adulthood (19–40 yrs)	Intimacy vs isolation	Affiliation and love	personal relationships Establishes mature relationship with a member of the opposite sex, chooses a suitable marital partner, performs work and social roles in a socially acceptable manner	Self-imposed isolation, emotionally immature, jealous, possessive
Middle adulthood (41–64 yrs)	Generativity vs stagnation	Productivity and ability to care for others	Spends times wisely by engaging in helpful activities such as teaching, counseling, community activities, and volunteer work. Displays creativity	Egocentric, disinterested in others, overinvolved in activities
Late adulthood or maturity (65 yrs to death)	Ego integrity vs despair	Renunciation or "letting go," and wisdom	Reviews life realistically, accepts past failures and limitations, helps members of younger generations view life positively and realistically, accepts death with dignity	Feels hopeless, helpless, fears death, dwells on past failures, disappointments, unable to adjust to aging process

childhood, with emphasis on how a child learns and adapts what is learned from the adult world. The four stages are sensorimotor, preoperational, concrete operational, and formal operational.

During the sensorimotor stage (0–2 yrs), the infant uses the senses in learning about self and the environment by exploration of objects and events, and by imitation. The infant also develops schemata, or methods of assimilating and accommodating incoming information; these include looking schema, hearing schema, and sucking schema.

The preoperational thought stage (2–7 or 8 yrs) is subdivided into the pre-conceptual and intuitive phases. Learning to think in mental images and the development of expressive languages and symbolic play occur between the ages of 2 and 4. During the ages of 4 to 7 the child exhibits egocentrism, seeing things from his or her own point of view. The child is unable to comprehend the ideas of others if they differ from his or her own. As the child matures, he or she realizes that other people see things differently.

The concrete operational stage begins at about age 8 and lasts until age 12. The child is able to think more logically as the concepts of moral judgment, numbers, and spatial relationships are developed.

The formal operational stage occurs during age 12 and lasts to adulthood. The person develops adult logic and is able to reason, form conclusions, plan for the future, think abstractly, and build ideals.

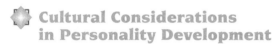 Cultural Considerations in Personality Development

Culture is an important variable in the assessment of individuals in addition to the structural and functional aspects of the family. To understand an ethnic group and to be able to work with individuals or family members, the nurse must be aware of a culture's distinctive qualities and the variety of life-styles, values, and structures within a given group that influence the development of a person's personality. Cultural differences are often the cause of poor communication, interpersonal tensions, inability to work effectively with others, and the poor assessment of health problems. Therefore, the racial identity, religious preferences, and unique cultural experiences of members of minority cultures cannot be ignored in mental health nursing. Andrews and Boyle (1995) include a section on developmental considerations as part of a transcultural nursing assessment guide to be used when providing care to culturally diverse individuals (p. 444).

Cultural practices of Native Americans, African Americans, Hispanics, and Asian Americans will be discussed to assist the reader in developing an understanding of personality development in these minority families. It should be remembered that cultural practices vary within these ethnic groups. Native Americans, for example, represent many different tribes, each with distinctive qualities.

Native Americans

Cultural identity of Native Americans is no longer determined by physical appearance but rather by the classification of *functional* or *nonfunctional*. The functional Native American has an intimate understanding of heritage obtained through socialization from childhood and considers herself or himself to be Native American. The individual's behavior is dictated by accepted patterns of other Native Americans. The nonfunctional Native American may appear to be full-blooded but may have little or no knowledge of the traditions or culture of Native American people. This person follows the cultural practices of the white race and considers himself or herself a non–Native American.

Beliefs and practices that influence the personality of members of this minority population are summarized. Native Americans believe that illness is a result of an imbalance between a person and natural or supernatural forces rather than an altered physiologic state. Illness may result from abusing another person, thinking bad thoughts, or entertaining thoughts of jealousy or anger. Healing ceremonies referred to as "sings" or prayers are practiced to restore homeostasis. Children are highly valued. Family, relatives, and friends play an important part in their kinship structure and support system. Work and productivity are valued; however, time is not an important factor. Suicide, homicide, and mortality rates are greater than those of any other race. Less emphasis is placed on the future compared to other cultures. Direct eye contact is not maintained because it is a disrespectful practice and an invasion of one's privacy (Andrews & Boyle, 1995).

African Americans

During the era of slavery, the African American family was allowed to exist only by the consent of the slave owner and was not autonomous or self-sufficient. Today, African Americans are able to maintain two-parent nuclear families while they adapt to a larger society and become members of the middle class. Distinctive characteristics of African American families include the following: (1) households may have a larger number of extended family members living with them owing to strong kinship bonds; (2) children often are expected to assume responsible duties such as helping with housework, running errands, and caring for younger siblings; (3) young children often hold odd jobs to supplement family incomes; (4) poor families have survival needs that often supersede the resolution of health problems; and (5) poor African American families often experience feelings of discomfort and alienation toward white health care providers. Health practices and beliefs that may still exist to some extent include voodoo, witchcraft, and reliance on folk home remedies (Andrews & Boyle, 1995; Friedman, 1981).

Hispanics

Hispanic families exhibit a significant characteristic referred to as familism. The family is the single most important social unit, and individual needs are subordinated to familial needs. The father, who is the head of the family, will work long hours to keep his large family economically self-sufficient. The wife frequently is ambivalent about her marital role owing to sexual inhibitions and beliefs; thus, the marital relationship becomes formal and distant because the husband is free culturally to have extramarital affairs to prove his *machismo* (manliness). In response to this relationship, the wife often turns to her children and female relatives to meet her needs for affection and companionship.

Children often are expected to assist with household chores and jobs outside the home. They are taught to place family needs before individual ambitions. The world of the adolescent girl generally consists of the family and home, whereas adolescent sons are encouraged to gain worldly experience.

Family power is exhibited by men over women and the older order over the younger family members: therefore, the younger females have the least power in the family.

Hispanic beliefs about health practices are significant: (1) specific foods can cause good or poor health; (2) being in tune with God fosters good health; (3) health is described as being free of pain; (4) certain illnesses are considered to be hot or cold and are treated by eating particular herbs; (5) the hospital is a place to die; and (6) illness is a family affair, during which time many relatives gather around (Andrews & Boyle, 1995; Johnson, 1997).

Asian Americans

Because of the recent influx of immigrants from Asia, nurses must be aware of the personality traits and cultural practices of different groups of Asian Americans. In the past, traditional family structure was patriarchal, in which the members displayed respect for and obedience toward their ancestors and toward the men in the family in order of seniority. As Asians began immigrating to the United States, family ties continued to be strong, but traditional family practices and folk medicine became less dominant.

Chinese folk medicine, for example, proposes that health is regulated by two opposing forces, yin and yang. They must be in perfect balance for physical, mental, and social well-being to occur. Yang, the positive force, represents the male, as well as light, warmth, and fullness, whereas yin is the negative, female force characterized by darkness, cold, and emptiness. Excessive yin predisposes one to nervousness and digestive disorders, and excessive yang contributes to dehydration, fever, and irritability.

The Chinese use hot foods to treat yin illnesses and cold foods for yang disorders. They may contact an herb pharmacist or herbalist to treat yin and yang disorders or an acupuncturist to treat musculoskeletal disorders. Family customs may promote the use of herbs, pills, and food to treat mental or physical disorders. The nurse should be aware that Chinese patients may follow both Western and Asian medical advice simultaneously, resulting in double doses of medication (Johnson, 1997).

The nurse should also be aware of differences among the other cultures (*e.g.*, Japanese, Korean, and Vietnamese peoples) identified as Asian American.

 ## Implications for Nursing Interventions

A working knowledge of personality growth and development is important when the nurse cares for patients in the mental health setting. The nurse participates in the individual's treatment plan in several ways: (1) identifying developmental needs through close observation and assessment of developmental tasks that have or have not been resolved; (2) assisting the person in understanding problem areas; (3) planning interventions that will decrease the continuance of maladaptive behavior; (4) anticipating future developmental stressors; and (5) evaluating the patient's progress during the course of treatment.

In pediatric settings, the psychiatric nurse works with parents and significant others to assess the cognitive and behavioral development of children. The nurse generally focuses on assessing and evaluating opportunities for the child's growth and development; assessing and evaluating the outcome of a child's development related to life experiences; and making recommendations or providing teaching pertaining to ways in which positive cognitive and behavioral development can be fostered and enhanced.

Without knowledge of differences in cultural norms and patterns, the mental health nurse may be unable to recognize the meaning of a person's behavior or actions. Normal patterns of behavior are often labeled as deviant, immoral, illegal, or crazy, depending on the type of behavioral norm violated. Communication styles, the establishment of rapport, goal expectations, and the acceptance of ideas often are impaired because of cultural dissimilarity. Personal feelings, beliefs, and attitudes must be identified, discussed, and accepted before one can work effectively with people seeking assistance.

 ## Summary

The dynamics of personality development were discussed, as well as factors influencing psychological maturation. Various theories of personality development were presented: (1) Freud's psychoanalytic theory, (2) Erikson's psychosocial theory, and (3) Piaget's cognitive developmental theory. Cultural considerations pertaining to the personality development of Native Americans, African Americans, Hispanics, and Asian Americans were stated. Implications for nursing interventions focusing on personality growth and development were given.

Learning Activities

I. Clinical Activities
  A. Assess the developmental level of at least two assigned patients by applying one of the following theories of personality development:
    1. Freud's psychoanalytic theory
    2. Erikson's psychosocial theory
    3. Piaget's cognitive developmental theory
  B. Discuss the developmental tasks appropriate for each patient's chronologic age.
  C. List any tasks that may be stress producing for each patient.
  D. State nursing interventions appropriate to assist the patient in resolving any identified conflicts.
  E. Assess each patient's cultural background:
    1. Does the patient belong to a minority group?
    2. Identify feelings, behavioral patterns, or social considerations (as discussed in this chapter) that may impair nursing interventions.
II. Independent Activities
  A. Read one of the following to increase your knowledge base of personality development:
    1. E. H. Erikson, *Childhood and Society*, 1963
    2. M. Bloom, *Life Span Development*, 1980
    3. M. M. Andrews and J. S. Boyle, *Transcultural Concepts in Nursing Care*, 1995

Critical Thinking Questions

1. The theories of personality development discussed in this chapter were all developed by men. Discuss how a feminine perspective might be different.
2. Assess a family with a cultural background different from your own. Compare the family to the material presented in this chapter. What family strengths do they have?
3. Ask friends or classmates of varying cultural backgrounds how they have been treated by the health care system. Have they received culturally sensitive care? What can you incorporate from these conversations into your own care of culturally diverse patients?

Self-Test

1. Match the following
    1. Id   a. Censoring force of the
                                               personality
    2. Freud's psychoanalytic   b. Eight stages of one's life span
       theory   characterized by a central task
    3. Piaget's cognitive   c. Discusses organization,
       developmental theory   dynamics, and development
                                            of one's personality
    4. Ego   d. Integrator or mediator of the
                                            personality
    5. Erikson's psychosocial   e. Describes intellectual growth
       theory   and development
    6. Superego   f. Unconscious reservoir of
                                            primitive drives and instincts

2. Cite examples of failure to resolve the following conflicts:
    a. Trust versus mistrust
    b. Autonomy versus shame and doubt
    c. Initiative versus guilt
    d. Industry versus inferiority
    e. Identity versus role confusion
    f. Intimacy versus isolation
    g. Generativity versus stagnation
    h. Ego integrity versus despair

3. Compare cultural practices of Native Americans, African
   Americans, Hispanics, and Asian Americans as they relate to the
   following developmental stages by Erikson:
    a. Latency or middle childhood
    b. Young adulthood
    c. Late adulthood or maturity

4. Identify four cultural considerations to be taken into account
   during the nursing assessment process.

SELECTED REFERENCES

Andrews, M. M., & Boyle, J. S. (1995). *Transcultural concepts in nursing care* (2nd ed.).
    Philadelphia: J. B. Lippincott.
Bloom, M. (1980). *Life span development.* New York: Macmillan.
Boyle, J. S., & Andrews, M. M. (1989). *Transcultural concepts in nursing care.* Philadelphia:
    J. B. Lippincott.
Erikson, E. H. (1963). *Childhood and society* (2nd ed.). New York: W. W. Norton.
Erikson, E. H. (1968). *Identity: Youth and crisis.* New York: W. W. Norton.

Freud, S. (1960). *The ego and the id.* J. Strachey (Ed.). New York: W. W. Norton.

Friedman, M. M. (1981). Family nursing: Theory and assessment. Norwalk, CT: Appleton-Century-Crofts.

Johnson, B. S. (1997). *Psychiatric–mental health nursing: Adaptation and growth* (4th ed.). Philadelphia: Lippincott–Raven Publishers.

Maslow, A. M. (1970). *Motivation and personality* (2nd ed.). New York: Harper and Row.

Maslow, A. M. (1962). *Toward a psychology of being.* Princeton, NJ: D. Van Nostrand.

Piaget, J. (1963). *The child's conception of the world.* Ames, IA: Littlefield, Adams.

Schultz, D. P. (1990). *Theories of personality* (4th ed.). Pacific Grove, CA: Brooks-Cole.

Sue, D. W., & Sue, D. (1990). *Counseling the culturally different: Theory and practice* (2nd ed.). Somerset, NJ: John Wiley & Sons.

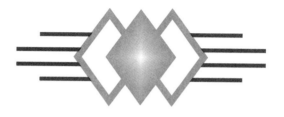

CHAPTER 14

EMOTIONAL RESPONSES TO ILLNESS AND HOSPITALIZATION

E ach person who is admitted to a general hospital brings with him not only a physical illness but also a definitive mental set that will influence both the manner in which he assumes his role as a patient and the course of his hospitalization.

Robinson, 1984

1 Explain the role of culture in an individual's response to illness and hospitalization.

2 Discuss why a person assumes the "sick role."

3 State the psychological or emotional needs of most people.

4 Explain the following emotional responses to illness:

   Anxiety

   Fear

   Loneliness

   Powerlessness

   Helplessness

   Hopelessness

5 State nursing interventions for each of the emotional responses listed in objective no. 4.

6 Discuss the concept of humor as it relates to illness.

7 Describe the impact of hospitalization on an adolescent.

Introduction

Change, such as illness and hospitalization, is a threatening experience that elicits various emotional responses from patients as well as from family members or significant others. A questionnaire developed by the author was distributed to approximately 200 patients in an attempt to obtain first-hand information about their responses to illness, hospitalization, and nursing care. The results revealed some important factors regarding the psychological or emotional needs of hospitalized patients, their emotional responses to illness, and their impressions of members of the health care team.

Of the 200 patients surveyed in 1985, 90% were hospitalized in a general community hospital; 60% were hospitalized for a week or less; 52% had a medical illness; and 35% underwent surgery.

Eighty-one percent of those surveyed felt they were treated as a person rather than as a patient with an illness, whereas 19% felt they were not. Ninety-one percent of the respondents stated they were permitted to maintain independence and participate in their own care, whereas 9% felt they were placed in a dependent position.

Of the persons asked, 84% stated that they were given a satisfactory explanation of treatment, equipment, and nursing care; 66% felt they were given the opportunity to make decisions regarding their treatment. Of the hospitalized patients responding, 44% felt that the nurses were aware of their spiritual needs; however, 56% did not. Fifty percent of the patients felt their need for privacy was respected. Forty-two percent felt the nursing personnel were aware of their fears during hospitalization.

Respondents also commented about the quality of nursing care they received. Most of the hospitalized persons stated they felt the nurses were friendly, competent, and professional, and took time to talk with them. Conversely, 65% of the patients felt their complaints were ignored, and 63% felt their family members were not informed of their progress. Only 37% of the patients were given an explanation of their illness or surgery.

Emotional responses to hospitalization varied. Most (52%) of the individuals experienced anxiety; 25% identified fear; 17% stated they were lonely and felt powerless or helpless; 15% admitted to feeling depressed; and 8% described feeling angry. Twenty-seven percent expressed a need for spiritual care.

Specific comments included the following:

"We were not informed that so many doctors would be caring for my mother. The doctors were not always available to let us know how she was doing."

"Most of my contact was with LPNs. The RNs were busy giving medication."

"The nurses were rude to me and my family. Two of them attempted to physically prevent me from leaving the floor, claiming my *bill* had to be paid first!"

"I learned to do anything to avoid being in that position [hospitalization] again!"

"Felt like I was in a business with no power over any solutions. Get in, get it done, don't ask questions, but make sure you pay."

"When he died there, all us were satisfied that everything that could be done for him had been done and he died in peace."

". . . completely satisfied with this hospital, personnel, treatment and everything pertaining to the patient–nurse relationship!"

"My minister provided me with *much* spiritual support. The chaplains in the hospital stopped by daily."

This chapter discusses psychological or emotional needs, behavioral or emotional responses, and nursing interventions as they pertain to the person who becomes a patient.

Hospitalization and the Sick Role

Various aspects of care occur within the hospital setting, such as diagnostic tests, medical treatment, surgical intervention, nursing interventions, rehabilitative care, and research. Holistic health care has emerged. Because it focuses on the physical, social, cultural, and spiritual needs of patients, it involves several disciplines.

Andrews and Boyle (1995) discuss cultural responses to illness. Several studies are cited regarding coping behaviors by African Americans, Mexican Americans, Anglo-Americans, Latinos, Americans, and Asians. "Health professionals should develop a respect for the cultural beliefs and practices of clients even when they run counter to scientific medical systems. . . . Attempting to change deeply held health beliefs through ridicule and skepticism not only may fail but also may alienate clients" (p. 250).

A hospitalized patient is influenced by several factors: (1) the extent or seriousness of the illness; (2) the manner of admittance to the hospital; (3) the patient's feelings, thoughts, and cultural attitudes about the hospital and personnel; and (4) information given by friends, acquaintances, and the attending physician. Experiences during childhood also influence a person's responses to hospitalization. If the parents have been matter-of-fact about visits to the doctor's office, the child is likely to accept the nurse, doctor, and other health caregivers as caring persons. The child learns to trust their judgment and cooperate with them while receiving care. If parents have used health care as a threat to reprimand a child, for example, "The nurse will give you a shot if you don't behave!" the child will expect the nurse or doctor to be punitive or sadistic in treatment approaches. These beliefs are carried into one's adult life, influencing responses to illness and hospitalization.

The sick role is assumed by people for many reasons. They may perceive themselves as helpless, requiring the assistance of others to meet their needs or modify their condition. Such persons often turn their lives over to the care of the nurse or doctor, expecting them to "fix" their problems and send them home when they have improved. One man acted unconcerned about his illness and treatment. He never questioned the attending physician about his condition or various medications and treatments that were ordered, nor did he mention going home. When the student nurse asked the patient if he were eager to get home, the patient stated that he would stay as long as the doctor thought he should. "He'll tell me when I'm ready to go home. That's his job." The student was amazed at the lack of concern displayed by the patient during hospitalization.

Illness relieves one of social responsibilities and often produces secondary gains, such as personal attention or disability benefits. The sick role may become a way of life. A 35-year-old man who had complained of an industrial back injury at 24 was able to collect industrial compensation and disability benefits. For 11 years he was unable to work but did manage to travel to attend sporting events, and to lead a relatively active life. When questioned by the student nurse whether he ever thought of trying another vocation, he informed her that he suffered "an industrial injury and the company is paying my way. I don't want to lose my benefits by becoming gainfully employed!"

The sick role may be a manipulative ploy when a person attempts to cope with various emotional conflicts. For example, a 54-year-old woman whose children had left home was hospitalized several times in one year for vague symptoms, including dizziness, heartburn, headaches, and chest pain. She was unable to work and was placed on sick leave. Her children and neighbors were quick to respond to her needs each time she was hospitalized. The attending physician explored the patient's vague complaints with her and identified underlying feelings of loneliness and depression. Her complaints were producing a secondary gain of attention and concern displayed by her children and neighbors. She was, to a degree, manipulating their lives because they planned their social and recreational activities around her needs while she assumed the sick role.

Psychological or Emotional Needs

Most people experience the following common emotional needs to some degree in their lives: to be loved and to love others, to feel secure, to feel important or good about themselves, to be self-sufficient, and to be productive or develop one's full potential. Consider the impact of illness or hospitalization on these needs.

A person with terminal cancer who is hospitalized over an extensive period experiences separation from loved ones at a critical time in life. It is difficult for family members or significant others to spend all of their time at the bedside of a seriously ill person. They may be absent at times when their presence would provide a feeling of security to the patient, particularly during bone marrow aspirations, chemotherapy treatments, and other serious procedures.

Cancer affects a person's self-concept, or the ability to feel good about oneself, especially if one's physical appearance is altered by weight loss or disfigurement. It can also cause a self-sufficient person to become dependent on others, producing feelings of helplessness and powerlessness as the person's physical condition deteriorates. Terminal cancer, usually accompanied by pain and weakness, interferes with one's ability to be productive or develop one's full potential.

The impact of cancer on a 26-year-old woman's emotional needs is an example. MJ, mother of three children, developed uterine cancer that was treated surgically, but not before it had metastasized to the lungs and brain. She had undergone chemotherapy and cobalt treatments, hoping to prolong her life. Her husband refused to visit her at the hospital; instead, he stayed home with the children waiting for "mommy to come home." As a result of her husband's decision, MJ was denied the presence of her loved ones during her last hospitalization. On one occasion, MJ told the student she felt like "an apple being peeled away one layer at a time." She was referring to the surgery, chemotherapy, and side effects of alopecia, nausea, vomiting, and weight loss. MJ also expressed concern that she would not be able to see her children go to school, become teenagers, and attend college. She felt that she was being denied the right to be a wife and mother. As her strength failed, MJ became dependent on the student nurse to bathe, feed, and turn her. She stated that she "hated to be dependent on others and wished she could at least wash her face and feed herself." MJ had become a lonely, insecure, dependent person with a negative self-concept. She was unable to develop her full potential as a wife, mother, and woman.

The role of a nurse is very important because the nurse plans interventions to meet these emotional or psychological needs of hospitalized people. Douville (1994) and Dumas (1996) cite personal experiences and practical tips to use while caring for individuals with the diagnosis of cancer. Box 14-1 summarizes the common emotional needs of individuals and the nursing interventions used to meet those needs.

If the nurse is aware that each person experiences the needs just described and implements nursing interventions to meet these needs, negative comments,

BOX 14-1 Nursing Interventions for Psychological and Emotional Needs of Patients

Need	Nursing Intervention
To be loved	Display a sincere interest in the patient by setting aside time each day to be with that person.
	Encourage the patient to verbalize feelings about loved ones.
	Identify significant others, such as family members, friends, and pastor.
	Assist the patient, family, or friends in planning scheduled visits whenever possible.

BOX 14-1 **Nursing Interventions for Psychological and Emotional Needs of Patients** (Continued)

Need	Nursing Intervention
To feel secure	Encourage verbalization of feelings about hospitalization.
	Explore feelings about security.
	Promote feelings of security by orienting the patient to the unit and explaining hospital policies, routines, and procedures.
	Answer questions honestly. Direct them to the attending physician whenever necessary.
To feel important or good about oneself	Convey to the patient that you care about him or her.
	Encourage verbalization of feelings about the self.
	Provide feedback by focusing attention on positive traits identified during hospitalization: (*e.g.*, nice voice, pretty hair, nice smile, interesting job).
To be self-sufficient and to have control	Promote independence by encouraging the patient to participate in self-care as much as possible.
	Encourage decision making regarding menu selection, treatment plan, which pain medication (if a choice is available), and so forth.
	Give positive recognition for any independence exhibited.
To be productive	Encourage patient to discuss feelings about role as an individual, spouse, parent, patient. Explore ways to be productive while hospitalized: oil painting, writing poetry, needlepoint, crewel work, planning household chores for family members, writing or dictating letters, reading, planning grocery list.

such as those elicited by the questionnaire described earlier, will become less common. Meeting such needs also influences a person's emotional responses to illness and hospitalization.

 ## Emotional Responses to Illness

Numerous books and articles have been written about emotional reactions to illness (see Selected References). Box 14-2 summarizes identified emotional responses to illness as described by various authors.

Anxiety

Over 30 descriptive words have been used to describe emotional responses manifested during illness, the most common being *anxiety*. Anxiety has been described as a fear of the unknown or unrecognized. The person experiences feelings of apprehension, tension, or uneasiness. Persons who assume the sick role cannot always identify the source of anxiety in their lives. They may experience anxiety as they (1) are told hospitalization is necessary, (2) arrive in a hospital setting, (3) undergo diagnostic tests, (4) face impending surgery, (5) undergo various treatment approaches, or (6) prepare to return home after hospitalization. One patient, a 44-year-old man, was playing basketball in the community center's gymnasium when he experienced severe chest pains. The emergency squad was called when his condition did not improve. He was rushed to the local community hospital to be admitted for treatment of a possible myocardial infarction. This *was* the first time that the man had experienced chest pains; as a result, feelings of anxiety occurred. He was uncertain what was contributing to his severe symptoms because he appeared to be in good physical health. Admission to the intensive care unit increased his anxiety because he was in unfamiliar surroundings, which included tubes, oxygen equipment, monitors, and personnel. As the student nurse cared for him, the patient told her that he had never been hospitalized before. She recognized his feelings of insecurity and, once the patient was stabilized, took time to explain why he was admitted to the unit. She also gave him a verbal orientation to the unit, described his treatment regimen, and asked if he had any questions. The patient thanked her for taking the time to discuss his illness, treatment, and nursing care.

Fear

Fear is another common response identified in hospitalized patients. "I'm afraid I might have cancer," "Ted's afraid of shots," "My husband's afraid to be put to sleep by the anesthesiologist" are some of the comments made by patients and their relatives in the hospital setting. They are referring to *recognized* sources of

BOX 14-2 Identified Emotional Responses to Illness

Lambert & Lambert	Robinson	Carlson & Blackwell	Barry
Behavioral reactions to physical illness:	*Psychological aspects of hospitalized patients:*	*Response change in health status:*	*Personality styles of general hospital patients:*
Anxiety	Anxiety	Alienation	Dependent
Denial	Crying	Hostility	Demanding
Ambivalence	Frightened	Restlessness	Controlled
Suspicion	Disoriented	Boredom	Orderly
Hostility	Depressed	Trust	Dramatizing
Regression	Demanding	Hope	Emotionally
Loneliness	Regression	Humor	Involved
Rejection	Dependency	Denial	Captivating
Depression	Helplessness	Privacy	Suspicious
Withdrawal	Hopelessness	Relaxation	Complaining
	Denial		Long-suffering
			Self-sacrificing
			Superiority
			Uninvolved
			Aloof
			Antisocial
			Inadequate

danger. Fear of such dangers can have an immobilizing or irrational influence on people during illness. Nurses can help patients to explore the reasons for their fears and plan appropriate interventions to alleviate them. An 18-year-old female patient was in labor for 10 hours, but her labor failed to progress. X-ray pelvimetry revealed cephalopelvic disproportion, and an emergency cesarean section was scheduled. She was quite upset and admitted that she was "scared." Before her cesarean section, the nurse and the anesthesiologist explained general anesthesia to the patient, how it is performed, and the nursing care that she would receive. After surgery, the student cared for the patient as she recovered from the general anesthetic. On recovery, the patient thanked the student for taking the time to "explain everything to me. I'm not so afraid now." The patient was discharged approximately a week after the cesarean section and voiced excitement about taking her newborn infant home. No evidence of fear was noted.

Loneliness

Everyone experiences loneliness at some time in life in this fast-paced, mobile, and changing society. Feelings of loneliness appear to increase during hospitalization. People feel lonely because of a need for contact with a person, place, or object. When hospitalized, the person is removed from the normal environment that contains familiar persons, places, and objects. The patient experiences a desire for contact but is unable to make it. Feelings of unexplained dread, desperation, or extreme restlessness may be noted in the patient as a result of inability to make contact. Loneliness, like fear, can immobilize a person.

During clinical rotation through a geriatric nursing home, student nurses were asked to assess assigned patients regarding loneliness. They observed the patients' rooms for familiar items brought from home, such as pictures, radios, televisions, items of furniture, or quilts and pillows. They also observed who visited the patients and how frequently. The results of their assessment revealed that most of the patients had brought personal items with them, but few patients had regular visitors such as family members, neighbors, or friends. Feelings of loneliness were voiced by many of the elderly patients as they spent much of their time sitting or sleeping, showing little interest in their environment, unless stimulated by others. Another group of students, in the medical–surgical setting, was instructed to observe patients' room for flowers, get-well cards, gifts, personal items brought from home, and visitors. It was interesting to note the students' reactions to the patients' rooms. One student stated, "Her room is so cold and barren looking. She looks so lonely." Other students commented, "It looks like everyone's deserted him since his surgery for cancer. Why doesn't his family visit?" and "Her room is so warm and friendly looking. She has flowers and cards all over the place." A discussion followed, pertaining to the influence of familiar items and visitors on the mood of hospitalized persons.

Powerlessness

Powerlessness occurs in the clinical setting owing to loss of control over oneself, one's behavior, and one's environment. It also can result when one lacks sufficient knowledge regarding illness and how it affects one's being, family, and future. Hospitalization encourages a person to be passive or dependent on the health care team, both for nursing care and for obtaining knowledge about one's illness. The patient is powerless to influence information obtained and recorded during the history-taking process when admitted; relinquishes the ability to make decisions; may become aggressive to compensate for the loss of power; and may become violent because of feelings of aggression and anger that are not expressed verbally.

Feelings of powerlessness, then, may result in withdrawn, demanding, or manipulative behavior as the person struggles to maintain control while hospitalized. A nurse was assigned to care for a patient who had undergone diagnostic tests for symptoms of dizziness, blurred vision, weight loss, weakness, chest pain, and insomnia. He had expected to be in and out of the hospital within three days, but inconclusive tests necessitated a longer stay. The patient asked his attending physician if the tests could be continued on an outpatient basis. After the physician informed him that he would need to stay at least two more days, the nursing staff noticed a change in this compliant patient's behavior. He became quite demanding and tried to manipulate the staff to persuade the doctor to discharge him early. The nurse spent time with the patient in an attempt to explore the meaning behind his change in behavior. He told her that he was the sole owner of a small business and felt that he was losing business while he was hospitalized. He was afraid that his business would fail if he wasn't at the office daily to oversee his office help.

Helplessness and Hopelessness

A person who believes that nothing more can be done is experiencing helplessness. Persons who are ill generally realize that they need help; whether they seek it depends on the presence of hope or the knowledge and feeling that there is an effective treatment for their illness. Helplessness can occur when a person is forced into the position of temporary or permanent dependency on others. Nurses working in rehabilitative units often see people express helplessness owing to dependency and the knowledge that nothing more can be done at present for their physical condition. Some persons refuse to give in to helplessness or hopelessness, a quality exhibited by two members of the 1984 Olympic team. A woman paraplegic qualified for the archery competition, and a young man diagnosed with Hodgkin's disease qualified for and won a gold metal in wrestling. Neither succumbed to feelings of helplessness; both maintained hope, used their inner strength or energy, and overcame their disabilities.

Helplessness or hopelessness may contribute to regressive behavior, ambivalence, and feelings of rejection, as well as to dependent behavior.

Family members or significant others also may experience feelings of helplessness when they hear the patient's prognosis. Comments such as, "I feel so helpless," "Please tell me what I can do to help," and "I've done everything I can think of. What more can I do?" all transmit the message of helplessness.

Nurses who maintain hope and inspire it in patients are a motivational force creating energy and the desire to achieve health. Lange (in Carlson & Blackwell, 1978, pp. 182–184) discusses the importance of hope in maternal–child nursing, medical–surgical nursing, and psychiatric–mental health nursing. She discusses the impact of hope on birth defects, chronic disabling illness, severe illness or injury, and psychiatric disorders that are emotional in origin. Seven coping skills and their impact on the degree of hope are presented by Lange.

1. Denying or minimizing the seriousness of an illness or disorder. People develop this skill to avoid facing the worst situation.
   Example: A diabetic refers to his illness as "just a little inconvenience."
2. Asking relevant questions about one's condition to relieve anxiety.
   Example: A woman experiencing tachycardia asks the nurse if "nerves" could be the cause of it.
3. Seeking reassurance and emotional support by reaching out to others. Family, friends, clergy, and health team members may be available to listen, thus lessening worry and uncertainty and reinforcing hope.
   Example: A woman asks her pastor to stop by to discuss her son's sudden change in behavior.
4. Learning an effective action to perform necessary procedures or provide self-care. Such coping instills a sense of pride in one's accomplishments.
   Example: A patient with chronic kidney failure is taught the portable dialysis technique.
5. Setting specific goals. The patient is encouraged to be as independent as possible, meeting one goal at a time.
   Example: The orthopedic patient is taught to "logroll" himself after surgery until he is able to increase his activity level.
6. Rehearsing alternative outcomes with staff and family. Hope is restored or maintained by considering previous successes or failures when faced with difficulties.
   Example: A patient scheduled to undergo surgery has a 50% chance of surviving. He shares his feelings with his family about his future *if* the surgery is successful.
7. Finding meaning in experiences such as crisis, illness, or prognosis of an illness.
   Example: A woman undergoing frequent bone marrow aspirations during hospitalization for leukemia stated that she hoped the research findings would help other patients as well as herself.

Clinical Examples of Emotional Responses to Illness

The following are clinical examples denoting regression, dependency, a struggle to maintain independence, withdrawal due to fear, and hope.

Regression

A 32-year-old woman was admitted for an emergency cholecystectomy. During her postoperative period, the patient became whining, demanding, and manipulative. When interviewed, the patient revealed ambivalent feelings toward her mother. She stated that she loved her but did not get along with her. (Her mother had been staying with her during the recovery period.) She also stated that she was afraid she would continue to have pain when she returned home. She had regressed to a developmental level of a 10- or 11-year-old child assuming the sick role. This regression relieved her of any social responsibilities that she might have. It also produced a secondary gain: her mother's attention and concern about her pain.

Dependency

A 59-year-old woman, newly diagnosed with diabetes, was identified as being "overly" dependent on the staff. She was quite obese and did not participate in her care. During an interview she confided in the student nurse that her husband washed and set her hair, did the housework, and prepared the meals. She stated that she had been sick and unable to work for a long time and enjoyed being taken care of by her family. She had assumed the sick role to relieve herself of social responsibilities and to allow her husband and family to meet her needs.

Independence or Maintaining Power

A 71-year-old woman with the diagnosis of angina refused to have student nurses assigned to her. She was active in her community, was very independent, had never been hospitalized, and was "capable of caring for herself." When procedures were scheduled, the patient became upset if they were not done "on time" and insisted on knowing why they were delayed. She would complain that the hospital was not run efficiently. When staff personnel entered her room she would dismiss them verbally and state that she would let them know "if and when she needed anything." On the second day of hospitalization the patient was observed to have tears in her eyes. She related that she was scared, saying she had never had "anything like this happen to me before" and she didn't like being sick. She further stated that she had "tons of work waiting for me at home." This patient demonstrated a valiant attempt to reject the sick role rather than to assume it. The passive manipulation and demanding behavior exhibited by this patient were her attempts to maintain control and independence during her hospitalization.

Withdrawal Due to Fear

A 62-year-old man, admitted to the hospital for gastritis, spent much of the time in his room, even though he was permitted and encouraged to walk in the halls. He responded briefly when spoken to and never initiated conversation with the staff. On the second day he disclosed to a student nurse that his wife had Parkinson's disease and he was having difficulty watching her symptoms progress. He had kept his emotions to himself, in an attempt to reassure his wife that she would be okay. During the interview his fear of the unknown (his wife's prognosis) was identified, and the patient appeared relieved that he was able to discuss his wife's illness with someone.

Hope

During her third month of pregnancy, a 16-year-old girl was in an auto accident that left her comatose as a result of her injuries. When she was eight months pregnant, she delivered by cesarean section a premature infant weighing 5 lb 6 oz. Immediately after the accident, her husband, who was in the service, was transferred to the city where she was hospitalized. He kept a daily vigil throughout his wife's hospitalization. After the birth of his daughter, the young serviceman stated that he would be waiting for "the second miracle to happen, my wife's return to good health." He stated, "All I have left is hope and a lot of prayers."

✦ Hospitalized Adolescents: Special Needs

Adolescent behavior during hospitalization can be frustrating as well as challenging to the care-giver. Common health problems contributing to the hospitalization of the adolescent include (1) auto accidents, sports-related accidents, or accidents that result from unsuccessful suicide attempts; (2) obesity; (3) teenage pregnancy; (4) alcoholism; (5) drug abuse; (6) depression; (7) venereal diseases; and (8) acne vulgaris. Anorexia nervosa and bulimia, indirect self-destructive behaviors, are adolescent health problems that often are treated on an outpatient basis, unless a life-threatening situation occurs.

During adolescence, the teenager faces two major conflicts: identity versus role confusion and independence versus dependence as he or she attempts to establish a stable self-concept, make a career or vocational choice, and adjust to a comfortable sexual role.

Psychological needs that must be met during hospitalization include peer interactions, privacy, autonomy, and the opportunity to verbalize concern about body image, sexual identity, and self-worth. Such concerns often result in the following emotional reactions: anger or hostility, resentment, fear, guilt, dependency, regression, and embarrassment. The hospitalized adolescent may reject hospital rules and regulations and even physical care because of fear of losing control. Illness often interrupts school and social life, resulting in behavior such as resentment, hostility, anger, manipulation, or aggressiveness. Fear and guilt may occur as the adolescent is overwhelmed by the disease process or illness. A 15-year-old girl diagnosed with diabetes thought she was being punished for her promiscuous behavior. She felt guilty and "confessed" her behaviors to the student nurse. The same patient also expressed a fear of diabetes and how it would affect her life. Another teenaged patient displayed fear and embarrassment because he was scheduled for an inguinal herniorrhaphy. He was concerned about his self-image and sexual role identity. A nurse explained the surgery to the young man and allayed his fears.

Homesickness also may occur if the teenager has never been separated from parents or family. Such feelings may result in undue dependency needs or regressive behavior.

If an adolescent is admitted to an adult unit, the nurse should be aware of the following effects of hospitalization:

1. Emotional trauma may occur owing to erroneous advice or information given by adult patients.
2. The adolescent's imagination may result in fear because he or she exaggerates sights and sounds.
3. The adolescent's need for peer interactions may not be met if placed in a room with an adult patient.
4. Strict visiting regulations may not allow visitors under age 16 on an adult unit.
5. Defense mechanisms commonly seen include denial, projection, displacement, regression, and isolation.

Nursing interventions for emotional responses and common behaviors of adolescents during hospitalization are listed in Box 14-3 (on pp. 250–251).

Impact of Physical Illness

Lambert and Lambert (1979) use a unique approach to emotional or behavioral responses to illness. Alterations in body structure and life-sustaining functions are discussed with specific attention to emotional, somatic, sexual, occupational, and social impact on the person. A patient undergoing a mastectomy may cry frequently owing to depression (emotional impact of a mastectomy); express concern about her body image because of the need to wear a prosthesis (somatic impact); avoid sexual contact with her husband owing to a poor self-concept (sexual impact); express feelings of incompetency in her vocation (occupational impact); and refuse to socialize owing to feelings of embarrassment or shame (social impact). Nursing care plans focus on the various impacts due to physical illness.

Barry (1996) devotes three chapters to the areas of personality styles of hospitalized patients, psychosocial aspects of illness, and coping challenges in chronic illness. She discusses the development of trust; the impact of illness on the patient's self-esteem; alteration in body image during various developmental

(*text continued on page 252*)

BOX 14-3 Nursing Interventions for Emotional Responses and Behaviors of Hospitalized Adolescents

Adolescent Emotional Responses/Behaviors	Nursing Interventions
Fear	Accept defenses or behavior used to retain control. Discuss with the patient when able. Give detailed explanations regarding treatment, nursing care, and progress.
	Encourage participation in care.
	Encourage questions and discuss concerns.
	Interpret medical terminology to decrease fears.
	Maintain consistency in care to discourage manipulative behavior.
Resentment	Explore feelings of resentment to identify underlying cause.
	Encourage visits with peers.
	Allow young siblings to visit.
	Permit flexible visiting hours when appropriate.
	Make arrangements for school work to continue.
	Do not "side" with parents if the adolescent displays hostility.
Embarrassment	Explain and maintain confidentiality.
	Provide an opportunity to discuss concerns, without family present if necessary.
	Be alert to feelings regarding body image and need for privacy.
	Encourage as much self-care as possible.
	Provide for personal space and minimal body exposure during care.
	Explain treatments, procedures, or surgery and impact on the body.
Homesickness	Provide, if possible, for home conveniences such as TV, telephone, and snacks.
	Arrange for dietary preferences when appropriate.

BOX 14-3 **Nursing Interventions for Emotional Responses and Behaviors of Hospitalized Adolescents** (Continued)

Adolescent Emotional Responses/Behaviors	Nursing Interventions
	Allow family members to bring in favorite foods if they are part of the diet prescribed by the attending physician.
	See that the patient is kept informed of news at home.
Guilt	Give appropriate detailed explanations regarding illness and causative factors.
	Be positive in approaches and comments to reinforce interest in the patient.
	Explain that hospitals are to help people, not punish them.
Manipulative behavior	Be consistent in expectations regarding rules and regulations for all patients.
	State the limits and behaviors expected from the patient.
	Explore the patient's perceptions and feelings.
	Avoid arguing, debating, or bargaining with the patient.
	Confront the patient, if necessary, regarding any manipulative ploys.
	Avoid a personal relationship.
Hostile, aggressive behavior	Be firm and consistent in treatment approaches.
	Accept the patient but make it clear that certain behaviors are unacceptable.
	Try to determine what precipitated these feelings.
	Assist the patient to explore alternative ways in handling feelings.
	Inform the patient that he or she is to take responsibility for his or her actions.
	Be supportive and provide positive feedback when the patient controls hostile or aggressive behavior.

stages and illness; the ability to be in control of one's environment, especially during illness, and the issues of loss, guilt, and intimacy as underlying dynamics in the patient's attempts to adapt to illness. Nursing approaches are given for specific physical conditions, such as menopause, amputation, mastectomy, severe burns, isolation due to immunosuppressive conditions, and congenital anomaly.

Nursing Interventions for Emotional Responses of Adults

Nursing interventions for emotional responses to illness, including anxiety, fear, loneliness, powerlessness, helplessness, and hopelessness, are presented in Box 14-4. (The emotional responses of denial, anger or hostility, and depression as well as spiritual needs of hospitalized patients are discussed in the chapter on loss and grief.)

Humor as a Nursing Intervention

"To be able to joke may spell the difference between sinking and swimming, psychologically. The capacity to laugh about things, including ourselves at times, means that we are still masters of our fate" (Harrower, 1971).

Norman Cousins used the concept of humor to overcome a chronic debilitating illness. When his condition did not respond to traditional treatment, he decided to view movies by comedians such as Laurel and Hardy, read humorous articles and books, and tell jokes. Journal articles, a book, and a movie describe Cousins' controversial method for treating his illness and his recovery.

Humor has been called a coping mechanism or outlet for feelings of tension, anger, aggression, and embarrassment. It serves as a tool for communication, illustrated in the following example. A student nurse was caring for a patient who had just returned from physical therapy. She wanted to straighten the linens before he returned to bed. Innocently, she stated to the patient, "Let me tighten your drawstrings before you get into bed." The patient and his roommate responded with laughter while the student nurse's face turned several shades of red. Later the patient apologized for his response and told the student he hadn't been able to laugh since he was admitted to the hospital. Although the student had not planned to be funny, the situation provided the patient with an opportunity to relate his feelings. He discussed a problem that was bothering him at work during his hospitalization. Other nurses have related humorous situations that "broke the ice" in their nurse–patient relationships.

BOX 14-4 Nursing Interventions for Adult Emotional Responses to Illness

Adult Emotional Responses	Nursing Interventions
Anxiety and fear (anxiety disorders are discussed in a separate chapter)	Accept the patient.
	Display a nonjudgmental attitude.
	Assess the patient's level of anxiety according to behavioral and physiological responses. (See Chapter 16 for classification of levels of anxiety as well as symptoms of anxiety.)
	Recognize the patient's feelings by readily encouraging verbalization of feelings.
	Assess and support the patient's strengths.
	Be readily available to assist the patient in meeting her or his needs.
	Explain procedures, treatments, and nursing care to decrease anxiety. Give only necessary details because too many make the procedure appear complicated and may frighten the patient. Increasing awareness and control of a situation generally reduce anxiety and fear.
	Use relaxation techniques to decrease anxiety.
Loneliness	Encourage verbalization of feelings about hospitalization.
	Recognize the need for contact with others.
	Be readily available by making routine periodic visits.
	Use touch as a therapeutic intervention when appropriate.
	Identify significant others and encourage visitation.
	Extend visiting hours or provide for special visitation if the situation warrants

(continued)

Adult Emotional Responses	Nursing Interventions
	the presence of a family member or significant other. Minimize physiologic pain because loneliness usually increases when pain is present.
Powerlessness and helplessness	Promote independence as the patient's physiologic or psychological problems subside by encouraging (1) verbalization of feelings such as frustration, anger, hostility, and fear; (2) participation in self-care; (3) decision making; and (4) participation in organizing and controlling the environment when appropriate, for example, placement of call light and bedside table, and bringing personal items from home.
	Educate the patient about the illness and treatment, promote self-care, and encourage a return demonstration when appropriate.
Hopelessness	Assess the patient's behavior for signs of suicidal ideation owing to feelings of doom, failure, and poor self-concept, and then intervene accordingly.
	Express a sincere interest in wanting to help the patient.
	Encourage the patient to relate to other patients such as roommates, or people with similar conditions such as those in the Reach for Recovery program and ostomy clubs. Recovered mastectomy patients visit hospitalized patients shortly after surgery. Ostomy patients are encouraged by members of ostomy clubs to participate in self-care.

Robinson (in Carlson & Blackwell, 1978) states that humor is a "natural phenomenon within the humanistic approach to patient care" and lists the following nursing situations in which humor may be used by patients or staff (p. 175): (1) to establish interpersonal relationships; (2) to relieve or release feelings of tension, anxiety, anger, hostility, and aggression; (3) to cope with feelings that are too painful or stressful to handle at that moment; and (4) to promote the learning process.

The following headline appeared in a local newspaper: "Laughter Cures Patients' Blues, Therapist Finds." An occupational therapist in Seattle, Washington, uses various humorous techniques to "heal emotional wounds." Patients who have difficulty expressing their feelings are encouraged to draw cartoons and wear Halloween masks that depict their mood for the day. Persons who have difficulty with interpersonal relationships watch a daytime soap opera that "borders on humor" and discuss how the characters interact with each other. The patients are able to identify with various humorous or stressful situations and coping behaviors used by the actors and actresses.

Humor occurs in the general hospital setting in various ways. The patient may receive amusing get-well cards, joke with people about hospitalization, or receive cheery gifts, such as balloon flower bouquets, smiling chrysanthemums, or singing telegrams. Rooms are decorated by family members in an attempt to "cheer up" patients. One patient displays a cartoon and joke scrapbook given to her by a friend. It is the topic of many conversations among the hospital staff and patients. Students walk into rooms on several occasions while patients are watching cartoons or situation comedies. Such television shows serve as coping mechanisms for the hospitalized patient who is lonely, depressed, or needs to be distracted from everyday conflicts.

Robinson discusses the use of humor in the nursing care plan for an elderly widow, who became depressed after major surgery. She attributes the success of humor to the patient's life-style and the tone of the ward. The patient was referred to as a person "with a good sense of humor who was the cut-up of the senior citizen's club" (in Carlson & Blackwell 1978, p. 203). The health care team was able to use humor therapeutically by creating a warm climate and promoting positive interpersonal relationships.

Humor is to be used cautiously because not all people are able to respond to this approach. They may not possess a sense of humor, or the timing may be inappropriate. Approaching problems from "the bright side" does not always work, at least not immediately.

🔶 Summary

Illness and hospitalization can be a life-threatening situation when a person undergoes diagnostic tests, medical treatment, surgical intervention, nursing intervention, rehabilitative care, and participates in research. Several factors influence the patient's behavior during hospitalization, including the extent or seriousness of the illness; the manner in which hospitalization occurs; personal feelings, thoughts and cultural attitudes; and information given by others. Childhood experiences also influence one's response to hospitalization and to members of the health care team. People assume the sick role for various reasons, among them a perception of helplessness, relief of social responsibilities, and manipulation of one's environment. Most people experience common emotional needs that are influenced by illness and hospitalization. These include the need to love and be loved, to feel secure, to feel good about oneself, to be self-sufficient, and to be productive. Examples of nursing interventions to meet these needs were discussed. An explanation of the more common emotional responses to illness, as well as appropriate nursing interventions, was given. These include anxiety, fear, loneliness, powerlessness, helplessness, and hopelessness. Clinical examples of regression, dependency, struggle to maintain independence, withdrawal due to fear, and hope also were given. The concept of humor as it relates to illness was discussed. Special attention was given to the psychological needs, emotional responses, and coping behaviors of hospitalized adolescents, as well as nursing interventions for fear, resentment, embarrassment, homesickness, guilt, manipulative behavior, and hostile, aggressive behavior.

Learning Activities

I. Clinical Activities
  A. Identify the following pertaining to one of your assigned patients:
    1. Psychological needs during hospitalization.
    2. Emotional responses to illness. Consider the somatic, sexual, occupational, and social impact of the patient's physical illness.
  B. Plan nursing interventions for each need and emotional response identified.
  C. Observe your patient for any expressions of humor. If such responses do occur, what purpose do you think they serve?
II. Independent Activities
  A. Read one or more of the following books listed in the Selected References:
    1. H. T. Ireys, et al. "Self-Esteem of Young Adults With Chronic Health Conditions: Appraising the Effects of Perceived Impact," 1994.
    2. L. M. Douville. *The Power of Hope*, 1994.
    3. B. McKinney. "COPD & Depression: Treat them Both," 1994.
    4. C. Simms. "How to Unmask the Angry Patient," 1995.
    5. C. Roye, "Breaking Through to the Adolescent Patient," 1995.
  B. List nursing interventions for a demanding, manipulative adolescent.

C. State nursing interventions to reduce fear in the surgical patient.

D. Plan nursing interventions for a 55-year-old woman who has never been hospitalized and politely tells you that she can take care of herself. (Diagnosis: Possible myocardial infarction.) Focus on possible emotional responses and psychological needs.

Critical Thinking Questions

1. As you admit Nancy, a 32-year-old new mother who has multiple sclerosis, you sense despair and lack of hope. Develop a series of questions so that you may ascertain Nancy's coping skills as related to hope. Which of Lange's seven coping skills might you help Nancy develop? How might you go about implementing this help?

2. A 1985 survey reminds us that 27% or one patient in three feels a need for spiritual care. Review the last three patients you cared for. How might you better assess their need for spiritual care? What interventions might you include on their plan of care?

3. You have a budget of $100 to create a Humor Bag to be used on the nursing unit. This Humor Bag will be available to patients, family, and staff alike. What will you put in it, and why?

Self-Test

1. Explain why a person assumes the sick role.
2. List the common emotional needs experienced by most individuals.
3. State nursing interventions for each of the needs listed in question no. 2.
4. Discuss how illness and hospitalization can create anxiety.
5. List nursing interventions to alleviate fear in a 12-year-old boy hospitalized for an emergency appendectomy.
6. List nursing interventions to decrease loneliness in a nursing home resident with emphysema.
7. Discuss how feelings of powerlessness can occur during hospitalization.
8. Differentiate between helplessness and hopelessness.
9. Explain how humor can be therapeutic in the hospital setting.
10. List the five impacts of physical illness as described by Lambert.
11. Explain the importance of understanding cultural beliefs and attitudes regarding illness.

SELECTED REFERENCES

Andrews, M. M., & Boyle, J. S. (1995). *Transcultural concepts in nursing care* (2nd ed.). Philadelphia: J. B. Lippincott.

Barry, P. D. (1996). *Psychosocial nursing assessment and intervention* (3rd ed.). Philadelphia: Lippincott–Raven Publishers.

Carlson, C., & Blackwell, B. (Eds.). (1978). *Behavioral concepts and nursing intervention.* Philadelphia: J. B. Lippincott.

Douville, L. M. (1994, December). The power of hope. *American Journal of Nursing.*

Dumas, M. A. S. (1996, April). What it's like to belong to the cancer club. *American Journal of Nursing.*

Harrower, M. (1971). *Mental health and M. S.* (pamphlet). New York: National Multiple Sclerosis Society.

Ireys, H. T., Gross, S. S., Werthamer-Larsson, L. A., & Kolodner, K. B. (1994, December). Self-esteem of young adults with chronic health conditions: Appraising the effects of perceived impact. *Journal of Developmental and Behavioral Pediatrics.*

Kimball, M. J., & Williams-Burgess, C. (1995, April). Failure to thrive: The silent epidemic of the elderly. *Archives of Psychiatric Nursing.*

Lambert, V., & Lambert, C. (1979). *The impact of physical illness and related mental health concepts.* Englewood Cliffs, NJ: Prentice Hall.

McKinney, B. (1994, April). COPD & depression: Treat them both. *RN.*

Robinson, L. (1984). *Psychological aspects of the care of hospitalized patients.* Philadelphia: F. A. Davis.

Roye, C. F. (1995, December). Breaking through to the adolescent patient. *American Journal of Nursing.*

Simms, C. (1995, April). How to unmask the angry patient. *American Journal of Nursing.*

Simon, J. (1988, April). Therapeutic humor: Who's fooling who? *Journal of Psychosocial Nursing and Mental Health Services.*

Twerski, A. J. (1988). *When do the good things start?* New York: Tapper Books.

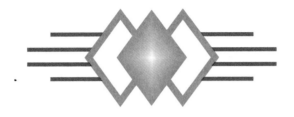

CHAPTER 15

LOSS AND GRIEF

I n this sad world of ours, sorrow comes to all. . . . It comes with bittersweet agony. . . . [Perfect] relief is not possible, except with time. You cannot now realize that you will ever feel better. . . . And yet this is a mistake. You are sure to be happy again. To know this, which is certainly true, will make you feel less miserable now.

Abraham Lincoln

1 Discuss the concept of loss.

2 State the types of losses an individual can experience.

3 Discuss the importance of understanding religious and cultural perspectives on death and dying.

4 Explain the stages of grief identified by Westberg.

5 Differentiate between normal and pathologic or dysfunctional grief.

6 Describe Kübler-Ross's five stages of the grieving process.

7 List the needs of dying persons and their survivors.

8 Explain the purpose of the Living Will.

9 State the rationale for "The Dying Person's Bill of Rights."

10 Discuss the role of a chaplain or member of the clergy in the hospital setting.

11 Compare the perceptions of death by children during various growth stages.

12 Plan nursing interventions for the emotional and spiritual needs of a terminally ill patient.

Introduction

Everyone has experienced some type of major loss—such as a spouse, relative, friend, job, pet, home, or personal item—at one time or another. The following definitions have been selected to familiarize the reader with the concept of loss:

1. Change in status of significant object
2. Any change in an individual's situation that reduces the probability of achieving implicit or explicit goals
3. An actual or potential situation in which a valued object or person is inaccessible or changed so that it is no longer perceived as valuable
4. A condition whereby an individual experiences deprivation of, or complete lack of, something that was previously present

A loss may occur suddenly or gradually, be predictable or unexpected, and be viewed as traumatic or temperate. For example, a 35-year-old man with cancer has been told he has approximately two years to live. He is experiencing the gradual loss of self that has been predicted by his physician. Whether the loss is traumatic or temperate to the patient and significant others depends on past experiences with loss; the value placed on the lost object; and the cultural, psychosocial, economic, and family supports available.

Loss also has been referred to as actual, perceived, anticipatory, temporary, or permanent. The death of a spouse is obvious to others and therefore is considered an *actual* loss. A recent college graduate who is unable to find employment and returns home may be experiencing a loss of freedom or independence. Unless the student shares his or her feelings with others, such loss of freedom or independence cannot be identified or verified by others and, therefore, is considered a *perceived* loss. *Anticipatory* loss is experienced before the time a loss occurs. Family members of a chronically or terminally ill person may anticipate the loss of a loved one before her or his death owing to the prognosis or severity of the person's illness. The wife of a cancer patient stated that she was "relieved that he doesn't have to suffer anymore. I knew it was just a matter of a week or two so I told my children not to be surprised if I called and told them he had died." She had anticipated the permanent loss of her husband. Temporary loss can occur in numerous ways, such as misplacing one's wedding ring or watch while working in obstetrics or the nursery, a child wandering off to a neighbor's house without letting the mother know, being laid off from work for a specific period because of a decrease in sales, or being hospitalized for emergency surgery. Such losses represent a condition in which the person is deprived temporarily of something that was previously present.

Student nurses were instructed to assess their assigned patients for any losses before or during hospitalization. They identified these examples:

1. Loss of body image and social role because of a below-the-knee amputation. The patient was a 19-year-old girl who was involved in a motorcycle accident. She had shared her feelings with the student nurse about her body image and dating after hospitalization.
2. Loss of a loved one owing to fetal demise or intrauterine death. The student nurse had been assigned to a young woman, who was in her twenty-eighth week of pregnancy. The following day, the patient expressed a sincere thanks to the student nurse for supporting her during such a difficult time in her life.
3. Loss of a job, as well as of body image and social role. The patient had lost his right arm in a farming accident and would be unable to return to his job as a telephone lineworker. He had been recently married and was concerned about the impact of his accident on his relationship with his wife. The student nurse encouraged the patient to verbalize his feelings about his accident and to discuss his concerns with his wife. A few days later the wife told the student nurse that she was glad that her husband was able to talk to her about his feelings and that the accident had drawn them "closer together."

4. Loss of physiologic function, social role, and independence because of kidney failure. One student cared for a 49-year-old woman who was undergoing renal dialysis every other day. She was admitted to the hospital for improper functioning of a shunt in her left forearm. The woman was depressed and asked that no visitors be permitted in her private room. She shared feelings of loneliness, helplessness, and hopelessness with the student nurse as she described the impact of kidney failure and frequent dialysis treatment on her life-style. Once an outgoing, independent person, she was housebound because of her physical condition and "resented what her kidneys were doing to her."

 ## Grief and Bereavement

Various emotional or psychological responses occur when one experiences a loss. These emotional experiences are referred to as grief and may result in maladaptive behavior or pathologic grief if the person is unable to work through the grieving process after a reasonable time. Mourning occurs when an individual expresses sorrow with outward signs of grief as a result of a loss.

Andrews and Boyle (1995) discuss grief and bereavement observed in culturally diverse clients such as Native Americans, Buddhists, Mexican Americans, Puerto Ricans, and Eurasians. "The contemporary bereavement practices of various cultural groups . . . demonstrate the wide range of expressions of bereavement. . . . Once nurses understand this, they can better appreciate their role in promoting a culturally appropriate grieving process. Conversely, hindering or interfering with practices . . . can disrupt the grieving process" (p. 369).

The term "bereavement" is described in the *Diagnostic and Statistical Manual of Mental Disorders* (1994) as a reaction to the death of a loved one in which an individual complains of feelings of sadness and associated symptoms such as insomnia, poor appetite, and weight loss. The duration and expression of "normal" bereavement vary among different cultural groups. If the symptoms persist two months after the loss, the diagnosis of Major Depressive Disorder may be given (p. 684).

Many articles and books have been written about the subject of grief. *Good Grief* (Westberg, 1979) discusses what happens to people when they lose someone or something important (*e.g.*, health, security, money, material comforts, a home, a job, or a spouse). Westberg states that there are healthy and unhealthy ways to grieve and that people should be familiar with the good aspects of grief. He contends that people who handle daily "little griefs" in a positive manner prepare themselves for healthy reactions to larger griefs when they occur. The following sections summarize the 10 stages of grief as described by Westberg. Not everyone passes through these stages in chronological order, but it is hoped each person will reach stage ten.

Stage One: State of Shock

During the first stage the grieving person experiences a state of temporary anesthesia that may last anywhere from a few minutes to a few days. If the state of shock lasts over a week or two, it is a sign of unhealthy grief and professional help should be obtained before maladaptive behavior occurs. For example, a woman whose husband was killed in an automobile accident appears "cool, calm, and collected" at the funeral home while greeting people who have come to offer their sympathy. If within a week or two she does not openly express feelings such as disbelief, anger, or loneliness, she may need support and encouragement to verbalize her emotions. Care-givers should be near and available during this stage of grief but are advised not to take over tasks that the person can perform. Self-care is therapeutic and enables the person to proceed to the next stage.

Stage Two: Expressing Emotion

People are encouraged to express pent-up emotions after a significant loss occurs. Westberg (1979) states, "We have been given tear glands, and we are supposed to use them when we have good reason to use them" (p. 26). Men may have difficulty expressing emotion because they have been conditioned not to cry; it is looked on as a sign of weakness. Members of the health care team should encourage the expression of emotions and should not be ashamed to cry with the patients.

Stage Three: Depression and Loneliness

During the third stage, the person experiences feelings of utter depression and isolation. The care-giver is advised to stand by in quiet confidence and reassure the grieving person that loneliness and depression are normal reactions and eventually do pass.

Stage Four: Physical Symptoms of Distress

Physical symptoms such as insomnia, chest pain, abdominal pain, and shortness of breath may occur when someone stops at one of the stages of the grief process. If no one helps the person to explore the reason for emotional and physical complaints associated with unresolved grief, an illness can develop. The classic example is the death of a widow or widower within a year of the spouse's death. Such persons are said to have died of "broken hearts," or they just gave up because they were unable to live without their mate. The physical consequences of distress resulted in death.

Stage Five: Panic

During the fifth stage the person is unable to think of anything except the loss. Concentration and productivity are impaired because of obsessive thoughts, causing the person to think she or he is "losing the mind." The helping person should encourage the grieving person in this stage to develop new and different interests and interpersonal relationships rather than to stay at home and prolong grief work.

Stage Six: Guilt Feelings

Normal guilt is guilt that we feel when we have done something or neglected to do something for which we ought, by the standards of society, to feel guilty. On more than one occasion survivors of deceased persons have made comments such as "If only I had insisted he see a doctor" or "I should have realized she was sicker than she looked." Such statements express guilt feelings. Persons who say that they will "never forgive themselves" and continually berate themselves for their actions, out of proportion to the real situation, are exhibiting symptoms of guilt. Such people should be encouraged to talk about guilt feelings so that they begin to handle them effectively and resume living.

Stage Seven: Anger and Resentment

Once the grieving person overcomes guilt feelings and is able to express emotions, stronger feelings such as anger and resentment may emerge. (Repressed or buried feelings of anger and resentment are unhealthy and can be very harmful to a person's personality.) During this stage the person may blame anyone or everyone for the loss. Most nurses have heard family members on at least one occasion question whether the attending physician did everything possible for the patient. "If only he had operated sooner. He waited too long," or "He should have called in a consultant when my husband didn't respond to treatment." These are examples of comments made by angry family members who resented the loss of a loved one. Such feelings are a normal part of grief and can be overcome in time.

Stage Eight: Resistance

During this stage, grieving persons resist returning to normal daily living. They are intent on keeping the memory of a loved one or thing alive. Returning to normal activities may be too painful for some people because they experience an emptiness in the world about them. Too many times grieving persons are forced to carry all the grief within themselves because they find it difficult to grieve in the presence of others. Society says "Okay, you had time to grieve. Now get back to work!" and expects the person to return to a normal state very shortly after a loss has occurred. Friends and relatives are encouraged to help keep the memory of the loss alive because this facilitates progress toward the stage of hope.

Stage Nine: Hope

After a few weeks or many months of grief, hope usually emerges. Life does go on; opportunities do exist for change or improvement in one's life in spite of the recently experienced loss. New friends can gradually help one find meaning again in life.

Stage Ten: Affirming Reality

Grieving persons usually realize that life will never be the same again, but they begin to sense that there is much in life that can be appreciated and enjoyed. To affirm something is to say that it is good and worth living for.

People who have a mature faith or belief in God often demonstrate an inner strength that helps them to face a serious loss without feeling that they have lost everything. Nurses must be aware of the religious beliefs and spiritual needs of their patients so that nursing interventions can address these areas. As stated in Chapter 14, 27% of those patients surveyed felt they had a need for spiritual care as well as physical care. Fifty-six percent did not feel nurses were aware of their spiritual needs during hospitalization.

 ## Pathologic or Dysfunctional Grief

The cause of pathologic or dysfunctional grief is usually an actual or perceived loss of someone or something of great value to a person. Clinical features or characteristics include expressions of distress or denial of the loss; changes in eating and sleeping habits; mood disturbances, such as anger, hostility, or crying; and alterations in activity levels, including libido. The person experiencing dysfunctional grief idealizes the lost person or object, relives past experiences, loses the ability to concentrate, and is unable to work purposefully because of developmental regression. The grieving person may exhibit neurotic or psychotic symptoms in an attempt to cope with stress and anxiety owing to the actual or perceived loss. Examples of such behavior include development of physical symptoms similar to those experienced by the deceased person before death; progressive social isolation and interrupted interpersonal relationships with friends and relatives; extreme anger or hostility, directed at people associated with the lost person or object; agitated depression; or activities that are detrimental to social or economic existence. Nursing interventions include teaching about the stages of grief and encouraging verbalization of feelings.

 ## Death and Dying

Kübler-Ross (1969) has identified five stages of the grieving process. The following basic premise has evolved as a result of her work with dying persons. Patients know when they are dying (with the exception of the patient who is seriously ill and dies within a very short time or is the victim of a fatal accident). She feels that the helping persons experience two reactions as they care for dying patients: (1) gut reactions and (2) mental reactions. Gut reactions are spontaneous thoughts and ideas that occur such as "I hope he doesn't die on me," or "Please let him live until my shift is over," or "What will I do if she dies on me?" The mental reactions that nurses experience depend on whether they are able to comprehend the patient's feelings about death and dying and whether they have resolved any feelings about their own mortality or death. Many times caregivers attempt to satisfy their own needs when talking with the patient. To work effectively with the dying patient, nurses must be aware of their own feelings regarding death and the patient's condition. Kübler-Ross has stated that the higher the education, the less capable we are of dealing with dying because too many educational responses have been learned, thereby blocking individual responses. In addition, nurses cannot help a dying patient to work through the grieving process if they push the patient to communicate when the patient isn't ready to talk; push themselves on the patient although the patient does not want the support; or genuinely do not like the patient. A summary of Kübler-Ross's well known stages of the grieving process follows.

Denial

During this stage the person displays a disbelief in the prognosis of inevitable death. This stage serves as a temporary escape from reality. Fewer than 1% of all dying patients remain in this stage. Typical responses are "No, it can't be true," "It isn't possible," and "Not me." Denial usually subsides when the person realizes that someone will help him or her to express feelings while facing reality.

Anger

"Why me?" "Why now?" and "It's not fair!" are a few of the comments commonly expressed during this stage. Nurses must remember that they represent a picture of health whenever they enter the patient's room and should be prepared for hostile responses or complaints. The patient appears to be difficult, demanding, and ungrateful during this stage.

Bargaining

"Just one more chance, please!" "If I get better, I'll never miss church again." or "If I promise to take my medicine, will I get better?" are all examples of attempts at bargaining to prolong one's life. The dying person acknowledges her or his fate but is not quite ready to die at this time. The person is ready to take care of unfinished business, such as writing a will, deeding a house over to a spouse or child, or making funeral arrangements.

Depression

"The dying patient is about to lose not just one loved person but everyone he has ever loved and everything that has been meaningful to him" (Kübler-Ross, 1971, p. 58). This stage is also a very difficult period for the family and physician because they feel so helpless watching the depressed patient mourn present and future losses. Treatment should not be forced on the depressed person. The patient should be supported and encouraged to voice feelings *if* he or she feels comfortable doing so.

Acceptance

At this stage, the dying person has achieved an inner and outer peace owing to a personal victory over fear: "I'm ready to die. I have said all the goodbyes and have finished unfinished business." During the acceptance stage, the patient may want only one or two significant people to sit quietly by the patient's side, touching and comforting her or him. Kübler-Ross states that during this stage, little physical pain and discomfort is felt. Tender loving care and compassion by one person generally meets the physical needs of the dying.

 ## Needs of the Dying and Survivors

Holst (1984) describes a list of needs experienced by dying persons as well as their survivors while they face conflicts and dilemmas during this critical time in their lives (Box 15-1 on p. 268). Holst states that families and patients may "die to many things before the disease finally takes life" (p. 11). Optimism, spontaneity, holidays, long-range planning, dreams, retirement, and grandparenthood are just a few of the many things that die as a person and her or his family live with a terminal illness.

Holst also shares the following six lessons learned while dealing with dying: (1) respect one another's needs for distance or spatial territory; (2) trust your feelings when expressing your emotions because there are few rights and wrongs; (3) respect the feelings each moment brings without deflating, defending, or defusing them; (4) respect each person's limits by not demanding more than a person can give; (5) respect and accept the life you share with others; and (6) accept the fact that as a human, who is capable of love, you are also vulnerable.

The rights of dying persons are listed in Box 15-2 (on p. 269), The Dying Person's Bill of Rights. Every nursing unit should have this bill of rights posted in a readily accessible area to remind members of the health care team of their responsibilities in providing holistic health care. If the nurse feels uncomfortable in planning care to meet these rights or needs, a team conference should be held to enlist suggestions or help from other members of the team.

 ## Living Wills

As noted in the Dying Person's Bill of Rights, the individual has the right to participate in decisions concerning care; the right to be free of pain; the right to die in peace and with dignity; and the right to maintain individuality. In an attempt to maintain control over the environment and remain as independent

BOX 15-1 Needs of Dying Persons and Survivors

Dying Person's Needs	Survivor's Needs
To vent anger and frustration	To provide a quality of life for the dying person while preparing for a life without that loved person
To share the knowledge that the end is near	To be available to offer comfort and care even though the survivor feels like running away to escape the pain of death
To ensure the well-being of loved ones who will be left behind, because the person resents the fact that life will go on without him or her	To hope that the loved one will somehow live in spite of obvious deterioration and inability to function. At this time, the survivor may pray for the peace of death.
To vent feelings or irritation at omissions or neglect although the person feels guilty over the pain this causes others	To vent feelings of irritation and guilt over the dying person's demands and increased dependency needs
To remain as independent as possible, fearing he or she will become unlovable	To live and appreciate each day as one plans for a future without the loved one
To be normal and natural at a time when nothing appears to be normal or natural. The dying patient generally experiences the fear of pain, loss of control, and dying alone. The patient has a need to maintain security, self-confidence, and dignity.	To reassure the dying person that the survivor will "continue in her or his footsteps" by holding the family together, raising the children, or managing the business, while knowing such talk about the future is painful to the dying person

Note: From Holst, L. (1984, April 6). To love is to grieve. *The Lutheran Standard*.

BOX 15-2 The Dying Person's Bill of Rights*

I have the right to be treated as a living human being until I die.

I have the right to maintain a sense of hopefulness however changing its focus may be.

I have the right to be cared for by those who can maintain a sense of hopefulness, however changing this might be.

I have the right to express my feelings and emotions about my approaching death in my own way.

I have the right to participate in decisions concerning my care.

I have the right to expect continuing medical and nursing attention even though "cure" goals must be changed to "comfort" goals.

I have the right not to die alone.

I have the right to be free from pain.

I have the right to have my questions answered honestly.

I have the right not to be deceived.

I have the right to have help from and for my family in accepting my death.

I have the right to die in peace and with dignity.

I have the right to retain my individuality and not be judged for my decisions, which may be contrary to beliefs of others.

I have the right to discuss and enlarge my religious and/or spiritual experiences, whatever these may mean to others.

I have the right to expect that the sanctity of the human body will be respected after death.

I have the right to be cared for by caring, sensitive, knowledgeable people who will attempt to understand my needs and will be able to gain some satisfaction in helping me face my death.

(Taken from the *American Journal of Nursing*, January, 1975, p. 99)

*The Dying Person's Bill of Rights was created at a workshop on "The Terminally Ill Patient and the Helping Person" in Lansing, Michigan, sponsored by the Southwestern Michigan Inservice Education Council and conducted by Amelia J. Barbus, associate professor of nursing at Wayne State University in Detroit, Michigan.

as possible during the progression of a terminal illness, patients have the alternative to implement a Living Will. This legal document communicates to family, friends, and professional staff the dying patient's wishes to be allowed to die and which support measures should or should not be used. State guidelines must be followed during the development and implementation of the Living Will. Such guidelines may vary from state to state.

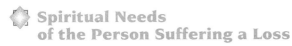 Spiritual Needs of the Person Suffering a Loss

As stated earlier, people suffer many types of loss, including loss of health. It is at this time in life that the person reaches out for support from significant others, such as friends, family, or the clergy.

Pumphrey (1977) discusses how patients search for an understanding listener and spiritual support by "sending out feelers," or making remarks such as "I haven't gone to church much lately" or "My pastor is so busy, I hate to bother him while I'm in the hospital." Pumphrey states, "Ideally, you (the nurse) should be able to respond to each patient's spiritual needs as naturally as you respond to his physical needs" (p. 64). Nurses need to familiarize themselves with the attitudes and requirements of various religious groups as described by Pumphrey. If uncomfortable with addressing various spiritual concerns, the nurse can suggest that the patient talk to the hospital chaplain, the patient's own clergy, members of her or his congregation, or other patients with similar religious beliefs. If none of these options seems appropriate, the nurse can provide quiet time for private meditation or prayer.

Andrews and Hanson (Andrews & Boyle, 1995) discuss assessing spiritual needs in culturally diverse clients. Four areas to be explored include the environment, behavior, verbalization, and interpersonal relationships (p. 358). For example, are religious objects visible? Do the patient or family members wear clothing that has religious significance? Are special dietary requests made? Such observations enable the nurse to address spiritual needs of the person suffering a loss.

Children and Death

Although children grow at varied paces, both physically and emotionally, books that discuss children and the impact of dying outline general growth stages, citing the needs and understanding of children in each phase of development. Preschool children between ages three and five years have a fear of separation from their parents and are unable to think of death as a final separation. They perceive death as a temporary trip to heaven or some other place in which the person still functions actively by eating, sleeping, and so forth. If a child displays guilt feelings because the child "wished something awful would happen when angry at mommy" he or she needs to be told that wishes do not kill. Conversely, the well adjusted child who appears to be a brave little girl or boy and displays little emotion while appearing to accept a parent's death should be seen by a professional counselor to be certain that no psychological problem is developing. Fear of death may occur due to parental expression of anger, stress, the use of physical restraints during an illness, or punishment for wrongdoing.

Children between the ages of five and six years see death as a reversible process that others experience; whereas children from six to nine years of age begin to accept death as a final state. It is conceptualized as a destructive force, a frightening figure, a bogeymonster, or an angel who comes during the night "to get bad people." Children of this age believe they will not die if they avoid the death figure. One dying child drew a picture of death as a tank with its gun barrel aiming directly at him, a destructive force he could no longer avoid.

By age 10 years, children begin to realize death is an inevitable state that all human beings experience because of an internal process. They also believe that the body of a dead person slowly rots until only bones remain as insects infest the coffin and prey on the body. Words such as afterlife, cremation, rebirth, and reunion may be verbalized by the child at this age.

Not all children think about death as described in basic textbooks. The following additional conceptions about death have been voiced by young children:

1. Parental death is a deliberate abandonment that the child caused, and the child will die next.
2. Death occurs while one sleeps; therefore, do not go to sleep or take naps.
3. The surviving parent caused the other parent to die.
4. Death is catching; don't associate with anyone who just lost a parent or relative or you will be the next person to die.

Factors other than age that influence a child's understanding of and responses to death include previous experience with death involving family, friends, or pets; knowledge of what is happening; and reactions of siblings, parents, families, and peers when death occurs.

Adolescents are able to intellectualize their awareness of death although they usually repress any feelings about their own death. As one adolescent commented, "My life is just beginning. I have a lot of years ahead of me before I need to think about dying." Death at this age is considered to be a lack of fulfillment; the adolescent "has too much to lose" by dying. Adolescents often hide the fact that they are mourning: they may listen to records, withdraw, or bury themselves in activities. They are inexperienced in coping with such a crisis and may not shed tears or voice emotions such as "I miss mom already," "I loved dad so much," "It hurts so much to lose someone you love," "I'm scared what will happen now that dad is dead. Who will take care of us?" or "It's not fair. He was too young to die." Children are capable of feeling the great loss of a loved person one moment and yet becoming fully absorbed in something funny the next. Adults need to be aware of this capability so that they do not misinterpret such behavior as disrespect or lack of love for the deceased person.

Assessment and Nursing Care of the Dying Patient

Perhaps we need to remind ourselves from time to time that patients who are dying are not just dying. They are also living. Whether or not they have the opportunity to live this final human experience to the fullest—each in his or her own way—is influenced in a great measure by those who take care of them (Browning & Lewis, 1972).

The philosophy of an institution about the dying process can be one of the most important factors in the quality of a patient's death (Barry, 1996).

Care-givers need to reflect on both of these views as they work with terminally ill persons. Nurses are conditioned to do all they can to help a patient recover to a state of wellness and have very little experience on how to cope with something beyond their control. They need to examine their own reactions to loss, grief, death, and dying before they can deal with the psychological needs of dying patients and survivors.

Adams (1984) discusses six variables that influence a nurse's reactions to dying patients: the patient's length of hospitalization; the frequency of admissions; the role of the family; the patient's condition on admission; coping styles exhibited by the patient; and the care-giver's subconscious. Each of these factors should be considered if the care-giver has difficulty working with a dying patient. The nurse may be responding to some aspect of the patient's personality or to subconscious memories of someone else. "Understanding the fascinating complexities of human interaction is a life-long process for most of us. . . . Each insight you gain allows you to give more empathetic, supportive care to a dying patient" (Adams, 1984, p. 43).

Dying persons provide a unique challenge to nurses. Consider the following questions raised by family, friends, and health care providers:

1. Should the patient be informed that he or she is dying? When? What if the family does not want the patient to know?
2. How much information should be given about the patient's condition? Should this take the form of minimal information or a description of how death will occur?
3. What can I say to comfort a dying patient?
4. What environment would be the best suited to a dying patient (*i.e.*, home, hospice, or hospital)?
5. How frequently should the patient be given pain medication? What if it depresses respirations or causes other untoward effects?
6. Should pastoral care be offered even if the patient indicates little or no interest in religion?

The nurse needs to assess the dying patient's knowledge about the illness and prognosis. Does the patient know what is wrong? How much longer does the patient think she or he will be hospitalized? What has the physician told the patient about the illness? How does the family feel about the hospitalization? As the patient responds to such questions, the nurse should observe for signs of the grieving process so that the nurse can plan appropriate interventions.

Nonverbal communication may provide a clue to the patient's emotions. The nurse also should observe the patient's interactions with family and friends, as well as the doctor and clergy. These people may constitute the task force to meet the patient's needs. The age of the patient needs to be considered because views toward death vary at different developmental stages. An adolescent may feel robbed of life, whereas an elderly cancer patient may welcome death as a release from pain. Mood swings may occur frequently as the patient wrestles with emotional responses such as denial, anger, fear, or depression. The patient's role in the family, marital status, and religious beliefs play an important part in providing support systems as the patient attempts to cope. The type of illness, symptoms the patient exhibits, and predicted type of death all influence the patient's reactions to dying. For instance, the patient who knows he or she will be medicated frequently to minimize pain and that he or she will slip into a deep sleep before death will probably face death more readily than will the patient who experiences excruciating pain and loss of body functions.

Several fears have been voiced by dying persons. The nurse needs to be cognizant of these fears so that nursing interventions will be planned to alleviate them. They are fear of the unknown, abandonment, loss of self-control or independence, pain, loss of identity, worthlessness or meaninglessness in one's life, and dying alone. Dolan (1983) discusses the importance of one's environment during death. Although the suggestions are for the patient who chooses to die at home, they are appropriate for a variety of settings and are worth mentioning at this time. Many of the patient's potential fears could be alleviated by altering the environment as follows:

1. Select a room with plenty of fresh air and sunshine.
2. Provide a readily accessible bathroom.
3. Decorate the room with familiar personal objects so that the patient can see them from the bed.
4. Provide access to music if the patient enjoys it.
5. Keep the room tidy and provide colorful bed linens as well as occasional fresh-cut flowers.
6. Keep medical supplies, bedside commode, and other sickroom items out of sight unless necessity dictates their presence.
7. Allow children to visit if the patient desires their company.
8. Allow pets to be enjoyed by the patient, if possible.

If the patient desires special snacks or food from home, the nurse should make every effort to grant this wish when possible.

There are privileges or rewards for nurses who care for terminally ill persons. Dying people often display dignity, courage, and an appreciation for life that one is unaccustomed to seeing. A simple telephone call, surprise anniversary or birthday party, or ride outdoors in a wheelchair constitutes a new quality of life for the dying person and survivors. The nurse matures while observing valiant efforts to sustain life in spite of pain, anxiety, or fear. Family interactions can teach helping persons a lot about support systems, family dynamics, and the will to live. Each family has its own unique way of relating and reacting to change or loss. Listening to the patient share emotions, being sensitive to and showing respect for the patient's needs, and providing privacy all constitute an atmosphere of love and concern that promotes successful grieving.

Nursing Care Plan 15-1 provides an example of a nursing diagnosis and goal-related nursing interventions for an individual experiencing loss.

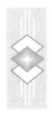

NURSING CARE PLAN 15-1
The Patient Experiencing Loss

Nursing Diagnosis: Grief related to actual loss

Goal: The individual will progress through the grieving process.

Nursing Interventions	Outcome Criteria
Assess individual's present coping skills (*e.g.*, denial, anger, bargaining, depression, or inability to grieve).	Individual will be able to identify factors that may hinder or delay any grief work.
Establish rapport by promoting a trust relationship.	Individual will be able to communicate needs openly.
Convey to the patient that although feelings may be uncomfortable, they are a normal and necessary part of the grief process.	Individual will be able to verbalize knowledge of the grief process.
Explain grief reactions.	Individual will be able to express feelings, verbally and nonverbally.
Encourage verbalization of feelings and exploration of reasons for behavior such as denial, anger, bargaining or depression (consider talking, writing, or drawing as methods of expression of feelings).	Individual will be able to verbalize acceptance of loss.

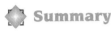 **Summary**

Loss is experienced by all of us at one time or another when we are deprived of something valuable that was previously present in our lives. Loss of one's health, spouse, home, job, or pet may occur suddenly or gradually, may be predictable or unexpected, and may be viewed as traumatic or temperate. The descriptive terms actual, perceived, anticipatory, temporary, and permanent loss were explained. Examples of loss of physiologic function or part of self, environment, or objects external to self, and loved or valued person were given. The terms "grief" and "bereavement" were defined. The ten stages of grief as described by Westberg, as well as Kübler-Ross's five stages of the grieving process, were discussed. Needs of the dying and their survivors as identified by Holst were stated. A copy of "The Dying Person's Bill of Rights" was included to familiarize the reader with this document. The purpose of a Living Will was explained. Spiritual needs of the person suffering a loss, as well as the role or tasks of the clergy on the health care team, were addressed. The understanding or perception of death by children at various growth stages was explained. Suggestions for nursing care of dying persons were listed with an emphasis on the nurse's need to examine personal reactions of loss, grief, death, and dying. The privileges and rewards for nursing personnel who care for terminally ill patients were noted.

Learning Activities

I. Clinical Activities
   A. Assess your assigned patient for any losses.
      1. Is the loss considered to be an actual, perceived, anticipatory, temporary, or permanent loss?
      2. Explain the type of loss. Is it physiologic, environmental, or the loss of a person?
      3. Identify which stage of the grieving process the patient is experiencing. Compare to the stages described by Westberg or Kübler-Ross.
      4. List any needs that your patient presents. Consider cultural diversity.
      5. Are the patient's rights being honored? (Review "The Dying Person's Bill of Rights.")
   B. Plan nursing interventions appropriate for the stage of grief identified, focusing on emotional and spiritual needs of the patient.
II. Independent Activities
   A. Read one or more of the following books about children and death:
      1. A. Gordon and D. Keass, *They Need to Know: How to Teach Children About Death*, 1979

2. P. Nelson, *Educating Children About Death as Well as Life*, 1989
3. T. S. Schoeneck, *Hope for Bereaved: Understanding, Coping and Growing Through Grief*, 1988
4. D. Edwards. *Grieving: The Pain and The Promise*, 1989

B. Plan therapeutic interventions for a nine-year-old child whose mother just died.

Critical Thinking Questions

1. Your best friend hasn't been herself lately; in fact, you are becoming increasingly worried about her. It has been 18 months since her father died of lung cancer. She is smoking more, missing class, and reacting angrily when questioned. You feel her grief is dysfunctional at this point. How might you help her?
2. Write a letter to a close family member who has died. Describe to that person how you felt as you moved through the different stages of grief according to Kübler-Ross. What helped you at those different stages? What have you learned that has application to your work with dying patients and their families?
3. Mrs. Kessler, a 78-year-old widow, has been under your care for several days. She has openly spoken about her wishes for a dignified death, with "none of that mechanical stuff, dearie." You have just overheard her son and doctor planning additional surgery for her without her involvement in the decision. What action should you take?

Self-Test

1. Differentiate between loss, grief, and bereavement.
2. List the emotional or behavioral reactions to loss as described by Kübler-Ross.
3. State the needs of a dying person.
4. List nursing interventions for each need identified in question no. 3.
5. State the survivor's needs.
6. Explain the purpose of "The Dying Person's Bill of Rights" and the Living Will.
7. Describe the tasks of the clergy as they relate to people experiencing a loss.
8. Discuss how the following age groups perceive death:
   Ages 3 to 5
   Ages 5 to 10
   Ages 10 to adolescence

9. You are assigned to a 21-year-old woman who has approximately two weeks to live and feel uncomfortable with this assignment. What would you do?
10. List ways to alter the environment of a dying patient to promote a homelike atmosphere.
11. State the rewards of caring for terminally ill persons.

SELECTED REFERENCES

Adams, F. (1984, June). Six very good reasons why we react differently to various dying patients. *Nursing '84*.

Amenta, M. O., & Bohnet, N. L. (1986). *Nursing care of the terminally ill*. Philadelphia: J. B. Lippincott.

Andrews, M. M., & Boyle, J. S. (1995). *Transcultural concepts in nursing care* (2nd ed.). Philadelphia: J. B. Lippincott.

Barry, P. (1996). *Psychosocial nursing assessment and intervention* (3rd ed.). Philadelphia: Lippincott–Raven Publishers.

Browning, M., & Lewis, E. (1972). The dying patient: A nursing perspective. *American Journal of Nursing*.

Dolan, M. (1983, April). If your patient wants to die at home. *Nursing '83*.

Edwards, D. (1989). *Grieving: The pain and the promise*. Salt Lake City: Covenant, Inc.

Gary, F., & Kavanaugh, C. K. (1991). *Psychiatric mental health nursing*. Philadelphia: J. B. Lippincott.

Gordon, A., & Keass, D. (1979). *They need to know: How to teach children about death*. Englewood Cliffs, NJ: Prentice Hall.

Holst, L. (1984, April 6). To love is to grieve. *The Lutheran Standard*.

Kübler-Ross, E. (1969). *On death and dying*. New York: Macmillan.

Kübler-Ross, E. (1971, January). What is it like to be dying? *American Journal of Nursing*.

Miles, A. (The Rev.) (1993, December). Caring for the family left behind. *American Journal of Nursing*.

Nelson, P. (1989, Spring). Educating children about death as well as life. *Thanatos*.

Pumphrey, J. (1977, December). Recognizing your patient's spiritual needs. *Nursing '77*.

Schoeneck, T. S. (1988). *Hope for bereaved: Understanding, coping, and growing through grief*. Syracuse, NY: Hope for Bereaved.

Taylor, P. B., & Ferszt, G. G. (1994, January). Letting go of a loved one. *Nursing '94*.

Westberg, G. (1979). *Good grief*. Philadelphia: Fortress Press.

Zerwekh, J. (1994, February). The truth-tellers: How hospice nurses help patients confront death. *American Journal of Nursing*.

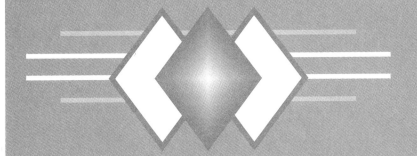

Nursing Interventions for Persons with Psychiatric Disorders

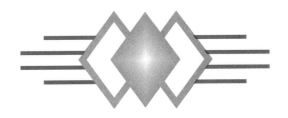

CHAPTER 16

ANXIETY DISORDERS

T he treatment of panic and other anxiety disorders has changed dramatically in the past 10 years primarily because of uniform diagnostic criteria, development of new pharmacological and cognitive therapies, and a general increase in research in this area.

The American Psychiatric Press Textbook of Psychopharmacology

American Psychiatric Press, Inc., 1995

1 Define anxiety.

2 Differentiate between anxiety and fear.

3 Define the following terms:

Signal anxiety

Anxiety trait

Anxiety state

Free-floating anxiety

Acute anxiety

Chronic anxiety

4 Discuss factors that contribute to the development of anxiety disorders.

5 List the common symptoms of anxiety.

6 Compare the levels of anxiety.

7 Differentiate between phobias, panic attacks, and obsessive–compulsive behavior.

8 Differentiate between post-traumatic stress disorder and acute stress disorder.

9 Explain the supportive role of the nurse in dealing with anxiety.

10 Formulate a nursing care plan for a patient with a generalized anxiety disorder.

Introduction

A student nurse had just completed the fundamentals course and was scheduled to begin her clinical laboratory experience. Her assignment was to care for a middle-aged patient with chronic obstructive pulmonary disease. The evening before her laboratory experience the nurse was unable to sleep. In the early morning as she dressed for clinical laboratory, she experienced dizziness, frequency of urination, abdominal cramping, and an increased heartbeat. When she arrived at the hospital and met with her instructor, the student nurse looked rather pale and was extremely quiet. During preconference the student shared her feelings and concerns with other students who were on the same clinical unit. With the help of the instructor, the student was able to discuss her nervous feelings and explore the reason for such a physiologic and emotional reaction. She was experiencing symptoms of anxiety or apprehension about the unknown (*i.e.*, her first clinical laboratory experience).

Have you ever experienced a lump in your throat, sweaty palms, dizziness, frequency of urination, diarrhea, insomnia, restlessness, or the inability to concentrate for some unknown reason? These are but a few of the symptoms of anxiety that are felt by each of us at one time or another because we live in a fast-paced, stressful society.

The concept of anxiety was first introduced to psychological theory by Freud. He referred to it as a danger signal a person exhibits in response to the perception of physical pain or danger. The term *anxiety* is used to describe feelings of uncertainty, uneasiness, apprehension, or tension that a person experiences in response to an unknown object or situation. A "fight-or-flight" decision is made by the person in an attempt to overcome conflict, stress, trauma, or frustration.

Fear differs from anxiety in that it is the body's physiologic and emotional response to a known or recognized danger. A person whose car stalls on the railroad crossing experiences fear of injury or death while the train rapidly approaches on the track. The patient who undergoes an emergency exploratory surgery may be afraid of the surgery and develop symptoms of anxiety because the patient is uncertain what the outcome will be.

Types and Severity of Anxiety

Types of anxiety are described as signal anxiety, anxiety trait, anxiety state, and free-floating anxiety. *Signal anxiety* is a response (anxiety) to an anticipated event. A mother who normally is relaxed exhibits tachycardia, dizziness, and insomnia when her child attends school for the first time; this is signal anxiety.

An *anxiety trait* is a component of personality that has been present over a long period of time and is measurable by observing the person's physiologic, emotional, and cognitive behavior. The person who responds to various nonstressful situations with anxiety is said to have an anxiety trait. For example, a 25-year-old secretary frequently complains of blurred vision, dizziness, headaches, and insomnia in a relatively stress-free job.

An *anxiety state* occurs as the result of a stressful situation in which the person loses control of her or his emotions. A mother who is told her son has been injured in a football game and has been taken to the emergency room may exhibit an anxiety state by becoming hysterical, complaining of tightness in the chest, and insisting on seeing her injured son.

Free-floating anxiety is anxiety that is always present and accompanied by a feeling of dread. The person may exhibit ritualistic and avoidance behavior (phobic behavior). A woman who is unable to sleep at night because she is certain someone will break into her home goes through a ritualistic behavior of checking all the windows and doors several times. She also avoids going out after dark because she fears coming back to a dark, empty home.

Severity of anxiety is described as normal, acute, chronic, or panic. Normal anxiety is anxiety that is present in a small degree, can motivate people, and is necessary for survival. Acute anxiety interferes with one's ability to think and is referred to as extreme nervousness. It usually occurs suddenly and lasts a short period of time. Chronic anxiety may be present over a period of months or years. The person appears to be stable but exhibits tremulous motor activity and rigid posture. Panic anxiety is a severe form of anxiety that causes disintegration of the personality, resulting in the inability to function normally. These categories of anxiety are discussed under the classification of anxiety disorders later in this chapter.

Etiology

Theorists have classified causes of anxiety as stress, childhood conflicts, faulty learning, and social or cultural factors. Psychodynamic theory states that unconscious conflicts of childhood, such as fear of losing a parent's love or attention, fear of losing security, competition with a parent of the same sex, resentment and anger, or fear of being considered a "bad person," may emerge and result in feelings of discomfort or anxiety in childhood, adolescence, or early adulthood.

Selye's biological theory (1956, 1974) focuses on the effect of stress on the body and is referred to as the general adaptation syndrome (GAS). Stress causes wear and tear (structural and clinical changes) on the body and requires some type of coping behaviors by the individual. Such behaviors may be adaptive or healing (positive) or maladaptive (negative), resulting in exhaustion and disintegration of the mind or body or both.

Behavioral theorists state that an individual's response to a stressful event is often the result of learned or conditioned behavior. If one experiences too many life changes over a short period of time, one does not have enough time to adjust or condition oneself to each change and may exhibit dysfunctional or maladaptive behavior.

Two people can react to the same stressful event with opposite responses. For example, college roommates both receive probationary notices because of failure to complete a required college course successfully. One student makes an appointment to discuss her grades with her advisor, whereas the other student is unable to sleep and complains of a headache, light-headedness, and shortness of breath. The first student has learned to be responsible for her actions and is seeking help, thereby showing a positive response to the stress of probationary action. The second student is exhibiting signs of anxiety. She is displaying a maladaptive response to the stress of probationary action. As a child she may have had limited opportunity to condition herself to stress, her parents may have fostered dependency by making decisions for her, or this may be her first experience with what she considers to be a failure.

Theorists who believe social or cultural factors cause anxiety explain that as a person's personality develops, his or her impression of self may be negative (low self-concept). The person experiences difficulty adapting to everyday social problems owing to this low self-concept and inadequate coping mechanisms. The stressful stimuli of modern society pose a psychological threat for such a person and can result in the development of maladaptive behavior and the onset of an anxiety disorder. For example, a 19-year-old man who had difficulty maintaining a C average in high school and did not fit in with the crowd works as a delivery person for a pizza company. As he makes a delivery he receives a traffic ticket for driving with a faulty muffler. The police officer informs him that if he has the defective muffler replaced within 24 hours he will not be fined. The young man makes an appointment to have his car fixed; however, his boss tells him he cannot allow him to take the time off. The young man becomes tense and experiences feelings of dizziness, tachycardia, and shortness of breath as he responds to his employer's comment. Owing to inadequate coping mechanisms, he is unable to consider alternative options, such as asking the employer to use the company car for one day or suggesting that he change work schedules with another employee. His low self-concept prevents him from pointing out to his employer that he has been a faithful employee with a good work record, and therefore his request should receive a special consideration owing to the nature of his problem. Unless this young man develops a positive self-concept and adequate coping mechanisms, he will continue to experience difficulty dealing with the stress of daily social or cultural problems.

Carpenito (1995) lists the following contributing risk factors or etiology for the nursing diagnosis of *anxiety.

1. Pathophysiologic factors, which interfere with the basic human needs
2. Situational factors, which result in an actual or perceived threat to self-concept or biologic integrity; actual or perceived loss of significant others; actual or perceived change in the environment or one's socioeconomic status; or the transmission of another person's anxiety to the individual.
3. Maturational factors, which encompass a threat to the developmental task(s) of infants, children, adolescents, adults, or the elderly

McFarland and Wasli (1997) list 16 contributing or causative factors in the development of anxiety, including threats to (1) self-concept, (2) personal security system, (3) beliefs, (4) stable environment, (5) role-functioning, (6) meaningful interpersonal relationships, and (7) health status.

*NANDA-approved nursing diagnosis.

Research Regarding Anxiety

Neuroreceptor imaging now plays a limited role in the research related to anxiety. Receptor sites for benzodiazepines have been studied in the medial occipital cortex; obsessive–compulsive disorder has been determined to be a genetic disorder; and selective serotonin reuptake inhibitors are now used to treat anxiety. Studies have also revealed abnormalities in glucose metabolic rates in individuals with obsessive–compulsive disorder (Holman & Devous, 1992).

Kawachi, Sparrow, Vokonas, and Weiss (1994) conducted a study examining the relationship between anxiety symptoms and the risk of coronary heart disease. The study concluded that there is a strong association between symptoms of anxiety and the presence of coronary artery disease.

Laboratory studies have shown that panic attack is characterized by a sudden increment in tidal volume rather than in respiratory frequency. A computerized, calibrated body suit (Respitrace) is used to allow 24-hour recordings. It has been shown that patients who have spontaneous panic attacks experience a tripling of respiratory tidal volume.

According to an article published in the November 29, 1996 issue of the *Orlando Sentinel*, researchers have found a gene that triggers anxiety. The gene, 5-HTTP, influences how the brain makes use of serotonin, a signaling molecule that affects the sense of well-being and basic attitudes of optimism and pessimism. Statistics indicated that the gene caused a 3% to 4% difference in the amount of anxiety or tension the subjects experienced. This finding is also considered to be important in the study of origins of normal and pathological personality variations. Research findings are to be published in the journal, *Science*, by Dr. Dennis Murphy and Dr. Dean H. Hamer of the National Institute of Mental Health.

 ## Clinical Symptoms of Anxiety

Clinical symptoms of anxiety are too numerous to list in detail. They are generally classified as physiologic, psychological or emotional, and intellectual or cognitive responses to stress, which may vary according to the level of anxiety exhibited by the patient. Some of the more common symptoms follow:

Physiologic symptoms
  Elevated pulse, blood pressure, and respiration
  Dyspnea or hyperventilation
  Diaphoresis
  Vertigo or light-headedness

Blurred vision
Anorexia, nausea, and vomiting
Frequency of urination
Headache
Insomnia or sleep disturbance
Weakness or muscle tension
Tightness in the chest
Sweaty palms
Dilated pupils
Psychological or emotional responses
Withdrawal
Depression
Irritability
Crying
Lack of interest or apathy
Hypercriticism
Anger
Feelings of worthlessness, apprehension, or helplessness
Intellectual or cognitive responses
Decreased interest
Inability to concentrate
Nonresponsiveness to external stimuli
Decreased productivity
Preoccupation
Forgetfulness
Orientation to past rather than present or future
Rumination

Symptoms of anxiety range from a state of euphoria to panic. A brief description of the levels of anxiety follows:

Level Zero: Euphoria This is an exaggerated feeling of well-being that is not directly proportionate to a specific circumstance or situation. Euphoria usually precedes the onset of level one: Mild anxiety.

Level One: Mild Anxiety This stage can be a positive experience in which the person has an increased alertness to inner feelings or the environment. During this level the person has an increased ability to learn, experiences a motivational force, may become competitive, and has the opportunity to be individualistic. Feelings of restlessness may also be present, and the individual may not be able to relax.

Level Two: Moderate Anxiety During this stage, a narrowing of the ability to perceive occurs. The person is able to focus or concentrate on only one specific thing. Pacing, voice tremors, increased rate of verbalization or talking, physiologic changes, and verbalization about expected danger occur.

Level Three: Severe Anxiety The ability to perceive is reduced, and focus is on small or scattered details. Inappropriate verbalization, or the inability to communicate clearly, occurs at this time owing to increased anxiety and decreased intellectual thought processes. Lack of determination or the ability to perform occurs as the person experiences feelings of purposelessness. Questions such as "What's the use?" or "Why bother?" may be voiced. Physiologic responses also occur at this time as the individual experiences a sense of impending doom.

Level Four: Anxiety, Panic State In this stage, complete disruption of the ability to perceive takes place. Disintegration of the personality occurs as the individual becomes immobilized, experiences difficulty verbalizing, and is unable to focus on reality. Physiologic, emotional, and intellectual changes occur as the individual experiences a loss of control.

Anxiety disorders are more prevalent during adolescence and young adulthood, but may begin during childhood.

 ## Classification of Anxiety Disorders

The fourth edition of the *Diagnostic and Statistical Manual of Mental Disorders* (DSM-IV) lists the following classifications of anxiety disorders: panic disorder, phobias, obsessive–compulsive disorder, post-traumatic stress disorder, acute stress disorder, generalized anxiety disorder, anxiety disorder due to medical condition, substance-induced anxiety disorder, and anxiety disorder not otherwise specified.

Panic Disorder with or without Agoraphobia

Panic disorder is a real illness with both a physical and a psychological component. At any given time, several million Americans may be afflicted by this disorder. Onset usually begins during late teens or early twenties, and although it can occur in both men and women, most individuals with panic disorder are women (approximately 75%). Panic attacks usually last between a minute and an hour. The intensity of the attacks may fluctuate considerably, even in the same person.

The diagnostic criteria for this category require that recurrent unexpected panic attacks occur. Symptoms include:

Dyspnea or shortness of breath
Palpitations
Chest pain or discomfort

Choking or smothering sensation
Vertigo or unsteady feelings
Diaphoresis
Feelings of unreality or depersonalization
Trembling or shaking
Syncope
Nausea or abdominal distress
Hot and cold flashes
Tingling in hands or feet (paresthesia)
Fear of losing control, going crazy, or dying

After a panic attack, the individual exhibits concern about having additional attacks, worries about implications of the attack or its consequences, or displays a significant change in behavior. The panic attacks are not due to the direct physiologic effects of a substance or a general medical condition, and they are not better accounted for by another mental disorder. Agoraphobia may or may not be present.

Symptoms of a panic attack develop suddenly and increase in intensity within minutes of awareness of the first sign; for example, chest pain occurs followed by three other symptoms that increase in intensity within 10 minutes of the onset of chest pain.

CLINICAL EXAMPLE 16-1
Panic Disorder

MJ, a 21-year-old woman who lived in New York, recently became engaged to a marine stationed in California. On four separate occasions two weeks after her engagement, MJ experienced episodes of dizziness, fainting, fatigue, chest pain, and choking sensations while at work. At the suggestion of her employer, she scheduled an appointment with her family physician to discuss her physical symptoms. After a negative physical examination, the family physician asked MJ if she was excited about her engagement. She hesitated at first, then stated that she loved her fiancé but was reluctant to leave her job, friends, and family to move to California. MJ was able to relate the onset of her symptoms to the time of her engagement. The family physician helped MJ to explore feelings of ambivalence about her engagement and suggested that she seek the help of a therapist. After several weeks of counseling, the panic attacks subsided and she was able to discuss her feelings with her fiancé.

Phobic Disorders

Phobias are the most common form of anxiety disorders. According to the National Institute of Mental Health, between 5.1% and 12.5% of Americans suffer from phobias. Phobia is described as "an irrational fear" of an object, activity, or situation that is out of proportion to the stimulus and results in avoidance of the identified object, activity, or situation. The person has unconsciously displaced the original internal source of fear or anxiety, such as an unpleasant childhood experience, to an external source. Avoidance of the object or situation allows the person to remain free of anxiety. The following is a brief discussion of agoraphobia, social phobia, and specific phobia.

Agoraphobia Recognized as the most common phobic disorder, agoraphobia is the fear of being alone in public places from which the person thinks escape would be difficult or help unavailable if the person were incapacitated. Normal activities become restricted and victims refuse to leave their homes. Two thirds of those exhibiting clinical symptoms are women in whom symptoms develop between ages 18 and 35 years. Onset may be sudden or gradual. Victims are likely to develop depression, fatigue, tension, and spontaneous obsessive or panic disorders. Some cultural or ethnic groups restrict the participation of women in public life. Such cultural practice must be considered before diagnosing an individual with agoraphobia.

Social Phobia This is a compelling desire to avoid situations in which a person may be criticized by others. The person experiences persistent, irrational fear of criticism, humiliation, or embarrassment. The person does realize that the fear is excessive or disproportionate to the activity or situation. Social phobia rarely is incapacitating but may cause considerable inconvenience. The abuse of alcohol and other drugs may occur as the person with social phobia attempts to reduce anxiety. Examples of social phobias are fears of public speaking, using public restrooms, or using public transportation. In certain cultures, such as Japanese or Korean, individuals may develop persistent and excessive fears of giving offense to others in social situations instead of being embarrassed themselves. Such fears may cause extreme anxiety and avoidance of social interactions.

Specific Phobia A specific phobia is defined as an excessive fear of an object, activity, or a situation, which leads a person to avoid the cause of that fear. The DSM-IV lists five subtypes of this disorder: animal, natural environment, blood–injection–injury, situational, and other (*i.e.*, fear of space, sound, or costumed characters).

The content of phobias as well as their prevalence varies with culture and ethnicity. The diagnosis of specific phobia should be given only if the fear is excessive in the context of the specific culture and the fear causes a significant impairment or distress.

There are approximately 700 identified phobias. Some of the more common ones are as follows:

Acrophobia—fear of heights
Androphobia—fear of men
Astraphobia—fear of storms, lightning, thunder
Ceraunophobia—fear of thunder
Claustrophobia—fear of enclosed places
Hematophobia—fear of blood
Hydrophobia—fear of water
Iatrophobia—fear of doctors
Nyctophobia—fear of night
Ochlophobia—fear of crowds
Pyrophobia—fear of fire
Zoophobia—fear of animals

Reactions by student nurses caring for patients with phobic symptoms include comments such as "Why do people have fears?" "How do fears develop?" "Can't the patient tell her fear is silly? Elevators can't hurt you," and "How did she survive, never leaving her house in five years? It must be terrible to experience so much fear that it controls your life!"

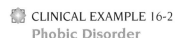 CLINICAL EXAMPLE 16-2
Phobic Disorder

MS, 19 years old, was attending a movie when she began to perspire profusely, tremble, breathe rapidly, and feel nauseated. She left the movie before it ended. Her symptoms became more common when she was around a group of people. As a result of these feelings, MS began to avoid crowds, and her daily activity consisted of going to work and returning home immediately after work. Within a month MS became housebound. She attempted to relieve her anxiety by using alcohol to relax but did not experience any relief. MS was encouraged by her family to seek psychiatric help. Counseling revealed that she had been lost in a crowd as a child while attending a circus and had been separated from her parents for several hours. Recently she had moved into an apartment. The therapist explored her feelings about moving away from the home. Memories of being separated from her parents as a child were identified as the underlying cause of her phobic reaction.

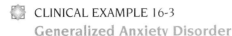

CLINICAL EXAMPLE 16-3
Generalized Anxiety Disorder

A 50-year-old woman was admitted to the psychiatric hospital for treatment of a generalized anxiety disorder. As the student nurse completed the initial assessment form, she noted that the patient was quite restless, sitting on the edge of her bed and fidgeting with her gown. She constantly rearranged her personal items on the bedside stand. Complaints of dizziness, an upset stomach, insomnia, and frequency of urination were noted. She appeared to be easily distracted as various people walked into the room to care for another patient and was rather impatient with the student nurse as she took the admitting vital signs. The patient's hands were cold and clammy and the radial pulse was 120 while the patient sat on the edge of her bed.

During clinical postconference, the student nurse shared her feelings of irritation about the patient. She also stated that the patient's anxiety was "infectious" and that she found herself becoming tense although she tried to remain calm during the admission procedure. Another student stated that she would have given the patient a sedative first to allow her to settle down and then would have attempted to carry out the initial assessment. The group discussed interpersonal reactions with persons who exhibit clinical symptoms of generalized anxiety and how easy it would be to avoid contact with the patient.

Generalized Anxiety Disorder

This disorder is characterized by unrealistic or excessive anxiety and worry occurring more days than not in a six-month period. The concern is about a number of events, such as job or school performance, and the individual is unable to control the worry. At least three of the following six symptoms are reported: restlessness, fatigue, impaired concentration, irritability, muscle tension, and sleep disturbance. The anxiety interferes with social, occupational, or other important areas of functioning and is not the direct result of a medical condition or substance abuse.

Obsessive–Compulsive Disorder

This disorder is characterized by two main clinical features, namely, recurrent obsessions or compulsions (or a combination of both) that interfere with normal life. Approximately 2% of all adults in all socioeconomic classes are afflicted with this disorder.

An *obsession* is a persistent, painful, intrusive thought, emotion, or urge that one is unable to suppress or ignore. Common obsessive thoughts include topics such as religion, sexuality, violence, the need for symmetry or exactness, and contamination. Everyone has experienced recurrent thoughts at one time or another. Lines of a song or poem may invade one's thoughts and continually run through one's mind. "I just can't seem to get this name off my mind," or "His words keep coming back to haunt me" are statements made by persons experiencing recurrent thoughts. The difference is that obsessions are considered senseless or repugnant, and they cannot be eliminated by logic or reasoning. A repetitive thought of killing one's mate is an example of a violent obsession.

A *compulsion* is the performance of a repetitious, uncontrollable, but seemingly purposeful act to prevent some future event or situation. Resistance to the act increases anxiety. Yielding to the compulsion decreases anxiety (primary gain). The person is aware of the senselessness of the behavior and does not derive pleasure from performing the act. Examples include repetitive touching, counting, checking, hoarding, and handwashing; such actions are not uncommon in children and adolescents.

✿ CLINICAL EXAMPLE 16-4
Obsessive–Compulsive Disorder

AY, a 56-year-old patient was observed performing the following ritualistic behavior continuously. The only time she would interrupt the activity was to go to the patients' dining room for meals, to attend to personal hygiene at the insistence of the staff, and to sleep. AY would begin by standing at the nurses' station for a few moments, mumbling incoherently at the staff, and then continue by starting on a ritualistic pathway. As she left the nurses' station she would walk 10 steps to the right, touch the wall with her right hand, flicker the light switch, and then proceed to her next objective, approximately 20 steps away. There she would touch another wall, do a 360° turn, and again mumble a few incoherent words. She then headed back to the nurses' station, repeating the behavior on the opposite side of the room. If there were any intrusions during this ritualistic performance, AY would exhibit signs of extreme anxiety. Needless to say, this behavior dominated her life and interfered with her role and social functioning.

Students who observed AY were amazed at the energy she possessed because she never seemed to tire. They were hesitant to approach her during this ritualistic activity because they were uncertain what she might do. One student stated, "I know this sounds foolish, but I'm afraid she might get upset and become hostile toward me." Another student said she felt foolish trying to walk with AY as she attempted to show AY she wanted to help her and be with her. A third student observed that the behavior was accepted by other patients on the unit and that no one seemed to interrupt AY.

Some people perform various rituals in the same sequence, and these have become a part of their daily routine. Washing clothes on Monday, ironing on Tuesday, shopping for groceries on Wednesday, and so forth, is an example of a weekly ritual. Getting up at the same hour each morning and following the same routine of showering, eating breakfast, and dressing is considered a daily routine. Leaving the house and returning to see if the gas burner is turned off or the door is locked is obsessive–compulsive behavior; however, normally it is not done to decrease anxiety and is not considered uncontrollable behavior.

The DSM-IV lists features such as depression, phobic avoidance, tics, and impaired social or role functioning as being present in patients with an obsessive–compulsive disorder.

Post-traumatic Stress Disorder

The DSM-IV reserves this category for persons who experience a psychological traumatic event that is considered to be outside the realm of usual human experience. Examples include rape or assault, military combat, natural disasters, serious physical injury as a result of a catastrophic event such as a fire, and torture. Vietnam War veterans have been one of the largest groups of persons to exhibit symptoms of this disorder.

Diagnostic criteria are as follows:

1. The person has been exposed to a traumatic event that involved actual or threatened death or serious injury, or a threat to the physical integrity of self or others.
2. The person's response involved intense fear, helplessness, or horror.
3. The traumatic event is persistently reexperienced through distressing recollections, recurrent distressing dreams, intense psychological distress, and the like.
4. The individual avoids stimuli associated with the traumatic event.
5. Persistent symptoms of increased arousal such as insomnia, irritability, inability to concentrate, hypervigilance, and exaggerated startle response occur.

The diagnosis of acute onset refers to symptoms that last less than three months. If symptoms persist beyond three months, the diagnosis of chronic onset is used. If the onset of symptoms occurs at least six months after the stressor, the diagnosis refers to delayed onset. Impaired role and social functioning may occur, as well as interference with occupational and recreational functioning. Low self-concept and suicidal ideation or thoughts may occur, along with substance abuse, because the individual has difficulty coping with the recollections of the traumatic experience.

CLINICAL EXAMPLE 16-5
Post-traumatic Stress Disorder

1. KW, a 35-year-old accountant, and his 5-year-old son were visiting his wife's family in Chicago when an electrical storm occurred during the early morning hours. KW awakened about 3:00 A.M. when he heard the loud cracking sound of fire in the hallway outside his second-floor bedroom. He attempted to reach his son, who was also sleeping on the second floor, but was driven back by the intense heat and smoke. KW managed to escape from the second story by climbing down an outdoor television antenna. He immediately attempted to enter the front door of the house in another effort to reach his son and in-laws, who were calling for help. He was unable to climb the stairway, which was engulfed in fire. When the fire department arrived, the fire fighters were able to revive KW's mother-in-law, but her husband and grandson had been burned severely and died of smoke inhalation. KW's wife arrived shortly after she received the news of the fire. As she and her husband slept in their motel room, he began to have nightmares about the fire and yelled out several times in his sleep. These nightmares recurred nightly for several months and began to interfere with KW's daily life. He repeatedly told his wife that he should have died instead of their son and his father-in-law. KW eventually was seen by a counselor, who was able to help him explore his feelings of guilt about having survived the fire.

2. Two student nurses had the opportunity to care for a Vietnam War veteran who was hospitalized for emergency surgery. During the initial assessment the patient revealed that he had tried marijuana and other drugs to help him forget some of the experiences he had had. He also stated he had expected a warm welcome when he returned to the United States but was shocked to find he was considered a murderer. His wife, who was present during the interview, stated that she learned very quickly not to awaken him from a deep sleep because he was "on guard" all the time and had "thrown a few punches." He also talked in his sleep frequently. The patient was somewhat bitter when he related that he had been unable to find a job since his discharge from the service. He stated, "Not only do I have horrible nightmares about Vietnam, but I am beginning to question my future as a human being."

The students stated that they felt helpless as they listened to the patient's feelings of rejection, hopelessness about the future, and anger toward those people who labeled him a murderer. During postconference they explored various interventions to help decrease the patient's anxiety and increase his self-esteem.

▢ CLINICAL EXAMPLE 16-6
Acute Stress Disorder

If, in the clinical example of post-traumatic stress disorder, the father exhibited dissociative symptoms such as detachment, derealization, and depersonalization for at least two days and no longer than four weeks, the clinical diagnosis may have been acute stress disorder. Other clinical symptoms include recurrent nightmares and the inability to function on a daily basis because of guilt feelings.

Acute Stress Disorder

This disorder is differentiated from post-traumatic stress disorder in that symptoms occur during or immediately after the trauma, last for at least two days, and either resolve within four weeks after the conclusion of the event or the diagnosis is changed. The individual exhibits dissociative symptoms, persistently reexperiences the traumatic event, avoids stimuli that arouse recollections of the trauma, and exhibits marked symptoms of anxiety or increased arousal. Significant impairment in social and occupational functioning occurs. The individual is unable to pursue necessary tasks.

Atypical Anxiety Disorder

The atypical category is a catchall for persons who exhibit signs of an anxiety disorder but do not meet criteria for any of the previously described conditions listed in this classification.

✦ Treatment of Anxiety Disorders

Learning to cope with and decrease anxiety by identifying the underlying conflict or frustration and by verbalizing concerns is a goal in the treatment of anxiety. Various techniques are used; the selection of a specific therapy depends on the particular situation.

Relaxation therapies or techniques have become quite popular because they can be used as therapeutic interventions in a variety of situations such as generalized anxiety and post-traumatic stress disorder.

Examples of such techniques used to decrease anxiety include

1. *Visual imagery:* This technique has been used effectively to reduce anxiety experienced by cancer patients. As patients relax they engage in a fantasy in which they visualize the identified cause of anxiety, such as pain due to cancer or the cancer itself. A person who has an unresolved conflict, such

as not attending the funeral of a loved one, could use this technique in an attempt to work through guilt feelings or unresolved grief.

2. *Change of pace or scenery:* Walking in the woods or along the beach, listening to music, caring for a pet, or engaging in a hobby are examples of ways to change pace or scenery in an attempt to decrease anxiety by removing oneself from the source or cause of stress.

3. *Exercise or massage:* Exercise can be a release or outlet for pent-up tension or anxiety. Massage is soothing and helps to relax one's muscles. Expectant mothers who practice the Lamaze technique for prepared childbirth use effleurage, or a massage of the abdominal muscles during uterine contractions, to promote relaxation.

4. *Transcendental meditation:* Four components of this relaxation technique include a quiet environment, a passive state of mind, a comfortable position, and the ability to focus on a specific word or object. Physiologic, psychological, and spiritual relaxation occur.

5. *Biofeedback:* The person is able to monitor various physiologic processes by auditory or visual signals. This technique has proven effective in the management of conditions such as migraine headaches, essential hypertension, and pain that is the result of increased stress and anxiety.

6. *Systematic desensitization:* Simply stated, this technique refers to the exposure of a person to a fear-producing situation in a systematized manner to decrease a phobic disorder. A behavioral therapist usually works with the person.

7. *Relaxation exercise:* Various methods are used to help people learn to relax. The common steps to relaxation include taking a deep breath and exhaling (similar to the cleansing or relaxing breathing of Lamaze technique); tensing and then relaxing individual muscles, starting with the head and progressing to the toes; and finally relaxing all parts of the body simultaneously. Some methods suggest that the person imagine a peaceful scene before doing the exercise.

8. *Therapeutic touch or "laying on of hands":* This technique is controversial and has not been accepted completely by the helping professions. Vivid examples are cited in the Bible, and faith healers use this technique.

9. *Hypnosis:* Some behavioral therapists use hypnosis to enhance relaxation or imagery. People have been taught self-hypnosis to decrease anxiety.

Other treatment modalities used to treat anxiety disorders include behavioral modification, cognitive therapy, exposure therapy, psychoanalysis, group therapy, family therapy, and environmental modification.

Antianxiety agents such as BuSpar, Ativan, Xanax, or Luvox may be prescribed; however, many therapists feel that these agents should be for short-term use only. Sedative-hypnotics may be prescribed to alleviate insomnia.

Antidepressants such as Paxil, Prozac, Desyrel, Zoloft, Serzone, or Effexor may be used when depression is an associated feature in an anxiety disorder. Beta-blockers may be used when physiologic symptoms such as rapid heart rate are present in social phobias. (See chapter on psychopharmacology regarding antianxiety agents.)

Nursing Intervention

People who exhibit signs of acute anxiety or a panic state may harm themselves or others and need to be supervised closely until the anxiety is decreased. Such individuals may need to be placed in a general hospital, mental health center, or psychiatric hospital to ensure a protective environment.

The person may be in severe distress or immobilized, or may be engaged in purposeless, disorganized, or aggressive activity. Feelings of intense awe, dread, or terror may occur. The patient may express the fear that he or she is "losing control."

After the patient is examined, a nursing care plan is initiated to correspond to the physician's or psychiatrist's treatment plan for an acute anxiety attack or panic state.

During the panic state the nursing interventions include

1. Staying with the patient at all times
2. Remaining calm. The patient will sense any anxiety exhibited by the nurse.
3. Speaking in short, simple sentences
4. Displaying firmness to provide external controls for the patient
5. Keeping the patient in a quiet environment to minimize external stimuli. The patient is unable to screen such stimuli and may become over whelmed.
6. Providing protective care because the patient may harm self or others. The patient's behavior also may elicit responses from other patients who are unable to tolerate her or his anxiety state.
7. Attempting to channel the patient's behavior by engaging the patient in physical activities that provide an outlet for tension or frustration
8. Administering antianxiety medication to decrease anxiety

Persons who exhibit symptoms of mild or moderate levels of anxiety may be treated as outpatients if the anxiety does not interfere with the ability to function. Unfortunately, most people with obsessive–compulsive disorder do not seek help because they are embarrassed or ashamed, and fear they will be viewed as "crazy."

Nursing interventions for mild-to-moderate anxiety levels include assessing the patient's anxiety level, reducing anxiety, providing protective care, encouraging verbalization of anxiety, meeting basic human needs, and setting realistic goals for patient care. The nurse provides supportive care by giving the patient a teaching checklist and by

1. Recognizing the patient's anxiety and helping him or her identify the anxiety and describe feelings
2. Reassuring the patient
3. Accepting the patient unconditionally. Do not pass judgment or respond emotionally to the patient's behavior.
4. Listening to the patient's concerns. Be available but respect the patient's need for personal space.
5. Protecting the patient's defenses (*e.g.*, ritualistic behavior). Any attempt to stop such behavior increases anxiety because the patient has no other defenses.
6. Encouraging verbalization of feelings. Answer questions directly.
7. Allowing the patient time to respond to nursing interventions. Set realistic goals for improvement. Allow the patient to set the pace.
8. Exploring alternative coping mechanisms to decrease present anxiety to a manageable level. Assist the patient in learning to cope with anxiety.

PATIENT TEACHING CHECKLIST

Anxiety

The following checklist has been developed to reinforce your knowledge about anxiety. Please inform the nurse if you are uncertain about any of the items listed below.

✔ Clinical symptoms I may experience include:
✔ The reasons I may experience anxiety include:
✔ Interventions I have learned to reduce anxiety are:
✔ Support persons I may contact include:
✔ The name of the medication I am taking is:
✔ Instructions regarding this medication
   - Take this medication as directed by your doctor
   - Do not drink alcohol while taking this medication
   - Do not take any over-the-counter medication without informing your nurse or doctor
   - Usual side effects include:
   - Report any unusual side effects promptly
   - Antianxiety agents are generally fast acting because onset occurs within 30 minutes, full effectiveness occurs in 1 to 2 hours, and effects usually last 4 to 6 hours
   - Dosage adjustment may be necessary
   - Do not discontinue taking this medication without first consulting your nurse or doctor

9. Identifying the patient's developmental stage and helping the patient to work through unmet developmental tasks.
10. Administering treatments or medications to reduce anxiety or other discomfort.

If hospitalization of the patient with an anxiety disorder is required, it is usually short-term and intensive. Outpatient follow-up care usually is recommended to continue with supportive therapeutic measures. Discharge planning includes an evaluation of the patient's present status, recommendations for outpatient referral, and instructions regarding drug therapy if a maintenance dose is necessary. The patient should be instructed about whom to contact if anxiety increases and panic or a crisis occurs.

Nursing diagnoses used to develop nursing care plans for individuals experiencing stress and anxiety include *anxiety, *ineffective individual coping, *high risk for injury, *impaired verbal communication, *impaired social interaction, *sleep pattern disturbance, *post-trauma response, *rape trauma syndrome, *hopelessness, *altered health maintenance, and *knowledge deficit regarding illness.

Nursing Care Plan 16-1 shows two examples of nursing diagnoses and goal-related nursing interventions and outcome criteria for patients with anxiety disorders.

Summary

Anxiety is defined as feeling of uncertainty, uneasiness, apprehension, or tension that a person experiences in response to an unknown object or situation. It is differentiated from fear, which is the body's physiologic and emotional response to a known or recognized danger. Clinical symptoms of anxiety may be manifested in physiologic, emotional, or intellectual (cognitive) responses. The types, severity, levels, and etiology of anxiety were discussed. The clinical symptoms of the DSM-IV classifications of anxiety disorders were discussed, including panic disorders, phobic disorders, generalized anxiety disorder, obsessive–compulsive disorder, post-traumatic stress disorder, acute stress disorder, and atypical anxiety disorder. Treatment of anxiety disorders, focusing on relaxation techniques, various types of psychotherapy, behavioral and environmental modification, and psychotropic drug therapy, was included. Nursing diagnoses used to develop nursing care plans for individuals experiencing stress and anxiety were listed. Examples of goals, nursing interventions, and outcome criteria for patients exhibiting moderate anxiety related to relocation and sleep pattern disturbance were cited.

*NANDA-approved nursing diagnosis.

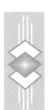

NURSING CARE PLAN 16-1

The Patient with an Anxiety Disorder

Nursing Diagnosis: Moderate *anxiety related to relocation

Goal: The patient will demonstrate decreased psychological and physiologic signs and symptoms of anxiety.

Nursing Interventions	Outcome Criteria
	Within 24 to 48 hours the patient will be able to do the following:
Educate regarding symptoms and causes of anxiety	Identify physiologic signs and symptoms of anxiety
Encourage verbalization of feelings	Describe own anxiety
	Identify one or two stressors contributing to anxiety
Explore coping skills	Describe own coping patterns
	Identify one or two alternative coping patterns
	Relate an increase in physiologic and psychological comfort

*NANDA-approved nursing diagnosis.

Nursing Diagnosis: *Sleep pattern disturbance related to stress and anxiety secondary to relocation

Goal: The patient will identify factors that promote restful sleep.

Nursing Interventions	Outcome Criteria
	Within 48 to 72 hours the patient will be able to do the following:
Promote development of a bedtime routine	Determine the desired number of sleeping hours required for restful sleep
	Identify an atmosphere conducive to restful sleep
Explore methods of relaxation	Identify one or two factors that promote relaxation
	Practice one or two relaxation techniques to facilitate sleep
Promote restful sleep by reducing or eliminating environmental distractions	Identify environmental distractions that inhibit sleep
	Identify sleep aids such as music, fan, night light

*NANDA-approved nursing diagnosis.

Learning Activities

I. Clinical Activities
   A. Care for a patient exhibiting clinical symptoms of anxiety.
   B. Describe symptoms of anxiety exhibited by the patient.
   C. Identify the level of anxiety being experienced by the patient.
   D. Identify coping mechanisms used in an attempt to decrease anxiety.
   E. Identify any situation or event that increases the patient's anxiety.
   F. Discuss the nursing interventions used to decrease the patient's anxiety.
II. Case Study: Generalized Anxiety Disorder
   A 24-year-old female patient was admitted to the hospital with complaints of dyspnea, chest pain, rapid pulse, and a feeling of "something stuck in her throat." The tentative diagnosis was acute respiratory infection.
   While caring for the patient, the student nurse was able to assess the patient's behavior and discuss various aspects of the woman's home life. The patient related feelings of a low self-concept and stated that she felt depressed at times as she attempted to work full-time and care for an invalid mother who lived with her. Nonverbal behavior included fingering the sheets as she talked, clearing her throat frequently, and shaking her right foot as she sat in the chair with her legs crossed.
   A. Identify the symptoms of a generalized anxiety disorder exhibited by the patient.
   B. Develop a nursing care plan listing the nursing diagnosis, goals, nursing interventions, and outcome criteria appropriate for this patient.
III. Independent Activities
   A. Select a television program that portrays stressful situations and discuss the reactions of the various actors and actresses.
   B. In a clinical agency emergency room, identify various stressful situations and discuss specific interventions that were used to reduce stress.
   C. Describe your nonverbal behaviors and physical symptoms experienced in your last stressful situation. How do you usually cope with situations? What changes could you make to cope more effectively?

Critical Thinking Questions

1. Assess your own feelings of anxiety. What causes you anxiety? What physical and cognitive responses occur when you are anxious? At what level do you experience most of your anxiety?
2. Interview a Vietnam veteran about his or her experiences during the war. Are symptoms of post-traumatic stress disorder evident? How might a veteran's experiences compare with those of an experienced inner city emergency room nurse? Is PTSD a disorder we should research related to its potential in nurses?

3. Pick four of the eight relaxation techniques discussed in this chapter and experience them yourself. Which provided you with the most relaxation? How might you incorporate some of these techniques into your own life?

Self-Test

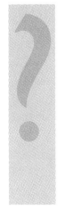

1. List examples of responses to stress in each of the following categories:
   Physiologic responses
   Psychological or emotional responses
   Intellectual or cognitive responses
2. Differentiate among the levels of anxiety:
   Euphoria
   Mild anxiety
   Moderate anxiety
   Severe anxiety
   Panic state of anxiety
3. List three causative factors (etiology) of anxiety and cite an example of each causative factor.
4. Define the following terms:
   Signal anxiety
   Anxiety trait
   Anxiety state
   Free-floating anxiety
5. Differentiate between a panic disorder and a generalized anxiety disorder.
6. Define obsession and state an example.
7. State an example of compulsive behavior and explain the purpose that it serves.
8. Define phobia and list three examples.
9. Explain why a post-traumatic stress disorder may develop in Vietnam War veterans.

SELECTED REFERENCES

Badger, J. M. (1995, September). 14 tips for managing stress on the job. *American Journal of Nursing*.

Carpenito, L. J. (1995). *Nursing diagnosis: Application to clinical practice* (6th ed.). Philadelphia: J. B. Lippincott.

French, M. S. (1996, November). The mind-body-spirit connection: An introduction to alternative therapies. *Advance for Nurse Practitioners*.

Furey, J. A. (1991, March). Women Vietnam veterans: A comparison of studies. *Journal of Psychosocial Nursing and Mental Health Services*.

George, M. S. (1993, September). Obsessive–compulsive disorder and Tourette syndrome. *Clinical Advances in the Treatment of Psychiatric Disorders.*

Holman, B. L., & Devous, M. D. (1992, October). Functional brain SPECT: The emergence of a powerful clinical method. *Journal of Nuclear Medicine.*

Karch, A. M. (1997). *Lippincott's nursing drug guide.* Philadelphia: Lippincott–Raven Publishers.

Kawachi, I., Sparrow, D., Vokonas, P. S., & Weiss, S. T. (1994, November). Symptoms of anxiety and risk of coronary heart disease: The normative aging study. *Circulation.*

Laria, M. T. (1995, December). Panic disorder. *Advance for Nurse Practitioners.*

McFarland, G., & Wasli, E. (1997). *Nursing diagnoses and process in psychiatric–mental health nursing* (3rd ed.). Philadelphia: Lippincott–Raven Publishers.

Peters, A. (1996, December). The unquiet mind: Treating obsessive-compulsive disorder. *Advance for Nurse Practitioners.*

Schatzberg, A. F., & Nemeroff, C. B. (Eds.). (1995). *The American Psychiatric Press textbook of psychopharmacology.* Washington, DC: American Psychiatric Press.

Selye, H. (1956). *The stress of life.* New York: McGraw-Hill.

Selye, H. (1974). *Stress without distress.* New York: New American Library.

Walley, E. J., Beebe, D. K., & Clark, J. L. (1994, December). Management of common anxiety disorders. *American Family Physician.*

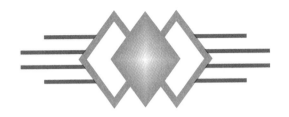

CHAPTER 17

ANXIETY-RELATED DISORDERS

T he sorrow which has no vent in tears may make other organs weep.

Henry Maudsley

LEARNING OBJECTIVES

1 Define the following terminology:

   Psychological factors affecting medical condition

   Somatoform disorder

   Dissociative disorder

   Personality disorder

   Anxiety disorder due to a general medical condition

   Culture-bound syndrome

2 Explain the Social Readjustment Rating Scale.

3 Discuss at least two theories commonly cited to explain the onset of stress-related disorders.

4 Differentiate between primary and secondary gain.

5 Differentiate between fugue and amnesia.

6 State the common characteristics shared by the various categories of personality disorders.

7 List the common nursing diagnoses identified in individuals exhibiting anxiety-related disorders discussed in this chapter.

 Introduction

Chapter 16 focused on factors that contribute to the development of the more commonly seen anxiety disorders. This chapter provides an overview of psychological factors affecting medical condition, somatoform disorders, dissociative disorders, personality disorders, anxiety disorder due to a general medical condition, and culture-bound syndromes.

 Psychological Factors Affecting
Medical Condition

The DSM-IV states that the essential feature of this category is the presence of one or more specific psychological or behavioral factors that adversely affect a general medical condition. They may influence the course of the general medical condition, interfere with treatment of the medical condition, constitute an additional health risk for the individual, or precipitate or exacerbate symptoms of the general medical condition. Psychological or behavioral factors such as anxiety, a "type A" personality trait, or stress-related physiologic responses may significantly affect the course of almost every major category of disease. This diagnostic category is intended for any medical condition caused by or influenced by psychological factors.

Etiology

Theories commonly cited to explain the role of stress or emotions in the development of or exacerbation of physical illness include Selye's general adaptation syndrome (1956), the emotional specificity theory, the organ specificity theory, the familial theory, and the learning theory.

According to Selye (1956), an individual who is unable to gain equilibrium or homeostasis after the "fight-or-flight" reaction to stress may experience the stage of exhaustion. Physical deterioration and death can occur as a result of continued stress in the presence of a weakened physical condition.

Contributors to the development of the emotional specificity theory include Shapiro and Crider (1969), who investigated the effects of different emotions on physiologic functioning. They found anger and hostility to be the underlying factors in the presence of essential hypertension. Friedman and Rosenman (1974) researched the "type A" personality, which is characterized by an excessive competitive drive, impatience, aggressiveness, and a sense of urgency. These individuals were found to have higher levels of serum triglycerides, cholesterol, adrenaline, and steroids than the more relaxed "type B" personalities. Because these substances have an adverse effect on the heart, causing the person to be at risk, the researchers concluded that a person with "type A" personality was more susceptible to the development of coronary heart disease.

Lacey, Bateman, and Van Lehn (1953) studied characteristic physiologic response patterns that they believed to be present since childhood. They concluded that a person responds to stress primarily with one specific organ or system, thereby showing susceptibility to the development of a specific disease. For example, whenever faced with an emotional conflict, a 25-year-old secretary would experience the sudden onset of midepigastric pain. The pain would persist until the conflict was resolved. She has the potential for development of an ulcer if she continues to experience frequent episodes of stress. Other persons may be prone to low back pain, asthmatic attacks, or skin rashes, depending on their susceptible organ or system. This theory is referred to as the organ specificity theory.

Proponents of the familial theory feel that dynamic family relationships influence the development of a medical disorder. A family therapist, Salvador

Minuchin (1974), believes that role modeling is an important factor in personality development. He identified the "psychosomatogenic family" as a group of individuals who develop physiologic symptoms rather than face or resolve conflict. Children of such families observe the coping mechanisms of their parents and other family members and develop similar behaviors when the need arises, to avoid conflict and experience positive reinforcement.

According to the learning theory, a person learns to produce a physiologic response to achieve a reward, attention, or some other type of reinforcement.

Lancaster (1980) states that the following dynamics occur during the development of a learned response:

1. The learning is of an unconscious nature.
2. There was a reward or reinforcement in the past when the person experienced specific physiologic symptoms.
3. Reinforcement can be positive or negative. Negative reinforcement is considered better than no reinforcement at all.
4. The person is not able to give up the disorder willfully.

For example, a child stays home from school when he is ill and receives attention from his mother as she reads to him, fixes his favorite meals, and monitors his vital signs. As a result of this experience, he unconsciously learns to produce physiologic symptoms of a migraine headache or an upset stomach as he feels the need for attention. This behavior may continue throughout his life as he attempts to satisfy unmet needs.

The Social Readjustment Rating Scale

Holmes and Rahe (1967), along with a group of other scientists, developed the Social Readjustment Rating Scale. This scale ranks 43 critical life events according to the severity of their impact on a person. Each event has a point value; the death of a spouse is considered to be the most significant critical life event, and minor violations of the law the least significant of the 43 events. The point values of events a person experiences for a single year are totaled, thus indicating the severity of environmental stressors and the potential for a health change within two years. For example, the individual could experience anxiety exacerbating asthma, stress-related exacerbation of an ulcer, or delayed recovery from a myocardial infarct if the rating score is above 200 (Box 17-1). A clinical example of the exacerbation of essential hypertension due to stress is presented on page 310.

BOX 17-1 The Holmes/Rahe Social Readjustment Rating Scale*

Instructions: Ask all questions in the order listed and score immediately. Record total number.

Life Event	Mean Value
1. Death of spouse	100
2. Divorce	73
3. Marital separation	65
4. Jail term	63
5. Death of close family member	63
6. Personal injury or illness	53
7. Marriage	50
8. Fired at work	47
9. Marital reconciliation	45
10. Retirement	45
11. Change in health of family member	44
12. Pregnancy	40
13. Sex difficulties	39
14. Gain of new family member	39
15. Business readjustment	39
16. Change in financial state	38
17. Death of close friend	37
18. Change to different line of work	36
19. Change in number of arguments with spouse	35
20. Mortgage or loan for major purchase (home, etc.)	31
21. Foreclosure of mortgage or loan	30
22. Change in responsibilities at work	29
23. Son or daughter leaving home	29
24. Trouble with in-laws	29
25. Outstanding personal achievement	28
26. Wife begins or stops work	26
27. Begin or end school	26
28. Change in living conditions	25
29. Revision of personal habits	24
30. Trouble with boss	23
31. Change in work hours or conditions	20
32. Change in residence	20
33. Change in schools	20
34. Change in recreation	19

(continued)

BOX 17-1 The Holmes/Rahe Social Readjustment Rating Scale* (Continued)

Life Event	Mean Value
35. Change in church activities	19
36. Change in social activities	18
37. Mortgage or loan for lesser purchase (car, TV, etc.)	17
38. Change in sleeping habits	16
39. Change in number of family get-togethers	15
40. Change in eating habits	15
41. Vacation	13
42. Christmas	12
43. Minor violations of the law	11

*From Holmes TH, Rahe RH (1967). The social readjustment rating scale. *Journal of Psychosomatic Research, 11*, 213–218.

The rating scale is scored as follows:

A 150–199 point value places the person at a mild risk for a health change in the next two years (25%–37% chance).

A 200–299 point value indicates that the person is at a moderate risk for a health change within the next two years (50% chance).

A 300 or greater point value indicates that the person is at a major risk for a health change within the next two years (79%–90% chance).

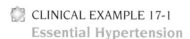 CLINICAL EXAMPLE 17-1
Essential Hypertension

JB, a 54-year-old executive, was seen by the company's attending physician for his annual physical examination. As the office nurse assessed him, she noted that his face was flushed, his blood pressure was 160/110, and he stated that he only had 30 minutes until he had to attend an executive meeting. After his physical examination was completed, the physician instructed JB to return to his office twice a week to have his blood pressure monitored and placed him on antihypertensive medication. The next few weeks JB returned faithfully as directed, continuing to present symptoms of hypertension. Although the nurse continued to stress preventive measures, JB did not change his life-style. Approximately four months later JB was admitted to the intensive care unit of the local community hospital with the diagnosis of a cerebral vascular attack. As a result of this condition, JB is a right-sided hemiplegic, with expressive aphasia. He has had to retire early and currently is engaged in a rehabilitative program.

(continued)

A student nurse caring for JB commented, "He could be my father. He's so young to spend the rest of his life as a disabled person." After reading the history and admission forms, the same student stated, "Why didn't he follow his doctor's advice to prevent his attack? Didn't he care what happened?" JB eventually answered this question, stating, "I didn't think this would happen to me. I never lost my temper when I was upset. Maybe I should have said what I thought rather than worry about hurting the other guy's feelings."

Treatment of Psychological Factors Affecting Medical Condition

The medical problem is treated before focusing on the emotional needs exhibited by the patient. Treatment is an individualized approach that considers the following factors:

1. Severity of clinical symptoms, both physical and psychological (*i.e.*, life-threatening structural changes requiring immediate medical attention or psychiatric care)
2. Type of psychophysiologic reaction, including presenting symptoms (*e.g.*, elevated blood pressure, tachycardia, skin rash, or gastric pain)
3. Emotional component of illness (*e.g.*, anxiety, anger, depression, or dependency needs)
4. Insight regarding illness displayed by patient (*i.e.*, awareness of stressors or conflict causing physical illness)

Many patients are admitted to the general hospital and receive traditional medical treatment such as bed rest, diet as tolerated, moist heat, antacids, and pain medication. Antianxiety agents, antidepressants, or sedative-hypnotic agents also may be prescribed. A decision may be made to refer the patient for counseling or psychiatric care. Referrals may be made for follow-up care by community counseling services after the patient is discharged.

Other treatments that may be prescribed include biofeedback for hypertension, irregular pulse, low back pain, tension, or migraine headache. The person is taught to relax so that he or she can control body processes in response to stress. Electrodes are connected to the hands, forehead, and chest as the person reclines in a comfortable chair. Heart rate, muscle tone, and brain waves are monitored. These factors influence a signal light that glows more intensely when the patient becomes tense. When the person relaxes, the glow diminishes. As a result of this conditioning process, the person is able to use biofeedback to relax and control physiologic responses to stress or anxiety.

Nursing Interventions for Psychological Factors Affecting Medical Condition

Nursing interventions should use the holistic health care approach by treating the patient's physical, psychological, and spiritual needs. Assessment of the patient includes collection of data regarding

1. Unmet psychological and physical needs
2. Present coping or defense mechanisms
3. Present self-concept
4. Available support systems
5. Developmental level
6. Strengths that the patient demonstrates
7. Insight regarding illness

These data can be used to develop an individualized nursing care plan to meet the patient's needs. When providing traditional medical treatment, give detailed explanations regarding the importance of taking medications, adhering to a specific diet, and following through with treatments such as physical therapy. Patient education should emphasize the importance of following medical treatment and reducing stress to prevent any further structural change.

The patient's role in the holistic approach is to attempt to identify any stressor(s) related to the present physical condition, discuss ways to modify or eliminate the stressor(s), and then state specific changes that can be made. Implementation of change by the patient is attempted with minimal supervision by the nurse. For example, a patient with peptic ulcer disease identifies the fact that he has dependency needs or is angry but has been unable to reveal his feelings in the past. He states that his supervisor expects too much of him and gives him unrealistic deadlines requiring long work hours. Once the stressors are identified, the patient is assisted in citing specific ways to modify or eliminate them, such as working fewer hours, setting priorities at work regarding deadlines, and discussing his feelings with his supervisor. Identified strengths are emphasized at this time to assist the patient in modifying or eliminating the stressor(s).

Other therapeutic interventions that may be considered individually include

1. Separating the person from a specific stressor; for example, visiting may be restricted if a family member causes emotional conflict. Independent housing may be considered as a long-term goal to reduce conflict and promote independence.
2. Assisting the patient to identify positive or alternative coping mechanisms
3. Assisting the patient in identifying support systems, such as a close friend, family member, professional counselor, or member of the clergy

4. Reviewing developmental tasks with the patient and exploring ways to handle difficult or unmet tasks successfully
5. Teaching the person relaxation techniques or exercises
6. Assisting with referrals for counseling, biofeedback technique, and other options
7. Administering prescribed medication for physical or psychological needs

Somatoform Disorders

According to the DSM-IV classification, somatoform disorders differ from psychological factors affecting medical conditions in that somatoform disorders are reflected in disordered physiologic complaints or symptoms, are not under voluntary control, and do not demonstrate organic findings.

This classification is subclassified into seven categories:

1. Body dysmorphic disorder (dysmorphophobia)
2. Somatization disorder
3. Conversion disorder
4. Pain disorder
5. Hypochondriasis
6. Undifferentiated somatoform disorder
7. Somatoform disorder, NOS

Clinical Types of Somatoform Disorders

A discussion of the categories of somatoform disorders follows. These disorders are often encountered in general medical settings.

Body Dysmorphic Disorder (Dysmorphophobia) The most common age for the onset of this disorder is from adolescence through the third decade, and the disorder can persist for several years. The individual is preoccupied with an imagined defect in appearance. If a slight physical abnormality exists, the person displays excessive concern. Common complaints focus on facial flaws for which a plastic surgeon or dermatologist usually is consulted. Preoccupation causes clinically significant distress or impairment in social, occupational, or other important areas of functioning. Obsessive–compulsive traits and a depressive syndrome are frequently present.

Somatization Disorder A somatization disorder is a free-floating anxiety disorder in which a person expresses emotional turmoil or conflict through a physical system, usually with a loss or alteration of physical functioning. Such a loss or alteration of physical functioning is not under voluntary control and is not explained as a known physical disorder. The onset usually begins before age 30 years and is considered to be a chronic illness in persons who demonstrate a dramatic, confusing, or complicated medical history, because they seek repeated medical attention. The physical symptoms or complaints that occur in the absence of any medical explanation govern the person's life by influencing her or him to take medication, to alter life-style, or to see a physician.

The symptoms are not intentionally produced or feigned. When there is a related general medical condition, the physical complaints or resulting social or occupational impairment are in excess of what would be expected from history, physical examination, or laboratory findings.

The type and frequency of somatic symptoms differ across cultures; therefore the symptom reviews should be adjusted to the culture. For example, there is a higher reported frequency of somatization disorder in Greek and Puerto Rican men than men in the United States.

Anxiety and depression frequently are seen, and the patient may make frequent threats or attempts at suicide. The person also may exhibit antisocial behavior or experience occupational, interpersonal, or marital difficulties. Because the patient constantly seeks medical attention, he or she frequently submits to unnecessary surgery.

Conversion Disorder A conversion disorder is a psychological condition in which an anxiety-provoking impulse is converted unconsciously into functional symptoms. There are four subtypes based on the nature of presenting symptoms or deficit. They include:

1. Motor symptom or deficit such as impaired balance, paralysis, dysphagia, or urinary retention
2. Sensory symptom or deficit such as loss of touch or pain sensation, double vision, blindness, or hallucinations
3. Seizures or convulsions with voluntary motor or sensory components
4. Mixed presentation if symptoms of more than one category are present

Conversion disorder occurs more frequently in the rural population, in individuals of lower socioeconomic status, and in individuals less knowledgeable about medical and psychological concepts. Higher rates are also reported in developing regions. Although the disturbance is not under voluntary control, the symptoms occur in organs that are voluntarily controlled, serve to meet the immediate needs of the patient, and are associated with a secondary gain.

Patients with conversion disorder benefit by primary and secondary gain. *Primary gain* is obtaining relief from anxiety by keeping an internal need or conflict out of awareness. *Secondary gain* is any other benefit or support from the environment that a person obtains as a result of being sick. Examples of secondary gain are attention, love, financial reward, and sympathy.

Conversion disorders can be seen clinically as motor symptoms or sensory disturbances. Examples include muscular weakness or analgesia (a diminished ability to feel pain).

The term *la belle indifference* is used to describe patient reactions such as showing indifference to the symptoms and displaying no anxiety. This is because the anxiety has been relieved by the conversion disorder.

Malingering should be differentiated from conversion disorder. *Malingering* is a conscious effort to simulate or feign the symptoms of an illness to avoid an unpleasant situation. It is done for a selfish gain. An example is a person complaining of a back injury after an auto accident, with the intent to sue for financial gain.

Age of onset for conversion disorder is usually late childhood or early adulthood, but it may occur for the first time during middle age or in later maturity. Such a disorder frequently impairs normal activities and may promote the development of a chronic sick role.

Pain Disorder The DSM-IV lists two subtypes of pain disorder to clarify further the factors involved in the etiology of pain:

1. Pain disorder associated with psychological factors. Psychological factors are judged to have a major role in the onset, severity, exacerbation, or maintenance of pain. General medical conditions play either a minimal or no role in the onset of this disorder.
2. Pain disorder associated with both psychological factors and general medical condition

Diagnostic criteria state the pain is the predominant focus of the clinical presentation and is severe enough to warrant clinical attention. It causes distress or impairment in social, occupational, or other important areas of functioning. Psychological factors play a role in the onset, severity, exacerbation, or maintenance of pain.

Although pain disorder may occur at any stage of life, it is more frequently seen in women who complain of chronic pain such as headaches and musculoskeletal pain. Approximately 10% to 15% of adults in the United States have some form of work disability due to back pain.

Hypochondriasis *Hypochondriasis* is a term used to describe a condition in which the person presents unrealistic or exaggerated physical complaints. The person becomes preoccupied with the fear of developing or already having a disease or illness in spite of medical reassurance that such an illness does not exist. Minor clinical symptoms are of great concern to the person and often result in an impairment of social or occupational functioning. Preoccupations usually focus on bodily functions or minor physical abnormalities. Such persons are commonly referred to as "professional patients" who shop for doctors because they feel they do not get proper medical attention. These people often elicit feelings of frustration and anger from health care providers. Approximately 4% to 9% of patients seen in general medical practice present with hypochondriasis.

This disorder usually is accompanied by anxiety, depression, and compulsive personality traits. It generally occurs in early adulthood and usually becomes chronic, causing impaired social or occupational functioning. The person may adopt an invalid's life-style and actually may become bedridden. This disorder is found equally in men and women.

Undifferentiated Somatoform Disorder This DSM-IV diagnosis is used when one or more physical complaints such as fatigue, loss of appetite, or urinary complaints last six months or longer, and after appropriate evaluation cannot be explained by a known general medical condition or the direct effects of a substance. If a medical condition exists, the complaints or resulting social or occupational impairment are in excess of what should be expected based on a comprehensive physical examination. This is a residual category for presentations that do not meet the full criteria for the disorders previously discussed.

Somatoform Disorder Not Otherwise Specified (NOS) This category is used to diagnose somatoform symptoms that do not meet the criteria for any specific somatoform disorder. Examples include pseudocyesis or a false belief that one is pregnant; nonpsychotic hypochondriasis of less than six months; and unexplained physical complaints of less than six months not due to another mental disorder.

Treatment of Somatoform Disorders

Treatment for persons with somatoform disorders is considered both challenging and frustrating owing to the chronicity of these disorders. Before having the patient pursue psychiatric care, establish trust with the patient and eliminate the possibility of any physical disease. A person who frequently complains of being ill may be unable to convince a member of the health team when an illness does occur.

The person and the family should be told after a thorough, essentially negative physical examination that the patient has no life-threatening or severe illness, although the patient does continue to exhibit symptoms. Antidepressants may be prescribed, as well as antianxiety agents. These drugs are effective in the treatment of moderate to marked depression with variable degrees of anxiety.

Psychotherapy directed at emotional support is the most common form of therapy. Modification of the environment, as well as the use of behavior modification, may be necessary.

Nursing Interventions for Somatoform Disorders

Health care-givers must remember that physical symptoms are quite real to the hypochondriacal patient, as well as to the person with a conversion disorder, pain disorder, or somatization disorder. Nurses must be aware of verbal and nonverbal responses to the patient so that they do not appear judgmental.

Patients with somatoform disorders do not produce their symptoms intentionally. Nurses should avoid reinforcing complaints by ignoring the symptoms but never the patient. They should assess the patient's physical condition carefully, refer physical complaints to the medical staff, and attempt to understand the purpose that may be served by blindness, deafness, itching, paralysis, numbness, or whatever the complaint. The person may be using such complaints to avoid certain responsibilities (*e.g.*, educational, vocational, or familial), to receive attention, to manipulate others, to handle conflict, or to meet dependency needs.

Common behaviors or problems the hypochondriacal patient may exhibit include (1) denial of any emotional problem; (2) self-preoccupation; (3) difficulty expressing self and feelings; (4) numerous somatic complaints; (5) reliance on medications; (6) history of repeated visits to physicians, visits to emergency rooms, admissions to hospitals, or surgeries; (7) anxiety; or (8) ritualistic behaviors. Patients with conversion disorders usually experience feelings of guilt, anxiety, or frustration; physical limitations due to paralysis, blindness, and so forth; low self-esteem; or difficulty dealing with anger, frustration, or conflict.

Nursing Care Plan 17-1 presents a nursing diagnosis and goal-related nursing interventions for a patient with somatoform disorder.

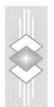

NURSING CARE PLAN 17-1
The Patient with Somatoform Disorder

Nursing Diagnosis: *Ineffective individual coping exhibited by numerous unfounded somatic complaints due to stress and anxiety

Goal: Before discharge, the patient will demonstrate a decrease in somatic complaints.

Nursing Interventions	Outcome Criteria
	Within 48 to 72 hours the patient will begin to do the following:
Establish rapport.	Demonstrate trust toward staff
Encourage verbalization of feelings rather than physical complaints.	Describe feelings to staff Demonstrate insight regarding the relationship of stress and anxiety, and unfounded somatic complaints
Explore alternative coping skills.	Identify one or two stressors contributing to anxiety Explore and use one or two effective coping skills to reduce identified stress or anxiety

*NANDA-approved nursing diagnosis.

Dissociative Disorders

The DSM-IV lists five clinical types of this category: dissociative amnesia, dissociative fugue, dissociative identity disorder, depersonalization disorder, and dissociative disorder not otherwise specified. The essential feature is a disruption of integrated functions of consciousness, memory, identity, or perception of the environment. Onset may be sudden, gradual, transient, or chronic. A summary of each clinical type follows.

Dissociative Amnesia (Formerly Psychogenic Amnesia)

Dissociative amnesia is a disorder described as the inability to recall an extensive amount of important personal information because of physical or psychological trauma. It is not the result of an organic mental disorder. Examples of predisposing factors include an intolerable life situation, unacceptability of certain impulses or acts, or a threat of physical injury or death. Amnesia can be described as

1. *Circumscribed or localized:* occurring a few hours after a traumatic experience or major event
2. *Selective:* inability to recall part of the events of a specific time
3. *Generalized:* inability to recall events of one's entire life
4. *Continuous:* inability to recall events after a specific event up to and including the present

Clinical features include perplexity, disorientation, and purposeless wandering. Although the person may experience a mild or severely impaired ability to function, it is usually temporary because rapid recovery generally occurs. The condition is more common during natural disasters or wartime. There has been an increase in reported cases related to previously forgotten early childhood trauma such as incest or sexual abuse.

Suggested treatment measures include hypnosis or narcoanalysis. Narcoanalysis is the injection of barbiturates before therapy, during which the patient's fantasies or memories are explored.

Dissociative Fugue (Formerly Psychogenic Fugue)

Fugue differs from psychogenic amnesia in that the person suddenly and unexpectedly leaves home or work and is unable to recall the past. Assumption of a new identity, partial or complete, may occur after relocation to another geographic area where the person is unable to recall his or her previous identity. Fugue is a rare occurrence that may be seen during times of extreme stress such as war, severe conflicts, or natural disasters, and may last days or months. Excessive use of alcohol may contribute to the development of this rare disorder.

The person generally must receive psychiatric care because of amnesia for recent events or lack of awareness of personal identity. Rapid recovery can occur.

Dissociative Identity Disorder (Formerly Multiple Personality Disorder)

Sybil and *The Three Faces of Eve* are popular media representations of multiple personality in which the person is dominated by at least one of two or more definitive personalities at one time. Emergence of various personalities occurs suddenly and often is associated with psychosocial stress and conflict. When two or more subpersonalities exist, each is aware of the others to varying degrees. One personality can interact with the external environment at any given moment; however, one or any number of the other personalities actively perceive all that is occurring. The individual personalities are usually quite discrepant and frequently appear to be opposites. Each is complex and integrated with its own unique behavior patterns and social relationships. For example, a shy, middle-aged bachelor may present himself as a gigolo on weekends. Passive identities tend to have more constricted memories. Controlling, hostile, or protective identities have more complete memories.

This disorder may occur in early childhood or later but rarely is diagnosed until adolescence. The degree of impairment may vary from moderate to severe, depending on the persistence, number, and nature of the various subpersonalities. This disorder can be difficult to identify unless the person is observed closely. It is seen more frequently in adult women than in adult men.

Psychiatric treatment of these rare complex personalities is quite challenging and requires the services of an experienced psychiatrist. Intermittent periods of hospitalization may be appropriate while attempting to integrate the personalities. If legal issues are raised, the person is referred to a forensic expert.

Depersonalization Disorder

The person who exhibits symptoms of this disorder experiences a strange alteration in the perception or experience of the self, often associated with a sense of unreality. This temporary loss of one's own reality includes feelings of being in a dreamlike state, out of the body, mechanical, or bizarre in appearance. Predisposing factors include fatigue, meditation, hypnosis, anxiety, physical pain, severe stress, and depression.

Clinical diagnosis includes documentation of frequent prolonged episodes that impair occupational and social functioning. Dizziness, depression, anxiety, fear of "going insane," and a disturbance in the subjective sense of time are common associated features. Adolescents and young adults are more likely to experience this disorder; it is considered rare after age 40 years.

Voluntarily induced experiences of depersonalization occur in meditative and trance practices in many cultures and religions and should not be confused with this disorder.

Although prognosis of an acute onset is good, the person may need to be removed from a threatening situation or environment to prevent the development of a chronic disorder.

Treatment similar to that listed for a conversion disorder is suggested. Psychoanalysis is also effective.

Nursing Interventions for Dissociative Disorders

Although care of patients with dissociative disorders is administered by psychiatrists or law enforcement officers to establish identity, nursing intervention may occur in such settings as the emergency room, a crisis center, or in-patient settings.

A thorough physical assessment should be done to eliminate organic causes (*e.g.*, a brain tumor). A psychosocial assessment is used to identify behavioral changes such as degree of orientation, level of anxiety, depth of depression, degree of impaired social and occupational functioning, and amount of amnesia present, if any. Environmental manipulation may reduce anxiety and make the patient feel safe and secure. People who experience feelings of being mechanical or in a dreamlike state may require assistance with their activities of daily living. Family counseling may be necessary to help family members learn new ways to deal with the patient. Common nursing diagnoses include *altered thought processes, *self-care deficit, *impaired verbal communication, and *anxiety.

 Personality Disorders

During the process of personality development, the person establishes certain traits that enable him or her to observe, interact with, and think about the environment and self. If the person develops a positive self-concept, body image, and sense of self-worth and is able to relate to others openly and honestly, she or he is said to have characteristics of a healthy personality. Should the person develop inflexible, maladaptive behaviors (*e.g.*, manipulation, hostility, lying, poor judgment, and alienation) that interfere with social or occupational functioning, the person exhibits signs and symptoms of a personality disorder.

Personality disorder is described as a nonpsychotic illness characterized by maladaptive behavior, which the person uses to fulfill his or her needs and bring satisfaction to self. These behaviors begin during childhood or adolescence as a

NANDA-approved nursing diagnosis.

way of coping and remain throughout most of adulthood, becoming less obvious during middle or old age. As a result of inability to relate to the environment, the person acts out his or her conflicts socially. Emotional, economic, social, or occupational problems are often seen as a result of such conflicts due to anxiety.

Characteristics of a personality disorder are as follows:

1. The person denies the maladaptive behaviors he or she exhibits; they have become a way of life.
2. The maladaptive behaviors are inflexible.
3. Minor stress is poorly tolerated, resulting in increased inability to cope with anxiety.
4. Ego functioning is intact but may be defective; therefore, it may not control impulsive actions of the id.
5. The person is in contact with reality although she or he has difficulty dealing with it.
6. Disturbance of mood, such as anxiety or depression, may be present.
7. Psychiatric help rarely is sought because the person is unaware or denies that his or her behavior is maladaptive.

There are 11 diagnoses grouped into three clusters or descriptive categories of personality disorders. Persons who exhibit paranoid, schizoid, and schizotypal personality disorders are considered "odd" or eccentric in the vernacular. Persons with disorders in the second cluster—histrionic, narcissistic, antisocial, and borderline personality disorders—are considered to be emotional, erratic, or dramatic in behavior. Anxious or fearful behaviors are often present in the third cluster, which includes avoidant, obsessive–compulsive, dependent, and personality disorder not otherwise specified.

Etiology of Personality Disorders

Theorists state the following etiologic factors in the development of personality disorders:

1. The person is biologically predisposed or more subject to develop the disorder. Examples of biologic predispositions include improper nutrition, neurologic defects, and genetic predisposition.
2. Childhood experiences foster the development of maladaptive behavior.

Receiving reward for behavior such as a temper tantrum encourages acting out (*i.e.*, the parent gives in to a child's wishes rather than setting limits to stop the behavior).

Creativity is not encouraged in the child; therefore, the child does not have the opportunity to express self or to learn to relate to others. The ability to be creative would provide the child with the opportunity to develop a positive self-concept and sense of self-worth.

Rigid upbringing also has a negative effect on the development of a child's personality because it discourages experimentation and promotes the development of low self-esteem. It may also cause feelings of hostility and alienation in the child–parent relationship.

Fostering dependency discourages personality development and allows the child to become a conformist rather than an independent being with an opportunity to develop a positive self-concept.

A child identifies with parents or authority figures who display socially undesirable behavior. As a result of this identification process, the child imitates behavior that he or she believes to be acceptable by others. Such behavior frequently puts the child in direct conflict with society.

3. Socially deviant persons have defective egos through which they are unable to control their impulsive behavior.
4. A weak superego results in the incomplete development of or lack of a conscience. Persons with immature superegos feel no guilt or remorse for socially unacceptable behavior.
5. The drive for prestige, power, and possessions can result in exploitative, manipulative behavior. Such is the case in prostitution, embezzlement, and gambling.
6. Urban societies, such as inner cities, are characterized by a low degree of social interaction, thereby fostering the development of deviant behavior.

Clinical Types of Personality Disorders

Following is a brief description of each of the categories of personality disorders.

Cluster A

Paranoid Personality Disorder Theorists believe that the person who develops a paranoid personality has chronic hostility that is projected onto others. This hostility develops in childhood owing to poor interpersonal family relationships. As a result, the person who has experienced much loneliness becomes unwarrantedly suspicious and mistrusts people. The person may suspect attempts to trick or harm him or her, question the loyalty of others, display pathologic jealousy, observe the environment for any signs of threat, display secretiveness, become hypersensitive, or display excessive feelings of self-importance. The person also may appear to be unemotional, lack a sense of humor, and lack the ability to relax. Features such as delusions and hallucinations may be absent. Interpersonal relationships are poor, especially when relating to authority figures or coworkers. This disorder is seen more frequently in men.

Reactions by student nurses to patients with unwarranted thoughts of suspicion include feelings of frustration, helplessness, anger, or disgust. If the patient exhibits signs of hostility, the nurse may fear aggressive behavior.

Schizoid Personality Disorder Synonyms for someone with a schizoid personality include introvert, loner, and lone wolf because the person has no desire for social involvement. The clinical symptoms include a pervasive pattern of detachment from social relationships and a restricted range of expression of emotions in interpersonal settings. The individual avoids close relationships with family or others, chooses solitary activities, has little interest in sexual experiences, does not take pleasure in activities, lacks close friends or confidants, appears indifferent to praise or criticism, and exhibits emotional coldness such as detachment or flattened affect. Attention is usually focused on objects such as books and cars rather than people. He or she may function well in vocations in which one generally works alone.

Schizotypal Personality Disorder The schizotypal classification is used to diagnose persons whose symptoms are similar to but not severe enough to meet the criteria for schizophrenia. Diagnostic criteria include

1. Disturbance in thought process (referred to as magical thinking), superstitiousness, or telepathy (a "sixth sense")
2. Ideas of reference
3. Social isolation (the person limits social contacts to those involved in the performance of everyday tasks)
4. Perceptual disturbance, such as recurrent illusions or depersonalization
5. Peculiarity in communication (noted as "odd" speech) but no loosening of association, as seen in the schizophrenic patient
6. Inappropriate affect that interferes with face-to-face interaction. The person is referred to as aloof or cold.
7. Paranoid ideation or suspiciousness
8. Odd or eccentric behavior or appearance
9. Excessive social anxiety that does not diminish with familiarity and tends to be associated with paranoid fears rather than negative judgments about self

This disorder may be first apparent in childhood or adolescence. It has been reported in about 3% of the population. Only a small percentage of individuals with this disorder develop schizophrenia or other psychotic disorders.

Cluster B

Antisocial Personality Disorder Synonyms for this personality disorder include sociopathic, psychopathic, and semantic disorder.

Several theories have been proposed to explain the development of the antisocial personality, although the exact cause is not really known. They are as follows:

1. Genetic or hereditary factors interfere with the development of positive interpersonal relationships during childhood. The child therefore does not learn to respect the rights of others. The child may become self-indulgent and expect special favors from others, but does not display appreciation or reciprocal behavior.
2. Brain damage or trauma can precipitate the development of antisocial behavior.
3. Low socioeconomic status encourages the development of an antisocial personality. People may turn to maladaptive behaviors, such as stealing, lying, and cheating, just to survive.
4. Faulty family relationships in a single-parent home inhibit normal personality development during childhood.
5. Parents unconsciously foster antisocial behavior in children during developmental years. If parents are too involved in their own personal problems or life-styles and neglect to spend time with the child or be available when help is needed, the child learns to fend for him- or herself. Any behavior that will result in a secondary gain of attention, security, or love is tried. If desirable results are obtained, the child continues to use the maladaptive behavior to meet his or her needs.

Antisocial behavior is usually seen in persons between the ages of 15 and 40 years. If diagnosed before age 18, the term, according to the DSM-IV, is *conduct disorder*. Symptoms may be evident before age 15 and include behaviors such as truancy, misbehavior at school resulting in suspension or expulsion, delinquency, substance abuse, vandalism, cruelty, and disobedience.

The DSM-IV states that the diagnosis of an antisocial personality is reserved for people age 18 years or older who exhibited signs of antisocial behavior before age 15. They also must exhibit three or more of the following clinical symptoms at age 18 years or older:

1. Lack of remorse, exhibiting indifference to persons from whom one has stolen, hurt, or mistreated
2. Expectation of immediate gratification and failure to accept social norms, resulting in unlawful behavior

3. Impulsive actions such as relocating without making specific plans for employment or living arrangements
4. Consistent irresponsibility
5. Aggressive behavior that results in fighting or assault of strangers as well as abuse of significant others
6. Lack of respect for the truth, resulting in repeated lying and similar behavior
7. Reckless behavior showing disregard for the safety of others

Cessation of criminal activities tends to occur around age 40 years. Statistics show that 80% to 90% of all crime is committed by antisocial people. Statistics also show that the diagnosis is more prevalent in men.

Borderline Personality Disorder Latent, ambulatory, and abortive schizophrenics are examples of previous labels for this DSM-IV classification. The person has symptoms that fall between moderate neurosis and frank psychosis, yet usually remains quite stable.

Theorists state that borderline disorders may be a result of a faulty parent–child relationship, in which the child does not experience a healthy separation from mother and therefore is unable to interact appropriately with the environment. Negative feelings are shared by parent and child, who are bound together by mutual feelings of guilt. Trauma experienced at a specific stage of development, usually 18 months, weakening the person's ego and ability to handle reality, is another possible cause. A third theory states that the person experiences an unfulfilled need for intimacy. As a result of attempting to establish an ideal relationship, the person becomes disillusioned and experiences feelings of rage, fear of abandonment, and depression.

According to the DSM-IV, clinical symptoms may include

1. Unstable and intense interpersonal relationships
2. Impulsive, unpredictable behavior that may involve gambling, shoplifting, and sex. Such a person tends to use and can tolerate large amounts of drugs and alcohol
3. Inappropriate, intense anger and inability to control anger
4. Disturbance in self-concept, including gender identity
5. Unstable affect that shifts from normal moods to periods of depression, dysphoria (unpleasant mood), or anxiety
6. Transient stress-related paranoid ideation or severe dissociative symptoms
7. Masochistic behavior (self-inflicted pain) and thoughts of suicide
8. Frantic efforts to avoid real or imagined abandonment
9. Chronic feelings of emptiness

Other features include feelings of overwhelming loneliness, inability to experience pleasure, and inability to maintain an occupation. This disorder is seen more frequently in women.

The main defense mechanisms identified in the borderline personality include denial, projection, splitting, and projective identification.

Rowe (1989) describes splitting and projective identification as primitive defenses. He defines *splitting* as the inability to integrate and accept both positive and negative feelings at the same moment. The person can handle only one type of feeling at a time, such as pervasive negativism or anger. This characteristic is the opposite of the feeling of ambivalence, in which a person can simultaneously experience feelings of love and hate for another person.

Projective identification is described as the ability to project uncomfortable or aggressive aspects of one's own personality onto external objects. The person is then able to protect self from the danger or threats the person perceives in the external object by attempting to control it. Examples of uncomfortable aspects of oneself include hostility, helplessness, guilt, and suspiciousness.

Histrionic Personality Disorder   The classification of a histrionic personality is characterized by a pattern of theatrical or overly dramatic behavior. The DSM-IV criteria states the individual exhibits at least five of the following behaviors:

1. Discomfort in situations in which he or she is not the center of attention
2. Inappropriate sexually seductive or provocative behavior
3. Rapid shifting and shallow expression of emotions
4. Uses physical appearance to draw attention to self
5. Exhibits a style of speech that is excessively impressionistic and lacking in detail
6. Self-dramatizes, is theatrical, and exaggerates emotions
7. Is easily influenced by others or circumstances
8. Considers relationships to be more intimate than they really are

Although the person may be creative and imaginative, feelings of dependence and helplessness exist. This condition is diagnosed more frequently in women and occurs in approximately 2% to 3% of the general population.

Students usually react with comments such as "I have a relative who acts like that" or "One of the girls in our class is always exaggerating things. Is that what's wrong with her?" One student commented that it was impossible to identify the patient's true feelings because of overall exaggerated responses when the student attempted interaction. The student felt that the patient was "pulling my leg, wanting me to believe everything she said."

Narcissistic Personality Disorder The main characteristic of a narcissistic disorder is an exaggerated or grandiose sense of self-importance. Clinical symptoms are usually seen by early adulthood. The individual exhibits five or more of the following diagnostic criteria stated in the DSM-IV:

1. Displays a grandiose sense of self-importance
2. Is preoccupied with fantasies of unlimited success, power, beauty, and the like
3. Believes he or she is unique and should associate with other high-status persons
4. Requires excessive admiration
5. Displays a sense of entitlement
6. Exploits others
7. Lacks empathy
8. Envies others and believes they are envious of him or her
9. Displays arrogance, haughty behaviors or attitudes

This disorder is prevalent in less than 1% of the general population and occurs predominantly in men.

Cluster C

Obsessive–Compulsive Personality Disorder Individuals who are obsessive–compulsive usually are preoccupied with rules and regulations, are overly concerned with organizational and trivial detail, and are excessively devoted to their work and productivity. The DSM-IV criteria list eight symptoms or behaviors exhibited by individuals with this disorder. Diagnosis is made if the individual exhibits four or more of the stated criteria:

1. Preoccupation with details, lists, and rules to the extent that the major point of the activity is lost
2. Perfectionism that interferes with task completion
3. Excessive devotion to work and productivity, thus excluding leisure activities and friendship
4. Overconscientious, scrupulous, and inflexible
5. Inability to discard worn-out or worthless objects that have no sentimental value
6. Reluctant to delegate duties to others
7. Adopts a miserly spending style
8. Displays rigidity and stubbornness

Depression is common. Interpersonal relationships are affected when feelings of resentment or hurt are experienced by a significant other. Men are affected more frequently than women.

Dependent Personality Disorder Dependent persons lack self-confidence and are unable to function in an independent role. Such persons allow others to become responsible for their lives. Following is a list of the DSM-IV diagnostic criteria for this disorder:

1. Difficulty making everyday decisions
2. Relies on others to assume responsibility for most major areas of life
3. Difficulty expressing disagreement with others
4. Difficulty initiating projects or doing things independently
5. Goes to excessive lengths to obtain nurturance and support from others
6. Feels uncomfortable or helpless when alone
7. Urgently seeks another relationship when a close relationship ends
8. Is unrealistically preoccupied with fears of being left to care for himself or herself

This diagnosis is made if the individual exhibits five or more of the criteria listed previously. According to the DSM-IV, this disorder is among the most frequently seen disorder in mental health clinics.

Avoidant Personality Disorder The avoidant personality is so sensitive to rejection, humiliation, or shame that the person appears devastated by the slightest amount of disapproval. Diagnostic criteria, according to the DSM-IV, include

1. Avoids occupational activities because of hypersensitivity to rejection, criticism, or disapproval
2. Unwillingness to enter into interpersonal relationships unless given a guarantee of uncritical acceptance
3. Social withdrawal to avoid shame or ridicule
4. Preoccupation with being criticized or rejected
5. Inhibited in new interpersonal relationships because of feelings of inadequacy
6. Views self as socially inept, personally unappealing, or inferior to others
7. Unusually reluctant to take personal risks or to engage in new activities because they may prove embarrassing

Diagnosis is based on the presence of four or more of the criteria listed above.

Feelings of anxiety, anger, and depression are common. Social phobia may result if clinical symptoms of social withdrawal and hypersensitivity persist over a period of time. This disorder is prevalent in about 10% of out-patients seen in mental health clinics.

Treatment of Personality Disorders

Management of a patient displaying a specific personality disorder is very difficult because the person is basically comfortable with her or his personality and lacks any motivation for change. A person cannot be sentenced to therapy. If treatment is sought, it is usually the result of increased anxiety that disrupts social interaction, increased awareness by the person of an unsatisfactory life-style, or the insistence of a significant other that psychiatric care be sought.

The first step in treatment is a throrough evaluation to ascertain the presence of a comorbid diagnosis such as depression, phobia, or delusional disorder. Treatment approaches include therapy that focuses on restructuring the personality, assisting the person with developmental levels and tasks, and setting limits for maladaptive behavior such as acting out.

Cognitive therapists present an information processing model to aid patients in understanding how they incorporate data that support their belief about self while excluding or discounting data that are contrary (Beck, 1996). Cognitive and behavioral therapy relate to current distressing situations and childhood experiences. Group therapy is used to reinforce the patient's realization that he or she is not unique and to discuss alternative ways to respond to stress. Reality therapy and intensive psychoanalysis are also used. Personality disorder patients can learn to think about themselves in more realistic functional ways.

Psychotropic drugs may be selected and prescribed for specific clinical symptoms or behaviors such as depression, paranoid thoughts, or aggression, and are individualized according to the patient's needs.

Treatment of any of the described disorders tends to be long-term and does not guarantee recovery. Many of the patients become semi-independent and have recurrent acute episodes.

Nursing Intervention for Personality Disorders

The nursing care of a person who is diagnosed as having a personality disorder is directed at the specific behavior, characteristics, and symptoms that are common to the identified disorder.

Maladaptive behaviors such as acting out, stubbornness, procrastination, overexaggeration, manipulation, and complete dependency can elicit negative responses from nursing personnel. A friendly, accepting environment should be established in which the patient, but not the maladaptive behavior, is accepted. It is imperative that nurses examine their own feelings about such behavior so that they do not allow such feelings to interfere with therapeutic nursing interventions.

The individual needs to be given an opportunity to develop ego controls such as the superego or conscience that is lacking or underdeveloped.

This can be achieved by consistent limit setting that is enforced 24 hours a day.

Common nursing diagnoses frequently used when planning care for individuals with personality disorders include *noncompliance, *ineffective individual coping, *altered thought processes, *impaired verbal communication, and *impaired social interaction.

Psychotropic drugs such as antianxiety or antidepressant agents and anticonvulsant medication (Tegretol, Depakene, Klonopin) to manage aggressive behavior are discussed in the chapter on psychopharmacology.

Anxiety Disorder Due to a General Medical Condition

This diagnosis was added to the DSM-IV and is used when an individual exhibits significant anxiety due to the direct physiologic effects of a general medical condition. Specifiers used to describe which symptom presentation predominates include with generalized anxiety, with panic attacks, or with obsessive–compulsive symptoms. This diagnosis is frequently seen in the general hospital, subacute units, and in long-term care facilities. For example, an individual with mitral valve prolapse may seek medical attention because of shortness of breath, increased heart rate, dizziness, and numbness and tingling in the upper extremities. If there are no abnormal physical or laboratory findings, the diagnosis would be anxiety disorder due to mitral valve prolapse.

DSM-IV criteria state that the anxiety is not better accounted for by another mental disorder, the disturbance does not occur exclusively during the course of a delirium, and there is significant distress or impairment in social, occupational, or other important areas of functioning.

Several medical conditions may cause anxiety, such as hyperthyroidism or hypothyroidism, chronic obstructive pulmonary disease, cerebral vascular accident, or arrhythmias.

Some drugs may cause anxiety-like symptoms. Examples include alcohol, caffeine, digitalis, narcotics, nonsteroidal anti-inflammatory agents, oral hypoglycemics, steroids, theophylline, and thyroid hormone. The diagnosis of substance- or alcohol-induced anxiety is also listed in the DSM-IV.

Treatment focuses on stabilizing the medical condition and providing anxiolytics as well as supportive individual or group therapy.

The nurse also supplies supportive care by giving the patient the following teaching checklist.

*NANDA-approved nursing diagnosis.

=========================== PATIENT TEACHING CHECKLIST ===========================
Anxiety

The following checklist has been developed to reinforce your knowledge about anxiety. Please inform the nurse if you are uncertain about any of the items listed below.

✔ Clinical symptoms I may experience include:
✔ The reasons I may experience anxiety include:
✔ Interventions I have learned to reduce anxiety are:
✔ Support persons I may contact include:
✔ The name of the medication I am taking is:
✔ Instructions regarding this medication
  ▪ Take this medication as directed by your doctor
  ▪ Do not drink alcohol while taking this medication
  ▪ Do not take any over-the-counter medication without informing your nurse or doctor
  ▪ Usual side effects include
  ▪ Report any unusual side effects promptly
  ▪ Antianxiety agents are generally fast acting as onset occurs within 30 minutes, full effectiveness occurs in 1 to 2 hours, and effects generally last 4 to 6 hours
  ▪ Dosage adjustment may be necessary
  ▪ Do not discontinue taking this medication without first consulting your nurse or doctor

❖ Culture-bound Syndromes

Kavanaugh (Andrews & Boyle, 1995) introduces the term *culture-bound syndromes*. For example, anorexia nervosa occurs only where food is abundant. Other conditions exist within specific cultural groups and may represent labeling differences. In China, the term *neurasthenia* is used to describe clinical symptoms similar to what Western medicine refers to as depression (p. 257). Following are examples of culture-bound anxiety-related syndromes described by Kavanaugh:

1. *Malignant anxiety*: Acute anxiety states associated with criminality and loss of stable culture due to colonialism
2. *Pibloktog*: Hysteria among Polar Eskimos such as running naked through the snow

3. *Susto:* Traumatic anxiety-depressive state that occurs throughout Latin America. Symptoms include anxiety, insomnia, listlessness, loss of appetite, and social withdrawal.
4. *Trance dissociation:* Possession syndromes believed to be caused by disease, the loss of one's soul, or the invasion of a benign or evil spirit. Occurs in various parts of the world

Treatment of such disorders also differs according to cultures. Home remedies, prayers, physical manipulation, trips to religious shrines, visiting "healers," or body massage may be used to decrease anxiety.

Summary

This chapter provided an overview of psychological factors affecting medical condition, somatoform disorders, dissociative disorders, personality disorders, anxiety disorders due to medical condition, and culture-bound syndromes. Etiology and diagnostic criteria for each category as denoted in the DSM-IV were included. Attention was given to the Social Readjustment Rating Scale developed by Holmes and Rahe, terminology related to specific disorders, and treatment or management of each disorder. Specific nursing interventions were cited. Nursing diagnoses commonly used when planning care for individuals with anxiety-related disorders were listed.

Learning Activities

I. Clinical Activities
   A. Identify patients in the clinical setting who have the diagnoses of anxiety-related disorders.
   B. Compare nursing care plans to differentiate nursing diagnoses and treatment goals.
   C. Discuss the rationale for specific nursing interventions.
   D. Compare psychopharmacologic approaches in the treatment of each disorder.
II. Situation for Discussion: Dissociative Disorder
   MJ, a 52-year-old treasurer of a large accounting firm, is suspected of having embezzled money for several years. An audit of the books substantiates the employer's suspicions. MJ is relieved of his duties and is scheduled to appear at a court hearing regarding his employer's charges. The day of the court hearing MJ is interrogated by the attorney representing his employer. MJ states that he cannot remember anything that happened during the time he worked as treasurer of the firm. The judge postpones the hearing pending the results of psychiatric testing. The tentative diagnosis is dissociative amnesia.

    A. Describe the clinical symptoms MJ is exhibiting.

    B. Discuss your role as a psychiatric nurse when caring for MJ during his psychiatric evaluation.

III. Independent Activities

    A. Read one of the following: *In Cold Blood* by Truman Capote, *Helter Skelter* by Vincent Bugliosi and Curt Gentry, or *"Son": A Psychopath and His Victims* by Jack Olsen. Evaluate your feelings about the characters who display antisocial behavior.

    B. View a prime-time television show that presents examples of maladaptive behavior (*e.g.*, police or crime shows). Identify the following behaviors:

      1. Manipulation
      2. Acting out
      3. Hostility
      4. Lying
      5. Excessive daydreaming
      6. Impulsive actions
      7. Aggressiveness

Critical Thinking Questions

1. Have three of your patients with recent health changes take the Holmes and Rahe Social Readjustment Rating Scale. How does their score relate to the timing of their illness? How can you promote their understanding of the effect that life events may have on health?

2. It is generally recommended that nursing interventions for somatoform disorders consist of a holistic approach. How "holistic" are you with any patient? How holistic are you in your own health maintenance routines? How might a holistic approach reduce health care costs?

Self-Test

1. State how Selye's general adaptation syndrome applies to the onset of an anxiety-related disorder.

2. State three methods of medical treatment for patients with the diagnosis of psychological factors affecting medical condition.

3. Discuss the assessment of patients with physical disorders resulting from stress.

4. Explain how the Holmes and Rahe Social Readjustment Rating Scale could be used to develop nursing interventions for persons with anxiety-related disorders.

5. Differentiate between hypochondriasis and somatization disorder.

6. Give examples of a secondary gain.
7. Define dissociative amnesia.
8. _____ amnesia occurs within a few hours after a traumatic experience.
9. State a situation in which dissociative fugue may occur.
10. Define multiple personality.
11. Describe depersonalization disorder.
12. Which personality disorder is considered the most common?
13. Describe narcissistic behavior.
14. List three examples of treatment prescribed for personality disorders.
15. Give an example of an anxiety disorder due to a medical condition.
16. Explain the term *culture-bound syndrome*.

SELECTED REFERENCES

American Psychiatric Association. (1994). *Diagnostic and statistical manual of mental disorders* (4th ed.). Washington, DC: Author.
Andrews, M. M., & Boyle, J. S. (1995). *Transcultural concepts in nursing care* (2nd ed.). Philadelphia: J. B. Lippincott.
Batson, R. (1992, July). Multiple personality disorder: Conceptual therapeutic resolutions. *Highland Highlights*.
Beck, J. S. (1996, February). Cognitive therapy for personality disorders. *Psychiatric Times*.
Carpenito, L. J. (1995). *Nursing diagnosis: Application to clinical pratice* (6th ed.). Philadelphia: J. B. Lippincott.
Friedman, M., & Rosenman, R. (1974). *Type A behavior and your heart*. New York: Knopf.
Hare, R. D. (1996, February). Psychopathy and antisocial personality disorder: A case of diagnostic confusion. *Psychiatric Times*.
Holmes, T. H., & Rahe, R. H. (1967, November). The social readjustment rating scale. *Journal of Psychosomatic Research*.
Lacey, J., Bateman, D., & Van Lehn, R. (1953, August). Autonomic response specificity. *Psychosomatic Medicine*.
Lancaster, J. (1980). *Adult psychiatric nursing*. New York: Medical Examination Publishing.
Minuchin S. (1974). *Families and family therapy*. Cambridge: Harvard University Press.
Rey, J. M. (1996, February). Antecedents of personality disorders in young adults. *Psychiatric Times*.
Ronningstam, E., & Gunderson, J. (1996, February). Narcissistic personality: A stable disorder or a state of mind? *Psychiatric Times*.
Rowe, C. J. (1989). *An outline of psychiatry* (9th ed.). Dubuque, IA: William C. Brown.
Selye, H. (1956). *The stress of life*. New York: McGraw-Hill.
Shapiro, D., & Crider, A. (1969). Psychophysiological approaches in social psychology. In: *The handbook of social psychology* (2nd ed.). Reading, MA: Addison-Wesley.
Smith, G. R. (1991). *Somatization disorder in the medical setting*. Washington, DC: American Psychiatric Press.

CHAPTER 18

HUMAN SEXUALITY AND SEXUAL DISORDERS

T he concept of sexual identity involves a sense of masculinity and femininity that is derived not only from biological sex drives but also from the individual's perception of his or her sexual being. This perception is partially based on experiences and interests and the attitudes of society, the culture, family, and friends.

Haffner, 1994

1   Differentiate among the terms *sex, sexual acts,* and *sexuality.*

2   Discuss the three categories of sexual and gender identity disorders as described in the DSM-IV.

3   Describe treatment modalities for various sexual disorders.

4   List common nursing diagnoses for individuals in sex therapy.

5   Discuss nursing interventions for patients who

> Make verbal comments with sexual overtones
>
> Aggressively attempt to make physical contact

Introduction

The terms *sex, sexual acts,* and *sexuality* are often used interchangeably. Trieschmann (1975) believes the terms should be differentiated. Sex is described as one of four primary drives that include thirst, hunger, and avoidance of pain. Sexual acts occur when behaviors involve the genitalia and erogenous zones. Sexuality is described as the combination of sex, sexual acts, and the psychosocial aspects of emotions, attitudes, and relationships.

Other definitions state that human sexuality is the result of biologic, chemical, and psychosocial influences on a person. Sexuality can be expressed verbally while talking to a significant other; it can be communicated in written form such as letters, poetry, or songs; and it can be expressed artistically. Behavioral expressions of sexuality include looking, touching, handholding, kissing, and so forth. Sexuality can be expressed in various ways during the development of an intimate interpersonal relationship.

The expression of sexuality may be influenced by cultural or ethnic factors, religious views, health status, physical attributes, age, environment, or personal choice as a result of one's personality development. "Normal" sexual behavior is generally described as a sexual act between consenting adults, lacking any type of force, and performed in a private setting in the absence of unwilling observers. Abnormal and unwanted sexual behavior therefore would be considered as any act that does not meet the criteria set forth in this definition.

Various sexual practices have been viewed as "normal" throughout the course of human history. The Greeks practiced homosexuality to teach young boys the attributes of manhood; Roman men openly practiced bisexual relations and frequently solicited the attention of married women. Polygamy has been practiced by various racial, religious, and cultural groups in the United States and abroad.

To work effectively with people who exhibit symptoms of sexual disorders, the nurse must examine any personal feelings about human sexuality. The nurse will come in contact with a variety of patient concerns regarding sexual identity or activity. The following examples may be experienced by any nurse. The mastectomy patient is concerned that her husband will no longer find her sexually attractive. A cardiac patient expresses a fear of resuming sexual activity after discharge from the hospital. Sexual intimacy is a concern of the colostomy patient who fears rejection owing to a change in body image and possible repugnant odors from the stoma. The paraplegic client is afraid to ask his doctor questions about sexual activity and relates his concerns to the nurse. A young man discloses his gay identity and fear of contracting acquired immunodeficiency syndrome (AIDS). The chemotherapy patient who is terminally ill requests privacy during visits by a significant other. Elderly patients of the opposite sex may ask permission to share a room in the nursing home. A teenaged girl admits to having several sexual encounters and fears having contracted a sexually transmitted disease. A middle-aged man makes sexual advances while being bathed and attempts to expose his genitals to a nurse. A young male patient asks a young nurse for her address and telephone number.

Sexuality has become a part of the nursing process in planning holistic health care. If nurses are uncomfortable with or confused about their own sexuality, they will be unable to establish a therapeutic relationship with any of the persons just mentioned. Their role as educators and their ability to discuss issues of sexuality will be ineffective if they are unaware of their own attitudes.

Formal sex education courses are available for those people who feel the need to explore the topic of sexuality. Masters and Johnson's books *Human Sexual Response* and *Human Sexual Inadequacy* are excellent reference sources. Other useful books are listed at the end of this chapter.

Classifications

This DSM-IV classification lists two new categories under Sexual and Gender Identity Disorders. They include sexual dysfunction due to a general medical condition and gender identity disorders. Sexual dysfunctions and paraphilias complete the disorders in this classification. A brief overview of each of the categories is presented.

Sexual Dysfunctions

Characteristics of this category include a disturbance in the processes that characterize the sexual response cycle or the presence of pain during sexual intercourse. The phases of the response cycle are identified as desire, excitement, orgasm, and resolution. Subtypes are used to indicate the etiology and context in which the disorder occurs. For example, the dysfunction may occur at the onset of sexual functioning, or it may develop after a period of normal functioning. It may be the result of inhibitions, psychological factors, impaired communication between partners, or certain types of stimulation.

The classification of sexual dysfunctions includes nine categories. The psychologically induced inability to perform sexually may result in

1. Hypoactive sexual disorder—This diagnosis is used only if the lack of desire causes distress to the person or the person's partner. Factors such as age, health, frequency of sexual desire, and life-style are considered when one is interviewing the person seeking help.
2. Sexual aversion disorder—Anxiety, fear, or disgust occurs when confronted with a sexual opportunity.
3. Female sexual arousal disorder—The woman may experience little or no subjective sense of sexual arousal.
4. Male erectile disorder—The inability to attain or maintain an adequate erection.
5. Female orgasmic disorder.
6. Male orgasmic disorder
    (These two categories are used to diagnose recurrent, persistent inhibited orgasm following an adequate phase of sexual excitement in the absence of any organic cause.)
7. Premature ejaculation—Ejaculation occurs before the person wishes owing to the absence of reasonable voluntary control during the sexual act.
8. Dyspareunia—This diagnosis is used to describe recurrent, persistent genital pain in the male or female not due to a general medical condition.
9. Vaginismus—Spasms of the musculature of the outer third of the vagina are recurrent, persistent, and involuntary, thus interfering with the sexual act.

Sexual Dysfunctions Due to a General Medical Condition

This disorder is distinguished from the previous disorder by the presence of clinically significant sexual dysfunction that is due to the direct physiologic effects of a general medical condition. Marked distress or interpersonal difficulty occurs during sexual activity. The subtypes of this disorder include

1. Female hypoactive sexual desire disorder due to . . .
2. Male hypoactive sexual desire disorder due to . . .
3. Male erectile disorder due to . . .
4. Female dyspareunia due to . . .
5. Male dyspareunia due to . . .
6. Other female sexual dysfunction due to . . .
7. Other male sexual dysfunction due to . . .
8. Substance-induced sexual dysfunction

Some common physical disorders that could cause difficulty with sexual activity are arteriosclerosis, liver disease, hypertension, thyroid disorder, and sexually transmitted diseases.

Medications that interfere with sexual activity have been identified as alcohol, antihypertensive drugs, cortisone, narcotic analgesics such as morphine and codeine, antihistamines, and sedatives. The presence of these conditions would need to be investigated before a diagnosis of sexual dysfunction is made.

Paraphilias

The DSM-IV describes paraphilia as a disorder in which unusual or bizarre sexual acts or imagery are enacted to achieve sexual excitement. An example would be simulated bondage, in which pain is inflicted with materials such as leather straps, handcuffs, whips, and chains. Paraphiliac imagery is subclassified further as severe sexual sadism when the imagery involves a nonconsenting partner who is injured as a result of such activity. Sexual masochism describes the injury of self during imagery.

Paraphiliacs generally are not seen by mental health professionals unless their behavior has created a conflict with society. Nonconsenting partners may report such activity to the legal profession. Concerned neighbors may suspect that children are the object of sadistic sexual behavior and inform the police or the child welfare bureau of such abuse. Voyeurism, exhibitionism, and pedophilia are three subclassifications of behavior that usually result in arrest and incarceration.

A list of paraphilias addressed in the DSM-IV follows.

Bestiality or Zoophilia Sexual contact with animals serves as a preferred method to produce sexual excitement. It is rarely seen.

Exhibitionism An adult male obtains sexual gratification from repeatedly exposing his genitals to unsuspecting strangers, usually women and children who are involuntary observers. He has a strong need to demonstrate masculinity and potency.

Fetishism Sexual contact with inanimate articles (fetishes) results in sexual gratification. Most often it is a piece of clothing or footwear. Parts of the body may also take on fetishistic significance. Its occurrence is almost exclusive with men who fear rejection by members of the opposite sex.

Frotteurism Sexual excitement is achieved by touching and rubbing against a nonconsenting person.

Masochism Sexual pleasure occurs while one is experiencing emotional or physical pain. The willing recipient of erotic whipping is considered to be masochistic.

Necrophilia Sexual arousal occurs while the person is using corpses to meet sexual needs. This disorder is classified as an atypical paraphilia.

Pedophilia The use of prepubertal children is needed to achieve sexual gratification. Pedophilia can be an actual sexual act or a fantasy.

Sadism Sexual gratification is experienced while the person inflicts physical or emotional pain on others. Severe forms of this behavior may be present in schizophrenia.

Telephone Scatologia Sexual gratification is achieved by telephoning someone and making lewd or obscene remarks.

Transvestism A heterosexual male achieves sexual gratification through wearing the clothing of a woman (cross-dressing). It is a learned response due to encouragement by family members. As a child, the person was considered more attractive when dressed up as a girl.

Voyeurism The achievement of sexual pleasure by looking at unsuspecting persons who are naked, undressing, or engaged in sexual activity. Individuals engaging in voyeurism are commonly called "Peeping Toms."

Characteristics of Paraphiliacs

A person may experience more than one paraphiliac disorder at the same time or may exhibit clinical symptoms of other mental disorders (*e.g.*, a personality disorder or schizophrenia).

Characteristics or associated features of persons who are classified as paraphiliacs include

1. Emotional immaturity (seen in the pedophiliac or "Peeping Tom," who is unable to engage in a mature heterosexual relationship owing to feelings of inadequacy)
2. Fear of a sexual relationship that could result in rejection
3. Shyness (seen in the voyeur who views others from a distance)
4. The need to prove masculinity, demonstrated by the exhibitionist
5. The need to inflict pain on another to achieve sexual satisfaction (seen in sadistic behavior)
6. The need to endure pain to achieve sexual satisfaction (experienced by the masochist)
7. Low or poor self-concept
8. Depression

Not all of these characteristics are present in each paraphiliac. Theorists state that the way a paraphiliac expresses himself or herself sexually affords a clue to the paraphiliac's self-concept. For example, the fetishist who has a very low self-concept chooses inanimate objects to satisfy sexual needs and therefore does not have to fear rejection by a partner.

If nurses understand the dynamics of paraphiliac behavior and are able to separate the behavior from the person, they are prepared to handle feelings of repulsion, anger, and frustration. To give therapeutic care, nurses need to be nonjudgmental and display a genuine interest in the person as they deal with their own ethical and moral values.

Gender Identity Disorders

The diagnostic features for this disorder are twofold. The DSM-IV states there must be evidence of a strong and persistent cross-gender identification in which one expresses the desire to be or the insistence to be of the opposite sex. The individual also experiences persistent discomfort about his or her assigned sex or feels inappropriate in the role of the assigned sex. Impairment occurs in social, occupational, or other important areas of functioning.

Boys identify with girls or women and are preoccupied with feminine activities. Girls display intense negative reactions when parents attempt to feminize them. They polarize to male attire and activities and prefer to associate with boy playmates.

Adult men and women who are preoccupied with their wish to live as the opposite sex may act on their desires by adopting behavior, dress, and mannerisms of the opposite sex. Cross-dressing and hormonal treatment may be attempted to pass convincingly as the other sex.

European statistics cited in the DSM-IV indicate that approximately 1 per 30,000 men and 1 per 100,000 adult women seek sex-reassignment surgery. There are no statistics available for the United States.

Transcultural Considerations

As stated earlier, an individual's ethnic, cultural, religious, and social background may influence sexual attitude, desire and expectations. Andrews (in Andrews & Boyle, 1995) comments about cultural norms related to appropriate male–female and same-sex relationships. Failure to adhere to cultural code is considered to be a serious transgression. In some cultures, sexual desires of the woman are not considered relevant; fertility is the primary function of the woman. What is considered deviant sexual behavior in one cultural setting may be an acceptable practice in another culture.

Research Regarding Sexual Orientation

According to D. Hamer, author of a study on sexual orientation, new evidence indicates that a gene from mothers influences male sexual orientation. The 1993 study also states that there probably are additional biologic factors at work, such as hormones and other variables unknown at this time. Another study, similar to Hamer's, suggests such a gene resides in a particular region of the X chromosome that men inherit from their mothers. (Hamer's research is included in the November, 1995 issue of the journal *Nature Genetics*.)

Treatment of Sexual Disorders

Treatment is individualized according to the type of disorder, underlying causative factors, and presenting symptoms. Jacobson, in her article "Illness and Human Sexuality" (1974), describes a bill of rights to guarantee sexual freedom and promote sexual health. These seven rights include the patient's right to express his or her sexuality, to become the person he or she desires to be, and to select a sex partner of choice, regardless of the partner's sex.

Persons in the health care field need to familiarize themselves with this type of philosophy because it provides an excellent reference when one is handling various sexual issues. Sexual acting-out may occur in the general hospital setting as the patient attempts to test sexuality owing to the loss of independence, low self-esteem, loss of a body part, loneliness, fear, anxiety, or loss of control.

Behavior frequently seen includes flirting, deliberate exposure of the genital area, dressing in seductive attire, touching the care-giver inappropriately, using profanity, or making provocative comments. Some patients use a shock approach by blatantly discussing promiscuous sexual activity or telling jokes that center on sexual contact.

The nurse is better able to handle such behavior by remembering that all behavior has meaning. Reactions such as verbal chastisement, shunning or ignoring the patient, or judging the patient's behavior are negative responses that should be avoided. Exploration of feelings, evaluation of the appropriateness of touch, and encouragement of normal sexual behavior are imperative if the nurse hopes to help the patient to express sexuality in a positive manner.

Treatment of paraphiliacs focuses on individual or group therapy to explore feelings of sexuality, anxiety, depression, and frustration. Methods of coping are also discussed.

Behavioral therapy, group therapy, and aversive therapy all focus on altering or managing unacceptable or undesirable behaviors. In aversive therapy, negative stimuli (*e.g.*, electric shock or an emetic) are used to condition the person each time an undesirable sexual act occurs. The undesirable behavior decreases because the person wishes to avoid the punishment associated with the negative stimuli. Loomis (1996) discusses behavior therapy in relation to paraphilia and sexual dysfunction.

Hormonal therapy to reduce sex drive has been reported in professional literature. Drugs used include Androcur, Provera, and Depo-Provera. Stilbestrol has been used as adjunctive therapy to reduce incidents of cross-dressing or transvestism. SSRIs (e.g. Paxil, Zoloft) are prescribed to reduce libido.

Environmental manipulation also has proven effective in relieving anxiety and altering undesirable behavior. Incarceration may be imposed legally in an effort to protect the public, especially children, from being victimized by persons such as pedophiles. The prisoner may then be interviewed and accepted into a special program using one or more of the therapies mentioned.

 ## Nursing Intervention

As stated earlier, nurses must examine feelings about their own sexuality before they are able to care for paraphiliacs who sexually act-out or present symptoms of psychosexual disorders. Nurses are not immune to the development of psychosexual dysfunction. Feelings of disgust, contempt, anger, or fear need to be identified and explored so that they do not interfere with the development of a therapeutic relationship. This is one of the reasons patients do better with a team approach rather than with individual therapy. If the nurse is unable to be objective while giving care, the nurse should have another member of the health team care for the patient. The quality of nursing care depends on the

BOX 18-1 Basic Principles of Sexual Assessment

1. Be comfortable and at ease.
2. Establish empathy.
3. Avoid personal values and biases during the interview.
4. Ensure a thorough knowledge base.
5. Ask specific rather than general questions.
6. Approach emotional or more sensitive questions gradually.
7. Progress from how information was learned, to attitudes, then behaviors.
8. State that certain sexual behaviors are common before asking questions about them.

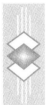

NURSING CARE PLAN 18-1

The Patient Demonstrating Impulsive Sexual Activity

Nursing Diagnosis: *Altered sexuality patterns: Impulsive sexual actions resulting in physical contact with staff and peers

Goal: Before discharge, the patient will exhibit socially acceptable behavior in the presence of peers and staff.

Nursing Interventions	Outcome Criteria
	Within 24 to 48 hours the patient will begin to do the following:
Explain to the patient that touching makes you feel uncomfortable. Explain to the patient that he or she must respect the rights of others.	Demonstrate respect for the rights of others by attempting to control impulsive physical contact
Ask the patient to explain his or her feelings when the patient acts impulsively.	Demonstrate trust toward staff Verbalize feelings to staff regarding impulsive behavior Demonstrate insight into own behavior
Be firm but nonjudgmental when setting limits.	Demonstrate an understanding of rationale for limit setting
Be consistent. Intervene in any overt acts toward other patients.	Agree to limit setting and specified consequences
Provide protective isolation from other patients if necessary because his or her overt behavior may provoke hostility. Avoid placing the patient in activities requiring physical contact.	Demonstrate socially acceptable behavior while participating in scheduled unit activities

*NANDA-approved nursing diagnosis.

344

nurse's ability to be nonjudgmental and to understand the behavior of a patient who is sexually acting-out. The nurse needs to be supportive yet set limits, so that the patient's behavior is socially acceptable.

Lief and Berman (1981) discuss eight basic principles to guide sexual assessments. They are listed in Box 18-1. Schultz and Videbeck (1994) also address nursing interventions related to issues of sexuality and homosexuality in the clinical setting.

Nursing interventions for patients who exhibit symptoms of sexual disorders also include planning care to meet the basic human needs, providing a structured environment, providing protective care for the patient, exploring methods to rechannel sexually unacceptable behavior, and participating in a variety of therapies, including behavior therapy, aversive therapy, and psychotherapy. The nurse must also assume the role of patient advocate to ensure the promotion of sexual health when the opportunity occurs.

Nursing diagnoses that are commonly used while implementing care include *altered sexuality patterns, *sexual dysfunction, *self-esteem disturbance, *body image disturbance, *anxiety, *fear, and guilt. Nursing Care Plan 18-1 presents a nursing diagnosis and goal-related nursing interventions for the individual demonstrating impulsive sexual activity.

 Summary

The concept of human sexuality was discussed. The DSM-IV categories of sexual and gender identity disorders were explained. Sexual acting-out behavior of hospitalized patients as well as the responses of nursing personnel were explored. Diagnostic criteria, associated features, and treatment methods were presented. Nursing diagnoses commonly used while implementing care were listed. Nursing interventions for patients exhibiting symptoms of sexual disorders were cited. Basic principles of sexual assessment were stated.

Learning Activities

I. Clinical Activities
  A. Assess your patient's sexual role satisfaction or sexuality while giving care.
  B. Evaluate the treatment plan for appropriateness. If indicated, plan and implement nursing interventions. List any additional suggestions regarding the care of this patient.

---

*NANDA-approved nursing diagnosis.

II. Clinical Situation for Discussion: Sexual Dysfunction

JK, a 36-year-old executive, was admitted to ICU with the diagnosis of myocardial infarction. The father of two children, JK has confided in the nurse that he is afraid to resume his duties as husband and father. He also stated that he is afraid to play golf even though the attending physician assured him he would eventually be able to lead a normal life if he adhered to the doctor's orders. After a visit by his wife, JK appeared withdrawn and apprehensive. As the nurse made evening rounds, JK complained of chest pain and stated that he thought his doctor was sending him home too early. Later that evening Mrs. K called the nurses' station and asked to talk to the head nurse. She expressed concern over her husband's withdrawal, lack of interest in visiting with her, and fear of going home. A week later JK was discharged. When he arrived home, he informed his wife that they should sleep in separate bedrooms so that he could get adequate rest. After two months of recuperation, JK was still unable to have sexual relations with his wife.

A. What behavior did JK exhibit that might indicate the onset of symptoms of sexual dysfunction? Note that the doctor feels that JK will be able to lead a normal life.

B. State nursing interventions that would have been appropriate to help JK express concern about his sexual role satisfaction while he was hospitalized.

C. What community services are available to help couples like JK and his wife understand the dynamics of their sexual relationships?

III. Independent Activities

A. Examine your feelings about your own sexuality.

B. Discuss or evaluate your feelings in response to the following situations:

1. A 22-year-old female college student is admitted to your unit for an emergency appendectomy. Following surgery you notice that the patient is visited by a "close friend," a woman who holds the patient's hand and strokes her hair. The visitor hugs the patient quite affectionately each time upon leaving.

2. A 29-year-old man is admitted to your unit to undergo tests before surgery for sex reassignment (transsexual surgery). You are assigned to care for this patient.

3. A 31-year-old man is admitted for gallbladder surgery. As you prepare the patient's room for his return from surgery, you notice he has several "skin" magazines and a woman's undergarment tucked under his pillow.

C. Refer to the works of Masters and Johnson (see Selected References) to familiarize yourself with their work.

Critical Thinking Questions

1. Team up with a classmate and interview each other concerning personal sexual history. After the interviews, discuss when you considered not telling the truth, when you became embarrassed, and what thoughts and feelings you experienced when evaluating how to answer each question. Could the interviewer tell when these feelings were occurring?
2. If you and your classmate, who know each other, felt embarrassed, how might a new patient feel? How might you make the patient more comfortable? How would you adjust the interview for a patient your own age? for a patient your father's age?
3. Prepare an inservice presentation on the anatomy and physiology of human sexual response. What did you learn? How will this information help you understand patients with sexual dysfunction?

Self-Test

1. Define paraphilia.
2. A person who desires to live, dress, and act out as a member of the opposite sex has the following disorder: _____.
3. A person who achieves sexual gratification by wearing the clothing of the opposite sex exhibits _____.
4. State four characteristics of paraphiliacs.
5. Cite an example of a sexual dysfunction.
6. List three examples of treatment of paraphiliacs.
7. Match the following:

   (1) Sadism   (a) Necrophilia
   (2) An example of masochism   (b) Self-inflicted pain
   (3) "Peeping Tom"   (c) Transsexualism
   (4) Sexual use of corpses   (d) Voyeurism
                                 (e) Erotic whipping of an unconsenting adult

8. List four nursing interventions for impulsive sexual actions that result in physical contact.
9. State the rationale for limit setting when caring for patients with sexual disorders.
10. List four reasons a patient may sexually act-out while hospitalized for a medical or surgical problem.

SELECTED REFERENCES

American Psychiatric Association. (1994). *Diagnostic and statistical manual of mental disorders* (4th ed.). Washington, DC: Author.

Andrews, M. M., & Boyle, J. S. (1995). *Transcultural concepts in nursing care* (2nd ed.). Philadelphia: J. B. Lippincott.

Cabaj, R. C. (1988, January). Gay and lesbian couples: Lessons on human intimacy. *Psychiatric Annals.*

Callanan, M. (1996, January). Sexual assessment and intervention for people with epilepsy. *Clinical Nursing Practice in Epilepsy.*

Carpenito, L. J. (1995). *Nursing diagnosis: Application to clinical practice* (6th ed.). Philadelphia: J. B. Lippincott.

Drench, M. E., & Losee, R. H. (1996, May/June). Sexuality and sexual capacities of elderly people. *Rehabilitation Nursing.*

Haffner, D. (1994, September). Sexuality and aging: The family physician's role as educator. *Geriatrics.*

Jacobsen, F. M. (1995, February). Managing sexual dysfunction and SSRIs. *Psychiatric Times.*

Jacobson, L. (1974, January). Illness and human sexuality. *Nursing Outlook.*

Katzin, L. (1990, January). Chronic illness and sexuality. *American Journal of Nursing.*

Kripke, C. C., & Vaias, L. (1994). The importance of taking a sensitive sexual history. *Journal of the American Medical Association 271*, p. 713.

Lief, H. I., & Berman, E. M. (1981). *Sexual interviewing throughout the patient's cycle: Sexual problems in medical practice.* Chicago: American Medical Association.

Loomis, M. E. (1996). Behavior therapy. In S. Lego (Ed.), *Psychiatric nursing: A comprehensive reference* (2nd ed.). Philadelphia: Lippincott–Raven Publishers.

Masters, W., & Johnson, V. (1966). *Human sexual response.* Boston: Little, Brown.

Masters, W., & Johnson, V. (1970). *Human sexual inadequacy.* Boston: Little, Brown.

Schultz, J. M., & Videbeck, S. D. (1994). *Manual of psychiatric nursing care plans.* Philadelphia: J. B. Lippincott.

Teets, J. M. (1990, December). What women talk about: Sexuality issues of chemically dependent women. *Journal of Psychosocial Nursing and Mental Health Services.*

Trieschmann, R. B. (1975). Sex, sex acts, and sexuality. *Archives of Physical Medicine and Rehabilitation 56*, pp. 8–9.

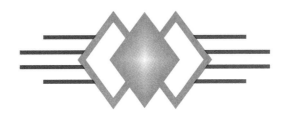

CHAPTER 19

ALTERED MOOD: DEPRESSION AND MANIA

T he high prevalence of depression in the general population, coupled with the disease's multifactorial etiology and extreme diverse presentation, makes diagnosis and treatment of this mood disorder a challenge for even the most astute clinician.

An Overview of Depressive Illness in Therapeutic Horizons, 1993

1 List five primary risk factors for depression.

2 Describe the causative factors pertaining to mood disorders.

3 Differentiate among the clinical symptoms of

Major depressive disorder

Bipolar I disorder

Bipolar II disorder

4 Differentiate between dysthymic disorder and cyclothymic disorder.

5 Discuss the rationale for each of the following modes of treatment in mood disorders: psychotherapy, chemotherapy, occupational or recreational therapy, phototherapy, and electroshock therapy.

6 State examples of nursing diagnoses frequently used in the clinical setting when providing care for individuals with mood disorders.

7 Construct a sample care plan for an individual exhibiting clinical symptoms of depression.

Introduction

Depression is the most common of the mental health disorders and the most treatable. It can manifest itself as "the blues" or sadness; grief; mourning; nonpathologic depression; pathologic or psychotic depression; or manic behavior.

Referred to as the "common cold" of psychiatry, approximately 5.2% of the United States population suffers from depression in any one month. Translated into numbers, approximately 9.5 million Americans are affected. These figures are based on estimates from the 1990 census of 182.6 million people aged 18 years and older. Estimates were provided by the National Institute of Mental Health. The lifetime risk of depression severe enough to require treatment may be as high as 20% or even higher. Women are at greater risk for depression than are men and they are more likely to seek treatment. Major depressive disorder is common in primary care outpatients (4% to 8%). According to various estimates, 50% of cases of depression may go undiagnosed and untreated (Angst, 1992; Wells et al., 1989).

Infants may exhibit signs of anaclitic depression or failure to thrive when separated from their mothers. School-aged children may experience depression along with anxiety and exhibit signs of hyperactivity. Teenage depression and suicide occur because of feelings of loneliness, low self-concepts, and drug abuse. Depression is common in older patients (*i.e.*, aged 60 years and older), particularly those living in long-term care facilities.

The DSM-IV still features two categories of mood disorders, depressive disorders and bipolar disorders; however, there has been a restructuring of the subtypes under bipolar disorders. Specific diagnostic criteria and symptoms are discussed within each category of mood disorders.

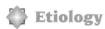 Etiology

In the past, causative factors were classified as genetic, biochemical, and environmental. There are a variety of medical illnesses that are highly correlated with depression. People of any age may experience depression as an adverse medication effect, although older adults are more likely than younger adults to experience medication-related psychiatric problems. A discussion of the causative factors as well as the primary risk factors for the onset of depression follows.

Genetic Predisposition Theory

According to statistics by the National Institute of Mental Health, various studies of adoptees have found higher correlations of depression between depressed adoptees and biologic parents than with adoptive parents. Studies of twins have shown that if an identical twin develops an affective disorder, the other twin has a 70% chance of also developing the disorder. The risk decreases to about 15% with siblings, parents, or children of the afflicted person. Grandparents, aunts, or uncles have about a 7% chance of developing an affective disorder.

Theorists also state that a dominant gene may influence or predispose a person to react more readily to experiences of loss or grief, thus manifesting symptoms of depression.

Biochemical Theory

Biogenic amines, or chemical compounds known as norepinephrine and serotonin, have been shown to regulate mood and to control drives such as hunger, sex, and thirst. Increased amounts of these neurotransmitters at receptor sites in the brain cause an elevation in mood; decreased amounts can lead to depression. This explanation is termed the *biogenic amine hypothesis.*

High levels of the hormone cortisol have also been observed in depressed persons. Normally, cortisol levels peak in the early morning, level off during the day, and reach the lowest point in the evening. Cortisol peaks earlier in depressed persons and remains high all day.

Environmental Theory

Financial problems, any type of loss, physical illness, perceived or real failure, and midlife crises are all examples of environmental factors contributing to the development of a depressive disorder. Examples of persons at risk or more prone to depression from environmental and psychosocial factors include

1. Separated, divorced, or widowed persons who lack companionship and usually suffer from loneliness
2. Young, poor mothers who are single heads of households. This group is faced with raising children and maintaining a household without emotional or financial support and is particularly prone to depression.
3. Young women who have been taught to be helpless. They are unable to assert themselves to face realities, solve problems, or make decisions.
4. Parents experiencing the "empty-nest syndrome." When children leave home, parents who have devoted their lives to raising them no longer feel needed and experience feelings of uselessness or loneliness.
5. Children who experience a real or perceived loss of a valued object. The dynamics of depression during childhood begin as the child develops a low self-esteem followed by a real or imagined loss such as parental love or attention. The child experiences ambivalent feelings toward the loss and develops guilt feelings as the negative or "hate" half of the ambivalence is experienced. Repression occurs as the child buries or hides such negative feelings. Any time negative feelings toward the valued object occur, the child becomes angry and experiences feelings of hostility and aggression turned inward.
6. People who think negatively. Norman Vincent Peale, author of *The Power of Positive Thinking*, and Aaron Beck, a noted psychiatrist, have both stated that a peron's mood can be influenced by the way she or he thinks. If a person is negative about self, the world, and the future, negative memories occur at the expense of positive experiences. Behaviorists and cognitive therapists propose that people become depressed because of having learned negative ways of acting and thinking. They believe that such persons need to reinterpret negative or distorted thoughts and actions more realistically and positively.
7. Elderly persons experiencing a decline in physical well-being or involuntary relocation such as long-term care placement.
8. Persons who abuse alcohol or other drugs. Alcohol is a depressant; many drugs depress the central nervous system (CNS) when they are abused.
9. Adverse medication effects can cause a depressive syndrome that may or may not remit when the medication is discontinued. Examples include histamine blockers, cardiac medications including antihypertensives, CNS depressants, antianxiety agents, antipsychotics, antiparkinson agents,

steroids, analgesics, nonsteroidal anti-inflammatory agents, antineoplastic agents, antimicrobials and oral hypoglycemics.

10. Persons with a chronic, debilitating, or terminal illness may experience feelings of loneliness, helplessness, or a low self-concept because of loss of independence. Several medical illnesses that are either mistakenly diagnosed as depression or are underlying causes of depression include nutritional deficiencies, CNS disorders, metabolic and endocrine disorders, fluid and electrolyte disturbances, and cardiovascular disturbances.

 ## Risk Factors for Depression

The following risk factors for depression have been established as clinical practice guidelines for primary care practitioners:

1. Prior episodes of depression
2. Family history of depressive disorder
3. Prior suicide attempts
4. Female gender
5. Age of onset younger than 40 years
6. Postpartum period
7. Medical comorbidity
8. Lack of social support
9. Stressful life events
10. Current alcohol or substance abuse
11. Presence of anxiety, eating disorder, obsessive–compulsive disorder, somatization disorder, personality disorder, grief, adjustment reactions. Depression may coexist with other psychiatric conditions.

 ## Diagnostic Categories

Depression has been categorized in many ways. One method is by placing depressive behaviors on a continuum from mild or transitory depression to severe depression. Mild depression is exhibited by affective symptoms of sadness or "the blues"—an appropriate response to stress. The person who experiences such depression may be less responsive to the environment and may complain of physical discomfort; however, the person usually recovers within a short period. For example, a person may become disappointed when told that he or she was not chosen as a representative to a conference that the person hoped to attend. During this time she or he may be unable to concentrate, may communicate less with coworkers, may appear less productive than normal, and may isolate self at work and at home.

Moderate depression is the depressive state that includes the DSM-IV sub-classifications of dysthymia and cyclothymia. Clinical symptoms are less severe than those experienced in a major depressive disorder and do not include psychotic features.

Severe depression is a category for persons with the DSM-IV subclassifications of major depressive disorder and bipolar disorder. Persons with severe depressive disorders can exhibit psychotic symptoms such as delusions and hallucinations. Major depressive disorders also are referred to as endogenous depression, a depression that appears to develop from within a person with no apparent cause or external precipitating factor. Depression caused by biochemical imbalance is such an example.

Clinical symptoms of moderate and severe depression can be classified as somatic, or physical, and as psychological. Somatic symptoms described by Rowe (1980), Donlon and Rockwell (1982), and Walker (1982) include

1. *Fatigue:* Approximately 80% of those persons complaining of fatigue, lethargy, the inability to perform normal tasks, or lack of energy, suffer from depression.
2. *Psychomotor retardation or pronounced reduced mental and physical activity:* The person may lack motivation, be indecisive, exhibit a slumped posture and awkward body movements, and appear lethargic. The person usually complains of an inability to concentrate and may exhibit slowed or muffled speech when communicating.
3. *Psychomotor agitation or pronounced agitated mental and physical activity:* These symptoms may occur as a result of increased anxiety experienced by the depressed person. Restlessness, pacing or constant walking, purposeless movements, or an inability to concentrate may occur.
4. *Chronic generalized or local pain:* The person is assessed to be apparently healthy, but complains of persistent headaches, back pain, or some other chronic pain.
5. *Sleep disturbances:* Depressed persons complain either of insomnia or of fatigue and lethargy that result in excessive sleeping. Sleep patterns may consist of difficulty falling asleep, difficulty staying asleep, difficulty sleeping soundly, or early morning awakening.
6. *Disturbances in appetite:* Persons who are depressed may experience symptoms of anorexia or loss of appetite, or they may be compulsive overeaters. Significant weight loss or weight gain occurs.
7. *Gastrointestinal complaints:* Nausea, diarrhea, and constipation are complaints frequently voiced by depressed persons.
8. *Impaired libido:* Decreased interest in sex or decreased responsiveness to sexual stimuli may be a concern of the depressed person.

9. *Anhedonia:* The inability to experience pleasure when participating in acts that normally produce pleasure may occur during depression.
10. *Lack of interest in self-care:* The person loses interest in personal appearance and neglects washing, grooming, and changing clothes.

Psychological symptoms of depression are as follows:

1. *Deep sense or feeling of sadness:* Characterized by crying, gloom, and a sad facial expression
2. *Anxiety:* Depressed persons may experience internal feelings of anxiety or psychomotor agitation that interfere with daily functioning.
3. *Unconscious anger or hostility directed inward:* Described in the dynamics of childhood depression. Such persons are irritable, restless, or easily annoyed.
4. *Guilt feelings:* Pertaining to real or imagined failures
5. *Indecisiveness:* Doubt about life and the future
6. *Lack of self-confidence:* A poor self-concept; this may result in thoughts of self-destruction.

Depressive Disorders

A comprehensive list of clinical symptoms of depression was presented in the discussion of diagnostic categories. Major depressive disorder, dysthymic disorder, and depressive disorder not otherwise specified are included in this category. A discussion of each follows.

Major Depressive Disorder

The DSM-IV diagnostic criteria state that persons with a major or severe depressive disorder do not experience momentary shifts from one dysphoric or unpleasant mood to another, as is seen in dysthymic and cyclothymic disorders. The individual must exhibit five or more of nine depressive symptoms during a two-week period and exhibits a depressed mood or loss of interest or pleasure. The symptoms interfere with social, occupational, or other important areas of functioning. The symptoms are not due to physiologic effects of a substance, nor are they due do a general medical condition.

Major depressive disorder may be coded as mild, moderate, or severe, with or without psychotic features, and as in partial or full remission. Reference is made as to whether this is a single or recurrent episode.

Dysthymic Disorder

Symptoms of dysthymia are similar to those of a major depressive disorder or severe depression; however, they are not as severe and do not include psychotic symptoms such as delusions, hallucinations, and impaired communication or

CLINICAL EXAMPLE 19-1
Major Depressive Disorder

AS, a 25-year-old professional basketball player, complained of fatigue during practice. He had a few episodes of vertigo the previous week and also stated he could not remember the different plays the coach recently designed. The team physician examined AS. During the examination, AS revealed that he didn't enjoy playing basketball anymore, had no interest in socializing with his peers or fiancée, and felt as if he "didn't belong" or fit in with other members of the team. The physician noted that despite no physiologic reason for a weight loss, AS had lost 15 pounds since his last physical examination. AS described a lack of appetite for approximately two weeks. The team physician was able to determine that AS was exhibiting clinical symptoms of a major depressive disorder without psychotic features or suicidal ideation, and subsequently prescribed an antidepressant and supportive psychotherapy.

incoherence. Clinical symptoms usually persist for two years or more and may be present all the time or may occur intermittently with normal mood swings present for a few days or weeks. Persons who develop dysthymic disorders are usually overly sensitive, often have intense guilt feelings, and may experience chronic anxiety.

According to DSM-IV criteria, the individual must exhibit, while depressed, two or more of six clinical symptoms, including poor appetite or overeating, insomnia or hypersomnia, low energy or fatigue, low self-esteem, poor concentration or difficulty making decisions, and feelings of hoplessness. Clinical symptoms interfere with various aspects of functioning and are not due to a medical condition or the physiological effects of a substance.

Depressive Disorder Not Otherwise Specified

This diagnosis is used to identify disorders with depressive features that do not meet the criteria for major depressive disorder, dysthymic disorder, adjustment disorder with depressed mood, or adjustment disorder with mixed anxiety and depressed mood.

Bipolar Disorders

This category includes bipolar I disorder, bipolar II disorder, cyclothymic disorder, bipolar disorder not otherwise specified. An overview of each disorder follows.

⚙ CLINICAL EXAMPLE 19-2
Dysthymic Disorder

KD, an elderly widow, was admitted to a nursing home with the diagnosis of depression. KD's husband had died four years earlier, when KD was 72 years old. At that time, she had moved into a senior citizens' apartment complex but was unable to care for herself because of crippling arthritis. She was transferred to a nursing home, where the staff noted that KD would become extremely agitated at times, complain of shortness of breath, and refuse to leave her room. Although the staff attempted to communicate with KD, she would tell them to leave the room. One of KD's nurses found her to be extremely apprehensive, crying, and complaining about nursing care. She confided in the nurse that she prayed every night that she would die. KD refused to participate in her care and dismissed the nurse from her room. The second day the same nurse noticed a change in KD's behavior as the patient apologized for her irritability and rudeness. She confided that various problems had been upsetting her. Later she agreed to take a walk with the nurse but was unable to tolerate the noise and activity of the hall and asked to return to her room.

The student nurse shared her experiences with KD in a multi-disciplinary team conference. KD had been diagnosed as having dysthymic depression three years before her admission. KD appeared to be depressed "most of the time," and frequently talked about death. The nurse shared her "innermost" feelings when she stated "I felt so helpless when she became upset and questioned why God didn't let her die." The next day the nurse was able to bring a volunteer's dog to KD's room and noticed that she responded with a smile while she petted the dog and talked to it. The staff commented that the only time KD appeared happy was when the dog visited twice a week. The conference focused on underlying emotions and psychological symptoms of depression that KD exhibited.

Bipolar I Disorder

At least two million Americans suffer from bipolar disorder. For those affected with the illness, it is extremely disruptive. Bipolar I disorder is a recurrent disorder in which the individual may experience one or more manic episodes or mixed episodes. During a manic episode, the individual exhibits an abnormal, persistently elevated, expansive or irritable mood that lasts for at least one week. Three of the following seven criteria must be present to a significant degree: inflated self-esteem or grandiosity, decreased need for sleep, pressure to keep talking, flight of ideas, distractibility, psychomotor agitation or

CLINICAL EXAMPLE 19-3
Bipolar I Disorder

MS, a 45-year-old housewife, was admitted to the psychiatric unit with the diagnosis of bipolar I disorder. The student nurse who assisted with the admission procedure noted that MS was wearing excessive rouge, eye shadow, and lipstick. Her purple dress was adorned with several necklaces, two neck scarves, and two belts. MS's fingernails and toenails were covered with purple nail polish. Every time the student attempted to question her, she would respond in a rapid, loud voice. The student noted that MS was easily distracted and appeared to jump from one idea to another while talking. She also described herself as an "indispensable" member of her church's governing board and stated, "I need to get home so that I can help the pastor make some important decisions." During the next several days, the student noted that MS was unable to sleep at night. Although she participated in numerous activities during the day, MS was not able to complete any projects successfully owing to a short attention span and distractibility. She would approach various patients and share intimate personal secrets with them.

During the postclinical conference, students who had attempted to relate to MS made various comments such as, "I can't believe someone really dresses like that," "Does she really believe she is needed by the pastor to make decisions?" and "How can I communicate with someone who talks so fast? I have difficulty understanding her."

increase in goal-directed activity, and excessive involvement in pleasurable activities that could result in painful consequences. Impairment in various areas of functioning, psychotic symptoms, and the possibility of self-harm exist.

Bipolar II Disorder

This disorder is characterized by recurrent major depressive episodes with hypomanic (a mood between euphoria and excessive elation) episodes. It is believed to occur more frequently in women than in men. Statistics cited in the DSM-IV indicate approximately 0.5% of the U. S. population will experience this disorder. Approximately 85% of those individuals are fully functional between episodes.

Diagnostic criteria require that the person have a presence or history of one or more major depressive episodes alternating with at least one manic episode. The symptoms cause significant impairment in areas of functioning.

CLINICAL EXAMPLE 19-4
Cyclothymic Disorder

WB, a 35-year-old plumber, was repairing a water heater when he began to talk rapidly and tell one joke after another to the homeowner. He laughed inappropriately and began to brag about his ability to "out-work" other employees. When WB returned to the company warehouse, his supervisor told him that the homeowner had called to inform him about WB's job performance and behavior. The supervisor expressed concern about WB's actions; the past several months he had noted that WB appeared to be either very happy or depressed. He described WB's mood as similar to the tracks of a roller coaster with several ups and downs. WB was advised to see his family physician before he would be permitted to continue to work.

Cyclothymic Disorder

This diagnosis is used when an individual displays numerous periods of hypomanic symptoms and depressive symptoms that do not meet the criteria for a major depressive episode. Such symptoms occur for at least two years, in which time they do not subside for more than two months at a time. The symptoms are not due to a general medical condition or the physiologic effects of a substance. Significant distress causes impairment in areas of functioning.

The subtypes used to describe this disorder include single manic episode or most recent episode mixed, hypomanic, depressed, and unspecified. During a mixed episode, clinical symptoms of both a manic episode and major depression last at least one week. A hypomanic episode occurs when the individual exhibits three of seven manic symptoms at least four days. The episode is not severe enough to cause marked impairment in various areas of functioning.

This disorder occurs equally in men and women. The lifetime prevalence is estimated to be 0.4% to 1.6% of the U.S. population. Approximately 90% of the individuals who experience this disorder experience recurrent episodes.

Mood Disorder Due to a General Medical Condition

As stated earlier in this chapter, depression can occur as the result of adverse medication effects or as the direct physiologic consequence of a medical condition. The individual exhibits a prominent and persistent disturbance in mood, which is depressed, markedly diminished, elevated, expansive, or irritable. History, physical examination, or laboratory findings confirm the diagnosis of

CLINICAL EXAMPLE 19-5
Mood Disorder Due to a Cerebral Vascular Accident (CVA)

CD, a 55-year-old woman, was admitted to a sub-acute unit in a long-term care facility for rehabilitation. Before the CVA, she had taught school for 30 years. During hospitalization, CD exhibited a flat affect, labile emotion, anger, loss of appetite, and insomnia, and would respond "I don't know" to questions posed by the staff. The clinical symptoms continued and appeared to interfere with physical therapy. A swallow study was conducted to rule out dysphagia. The results were negative. A psychiatric consultation was requested. The diagnosis confirmed the presence of a mood disorder secondary to a CVA.

depression in the absence of delirium. Symptoms cause clinically significant impairment in areas of functioning.

The DSM-IV cites the prevalence of this disorder as 25% to 40% of individuals with certain neurologic conditions.

Other Mood Disorders

Bipolar disorder not otherwise specified and mood disorder not otherwise specified are used to identify disorders that do not meet the criteria for bipolar I disorder, bipolar II disorder, cyclothymic disorder, or mood disorder due to a general medical condition.

Although substance-induced mood disorder is included in this classification, it is also discussed in substance-related disorders and coded as such.

Transcultural Considerations

Depressive symptoms differ in various cultures. Depression may be experienced in somatic terms. Culturally distinctive experiences may be misdiagnosed as psychotic symptoms. There appears to be no differential incidence of bipolar I disorder based on race or ethnicity. Clinicians may have a tendency to diagnose schizophrenia instead of bipolar disorder in some ethnic groups.

Research

Brown (1995) discusses research into herbal medicines for treatment of psychiatric disorders. The National Institute of Mental Health has funded a pharmacologic treatment research program. Approximately 146 natural products have been tested. A plant known as Saint-John's-wort has been found to act as an antidepressant. The World Health Organization recently completed a study of the use of ginkgo as an adjunct to Elavil in the treatment of depression.

Medina (1995) discusses the career of manic-depression research since 1987. He cites the various pseudogenetic studies dealing with the linkage between human genes and human behaviors. "No gene for bipolar disorder has been isolated. . . . There is strong disagreement as to the number of genes actually involved in the disease. The ups and downs of the published literature illustrate the enormous problems researchers encounter attempting to describe human behavior in terms of genetic sequence" (p. 30).

Holman and Devous (1992) review research regarding depression during the last 10 years. There are indications of reduced global blood flow or glucose metabolism occurring in patients with major depressive disorder. Studies cite a relationship between cerebral biochemistry and symptom severity. Conclusions are considered to be premature at this time.

Treatment of Depression and Mania

Hospitalization is recommended for those persons who are severely depressed, displaying suicidal ideation, or requiring medical care secondary to depression. Persons displaying symptoms of acute manic behavior require hospitalization as well.

Antidepressant drugs, when necessary, usually are started immediately because symptomatic relief usually is not achieved for approximately two to four weeks after therapy has been initiated. Tricyclic antidepressants may be prescribed for persons with symptoms such as decreased appetite, weight loss, decreased energy, or poor sleep habits. The advent of selective serotonin reuptake inhibitors has changed prescribing practices in the treatment of depression. (See Chapter 12 for additional information.)

Remeron (mirtazapine) is an antidepressant recently approved for use by the Food and Drug Administration. It is categorized as an atypical antidepressant that enhances central noradrenergic and serotonergic activity. Efficacy has not been established in the general psychiatric population. Initial clinical trials included 2,796 individuals.

Lithium also is started immediately to treat bipolar disorder because it is quite effective in controlling mania. It is considered a potentially dangerous drug because the therapeutic level is slightly less than the toxic level. Serum levels must be monitored for toxic level, and the patient should be observed for side effects. Patients usually respond to levels of 0.8 to 1.5 mEq/liter. Toxic levels occur above 1.5 or 2.0 mEq/liter. Because lithium takes approximately two weeks to effect change in the patient's symptoms, a major tranquilizer also is prescribed until the lithium is effective.

Stimulants such as Ritalin or Cylert are used clinically to treat treatment-resistant depression. Anticonvulsant drugs are used to treat patients whose mood swings are unusually rapid.

Individual, family, group, cognitive, or behavioral psychotherapy may be prescribed to treat depression. Manic persons should show some response to medication before therapy sessions, such as decreased agitation and restlessness, and an increased attention span.

In addition, occupational or recreational therapy is used to channel the activity level of persons exhibiting manic behavior or psychomotor agitation and to increase the self-esteem of depressed persons.

Phototherapy, or the exposure to bright artificial light, can markedly reverse symptoms of seasonal depression that occurs in the fall and winter (referred to as seasonal affective disorder or SAD). Phototherapy presumably works by shifting the timing or phase of the circadian rhythms of patients with depression. Morning light advances the timing, whereas evening light delays the timing of circadian rhythms. Thus, using artificial light to simulate morning light can be effective for persons with SAD (Lewy et al., 1987).

Antianxiety agents may be prescribed for persons who also manifest symptoms of anxiety. Sedative-hypnotics, such as barbiturates, may be ordered to treat underlying anxiety and sleep disturbances.

Psychotropic drugs may be prescribed to treat acute psychotic symptoms, such as hallucinations and delusions, as well as symptoms of agitation, overactivity, and combativeness in major depression.

Electroconvulsive (electroshock) therapy is effective in the treatment of depression, especially for persons who are nonresponsive to chemotherapy or who require a rapid remission of symptoms. (Electroconvulsive therapy is usually effective within a few days.)

Some types of depression are considered treatable by a family physician; however, persons exhibiting the following behaviors should be referred to a mental health care specialist: failure to respond to drug therapy, suicidal ideation, recurrent manic episodes, and irrational thinking.

The assessment, treatment, and nursing intervention for persons who express feelings of hopelessness, helplessness, worthlessness, and suicidal thoughts are discussed in Chapter 20.

 ## Nursing Interventions

Persons who are depressed may be difficult to communicate with or approach. Isolation, withdrawal, ambivalence, hostility, guilt, or impaired thought processes are but a few symptoms that can interfere with the development of a therapeutic relationship. The manic patient's hyperactivity, pressured speech, and manipulation also interfere with attempts at communication.

The nurse must be aware of personal vulnerability to depressive behavior. Working with such persons may cause one to react to the depressed atmosphere and in turn experience symptoms of depression. The following is a list of attitudes that the nurse should display toward depressed and manic persons:

1. *Acceptance.* The nurse should spend time with the patient and accept the patient for what he or she is. Depressed persons are not always able to express feelings and may exhibit peculiar behavior. Because depressed persons exhibit a low self-esteem, the care-giver should avoid acting in any manner that could be interpreted as rejection or criticism. The manic patient's manipulative, demanding behavior may elicit feelings of disgust and nonacceptance. The nurse should make the manic person aware that the nurse will accept the person but not the behavior. Limit setting is one way of displaying acceptance.
2. *Honesty.* The nurse should be truthful, not make promises that she or he is unable to keep, and not provide false reassurance. The depressed person is less able to tolerate disappointment.
3. *Empathy.* Any attempts to cheer up a depressed person will be viewed as an inability to understand her or his feelings or problems. Such an approach may cause further withdrawal, isolation, and depression. The care-giver should provide the person with an opportunity to express negative, painful feelings and respond in such a way as to convey the message that one recognizes and empathizes with the emotions, thoughts, or feelings of another.
4. *Patience.* Depressed persons may be unable to make decisions as simple as what to eat for breakfast or what items of clothing to wear. The nurse should be aware of the impact of psychomotor retardation on decision making. Psychomotor agitation also requires patience. Underlying anxiety in the depressed person may cause hyperactivity, anger, and hostile behavior. The nurse also must demonstrate patience while setting limits with the demanding, manipulative manic patient. Such persons can try one's patience, resulting in feelings of frustration, irritation, and anger on the part of the care-giver.

Assessment focuses on mood, affect, behavior, and appearance. Body language replaces communication skills because the person is unable to convey feelings of anger, hostility, and ambivalence.

Several assessment scales are used to determine the presence of depression. They include the Hamilton Rating Scale for Depression, Global Assessment of Functioning, Wakefield Questionnaire, Beck Depression Inventory, and Geriatric Depression Scale.

Questions the nurse can ask the patient to assess the level of depression, while observing facial expressions, body posture, tone of voice, and overall appearance, include the following:

1. Do you have difficulty falling asleep at night?
2. Do you experience middle-of-the-night awakening?

3. If so, are you able to return to sleep?
4. Do you awaken earlier than usual in the morning?
5. Are you alert or depressed when you get up in the morning?
6. Do you sleep excessively?
7. Have you been experiencing feelings of worthlessness, self-reproach, or inappropriate guilt?
8. Do you have difficulty concentrating or making decisions?
9. Can you watch an entire movie or television show?
10. Does your mood change or fluctuate during the day?
11. Has your sex drive lessened?
12. Are you frequently constipated?
13. Has your energy level decreased?
14. Have you lost interest in life?
15. Has there been a change in your appetite?
16. Do you feel alienated from those around you?
17. Have you ever considered or attempted suicide? (If so, ask the patient when, and whether he or she has a plan at present.)

Nursing intervention includes assisting the person in meeting basic human needs. The more severe the depression, the more important becomes physical care because the person loses interest in self-care. Patients who exhibit manic behavior also may neglect personal hygiene. The care-giver may need to assist the person with bathing and grooming, as well as with personal hygiene. Because appearance is neglected, the patient may need help with selecting the appropriate attire to wear, as well as with washing and pressing clothing.

Dietary needs should be monitored. The depressed person may be too uninterested to eat, whereas the manic person may be too hyperactive to eat. Intake and output (I & O) should be monitored until the patient is able to take the responsibility of meeting nutritional needs.

Periods of rest and activity need to be evaluated because depressed patients may sleep continuously in an attempt to avoid the problems and anxieties of reality. Dysthymic depression is characterized by increased feelings of depression as the day progresses. Such persons generally "feel better in the morning." Persons with major depressive disorders or psychotic depression fall asleep easily, awaken early, and feel better as the day progresses.

Simple activities are most effective for a person with a short attention span or an inability to concentrate. Completion of such tasks enhances the person's self-concept because he or she feels more worthwhile after the job is done. One also must consider the person's energy level; the more energy the task requires, the less energy the person will have to engage in hostile, aggressive behavior.

Protective care may be necessary for the manic as well as for the depressed person. Persons who exhibit manic behavior may injure themselves owing to excessive motor activity, inability to concentrate, distractibility, and poor judgment. Their destructive tendencies may include self-inflicting behavior and accidental injury. They also may provoke self-defensive actions unintentionally from others who fear injury.

Depressed persons may attempt self-inflicted harm or suffer injury owing to severe depression, lack of interest, psychomotor retardation, the inability to concentrate, or the inability to defend themselves against aggressive persons. The nurse should be aware of the potential for self-destructive behavior. Such an action may occur as the person's psychomotor retardation lessens, the ability to concentrate returns, and the person is able to formulate a plan of action.

Assisting with electroconvulsive or electroshock therapy is another nursing intervention while caring for depressed patients. Such persons are given a complete physical examination before treatment. The nurse's role before treatment is to withhold breakfast and to administer an anticholinergic medication to decrease or dry up body secretions to lessen changes of aspiration during treatment. The nurse must be available to answer any questions the patient may have, to provide supportive care, and to assist with the treatment and monitor the person's responses during a recovery period that usually lasts from a half hour to one hour. Care of the patient undergoing electroconvulsive therapy is described in detail in Chapter 8.

Observing for side effects of psychotropic drugs is another responsibility of the nurse. Tricyclic antidepressants may cause dry mouth, blurred vision, drowsiness, difficulty with urination, and constipation. Antipsychotic drugs may produce extrapyramidal side effects. (Refer to Chapter 12 for additional information.)

Monoamine oxidase inhibitors (MAOIs) require strict dietary adherence. Foods to be avoided include yogurt, cheese, wine, beer, pickled herring, chopped liver, sour cream, yeast extracts, and chocolate. Hypertensive crisis may occur after the administration of such drugs if the person combines the drug with food containing tyramine.

Lithium blood levels must be monitored frequently during an acute phase of bipolar disorder and on a routine basis during the maintenance phase because toxicity may occur in response to excessive doses of the drug or in the presence of a decreased serum sodium level. The therapeutic level is usually between 0.8 and 1.5 mEq/liter. Diuretics, profuse diaphoresis, a low-salt diet, or diarrhea may result in lowered serum sodium levels and higher lithium levels. Symptoms of lithium toxicity include vomiting, diarrhea, weight loss, excessive thirst, abnormal muscle movement, muscle twitching, slurred speech, blurred vision, dizziness, stupor, and an irregular heart beat.

Patient education is another nursing intervention for depressed and manic persons. Such persons should be informed about the importance of outpatient treatment as well as the continuation of prescribed drugs. They may be placed on longer-term maintenance levels of medication and could suffer a relapse if they discontinued the drugs. They should be taught to recognize the onset of side effects, as well as the recurrence of symptoms, to avoid rehospitalization. A person diagnosed as having bipolar disorder, mixed type, was able to describe the changes in affect and behavior in the initial phases of his illness.

He related to the student nurse that "I could feel the changes coming on." He had been instructed to notify his attending physician or psychiatrist whenever he experienced such changes so that his outpatient treatment could be reevaluated in an effort to prevent the development of severe symptoms.

Manic patients should be cautioned not to take on too many responsibilities or to overextend themselves. Depressed persons should be instructed to contact a support person if feelings of depression return or increase in intensity.

Another aspect of nursing care is that of being supportive during psychotherapy sessions. The person may have difficulty expressing feelings of hostility, ambivalence, and guilt. Feelings of anxiety may occur or increase as the person begins therapy sessions. Such sessions may be directed at exploring feelings about self and one's relationship with the environment in an attempt to improve the person's self-esteem and decrease feelings of helplessness, hopelessness, and powerlessness. The nurse can be supportive by supplying the teaching checklist, by being available to the patient, and by recognizing symptoms such as underlying anxiety.

 ## Nursing Diagnoses

Examples of nursing diagnoses frequently used in the clinical setting while providing care for individuals exhibiting symptoms of affective disorders include agitation, anger, *anxiety, *impaired verbal communication, *impaired social interaction, *self-esteem disturbance, manipulation, *altered nutrition (less than body requirements), *risk for injury, and *sleep pattern disturbance. Nursing Care Plan 19-1 (on pp. 368–369) describes nursing diagnoses and goal-related nursing interventions for a patient with suicidal ideation and manic behavior.

 ## Summary

Depression, an emotional state that most people experience at one time or another, can manifest itself along a continuum from feelings of sadness to psychotic depression. Depression also may manifest itself in the form of

NANDA-approved nursing diagnosis.

━━━━━━━━━━━━━━━━━ PATIENT TEACHING CHECKLIST ━━━━━━━━━━━━━━━━━
Depression

The following checklist has been developed to reinforce your knowledge about depression. Please inform the nurse if you are uncertain about any of the items listed below.

✔ Clinical symptoms I may experience include:
✔ The reasons I may be depressed are:
✔ Interventions I have learned to reduce depression are:
✔ Support persons I may contact include:
✔ The name of the medication I am taking is:
✔ Instructions regarding this medication
   ▪ Take this medication as directed by your doctor
   ▪ Antidepressant medication usually takes 2 to 3 weeks to reach a therapeutic level
   ▪ Dosage adjustment may be necessary
   ▪ Do not drink alcohol or take over-the-counter medication without informing your nurse or doctor
   ▪ Usual side effects include
   ▪ Report any unusual side effects promptly
   ▪ Do not discontinue taking this medication without consulting your nurse or doctor

hyperactivity and manic behavior. Theories pertaining to the causative factors of mood disorders were discussed. Risk factors indicating the potential for the development of mood disorders were listed. The diagnostic categories of mood disorders, including major depressive disorder, dysthymic disorder, depressive disorder not otherwise specified, bipolar I and II disorders, cyclothymic disorder, mood disorder due to a general medical condition, and substance-induced mood disorder were discussed. Transcultural considerations and current research were included. Treatment of depression and mania focused on the various psychotropic drugs as well as supportive therapies. Nursing interventions focused on nursing attitudes; assessment, including the use of assessment scales; implementation of care to meet physiologic and psychological needs; observation for side effects of prescribed drugs; and patient education. (The reader is referred to Chapters 8, 12, and 20 for information related to electroconvulsive therapy, the use of antidepressants, and the protective care of the suicidal patient.) Examples of nursing diagnoses frequently used in the clinical setting were stated. A sample nursing care plan was given focusing on the nursing diagnosis of *risk for injury related to suicidal

*NANDA-approved nursing diagnosis.

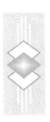

NURSING CARE PLAN 19-1
The Patient with Suicidal Ideation and Manic Behavior

Nursing Diagnosis: *Risk for injury related to suicidal ideation
("I want to die.")

Goal: The patient will remain free of injury during hospitalization.

Nursing Interventions	Outcome Criteria
	During hospitalization, the patient will do the following:
Use suicidal intention rating scale to assess lethality (see Chapter 20).	Agree to a suicide contract Notify staff of suicidal ideation
Implement suicide precautions (see Chapter 20 for protective care of the suicidal patient).	Demonstrate an understanding of the purpose of protective care Demonstrate compliance with unit rules and regulations
	Within 24 to 48 hours the patient will do the following:
Accept the patient as she or he is.	Feel accepted as a worthwhile individual
Assign the same staff members to work with the patient whenever possible.	Demonstrate trust toward staff; feel safe and secure in the therapeutic environment
Use therapeutic communication skills such as silence and active listening to encourage verbalization of feelings.	Begin to verbalize thoughts and feelings
Administer prescribed antidepressant medication.	Demonstrate compliance regarding prescribed medication
Educate the patient regarding purpose of medication and potential side effects.	Demonstrate an understanding of the purpose of antidepressant medication

Nursing Diagnosis: *Risk for injury related to manic behavior of hyperactivity, restlessness, and agitation

Goal: The patient will remain free of injury during hospitalization.

Nursing Interventions	Outcome Criteria
	Within 48 to 72 hours the patient will begin to do the following:
Limit or reduce environmental stimuli whenever possible	Exhibit a decrease in hyperactivity, restlessness, and agitation
Encourage verbalization of feelings	Verbalize feelings of stress or tension *(continued)*

NANDA-approved nursing diagnosis.

NURSING CARE PLAN 19-1 (Continued)

Nursing Interventions	Outcome Criteria
Limit participation in activities, in terms of group size and frequency, based on level of tolerance	Recognize the need to avoid overstimulation during periods of restlessness or agitation
Set goals to provide consistency and structure within the environment	Demonstrate compliance with goal-setting
Administer psychotropic medication (*e.g.*, Lithium) as prescribed to prevent injury to self or destructive behavior	Regain self-control

ideation and *risk for injury related to manic behavior of hyperactivity, restlessness, and agitation.

Learning Activities

I. Clinical Activities
   A. Begin a relationship with a person experiencing symptoms of a mood disorder.
      1. Identify the person's level of depression or manic behavior.
      2. List physiologic and psychological symptoms.
      3. Describe the person's appearance, behavior, and ability to communicate.
      4. Does the person exhibit any signs of suicidal intent?
      5. List any psychotropic drugs ordered, evaluate their action, and observe for any side effects. State what nursing management and health teaching should be done for each drug taken.
      6. List therapies being used and discuss value or effectiveness of each.
   B. Familiarize yourself with the agency's precautions for suicidal patients, as well as seclusion and restraint procedures.
   C. Chart your observations and interactions.
   D. Develop a nursing care plan for this person.
II. Mood Disorder Situation
   KJ, a 39-year-old widow, seen in the emergency room, complains of difficulty sleeping at night, headache, fatigue, and an uneasy feeling that she is unable to explain. These symptoms have persisted over the past several months and have become increasingly worse. She has lost approximately eight lbs owing to anorexia and is having difficulty with constipation. KJ is diagnosed as having a dysthymic disorder. Develop a brief but specific nursing care plan for this patient.

*NANDA-approved nursing diagnosis.

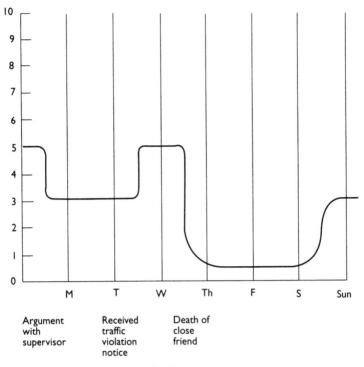

FIGURE 19-1 Sample Mood Self-Assessment

III. Independent Activities
  A. List at least three situations in which you have observed persons who appeared to be depressed. Was the cause of the mood change identifiable? Was the mood change appropriate to the cause? What coping mechanisms or support systems did the person use?
  B. Read *Darkness Visible: A Memoir of Madness* by William Styron.
  C. Assess your own mood states for 1 week by plotting a daily graph. Using a scale of 1 to 10, indicate feelings of sadness at the lower level of the scale and feelings of well-being or elation at the higher level, with 5 as the normal level. List those situations influencing any changes in your mood directly under the number and day of the week indicated on the scale. See Figure 19-1 for an example.

Critical Thinking Questions

1. As winter progresses, you notice that a classmate seems depressed and unmotivated. Attempts to discuss a mutual class project are met with disinterest. At first you are confused, but after several weeks, you notice she isn't dressed as

neatly as usual, is eating all the time, and is sleepy in class. What major depressive disorder do you suspect? What question should you ask her to ascertain if your conclusion is correct? What recommendations can you make to her?

2. Observe the population in a homeless shelter or community group home. What behaviors do you observe? Interview some of the staff. Are they prepared for managing client behaviors? What changes might improve their therapeutic effectiveness?

3. Your depressed patient confides in you that her new medication, Elavil, isn't working and she is going to stop taking it. On checking her medication Kardex, you notice she has been on Elavil for seven days. Prepare a patient education lesson plan to teach her about this drug.

Self-Test

1. State three theories pertaining to the development of a mood disorder.
2. List five examples of persons who are more at risk for development of depression.
3. State five somatic symptoms associated with depression.
4. Discuss four psychological symptoms associated with depression.
5. Differentiate between dysthymic disorder and major depression.
6. Differentiate between bipolar I disorder and bipolar II disorder.
7. Explain the criteria for the diagnosis of mood disorder due to a general medical condition.
8. Describe at least three treatment modalities used when providing care to individuals with the diagnosis of a mood disorder.
9. List five nursing interventions used during the care of an individual with bipolar I disorder.
10. State the rationale for monitoring serum lithium levels.
11. Compare the different types of antidepressants used to stabilize clinical symptoms of depression.

SELECTED REFERENCES

American Psychiatric Association. (1994). *Diagnostic and statistical manual of mental disorders* (4th ed.). Washington, DC: American Psychiatric Press.

Angst, J. (1992). Epidemiology of depression. *Psychopharmacology, 106.*

Beck, A. T., Ward, C., Mendelsohn, M., Mock, J., & Erbaugh, J. (1961, April). An inventory for measuring depression. *Archives of General Psychiatry.*

Brown, S. J. (1995, December), Mental health researchers explore Hindu herbs. *Clinical Psychiatry News.*

Carpenito, L. J. (1995). *Nursing diagnosis: Application to clinical practice* (6th ed.). Philadelphia: J. B. Lippincott.

Donlon, P., & Rockwell, D. (1982). *Psychiatric disorders: Diagnosis and treatment.* Bowie, MD: Robert J. Brady.

Fowler, L. F. (1992, March). Family psychoeducation: Chronic psychiatrically ill Caribbean patients. *Journal of Psychosocial Nursing and Mental Health Services.*

Holman, L., & Devous, M. D. (1992, October). Functional brain SPECT: The emergence of a powerful clinical method. *Journal of Nuclear Medicine.*

Karch, A. M. (1996). *Lippincott's nursing drug guide.* Philadelphia: Lippincott–Raven Publishers.

Kronberg, M. E. (1995, May). Down in the dumps: Depression in the primary care setting. *Advance for Nurse Practitioners.*

Lewy, A. J., Slack, R. L., Miller, S., et al. (1987). Antidepressant and circadian phase-shifting effects of light. *Science, 235,* 352–354.

Medina, J. (1995, February). Pseudogenetics, part II. *Psychiatric Times.*

Overview of depressive illness. (1993, May). In R. Spencer (Ed.). *Therapeutic Horizons.*

Rothschild, A. J. (1993, December). The dexamethasone suppression test in psychiatric disorders. *Psychiatric Annals: The Journal of Continuing Psychiatric Education.*

Rowe, C. J. (1980). *An outline of psychiatry.* Dubuque, IA: William Brown.

Sanders, S. L. (1996, June). A protocol for diagnosing and treating depression. *Advance for Nurse Practitioners.*

Styron, W. (1990). *Darkness visible: A memoir of madness.* New York: Random House.

Walker, J. I. (1982). *Everybody's guide to emotional well-being.* San Francisco: Harbor Publishing.

Wells, K. B., Hays, R. D., Rogers, W. H., et al. (1989). Detection of depressive disorder in prepaid and fee-for-service practices: Results from the medical outcomes study. *Journal of the American Medical Association, 262.*

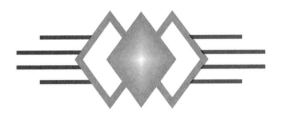

CHAPTER 20

RISK FOR SELF-DIRECTED VIOLENCE: SUICIDE

E very client has the potential for suicide which may be the culmination of self-destructive tendencies that have resulted from the client's internalizing his or her anger.

Schulz & Videbeck, 1994

LEARNING OBJECTIVES

1 State five causative factors or motives for self-destructive behavior.

2 Identify those persons considered to be at risk for or prone to self-destructive behavior.

3 State examples of verbal and behavioral suicidal clues.

4 Discuss cultural beliefs about suicide.

5 Differentiate between suicidal ideation, intent, threat, gesture, and attempt.

6 Differentiate among primary, secondary, and tertiary prevention in relation to nursing care of the suicidal patient.

7 Explain the importance of self-assessment when working with suicidal patients.

8 Define the term *postvention*.

9 Discuss the medical treatment of suicidal persons.

10 Describe the therapeutic milieu for a patient on suicidal precautions.

11 List therapeutic nursing interventions when caring for a person exhibiting self-destructive behavior.

Introduction

Suicide is the eighth leading cause of death in the United States, claiming approximately 30,000 lives each year. It is the third leading cause of death among people aged 15 to 24 years. The need to be loved and accepted, along with a desperate wish to communicate feelings of loneliness, alienation, worthlessness, helplessness, and hopelessness, often result in intense feelings of anxiety, depression, and anger or hostility directed toward the self. If no one is available to talk to or listen to such feelings of insecurity or inadequacy, a suicide attempt may occur in an effort to seek help or end an emotional conflict.

Statistics regarding the frequency of and mortality rate due to suicide vary according to which sources publish the data. The following information, therefore, is a summation of statistical data available from 1988 through 1993. Resources include the National Institutes of Health, the Harvard School of Public Health, the *American Journal of Epidemiology*, the Centers for Disease Control, the *Psychiatric Times*, and the *American Journal of Public Health*.

1. Suicide is the second leading cause of death among college students. Approximately 18 American adolescents commit suicide daily. Children

aged 10 to 14 years are killing themselves three times more often than they were 25 years ago.

2. There are approximately 500,000 attempts yearly.

3. One of every ten persons entertains recurrent or persistent thoughts of suicide (suicidal ideation).

4. Approximately 1% of the annual deaths in the United States are reported as suicide. A more realistic figure is 2% to 3%; however, such attempts generally are reported as accidents to spare families the stigmatizing impact of suicide and to facilitate insurance coverage that otherwise would not occur in the event of suicide.

5. Approximately 80% of those persons contemplating suicide consult their family physician about some other matter before such an attempt. Such a visit may be a cry for help because of feelings of ambivalence about suicide or part of a well planned scheme to obtain lethal material (*e.g.*, sleeping pills).

6. Approximately 39% of all suicides are persons 65 years of age and older.

7. Approximately 80% of those persons attempting suicide give clues. Such clues are categorized as verbal or behavioral. *Verbal clues* include talking about death, making comments that significant others would be "better off without" the person, and asking questions about lethal dosages of drugs. *Behavioral clues* include writing forlorn love notes, directing angry messages at a significant other who has rejected the person, giving away personal items, or taking out a large life insurance policy. A third category, *situational clues*, is used to describe those events or situations that present themselves when something happens either around or within the person, such as the unexpected death of a loved one, divorce, job failure, or diagnosis of a malignant tumor. Such situational clues may place the person at high risk for suicide.

8. Men accomplish suicide more often than women; however, women attempt suicide three times more often.

9. Suicide represents a loss of over 16 billion dollars each year considering lost productivity, medical care, and welfare payments to survivors.

10. Among the mentally ill, individuals with the diagnosis of schizophrenia have the highest suicide rate, followed by individuals suffering from major depression.

✿ Etiology

Suicide is defined by *Webster's* as the act of intentionally killing oneself. Risk for suicide infers the possibility that an individual will voluntarily and intentionally kill herself of himself. Why does a person contemplate such an act? Causative factors, or motives for attempting suicide, include

1. *A progressive failure to adapt.* The person no longer is able to cope in a world of stressors that are overwhelming.

2. *Feelings of alienation or isolation, especially in teenagers.* The isolation may occur gradually, resulting in a loss of all meaningful social contacts and relationships. Isolation can be self-imposed or can occur as a result of the inability to be assertive, express feelings, cope positively, or develop meaningful relationships with others.

3. *Feelings of anger or hostility.* A person may harbor feelings of intense hostility toward a significant other and intend to get revenge or manipulate the person. For example, a woman deserted by her husband may feel that her suicidal act will cause him to suffer guilt feelings and loss of esteem among friends and relatives or that perhaps the attempt will force him to return home. Feelings of hostility may also be directed inward owing to self-hatred. The suicide then is a form of self-punishment. For example, an army officer broods over the orders he gave to his company that resulted in killing several young children. Suicide would be a form of self-punishment and atonement for a sin or crime he feels that he committed.

4. *A reunion wish or fantasy.* A newspaper article described the death of an elderly man whose wife had just died. He left a note to his children stating that he did not want to live without his wife, and because of his belief in life after death, he planned to join his wife.

5. *A way to end one's feelings of hopelessness and helplessness.* Hope is a sense of the possible; it gives promise for the future and an expectation of fulfillment. Persons who experience hopelessness feel insecure and believe that there are no solutions to various problems. They experience a sense of the impossible. Helplessness is a feeling that everything that can be done has been done; there is nothing left to sustain hope.

6. *A cry for help.* Some people attempt suicide hoping to draw attention to themselves to receive help. For example, a 49-year-old woman in financial distress attempted suicide by taking a moderate overdose of sleeping pills, hoping that her boyfriend, who never displayed an interest in her business, would come to her rescue financially as well as emotionally.

7. *A deliberate gamble with death from feelings of frustration, self-hatred, or ambivalence.* Persons who are ambivalent harbor feelings of self-preservation and self-destruction. Such persons may threaten or attempt suicide and then seek help. Stunt performers, daredevil drivers, and persons who play such games as Russian roulette are deliberately gambling with death and may harbor feelings of ambivalence or self-hatred. Such persons appear to be living on "borrowed time" because they live with the risk of death frequently.

8. *An attempt to "save face" or seek a release to a better life.* Persons who were involved in the stock market crash of 1929 during the Great Depression

jumped from windows in suicide attempts caused by feelings of failure. These people had viewed themselves as competent, successful, and respected before the crash. The suicides were an effort to save face, relieving them of the responsibility of dealing with business failures.

9. *Terminal or chronic illness.* People with a terminal or chronic illness may attempt suicide as a last chance to maintain control of their lives or as a wish to be released from pain. Noncompliance, or refusal to follow the prescribed medical care, is a passive or indirect form of suicide seen among the chronically or terminally ill. For example, a patient with advanced emphysema refused to follow the doctor's advice to quit smoking although he was maintained on oxygen per nasal cannula. The patient died as a result of noncompliance.

10. *Impaired thought processes* (e.g., *delusions or hallucinations*). Persons who hallucinate or entertain delusional thoughts may respond to persistent thoughts or "voices" that tell them to follow through with life-threatening acts.

Individuals at Risk for Self-destructive Behavior

The following is a list of those persons considered to be at risk or prone to self-destructive behavior:

1. The elderly and adolescents
2. Older divorced, separated, or widowed persons
3. Unemployed persons
4. Professional workers such as physicians, dentists, and lawyers
5. People in poor physical health
6. Socially isolated individuals
7. Members of minority groups such as Native Americans

These groups of individuals may experience feelings of dependency, loneliness, and worthlessness as they attempt to care for themselves in a society that places much emphasis on youth, physical fitness, success, and independence.

Other at-risk groups include

8. Individuals with comorbid conditions such as alcoholism and substance abuse. Alcohol and certain drugs are known to cause central nervous system depression. The mixing of drugs and alcohol may cause a drug–alcohol interaction that could result in death. Many drugs cause psychological or physiologic dependency, thus creating emotional conflict and depression

as well as physiologic deterioration. Drug–drug interactions also increase the likelihood of death as a result of self-destructive impulses.

9. People such as air traffic controllers, whose occupations require selfless public service and dedication, and who work under high pressure. The lives of police officers also are often stressful because the long work hours and disruption of family and social life.

10. Chronically or terminally ill persons whose life-styles are disrupted by illnesses. Persons with anorexia nervosa or bulimia are definitely at risk. They are committing a passive form of suicide that could become acute and is caused by feelings of frustration, guilt, anger, or loss of control.

11. Accident-prone individuals. Such persons, who experience repeated accidents in which their lives are in jeopardy, may be attempting suicide unconsciously.

12. Previous attempters. Persons who have not developed adequate coping mechanisms or who lack sufficient support systems are at risk each time they experience increased stress.

13. Persons who engage in autoerotic sexual acts. The use of chains, shackles, ropes, or other devices to enhance autoerotic feelings often restricts or immobilizes the person and creates a level of semiconsciousness that could result in accidental death or suicide.

14. Persons with psychiatric diagnoses such as schizophrenia, organic mental disorders, personality disorders, anxiety disorders, and mood disorders. Command hallucinations, delusions of grandeur, lack of impulse control, manipulative behavior, overwhelming grief, or a chemical imbalance such as occurs in depressed persons may result in suicidal behavior.

Hatton, Valente, and Rink (1977) have developed a method of assessing a person's degree of suicidal risk, which is detailed in Table 20-1.

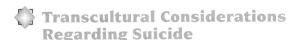

Transcultural Considerations Regarding Suicide

A review of the literature has revealed that minimal information is available pertaining to cultural beliefs about suicide. Suicide rates among white and African-American adolescents and young adults are discussed in Andrews and Boyle (1995). Both white and African-American young women have relatively lower suicide rates than young men. The suicide rate of young white men is twice that of African-American young adults. Suicide patterns among Native American youths vary among tribes, depending on group integration, cohesion, regulation, and physical environment.

Culturally sanctioned suicide has been practiced by the Japanese (hara-kiri) and Hindu widows (suttee). Members of militant groups in the Middle East still

TABLE 20-1 ASSESSING THE DEGREE OF SUICIDAL RISK

Behavior or Symptom	Intensity of Risk		
	Low	Moderate	High
Anxiety	Mild	Moderate	High, or panic state
Depression	Mild	Moderate	Severe
Isolation–withdrawal	Vague feelings of depression, no withdrawal	Some feelings of helplessness, hopelessness, and withdrawal	Hopeless, helpless, withdrawn, and self-deprecating
Daily functioning	Fairly good in most activities	Moderately good in some activities	Not good in any activities
Resources	Several	Some	Few or none
Coping strategies and devices being used	Generally constructive	Some that are constructive	Predominantly destructive
Significant others	Several who are available	Few or only one available	Only one, or none available
Psychiatric help in past	None, or positive attitude toward	Yes, and moderately satisfied with	Negative view of help received
Life-style	Stable	Moderately stable or unstable	Unstable
Alcohol and drug use	Infrequently to excess	Frequently to excess	Continual abuse
Previous suicide attempts	None, or of low lethality	None to one or more of moderate lethality	None to multiple attempts of high lethality
Disorientation and disorganization	None	Some	Marked
Hostility	Little or none	Some	Marked
Suicidal plan	Vague, fleeting thoughts but no plan	Frequent thoughts, occasional ideas about a plan	Frequent or constant thoughts with a specific plan

(Hatton, D., Valente, S., & Rink, A. [1977]. *Suicide assessment and intervention*. p. 56. New York: Appleton-Century-Crofts.)

practice culturally sanctioned suicide by attaching explosives to themselves and detonating them when approaching specific targets.

Suicide is forbidden under Islamic law and is considered shameful in the Filipino culture. Suicide of elderly Eskimos who could no longer participate as a productive members of a tribe was expected (Giger & Davidhazar, 1991). Some religions, such as Roman Catholicism, do not permit church funerals for suicide victims.

Suicide studies have been conducted in the United Kingdom and in Australia. Although no cultural aspects were addressed, findings revealed that the completed suicides were the result of diagnosable mental illnesses such as depression, chemical dependency, and alcoholism. The retrospective studies were described by Dr. G. Gabbard of the Menninger Clinic during his presentation at the 7th Annual U.S. Psychiatric and Mental Health Congress in Washington, DC.

Misconceptions About Suicide

Several misconceptions exist regarding the dynamics of suicide. They are presented in an attempt to inform the reader of such fallacies.

1. *Suicidal individuals give no warning of their intent.* Eight of 10 persons give some type of verbal or behavioral clue before a suicide attempt. All threats should be taken seriously.
2. *Suicidal persons want to die; therefore, once suicidal, always suicidal.* In reality the person is generally suicidal for a limited period termed the *suicidal crisis* period. During this crisis, the person is undecided about living and dying (ambivalent) and gambles with death. The person leaves her or his destiny or fate in the hands of others. Those saved are usually quite grateful.
3. *Once a suicidal attempt has failed, the suicidal risk is over.* Persons who attempt suicide remain at risk during the period of improvement because they experience increased energy levels and are able to put morbid thoughts and feelings into action. Persons recovering from a severe depression are considered to be at high risk for approximately 9 to 15 months.
4. *Suicidal tendencies are inherited.* There is no evidence to support this misconception. Suicide is an individual pattern of behavior.
5. *Only "crazy" people commit suicide.* Approximately 10% of all suicides occur as a result of major psychological breakdowns. Farberow and Shneidman (1961) state that studies of genuine suicide notes show that the people were depressed but not psychotic.
6. *Suicide occurs more frequently among the very rich or very poor.* Suicide occurs among all levels of society, regardless of socioeconomic status.

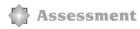 Assessment

Suicide is considered more preventable than any other cause of death. This statement is based on the assumption that all suicidal persons are ambivalent about life and therefore are never 100% suicidal.

Assessment of the person who is self-destructive includes the application of close observational and listening skills to detect any suicide clues, the specificity of the plan, and its degree of lethality. Badger (1995) lists commonly used assessment terminology to describe the range of suicidal thoughts and behavior. Referred to as "The Suicide Lexicon" the terminology includes:

1. Suicidal ideation or vague, fleeting thoughts about wanting to die
2. Suicidal intent or thoughts about a concrete plan to commit suicide
3. Suicidal threat or the expression of a person's desire to end his or her life
4. Suicidal gesture or intentional self-destructive behavior that is clearly not life-threatening but does resemble an attempted suicide
5. Suicidal attempt or self-destructive behavior by which an individual responds to ambivalent feelings about living

As stated previously, 80% of all potential suicide victims give some type of clue. Clues that might lead one to suspect that a patient is entertaining suicidal thoughts or is developing a concrete plan to commit suicide include any person who

1. Talks about death, suicide, and wanting to be dead, and appears to be in deep thought
2. Asks suspicious questions such as "How often do the night personnel make rounds?" "How many of these pills would it take a kill a person?" "How high is this window from the ground?" "How long does it take to bleed to death?" and so forth.
3. Fears being unable to sleep and fears the night
4. Is depressed and cries frequently
5. Keeps away from others owing to self-imposed isolation, especially in secluded areas or behind locked doors
6. Is tense and worried, and has a hopeless, helpless attitude
7. Imagines he or she has some serious physical illness like cancer or tuberculosis. The person may want to end the suffering or decrease the imagined burden to the family.
8. Feels very guilty about something real or imaginary or feels worthless. The person may feel she or he is not worthy to live.
9. Talks or thinks about punishment, torture, and being persecuted

10. Is listening to voices. (The voices may tell the person to try to take his or her life.)
11. Suddenly seems very happy, without any apparent reason, after being very depressed for some time. (The person may be happy now that she or he has figured out a method of committing suicide.)
12. Collects and hoards strings, pieces of glass, a knife, or anything else sharp that might be used for self-harm
13. Is very aggressive or very impulsive, acting suddenly and unexpectedly
14. Shows an unusual amount of interest in getting his or her affairs in order
15. Gives away personal belongings
16. Has a history of suicide attempts

During the assessment process, the nurse begins to establish a therapeutic relationship based on trust by displaying an attitude of acceptance, empathy, and support. Such a response is supportive to persons who experience feelings of worthlessness, helplessness, and hopelessness. The encouragement of verbalization of negative feelings is essential, as well as the direct questioning about suicidal intent.

A self-rating hopelessness form, the Beck Hopelessness Scale, is used in clinical practice to assess a person's level of optimism and pessimism (Beck, Steer, Beck, & Newman, 1993). Hopelessness is the best proven clinical predictor of eventual suicide other than a previous attempt. Suicidal intent may also be assessed by inquiring about symptoms of subjective intent and objective suicidal planning. The patient should be asked about the purpose of the suicide attempt, whether fatality is perceived, and how rescuable the individual thinks he or she would be if medical attention were immediately available. Most suicides are well planned, although they may ultimately be carried out impulsively (Malone & Mann, 1996).

Nursing Intervention

Nursing intervention focuses on prevention of self-destruction and is classified as primary, secondary, and tertiary prevention. Primary prevention focuses on the elimination of factors causing or contributing to the development of an illness or disorder. Secondary prevention is described as an attempt to identify and treat physical or emotional disorders in the early stages before they become disturbing to an individual. For example, a 24-year-old schoolteacher experiences feelings of increased anxiety and mild depression when told by her fiancé that he is breaking their engagement. Effective assessment or secondary prevention should alleviate such symptoms and prevent the onset of self-destructive behavior. Tertiary prevention is intervention aimed at reducing residual disability after an illness. A residential treatment center, halfway house, or rehabilitation center may be used to treat a recovering alcoholic patient who previously attempted suicide and is recovering from a severe depression, but needs the supervision and support of others as she or he handles the drinking problem.

Crisis intervention is performed in emergency situations in which a suicidal crisis exists. The nurse assesses the person and the problem, plans therapeutic interventions, intervenes, and assists the person in making realistic plans for the future while the person uses successful coping mechanisms to reduce anxiety and tension (see Chapter 9).

Self-assessment (autognosis) is imperative if the nurse expects to handle self-destructive persons effectively. Questions the nurse uses as a self-assessment guide should focus on

1. Values and belief about life versus death
2. Positive and negative feelings about the suicidal person
3. Ability to be nonjudgmental
4. Energy level, mentally and physically, when working therapeutically with a suicidal person
5. Ability to let the person assume the responsibility for his or her actions

Suicide precautions vary according to the person's intent on self-destruction. Bailey and Dreyer (1977) discuss a suicidal intention rating scale (SIRS) that provides a guide in the management of hospitalized persons considered to be self-destructive. A person who displays no evidence of past or present suicidal ideation is given a rating of 0. Nursing intervention consists of the normal hospital care. A person who shows evidence of suicidal ideation, has not made an attempt at self-destruction, and has not threatened suicide is given a rating of 1+. The nurse observes and evaluates the person for evidence of recurrent suicidal thoughts. Actively thinking about suicide or evidence of a previous attempt is given a rating of 2+. Such a person should be protected from self-destructive impulses. Personal items are made available for use but must be returned to the staff and kept under lock and key if they are potentially dangerous. These items include glass containers, sharp objects, hard plastics, belts, ties, pins, and any liquid cosmetics or deodorants that could be drunk and result in poisoning. A person who makes a suicide threat, such as "Leave me alone or I'll kill myself," is assigned a rating of 3+. Such a person should be searched at the time of admission for the possession of lethal instruments. Any carry-in items such as luggage also should be checked. Potentially dangerous items (*e.g.*, a razor, mirror, or nail file) are to be used only under the direct supervision of a hospital employee. Protective care includes periodic checks at least every 30 minutes, limited visits by family members only, and no privileges to leave the unit unless otherwise specified by the physician. If the person does leave the unit, she or he is to be accompanied by a member of the staff. A 4+ rating is reserved for the person who has actively attempted suicide or is hospitalized to prevent self-destructive impulses. Nursing interventions for a 4+ rating may include the following protective care. An explanation should be given to the patient so that he or she understands what is being done and why (because the nurse is legally bound to follow agency policies and procedures).

1. Confinement to a security room to observe the person's behavior more readily. The door is locked whenever the patient is left alone, and frequent, periodic checks are made at irregular intervals. The nurse can provide constant watchful care by staying with the person, and by listening and being supportive. The use of restraints, full or belt, is used as a last resort to immobilize agitated, self-destructive persons. Windows in the room should be locked, with screens covering the glass to prevent self-harm. Seclusion must be used judiciously because it can isolate a person further and enhance feelings of worthlessness, helplessness, and hopelessness. Documentation in verifying observation of suicidal precautions is imperative.
2. Removal of objects that could prove to be dangerous to the person. This is done by searching the person's clothing, carry-in items, and body in a dignified or professional manner. The body search includes checking any part of the body in which harmful objects might be stored, such as body orifices and the hair. One female patient concealed Librium in a plastic bag in her vagina, with the intent of overdosing at some future time during hospitalization.
3. Removing street clothes and placing the person in a seclusion gown, as well as removing bed linens. Suicide attempts have been made by using linen or clothing as a means to hang oneself.
4. Feeding the patient in the seclusion room. Food is served on paper dishes if one of the staff is unable to stay with the patient during meals. Sharp utensils are removed from the tray to prevent an impulsive attempt at self-destruction.
5. Direct supervision of the person whenever she or he is removed from the security room to prevent impulsive self-destructive behavior.
6. Restricted visitation privileges. Such visitors require special permission by the attending physician. After visitors have departed, the patient should be checked for items that may have been accidently left behind or innocently given to the patient.
7. Securing a verbal stated promise not to attempt suicide. Instead, the patient will seek out a staff member if he or she experiences suicidal thoughts.
8. Giving a message of hope by being optimistic that life can be better and the patient will receive help in an attempt to solve her or his problem.
9. Medicating, if necessary. Injections usually are given to persons in security rooms to facilitate rapid absorption and to prevent noncompliance, such as refusal to take medication or hoarding of it.

If a patient is admitted to a general hospital after a suicide attempt, 24-hour supervision is required at the expense of the family because seclusion rooms are not usually available.

Once the person has inner control over self-destructive behavior, he or she is removed from seclusion or the security room. The patient should be encouraged to engage in an activity that is an outlet for tension and hostility. Participating in an active sport like volleyball, working with sandpaper, or pounding wood are examples of such an outlet. The room assignment should be near the nurses' station to allow close observation. Having another patient in the same room offers support to the person and lessens feelings of loneliness.

The patient should be monitored while taking any prescribed medication because patients have been known to save medication for future suicide attempts. As the depression lessens, the person acquires energy to follow through with another self-destructive attempt.

Participation in group, individual, or family psychotherapy is encouraged. Providing the patient with the following teaching checklist may be helpful. As the patient recovers and discharge planning occurs, she or he is encouraged to identify agencies or support systems in the community that can be contacted to

---

PATIENT TEACHING CHECKLIST
Suicidal Ideation

The following checklist has been developed to reinforce your knowledge about suicidal ideation. Please inform the nurse if you are uncertain about any of the items listed below.

✔ Suicidal ideation is the consideration of a permanent solution to a temporary problem that usually can be resolved with professional help.
✔ The reasons I have felt suicidal include:
✔ Interventions I have learned to reduce suicidal thoughts include:
✔ Support persons I may contact include:
✔ The name of the medication I am taking is:
✔ Instructions regarding this medication
  ▪ Take this medication as directed by your doctor
  ▪ Do not drink alcohol while taking this medication
  ▪ Do not take any over-the-counter medication without informing your nurse of doctor
  ▪ Usual side effects include:
  ▪ Report any unusual side effects promptly
  ▪ Dosage adjustment may be necessary
  ▪ Do not discontinue taking this medication without first consulting your nurse or doctor

---

alleviate recurrent suicidal feelings. The patient and family should be educated about signs and symptoms of depression, warning signs of suicidal thoughts, and effects of medication, including any special precautions.

It would be wrong to suggest that closely supervised patients do not succeed in suicide attempts. A clinical example of a person who did succeed in a suicide attempt during hospitalization follows.

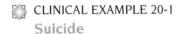

CLINICAL EXAMPLE 20-1

Suicide

SM, a 35-year-old engineer and father of three children, had been admitted to the neuropsychiatric unit of a state hospital with the diagnosis of depression. During the intake interview, SM exhibited symptoms of suicidal ideation because he made statements such as "I'd be better off dead," "My family would be better off without me," and "Yes, I have thought about killing myself." SM was placed on strict suicide precautions and antidepressant medication, and began attending therapy sessions on the unit. Within three weeks, the suicidal precautions were lifted, and SM was granted lawn privileges but was to be supervised by one of the hospital employees. SM appeared to be improving and was granted a day pass to visit his family four weeks after his admission. At approximately 3:00 the day after SM visited his family, he asked for lawn privileges to play tennis. Although SM was supervised by a hospital employee, he was able to run away and leave the hospital grounds. Later that evening SM's family notified the hospital that he had secured a handgun and committed suicide by firing the gun into his mouth.

Psychological Autopsy

The student nurse who had begun to develop a therapeutic relationship with SM was shocked by the news and immediately experienced guilt feelings. She stated, "Did I say something to upset him that much? Was it my fault he committed suicide?" She questioned whether there were some verbal clues that she should have noticed. The staff was quite helpful in explaining to the student that patients may commit suicide in spite of all the precautions taken during hospitalization. They further explained to her that in her capacity as a student, she was not with the patient 24 hours a day to observe him continuously as the three shifts did. She should therefore not blame herself for his actions.

This interaction with the staff, in which the staff review the patient's behaviors and suicidal act, is referred to as a psychological autopsy. It is a process used to examine what clues, if any, were missed to learn from the evaluation of a particular situation.

Postvention

Survivors of a successful suicide attempt are victims also. They initially experience feelings of confusion, shock, or disbelief. Once they recover from the psychological impact of a loved one's death, feelings of anger, ambivalence, guilt, grief, and possible rejection emerge. *Postvention*, a therapeutic program for bereaved survivors of a suicide, allows family members or other survivors to vent their feelings at a time of such trauma. This program provides immediate contact with the survivors (within 24 hours) to assist them in coping with their feelings of shock and grief. This is the first phase of postvention. During the second phase, survivors are given the opportunity to develop new coping methods in an effort to prevent the development of maladaptive or destructive behavior. The survivor learns to cope with feelings of lowered self-esteem, depression, and the fear of developing a close interpersonal relationship. The third phase focuses on helping the survivors view the grief experience as a growth-promoting experience and ends on the first anniversary of the suicide.

Special attention should be given to children who are survivors because they are quite vulnerable to the death of a parent. They may feel that they caused the death by "wishing mommy dead" or "telling mommy I hate her." As a result of such feelings, children may be unable to work through the grieving process, become preoccupied with the subject of suicide, develop self-destructive behavior, exhibit signs of depression, or have difficulty working through the developmental tasks of childhood.

The following interventions are helpful as preventive and postventive measures with children who are survivors:

1. Allow the child to express feelings.
2. Assist the child in the development of a meaningful relationship with others.
3. Encourage the development of positive coping skills.
4. Teach the child assertiveness.
5. Allow the child to develop ideas and values.
6. Expose the child to courses on psychologic principles and human behavior in the educational process.

Nursing Diagnoses and Sample Care Plan

Several examples of nursing diagnoses frequently used in the clinical setting while providing care for individuals exhibiting symptoms of mood disorders were cited in Chapter 19. Additional nursing diagnoses related to care of the individual at risk for suicidal behavior include *anxiety, *ineffective individual coping,

*NANDA-approved nursing diagnosis.

situational or maturational crisis, *decisional conflict, depression, emotional lability, *hopelessness, altered impulse control, and high risk for suicide. Nursing Care Plan 20-1 gives a nursing diagnosis and goal-related nursing interventions for an individual admitted to a psychiatric facility because of a suicide attempt.

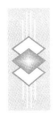

NURSING CARE PLAN 20-1
The Patient with a History of Suicide Attempts

Nursing Diagnosis: High risk for suicide: history of suicide attempt before hospitalization, related to poor self-concept

Goal #1: During hospitalization the patient will feel safe and secure and not attempt to harm self.

Nursing Interventions	Outcome Criteria
Assess current risk for suicide.	Verbalizes thoughts and feelings regarding suicide
Implement suicide precautions to provide a safe environment, observe patient's behavior, and maintain close supervision.	Demonstrates compliance with suicide precautions (*e.g.*, remains in visual contact)
Explain level of care to patient.	Understands rationale for present level of care
Secure a suicide contract.	Agrees to written contract
Prevent impulsive acts by discussing alternatives to suicide.	Verbalizes perception of present situation

Nursing Diagnosis: High risk for suicide: history of suicide attempt before hospitalization, related to poor self-concept

Goal #2: Before discharge, patient will develop a positive self-concept.

Nursing Interventions	Outcome Criteria
	Within 48 to 72 hours the patient will do the following:
Accept the patient for who he or she is.	Demonstrate a feeling of acceptance
Avoid judgmental statements about self-destructive behavior.	
Convey a caring attitude.	
Encourage verbalization of feelings.	Identify present stressors or issues related to suicidal ideation and attempt to harm self
	Identify one or two positive aspects of self
Provide opportunity for patient to succeed in simple minor tasks so that patient will receive positive feedback and sense of self-worth.	Verbalize absence of suicidal ideation
	Communicate feelings of self-worth
	Acknowledge need for continuing therapy once mood stabilizes to enhance self-esteem

NANDA-approved nursing diagnosis.

388

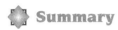 **Summary**

Suicide, one of the eight leading causes of death in the United States, often occurs as the result of intense feelings of anxiety, depression, anger, or hostility. Statistics pertaining to suicide were presented, as well as causative factors or motives for self-destructive behavior. Examples of persons considered to be at risk were cited, such as persons living alone, adolescents, the elderly, the chronically or terminally ill, and psychotic persons. Hatton, Valente, and Rink's method of assessing a person's degree of suicidal risk was presented. Transcultural considerations regarding suicide were discussed. Misconceptions about suicide were explored.

Assessment of suicidal intent and lethality were described. Nursing interventions, including primary, secondary, and tertiary prevention, were included. The importance of self-assessment or autognosis was stressed. A discussion of the suicidal intention rating scale was included, focusing on nursing interventions appropriate for each rating. A detailed explanation of protective care for strict suicide precaution was given. Psychological autopsy, a process for reviewing a successful suicide attempt, was described. Nursing measures, pertaining to the person removed from suicide precautions, were explained. Post vention, a therapeutic program for bereaved survivors of a suicide, was discussed, with special attention given to children who are survivors. Examples of common nursing diagnoses related to the care of the individual at risk for suicidal behavior were given. A sample care plan focusing on nursing interventions for the individual who attempted suicide was also presented.

Learning Activities

 I. Clinical Activities
   A. If possible, establish a therapeutic relationship with a suicidal patient.
   B. Rate the patient's suicidal ideation.
   C. Describe the type of protective care the patient is receiving.
   D. Using the nursing process, plan nursing care for the patient.
II. Independent Activities
   A. Identify what makes you feel happy and sad.
   B. How do you cope with sad or depressed feelings?
   C. State what you do to cheer yourself up.
   D. List one or two situations in your life that caused you to be depressed. Why and for how long did you feel depressed?

E. Discuss the effect of weather and music on your mood.

F. Make a list of those things you like best about yourself and state why you like those things.

G. Identify agencies in your community that provide support for persons contemplating suicide.

Critical Thinking Questions

1. Write a journal of your feelings, thoughts, stressors, and coping methods for several weeks. Review it for patterns; that is, identify events, situations, or individuals who are stressors (*e.g.*, what makes you mad or sad.) What do you do to cope? Are your coping methods healthy? Do they work?

2. Team up with a classmate and interview each other about your values and beliefs concerning life, death, and suicide. What differences and similarities do you have?

3. You notice that your 13-year-old neighbor always wears black, refuses to make eye contact, is often alone, and has a defeated posture. Your mother and the boy's mother are good friends. You are concerned about the teen's increasing isolation. Describe several interventions that might be appropriate in this situation and explain your rationale for selecting them.

Self-Test

1. State the classifications of clues to suicidal behavior and give examples of each.
2. List five causative factors that may lead to suicide.
3. State five categories of people considered to be at risk or prone to self-destructive behavior.
4. Discuss three misconceptions about suicide.
5. State the rationale for autognosis or self-assessment when working with suicidal patients.
6. State the purpose of the assessment process when admitting a self-destructive person to the hospital.
7. Explain the rationale for strict suicidal precautions.
8. List in detail those nursing interventions included in strict suicidal precautions.

9. Describe nursing care measures used once a patient has gained control over self-destructive behavior.
10. Describe the three phases of postvention for survivors or victims of a successful suicide attempt.
11. List nursing interventions for the nursing diagnosis of high risk for suicide.
12. Discuss two cultural beliefs about suicide.

SELECTED REFERENCES

Anderson, D. B. (1991, March). Never too late: Resolving the grief of suicide. *Journal of Psychosocial Nursing and Mental Health Services.*

Andrews, M. M., & Boyle, J. S. (1995). *Transcultural concepts in nursing care* (2nd ed.). Philadelphia: J. B. Lippincott.

Badger, J. M. (1995, March). Reaching out to the suicidal patient. *American Journal of Nursing.*

Bailey, D., & Dreyer, S. (1977). *Care of the mentally ill.* Philadelphia: F. A. Davis.

Beck, A. T., Steer, R. A., Beck, J. S., & Newman, C. F. (1993, February). Hopelessness, depression, suicidal ideation, and clinical diagnosis of depression. *Suicide and Life-Threatening Behavior.*

Beeber, L. S. (1996). The client who is suicidal. In S. Lego (Ed.). *Psychiatric nursing: A comprehensive reference* (2nd ed.). Philadelphia: Lippincott–Raven Publishers.

Buchanan, D., Farran, C., & Clark, D. (1995, October). Suicidal thought and self-transcendence in older adults. *Journal of Psychosocial Nursing and Mental Health Services.*

Cardell, R., & Horton-Deutsch, S. (1994, December). A model for assessment of inpatient suicide potential. *Archives of Psychiatric Nursing.*

Carpenito, L. J. (1995). *Nursing diagnosis: Application to clinical practice* (6th ed.). Philadelphia: J. B. Lippincott.

Cidylo, L. (1991, October). Gender plays a significant role in suicide. *Psychiatric Times.*

Conrad, N. (1991, March). Where do they turn: Social support systems of suicidal high school adolescents. *Journal of Psychosocial Nursing and Mental Health Services.*

Cugino, A., Markovich, E. I., Rosenblatt, S., Jarjoura, D., Blend, D., & Whittier, F. D. (1992, March). Searching for a pattern: Repeat suicide attempts. *Journal of Psychosocial Nursing and Mental Health Services.*

Farberow, N. L., & Shneidman, E. (1961). *The cry for help.* New York: McGraw-Hill.

Gabbard, G. O. (1994, November). Psychotherapy of the suicidal patient. Washington, DC: 7th Annual U.S. Psychiatric and Mental Health Congress.

Giger, J. N., & Davidhazar, R. E. (1991). *Transcultural nursing: Assessment and intervention.* St. Louis: Mosby Year Book.

Hatton, D., Valente, S., & Rink, A. (1977). *Suicide assessment and intervention.* New York: Appleton-Century-Crofts.

Malone, K. M., & Mann, J. (1996, March/April). Assessment and treatment of suicidal behavior in depression. *Clinical Advances in the Treatment of Psychiatric Disorders.*

Schultz, J. M., & Videbeck, S. D. (1994). *Manual of psychiaric nursing care plans* (4th ed.). Philadelphia: J. B. Lippincott.

Susser, M. (1993, February). Suicide: Risk factors and the public health. *American Journal of Public Health.*

Valente, S. M. (1991, December). Deliberate self-injury: Management in the psychiatric setting. *Journal of Psychosocial Nursing and Mental Health Services.*

Valente, S. M. (1993, September). Evaluating suicide risk in the medically ill patient. *Nurse Practitioner.*

Westreich, L. (1995, September 15). Assessing an adult patient's suicide risk: What primary care physicians need to know. *Postgraduate Medicine.*

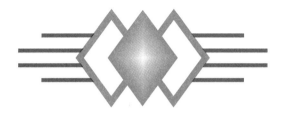

CHAPTER 21

ALTERED THOUGHT PROCESSES: DELUSIONAL OR PARANOID BEHAVIOR

Delusional disorder is relatively uncommon in clinical settings, with most studies suggesting that the disorder accounts for 1% to 2% of admissions to inpatient mental health facilities.

American Psychiatric Association, DSM-IV, 1994

LEARNING OBJECTIVES

1 Define the term *delusion*.

2 Describe the predominant theme of the following subtypes of delusional disorder:

Erotomanic

Grandiose

Jealous

Persecutory

Somatic

3 Differentiate among delusional disorder and shared psychotic disorder.

4 Discuss the importance of identifying the specific cultural and religious background of a patient diagnosed with a delusional disorder.

5 Describe the psychiatric management of delusional disorders.

6 State nursing interventions for the following nursing diagnosis related to delusional behavior: Altered thought processes because of inaccurate interpretation of environmental stimuli, resulting in feelings of suspicion and fear.

Introduction

Paranoid disorder was reclassified in the DSM-III-R and is referred to as delusional disorder in the DSM-IV. The term *paranoid* is commonly used to describe a person who exhibits overly suspicious behavior. Technically, the term is used to describe a wide range of behaviors, from aloof, suspicious, and nonpsychotic behaviors, to well systematized and psychotic symptoms. The descriptive terms *delusional* and *paranoid* are used interchangeably in this chapter and are based on the information provided by the DSM-IV and appropriate reference material.

Etiology

Several predisposing factors have been identified in the development of delusional disorders. They include relocation due to immigration or emigration; sensory handicaps, such as deafness or blindness; severe stress; low socio-economic status, in which the person may experience feelings of discrimination, powerlessness, or low self-esteem; and trust–fear conflicts.

Clinical Features

Delusional persons usually exhibit extreme suspiciousness, jealousy, and distrust, as well as being convinced that others intend to do them harm. They may exhibit persecutory delusions, in which they feel they are being conspired against, spied on, poisoned or drugged, cheated, harassed, maliciously maligned, or obstructed in some way. Conjugal paranoia or delusional jealousy, in which the person is convinced without due cause that his or her mate is unfaithful, may exist. Delusional persons refuse to acknowledge negative feelings, thoughts, motives, or behaviors in themselves, and project such feelings onto others by blaming others for their problems. Delusional persons spend much time confirming suspicions and defending themselves against imagined persecution. Such self-centered thoughts, in which everything is taken personally, are called ideas of reference.

An individual, usually an unmarried woman, exhibiting clinical symptoms of erotomania believes she is loved by a person of elevated social status. The delusion is usually of romantic or spiritual love rather than sexual love. Individuals such as movie stars or prominent television personalities have been victimized by such persons, who write letters, stalk the individuals, send gifts, or attempt to visit them.

Grandiose delusions are present when the individual believes he or she possesses unrecognized talent or insight, such as that of a religious leader, and seeks a position of power.

Preoccupation with the body by verbalizing unusual somatic complaints also occurs in persons with altered thought processes. They may complain of disfigured or nonfunctioning body parts, believe they are infested with insects, or believe they have a serious illness. A substantial suicide risk exists because some individuals believe death is imminent.

Delusional persons often exhibit resentment, anger, grandiose ideas, social isolation, seclusiveness, or eccentric behavior. Such people may resort to complaining about various injustices and frequently instigate legal actions. They rarely seek treatment and are brought to the attention of mental health professionals by friends, relatives, or associates who are concerned about their behavior. Social and marital functioning are often impaired, although the person preserves daily, intellectual, and occupational functioning.

 ## DSM-IV Criteria

The DSM-IV lists several disorders in which the clinical symptom of delusional thoughts may occur. They include dementia, alcohol-induced psychotic disorder, substance-induced psychotic disorder, schizophrenia, psychotic disorder due to a medical condition, mood disorder, shared psychotic disorder, paranoid personality disorder, and delusional disorder. This chapter focuses on shared psychotic disorder and delusional disorder. The remaining disorders are addressed within the text.

Shared Psychotic Disorder (*Folie à Deux*)

This disorder involves two individuals who have a close relationship and share the same delusion. The "inducer" or "primary case" has a psychotic disorder with prominent delusions that the other individual, usually passive and initially healthy, begins to believe. Such persons are often related by blood or marriage, have lived together for an extensive period of time, and may be socially isolated. Such a disorder has occurred within a group of individuals or in families in which the parent is the "primary case." Delusions may be bizarre or nonbizarre. They are not due to the direct physiological effects of a substance or medical condition.

Delusional Disorder

According to the DSM-IV criteria, this disorder is differentiated from schizophrenia in that delusions are not bizarre and audiovisual hallucinations do not generally occur. Delusions involve situations that can conceivably occur in real life, such as being poisoned or believing someone has tampered with the brakes in one's car. They are not due to any other mental disorders.

The five subtypes, erotomanic, grandiose, jealous, persecutory, and somatic were discussed earlier. Mood changes may occur, including irritability, anger, depression, and violence. Legal difficulties may arise. Such persons may be subject to unnecessary medical tests and procedures. Social, marital, or work problems are not uncommon; however, cognitive disorganization or emotional deterioration

---

🔅 CLINICAL EXAMPLE 21-1
Shared Psychotic Disorder

Mr. and Mrs. G. were brought to the local psychiatric receiving facility by the county sheriff. Neighbors had reported both individuals were observed boarding up their windows, chasing people off the sidewalk in front of their house, and accusing people of spying on them. Garbage was piled in the driveway, attracting rodents and stray cats. Mail was left uncollected in their mailbox.

During the interview, it was noted that the wife agreed with the bizarre story that the husband related. He described delusions of persecution in which he believed aliens were spying on them. They had moved several times because they feared for their safety.

When interviewed separately, they gave identical stories. It was determined that the husband was the "inducer."

CLINICAL EXAMPLE 21-2
Delusional (Paranoid) Disorder

A 45-year-old Cuban man who recently moved to Florida with his family suddenly becomes suspicious that Fidel Castro is "out to get him." He barricades the windows and doors of his home, has his telephone number unlisted, and warns his family to be careful whenever they leave the house. Although he displays this delusion of persecution and exhibits hypervigilance, he is able to function with minimal impairment. When questioned, his wife states that he has felt guilty about leaving his parents behind in Cuba.

Working with such a patient would be extremely difficult because his delusional system may have an element of truth in it. People who have emigrated to the United States from Cuba and other countries have related stories of persecution for crimes they did not commit, whereas others have fled to avoid persecution for crimes committed. Living in such an environment could predispose someone to the development of a highly suspicious thought process.

do not usually occur. The type of delusional disorder is based on the predominant delusional theme, because cases with more than one theme are frequent.

Transcultural Considerations

The content of delusions reflects cultural patterns. The content may be primarily psychological, religious or spiritual, moral or social, naturalistic or supernatural, or physical or medical (Kavanaugh in Andrews & Boyle, 1995). Some cultures have widely held and culturally sanctioned beliefs that might be considered delusional in other cultures; therefore, an individual's cultural and religious background must be considered during the evaluation process.

Treatment

The treatment of paranoid disorders is difficult because of the denial by the patient, the presence of suspicion, and resistance to therapy because of the paranoid delusions. The person is highly threatened by any personal contact required during treatment. Treatment depends on the severity of the disorder and the ability of the person to function outside the hospital setting. It may occur in private practice by a psychiatrist or in a mental health clinic, where symptoms are alleviated to the degree that is essential for continued employment and community living. If feelings of persecution persist, and the tendency toward impulsive, destructive behavior presents a problem to the family and community, hospitalization may be required.

The initial treatment plan is threefold: evaluate safety, provide symptom remission, and establish rapport. If the person is extremely belligerent, injectable neuroleptics are very effective in controlling distressing feelings. Once such feelings are alleviated and psychotherapeutic intervention begins, the therapist must be honest and straightforward while focusing on the patient's emotional response to the environment. The therapist also must convey to the patient that although she or he does not agree with any delusions, the therapist is interested in the patient's welfare. Confronting delusions directly may increase agitation and usually is not beneficial to the patient. Long-term management generally consists of low-dosage antipsychotic or neuroleptic drugs and individual psychotherapy.

Nursing Diagnoses and Interventions

Paranoid persons may make the nurse feel as if she or he were being attacked, assaulted, and belittled. The nurse may feel stupid because the paranoid person blames the nurse or others for his or her difficulties. The nurse should be aware that delusions protect patients from recognizing or coping with feelings that are often the opposite of those represented by the delusion, result from overwhelming anxiety, represent an exaggerated picture of what the person believes, and often result in the use of the defenses such as projection or intellectualization. Barile (Lego, 1984) lists five nonproductive reactions to delusional patients. These responses include (1) becoming anxious and avoiding the patient; (2) reinforcing delusions by actually believing the patient; (3) attempting to prove that the patient is mistaken by presenting a logical argument; (4) setting unrealistic goals that lead to disappointment, frustration, or anger; and (5) being inconsistent with nursing interventions.

Nursing care of paranoid patients focuses on establishing rapport; enhancing self-esteem; decreasing fears and suspicion; handling hostility, aggression, delusions, and ideas of reference; observing for suicidal ideation; and assisting the patient in the activities of daily living.

The following are goals for patients to correct delusional systems:

1. Identify ways to control thoughts such as distracting oneself from thinking the same thought repeatedly.
2. Identify signs, such as staring, that indicate thoughts are becoming disorganized.
3. Anticipate that a new situation may increase anxiety and think of a way to decrease anxiety.
4. Share thoughts and ideas with others to examine their appropriateness.
5. Establish thought-stopping techniques.

6. Engage in thought-switching techniques.
7. Identify and dispute irrational thoughts.
8. Use a problem-solving process.

Providing the patient with the following teaching checklist may also be helpful.

Long-term goals focus on assisting the patient in developing alternative ways to cope with stress and loss, developing feelings of trust toward family or close associates, and complying with a medication regime.

Examples of nursing diagnoses related to individuals exhibiting clinical symptoms of delusional thoughts or paranoid behavior include *altered thought processes, suspiciousness, *risk for violence, *noncompliance, *self-esteem disturbance, *ineffective individual coping, and altered perception. Nursing Care Plan 21-1 (on p. 400) provides an example of a nursing diagnosis and goal-related nursing interventions for the individual with the DSM-IV diagnosis of delusional disorder.

═══════════════ PATIENT TEACHING CHECKLIST ═══════════════
Delusional Disorder

The following checklist has been developed to reinforce your knowledge about your illness. Please inform the nurse if you are uncertain about any of the items listed below:

✔ Clinical symptoms I may experience include:
✔ The reasons I may feel suspicious, paranoid, or delusional include:
✔ Interventions I have learned to increase feelings of security:
✔ Support persons I may contact include:
✔ The name of the medication I am taking is:
✔ Instructions regarding this medication
  ▪ Take this medication as directed by your doctor
  ▪ Do not drink alcohol while taking this medication
  ▪ Do not take any over-the-counter medication without informing your nurse or doctor
  ▪ Usual side effects include:
  ▪ Report any unusual side effects promptly
  ▪ Dosage adjustment may be necessary if your symptoms do not respond positively to the present dosage
  ▪ Do not discontinue taking this medication without first consulting your nurse or doctor

Note: Not all patients with the diagnosis of delusional disorder respond to the first three interventions listed above, nor will all patients agree to take medication. This checklist is designed to assist the compliant delusional patient.

───

NANDA-approved nursing diagnosis.

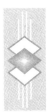

NURSING CARE PLAN 21-1

The Patient with Delusional Disorder

Nursing Diagnosis: *Altered thought processes related to misperception of environmental stimuli resulting in feelings of fear and suspicious thoughts

Goal #1: The patient will experience decreased feelings of fear and suspicious thoughts during hospitalization.

Nursing Interventions	Outcome Criteria
	Within 48 to 72 hours the patient will begin to do the following:
Establish rapport and a trusting relationship by listening, showing acceptance of the patient, and being consistently reliable.	Demonstrate a willingness to trust staff
Explore feelings of fear and suspicious thoughts.	Express feelings and report suspicious thoughts as they occur
Be genuine and honest.	State feelings in a given situation
	Report a decrease in suspicious thoughts

Nursing Diagnosis: *Altered thought processes related to misperception of environmental stimuli resulting in feelings of fear and suspicious thoughts

Goal #2: The patient will demonstrate socially acceptable behavior during hospitalization.

Nursing Interventions	Outcome Criteria
	Within 48 to 72 hours, the patient will begin to do the following:
Encourage patient to verbalize feelings about his or her environment.	Identify environmental stimuli that are perceived to be a threat
Avoid competitive, aggressive activities or close physical contact to minimize negative responses to environment, such as suspicions.	Exhibit positive responses to environmental stimuli
Discuss diversional activities to channel energy and maintain self-control.	Demonstrate an increase in self-control

* NANADA-*approved nursing diagnosis.*

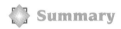 **Summary**

This chapter focused on the classification of delusional or paranoid disorders. The etiology or predisposing factors were stated and clinical features were discussed. The DSM-IV criteria for shared psychotic disorder and delusional disorder were given. Examples were cited. Transcultural considerations were discussed. Treatment approaches were addressed, focusing on the administration of neuroleptic medication and individual psychotherapy to control feelings of distress. Nursing interventions, including nonproductive reactions to delusional patients, were presented. Examples of nursing diagnoses and nursing interventions for an individual with the DSM-IV diagnosis of delusional disorder were given.

Learning Activities

I. Clinical Activities
   A. Focus on at least one patient who is demonstrating suspicious behavior.
   B. Identify the use of projection as you interact with the patient.
   C. Identify delusional thinking and the purpose it serves (*e.g.*, grandiose thinking to enhance one's self-esteem).
   D. Observe how the patient's behavior affects the staff.
   E. List specific activities aimed at establishing rapport and enhancing self-esteem.
   F. Does the patient express fear verbally or nonverbally, and in what situations?
   G. If possible, discuss with the patient ways to alter or cope with one situation that produces fear.
   H. Attempt to identify a person in the community who may become a support person and to whom this patient might relate on a continuing basis.
II. Independent Activities
   A. Review "The Client Who Is Delusional" by Linda Barile (Lego, 1984) and complete the following:
      1. Define paranoid, grandiose, sexual, religious, somatic, and inferiority delusions.
      2. Discuss the five examples of nonproductive reactions to delusional persons.
   B. Review the psychotropic drugs used to treat individuals with paranoid disorders and state the rationale for each.

Critical Thinking Questions

1. Newspapers and television news programs frequently report on celebrities being stalked by fans. Select a recent or current story. Using what you have learned about delusional disorders, analyze the stalker's behavior. What conclusions can you draw from this situation?
2. As you have learned, delusional disorder can occur in recent immigrants. Identify the immigrant population closest to where you live. Contact the community health department that services this population. What questions would you ask a community health nurse to determine if any of the immigrants show symptoms of delusional disorder?
3. Listen to your inner dialog to identify autonomic negative thoughts. Identify specific thought-stopping techniques and describe how you would use them to reduce these thoughts.

Self-Test

1. *Folie à deux* is a term used to identify _____.
2. Define delusional disorder.
3. Discuss the importance of considering cultural or religious background when providing care for a person with the diagnosis of delusional disorder.
4. State the reason a therapist is challenged when working with a patient who is paranoid.
5. Explain the rationale for administering neuroleptic medication to a person with persecutory delusions.
6. State why the behavior of a person with delusional thoughts may be unpredictable.

SELECTED REFERENCES

Abrams, A. C. (1995). *Clinical drug therapy: Rationales for nursing practice* (4th ed.). Philadelphia: J. B. Lippincott.

American Psychiatric Association. (1994). *Diagnostic and statistical manual of mental disorders* (4th ed.). Washington, DC: American Psychiatric Press.

Andrews, M. M., & Boyle, J. S. (1995). *Transcultural concepts in nursing care* (2nd ed.). Philadelphia: J. B. Lippincott.

Carpenito, L. J. (1995). *Nursing diagnosis: Application to clinical practice* (6th ed.). Philadelphia: J. B. Lippincott.

Gary, F., & Kavanagh, C. K. (1991). *Psychiatric mental health nursing*. Philadelphia: J. B. Lippincott.

Houseman, C. (1990, April). The paranoid person: A biopsychosocial perspective. *Archives of Psychiatric Nursing.*

Johnson, B. S. (1997). *Psychiatric mental health nursing: Adaptation and growth* (4th ed.). Philadelphia: Lippincott–Raven Publishers.

Kaplan, H. I., & Sadock, B. J. (1981). *Modern synopsis of comprehensive textbook of psychiatry* (3rd ed.). Baltimore: Williams & Wilkins.

Lego, S. (1984). *The American handbook of psychiatric nursing.* Philadelphia: J. B. Lippincott.

Newhill, C. E. (1990, February). The role of culture in the development of paranoid symptomatology. *American Journal of Orthopsychiatry.*

Rosenthal, T., & McGuiness, T. (1986, February). Dealing with delusional patients: Discovering distorted truth. *Issues in Mental Health Nursing.*

Schultz, J. M., & Videbeck, S. D. (1994). *Manual of psychiatric nursing care plans* (4th ed.). Philadelphia: J. B. Lippincott.

Sebastion, L. (1987, May). Psychiatric hospital admissions: Assessing patients' perceptions. *Journal of Psychosocial Nursing and Mental Health Services.*

Sideleau, B. F. (1987, March). Irrational beliefs and intervention. *Journal of Psychosocial Nursing and Mental Health Services.*

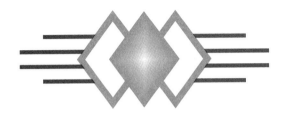

CHAPTER 22

ALTERED THOUGHT PROCESSES: SCHIZOPHRENIA AND OTHER PSYCHOTIC DISORDERS

A woman from Canaan who was living there came to him, pleading, "Have mercy on me, O Lord, King David's Son! For my daughter has a demon within her, and it torments her constantly."

Matthew 15:22

1 Discuss the latest research findings related to the development of schizophrenia.

2 Describe at least three theories regarding the development of schizophrenia.

3 Differentiate between positive and negative symptoms of schizophrenia.

4 Differentiate the five specific types of schizophrenic disorders by symptoms and developmental level of onset.

5 Differentiate between schizophrenic and schizophrenic-like disorders.

6 Compare clinical symptoms of brief psychotic disorder with psychotic disorder due to a medical condition.

7 Describe modes of treatment to aid the schizophrenic person with adaptation to stress.

8 State nursing diagnoses commonly used while planning care for individuals with the DSM-IV diagnosis of schizophrenia.

9 Describe therapeutic nursing interventions when planning care for patients with the diagnosis of psychotic disorder due to epilepsy.

 Introduction

Approximately two to four million individuals in the United States exhibit clinical symtoms of schizophrenia, the most complex and disabling type of mental illness. It continues to be poorly understood with regard to its diagnosis, etiology, course, and treatment. Because of the heterogeneity and complexities of this illness, training, research, and education in schizophrenia have been awarded the highest priority at the National Institute of Mental Health. The Department of Psychiatry at Albert Einstein College of Medicine maintains a strong dedication and commitment toward training and education, as well as toward clinical neuroscience research in the area of schizophrenia (Iqbal et al., 1993).

 Theories of Schizophrenia

Several theories have been proposed regarding the etiology or psychodynamics of schizophrenia, although the exact cause has not been identified. A brief summary of the theories follows.

Psychological or Experiential Theory

Proponents of this most common theory state that schizophrenia develops early in life because of various stressors. Among these are poor mother–child relationships, deeply disturbed family interpersonal relationships, impaired sexual identity and body image, rigid concept of reality, and repeated exposure to double-bind situations. A *double-bind situation* is a no-win experience in which there is no correct choice. An example might be when a mother tells a child who is dressed in good clothes that he may go out and play but not get dirty. At the same time, the mother's body language conveys the message that she prefers that the child stay indoors. The child does not know which message to follow.

The following is an example of a home situation that could contribute to the development of schizophrenia if therapeutic intervention does not occur.

A 10-year-old boy lives with his parents, two siblings, and an invalid grandmother. The mother works full-time and, because of physical disability, is unable to do the housework. The grandmother is unable to help with daily chores so the children are expected to help with various tasks such as sweeping, cleaning, ironing, and emptying the garbage. If the work is not done to the mother's satisfaction, the children are punished physically and are made to forfeit various privileges.

The mother does not communicate well with other family members. When she arrives home from work, she usually complains about work and the condition of the house. The children have learned to avoid her as much as possible.

The father is a traveling salesman and does not spend much time with the children. When the father is home, he and his wife argue about finances and disciplining the children. Because the father is gone frequently, the 10-year-old boy has not had a father figure with whom he can identify. He has begun to show an interest in cooking and playing with dolls.

The mother and grandmother do not get along well. Each tries to outdo the other with various somatic or physical complaints.

Because of his fear of punishment, the boy has begun to withdraw to his room whenever his parents argue or his mother complains about the housework. On occasion he has soiled the bed while sleeping and has resorted to babytalk.

Biologic Theory

Theorists have listed at least two subtypes under the biologic theory; these are genetic and biochemical predisposition to schizophrenic disorders.

The genetic (or hereditary) predisposition theory suggests that children of schizophrenic parents are more apt to develop schizophrenia than are other persons. Approximately 40% of children born to parents who are both schizophrenic will be affected. If only one parent is schizophrenic, approximately 10% of the children will be psychotic.

The biochemical or toxic psychosis theory lists possible contributive factors to the onset of schizophrenia. Substances similar to hallucinogens or mind-altering drugs, which accumulate excessively in the body and cause an elevated level of dopamine, are possible factors being considered. According to the theory, excessive dopamine allows nerve impulses to bombard the brain, resulting in schizophrenic symptoms. The administration of antipsychotic medication supposedly blocks the excessive release of dopamine. The cause of the release of high levels of dopamine has not yet been found.

Environmental or Sociocultural Theory

Theorists state that the person who develops schizophrenia has a faulty reaction to the environment and is unable to respond selectively to numerous social stimuli. Theorists also believe that persons who come from low socioeconomic areas or single-parent homes in deprived areas do not have the chance to experience achievement. An example of this theory can be seen in the following situation.

An 8-year-old girl lives in a two-room apartment infested with rats and roaches. Her mother, who is unwed, is on welfare and receives Aid for Dependent Children to support six children. The young girl is expected to babysit three younger children while her mother seeks employment and goes shopping for groceries. Consequently, she has missed much schooling and has been retained in the first grade for another year. Her occasional playmates consist of a 5-year-old boy and a 7-year-old girl, both of whom are also deprived children.

In response to this faulty environment, the young girl has learned to fantasize and to create her own play-world. She has created her own language so that others do not learn about her secret world. If this behavior continues without therapeutic intervention, the young girl could be presenting clinical symptoms suggestive of the development of schizophrenia.

Organic Theory

Those who suggest the organic theory offer hope that schizophrenia is a functional deficit, occurring in the brain and caused by such stressors as infection, poison, trauma, or abnormal substances. They also propose that schizophrenia may be a metabolic disorder.

Vitamin Deficiency Theory

The vitamin deficiency theory suggests that persons who are deficient in vitamin B—namely B_1, B_6, and B_{12}—as well as vitamin C may become schizophrenic as a result of a severe deficiency.

Although this theory, as well as other theories, has not been confirmed, research continues in hope of isolating a chemical that might be responsible for the development of schizophrenia.

Research Findings

Neuroimaging techniques are now being used in the research of schizophrenia. They include computed tomography (CT), magnetic resonance imaging (MRI), single photon emission computed tomography (SPECT), and positron emission tomography (PET). CT studies have indicated that ventricular enlargement, cortical atrophy, or cerebellar atrophy are present in individuals with the diagnoses of schizophrenia. The most consistently replicated findings indicate ventricular enlargement, especially of the lateral ventricles.

MRI is a relatively new psychiatric research technique that has identified the following abnormalities in the presence of schizophrenia: smaller frontal, temporal, hippocampal, thalamic, and cerebral areas, as well as ventricular enlargement.

SPECT findings suggest that a pattern of hypofrontality and increased blood flow in the basal ganglia may be present in schizophrenia. PET, the most elegant of the brain imaging techniques, has also identified patterns of relative hypofrontality.

Regional cerebral blood flow is a noninvasive technique used to measure cerebral metabolic activity. Xenon-133 is mixed with air, inhaled in a controlled environment, external brain detectors are applied, and the amount of xenon-133 clearance from the brain is measured. Baseline metabolic function of the frontal lobe and left hemisphere has been identified in some patients with the diagnosis of schizophrenia (Holman & Devous, 1992; Pfefferbaum et al., 1990; Sharif, Gewirtz, & Iqbal, 1993).

Kaufmann and Malaspina (1993) discuss the role of genetic factors contributing to the development of and vulnerability to schizophrenia. Research questions focus on whether schizophrenia is inherited, how is it inherited, what abnormal genes are involved, and what additional variables increase or decrease the chances of genetically predisposed individuals developing schizophrenia. Reference has been made to chromosome 6, according to findings published in the November, 1995 issue of the journal, *Nature Genetics*.

 Clinical Symptoms

The DSM-IV classification lists five subclassifications or subtypes of schizophrenic disorder: disorganized, catatonic, paranoid, undifferentiated, and residual. Five other psychotic disorders classified as schizophrenic-like disorders are schizophreniform disorder, brief psychotic disorder, schizoaffective disorder, psychotic disorder due to a general medical condition, and shared psychotic disorder. The latter disorder was discussed in the previous chapter.

Although schizophrenia usually occurs between the ages of 15 and 45 years, some theorists believe the onset is diagnosed primarily between the ages of 17

BOX 22-1 Positive and Negative Syndrome Scale (PANSS)

Positive Scale (P): Excess or distortion of normal functions
  Delusions (persecutory, referential, somatic, religious, or grandiose)
  Conceptual disorganization
  Hallucinatory behavior (auditory, visual, olfactory, gustatory,
    or tactile)
  Excitement
  Grandiosity
  Suspiciousness/persecution
  Hostility
Negative Scale (N): Diminution or loss of normal functions
  Blunted affect or affective flattening
  Emotional withdrawal
  Poor rapport
  Passive/apathetic social withdrawal or avolition
  Difficulty in abstract thinking (formerly "loosening of associations")
  Lack of spontaneity and flow of conversation or alogia
  Stereotyped thinking

and 27 years. Characteristic symptoms fall into two broad categories, positive and negative. The positive symptoms reflect an excess or distortion of normal functions; negative symptoms reflect a diminution or loss of normal functions. Box 22-1 lists the positive and negative symptoms of schizophrenia.

Following is a list of psychiatric terms not previously described in the text that are considered to be clinical symptoms of schizophrenia (referred to as general psychopathology): somatic concern, anxiety, guilt feelings, tension, mannerisms and posturing, depression, motor retardation, uncooperativeness, unusual thought content, disorientation, poor attention, lack of judgment and insight, disturbance of volition, poor impulse control, preoccupation, and active social avoidance.

Symptoms of schizophrenia are described in more detail as each clinical subclassification or subtype is presented.

 Transcultural Considerations

As stated in previous chapters, nurses must consider cultural differences when assessing clinical symptoms in persons with psychiatric disorders. Ideas that appear delusional in one culture may be acceptable in another. Visual or auditory hallucinations with a religious content may be a normal religious experience or considered to be a special sign to some individuals. The speaking in tongues that occurs in some religions could be assessed as delusional, hallucinatory, or disorganized speech.

According to the DSM-IV, clinicians have a tendency to overdiagnose schizophrenia in some ethnic groups. Catatonic behavior is more common in non-Western countries. Persons with the diagnosis of schizophrenia in developing nations tend to experience a more acute course with a better outcome than do individuals in industrialized nations.

Clinical Types of Schizophrenia

Disorganized Type

The classification of disorganized type (previously called hebephrenic) is considered to be the most severe type of personality disorganization. Clinical symptoms may occur because the person is unable to complete a transition from adolescence to maturity, thereby contributing to an early onset. Clinical symptoms include

1. Flat, inappropriate, or silly affect such as giggling or superficial sadness. An example would be to laugh when told someone had just been murdered.
2. Disorganized speech or the inability to make sense or be understood when talking. The person appears to be mumbling words rather than speaking clearly.
3. Behavioral disorganization or severe disruption in the ability to perform activities of daily living. The individual is not goal oriented.
4. Hallucinations and delusions are not well organized.
5. Absence of systematized or logically defined delusions.

Catatonic Type

Catatonic schizophrenia is differentiated from other types of schizophrenic disorders mainly by behavioral or psychomotor symptoms. Symptoms include

1. Abnormal or catatonic posturing, in which the person voluntarily assumes an unusual or bizarre position.
2. Catatonic stupor or withdrawal from the environment. Expressionless, the patient may stare into space. A decrease in spontaneous movements also may be noted, in which the person lies, sits, or stands still for long periods of time. Although the patient appears nonresponsive, he or she may still be in contact with the environment and aware of all that is happening. Catatonic patients have recalled detailed experiences after recovering from the stupor.
3. Catatonic rigidity. The patient assumes a position and will not move when efforts are made to change the position.
4. Catatonic negativism. The patient who is catatonic is resistant to all instructions or attempts to be moved.

5. Catatonic excitement. The person responds to stimuli from within and becomes extremely agitated. Movements may be purposeless or stereotyped. Such a person is to be considered potentially aggressive and capable of assault during this state.
6. Unexpected shifts from one behavioral state to another.
7. Waxy flexibility. The person will maintain the position in which she or he has been placed.
8. Two mannerisms occasionally exhibited by the catatonic patient: *echolalia* (repeats all words or phrases heard) and *echopraxia* (mimics actions of others).

⚙ CLINICAL EXAMPLE 22-1
Disorganized Type

MJ, a 19-year-old waitress, was seen in the admitting office of a psychiatric hospital. During the initial interview, she giggled inappropriately. Her long, uncombed hair fell over her face, concealing her facial expressions. She mumbled incoherently at times and displayed the behavior of a 13- or 14-year-old adolescent. She complained of numerous aches and pains and stated that voices told her she was being punished for not cleaning her room. MJ's mother stated that she remained in her room at home and did not socialize with friends. Her parents sought help when they noticed her behavior regressing during the past two months.

Because of the young age of most patients diagnosed as schizophrenic disorder, disorganized type, student nurses' reactions vary from shock to disbelief. Students may identify with the patient who is close to their age or resembles someone that they know. This reaction could interfere with the development of a therapeutic relationship. Such feelings should be shared and explored with the clinical instructor.

Once the initial reaction has been examined and resolved, nursing care can be initiated based on the assessment of the patient. With a patient such as MJ, who mumbles and giggles inappropriately owing to feelings of discomfort or inadequacy, communication must be established. Reality should be stressed when the patient discusses the voices that talk to her.

A physical examination should be done within 24 hours to rule out any organic cause of physical complaints. Once the results are known, reality can be stressed if the patient continues to complain. Limit setting may be used to discourage complaints by refusing to discuss somatic concerns with the patient if there is no pathologic basis for the complaints. Regressive behavior occurs as the patient reverts to a more comfortable developmental stage to decrease feelings of anxiety. Social withdrawal occurs as the patient becomes preoccupied with thoughts and fantasies.

⚙ CLINICAL EXAMPLE 22-2
Catatonic Type

CS, a 25-year-old engineer, was admitted to the hospital as result of dehydration because of refusing to eat. During his hospitalization, CS was negativistic, refusing nursing care, food, and medication. He rarely spoke and assumed uncomfortable positions in bed for long periods. When placed in various positions by the nurse during the morning bath or shower, CS remained in the positions until they were changed by the nurse. He also exhibited purposeless movements of his hands and feet while sitting in the chair.

The student nurse's reactions to catatonic behavior usually consist of fear and frustration. Fear of unpredictable, abnormal behavior is a normal response that results in the exercise of caution when one is working with catatonic patients. Frustration is heightened when the patient exhibits negativistic behavior such as refusal to eat or nonresponsiveness to the environment.

The sudden onset of catatonic behavior usually occurs between the ages of 15 and 25 years and is of short duration. Statistics show that more women than men are diagnosed as catatonic schizophrenics. The prognosis is good for an acute state, but many patients have recurrent episodes.

Basic human needs must be monitored to ensure adequate nutrition, elimination, activity, and rest. The patient may need to be protected during periods of unpredictable agitated behavior.

Paranoid Type

The main behavior identified in persons with paranoic schizophrenia is that of suspiciousness. Clinical symptoms include

1. Overuse of the defense mechanism projection. Persons may blame others for failures in their life or for their illness, or believe that people are talking about them because people do not like them. (Refer to *ideas of reference* in vocabulary list at the end of the chapter.)
2. Hostility and aggressiveness or violence. Persons may display impulsive, hostile behavior to defend themselves against suspected harm. Violence or suicide may be the result of auditory hallucinations (voices telling them to act in a certain way).
3. Argumentative behavior. Paranoid individuals are very defensive and prone to arguing owing to their suspicious nature.

4. Auditory hallucinations, which are persecutory or grandiose. Paranoid patients may state that voices are telling them that they must die or that a specific person is going to harm them. While experiencing a grandiose auditory hallucination, a patient may state that the President of the United States has asked him to attend the Inaugural Ball, for example.
5. Delusions of grandeur, persecution, jealousy, or religion. Examples of delusions were cited earlier. The delusions of paranoid schizophrenic patients are usually mystical and less organized than those seen in patients with the paranoid disorder, paranoia.

The onset of paranoid schizophrenia is usually seen in later adult life, between the ages of 30 to 35 years, but can occur at any age. Prognosis may be more favorable than for other types of schizophrenia with regard to capacity for independent living and occupational functioning.

It is not unusual for the student nurse to react to the paranoid patient with feelings of fear because of his or her hostile, aggressive, argumentative, or unpredictable behavior. It is difficult to communicate with a patient who expresses a delusion or talks about hearing voices. Nursing interventions for the paranoid schizophrenic patient focus on behaviors such as suspiciousness, hostility, and aggression.

Residual Type

The residual type can be described as the state of being in partial remission. The patient diagnosed as residual type has a history of at least one previous schizophrenic episode but no longer exhibits obvious or intense psychotic symptoms. The patient may exhibit clinical symptoms of social withdrawal, associative looseness, illogical thinking, or eccentric behavior. If the person is experiencing delusions or hallucinations, they are not readily discernible.

◈ CLINICAL EXAMPLE 22-3
Paranoid Type

BW, a 35-year-old mechanic, was brought to the admissions office by his wife because he had exhibited strange behavior for several months. He accused his wife of poisoning his food, spending all his money, having an affair with his boss, and telling stories about him. He displayed no facial expressions during his initial interview and became quite argumentative when questioned about his job. At the end of the interview, BW confided in the interviewer that he had been receiving messages from Jesus Christ while watching television.

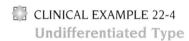 CLINICAL EXAMPLE 22-4
Undifferentiated Type

AB, a 52-year-old carpenter, was making a rocking chair in his workshop when he suddenly began to talk to the television set. When his wife stopped by to bring him supper she was shocked to find the rocking chair broken and the tools scattered on the floor. Her husband was huddled in the corner, curled up like a small child, talking to himself and singing Christmas carols. At times he mumbled incoherently. When Mrs. B attempted to talk to him, her husband did not recognize her or know where he was.

Undifferentiated Type

This category is used for a person who exhibits a mixture of psychotic symptoms such as delusions, hallucinations, grossly disorganized behavior and speech, and negative symptoms of schizophrenia but cannot be classified in any of the other categories.

The following is a clinical example of a patient diagnosed as schizophrenic disorder, undifferentiated type.

The more acute or sudden the onset of schizophrenic disorder, the more favorable is the prognosis. The earlier in life psychotic symptoms develop, the less favorable the prognosis.

 ## Schizophrenic-like Disorders

The five subtypes of schizophrenic-like disorders are (1) schizoaffective disorder, (2) schizophreniform disorder, (3) brief psychotic disorder, (4) psychotic disorder due to a general medical condition, and (5) shared psychotic disorder, which was discussed in the previous chapter.

Schizoaffective disorder is characterized by an uninterrupted period of illness during which, at some time, there is a major depressive, manic, or mixed episode concurrent with the negative symptoms of schizophrenia. During that same period of illness, in the absence of prominent mood symptoms, the individual exhibits delusions or hallucinations for at least two weeks.

The diagnosis of schizophreniform disorder is used when the person exhibits features of schizophrenia for more than one month but less than six months and impaired social or occupational functioning does not necessarily occur.

Brief psychotic disorder is a disturbance that involves the sudden onset of at least one of the positive symptoms of psychosis (hallucinations, delusions, disorganized speech, or grossly disorganized or catatonic behavior). The disturbance occurs for at least one day but less than one month, as the individual eventually exhibits a full recovery or return to former level of functioning.

Psychotic disorder due to a general medical condition is the diagnosis used to describe the presence of prominent hallucinations or delusions judged to be due to the direct physiologic effects of a specific medical condition. For example, olfactory hallucinations may be experienced in the presence of temporal lobe epilepsy. A right parietal brain lesion may cause an individual to develop delusions. There must be evidence from history, physical examination, or laboratory findings to confirm the diagnosis.

 ## Treatment

Four treatment methods have been identified as effective when treating the schizophrenic patient. The selection of the treatment method depends on the type of schizophrenic disorder and the severity of the psychotic behavior. All four methods may be combined at one time. They are

1. *Psychotherapy:* Individual, group, behavioral, supportive, or family therapy may be used. Selection of the specific type of therapy depends on presenting clinical symptoms, the person's ability to communicate, and the relationship with the family. The therapist also evaluates whether the patient will benefit more from an individual or a group approach.
2. *Milieu therapy:* A structured environment is used to minimize environmental and physical stress and to meet the individual needs of patients until they are able to assume responsibility for themselves.
3. *Chemotherapy:* Antipsychotic drugs (*e.g.*, Haldol, Clozaril, Risperdal, Mellaril, Prolixin, and Navane) may be prescribed. The choice of drug depends on the symptoms, the patient's tolerance and response to the drug, and expected outcome of drug therapy. If the patient is acutely disturbed, he or she may require an injectable form of Prolixin or Haldol. The cost of the drug also must be considered because the patient may discontinue taking the drug if she or he cannot afford it. Most schizophrenic patients receive drugs over an extended period and usually continue them after discharge from the hospital. Individuals on Clozaril are monitored closely because of possible agranulocytosis or leukopenia and abnormal liver function test results.

    Four investigational agents emulating the atypical antipsychotic pharmacology of Clozaril have successfully completed phase III trial results. They have not caused agranulocytosis and appear to exert fewer side effects than Haldol. They are olanzapine (Zyprexa), sertindole, quetiapine (Seroques), and ziprasidone (Bender, 1996).

There is a small population of patients with the diagnosis of schizo-phrenia who probably should not be treated with neuroleptic medication. This group includes persons whose illness is unaffected or worsened by medications, patients with a history of complete recovery in a brief time without the use of drugs, or persons at risk for severe adverse side effects. The risks may outweigh the benefits (Marder & Van Putten, 1995).

Antiparkinson agents may be prescribed to prevent or decrease the extrapyramidal side effects of psychotropic drugs. Examples of such drugs are Cogentin, Artane, Akineton, and Symmetrel. Refer to Chapter 12 for more information.

4. *Somatic or electroconvulsive therapy:* These therapies may be used as a treat-ment for severe schizophrenic disorders if the patient is unresponsive to tri-als of psychiatric medication. The use of electroconvulsive therapy has declined owing to the introduction of psychotropic drugs during the late 1950s and early 1960s.

 ## Nursing Diagnoses and Interventions

Nursing interventions focus on assisting the patient to meet the following goals: (1) establish a trusting relationship; (2) alleviate anxiety; (3) maintain biologic integrity; and (4) establish clear, consistent, and open communication.

The nurse must establish a therapeutic relationship to communicate effectively with the patient. Communication should be in simple or easy-to-understand terms and should be directed at the patient's present level of functioning. Supplying the patient with the teaching checklist (on p. 418) may be helpful in assessing the patient's knowledge and level of functioning. Schizophrenic patients may refuse to communicate or may communicate in-effectively as a result of

1. Self-contradictory or conflicting statements
2. Frequent changes in subject
3. Inconsistency in verbalization
4. Talking in incomplete or fragmented sentences
5. Presence of hallucinations and delusions

The nurse must remember that all behavior is meaningful to the patient, if not to anyone else.

Assessment of the schizophrenic patient includes identifying behavioral problems such as regression, disorientation, withdrawal, agitation, and acting-out. Assessment of the patient's ability to perform activities of daily living and meet basic human needs is imperative to maintain life. The patient's physical

================= PATIENT TEACHING CHECKLIST =================
Schizophrenia

The following checklist has been developed to reinforce your knowledge about schizophrenia. Please inform the nurse if you are uncertain about any of the items listed below.

✔ Clinical symptoms I may experience include:
✔ The reasons I may experience such symptoms include:
✔ Interventions I have learned to cope with or reduce such symptoms include:
✔ Support persons I may contact include:
✔ The name of the medication I am taking is:
✔ Instructions regarding this medication
  ▪ Take this medication as directed by your doctor
  ▪ Do not drink alcohol while taking this medication
  ▪ Do not take any over-the-counter medication without informing your nurse or doctor
  ▪ Usual side effects include:
  ▪ Report any unusual side effects promptly
  ▪ Dosage adjustment may be necessary
  ▪ Do not discontinue taking this medication without first consulting your nurse or doctor
✔ Lab work may be ordered to monitor your blood count, liver profile, or serum drug level. If you are not able to keep an appointment for lab work, please notify your nurse or doctor so that the test can be rescheduled.
✔ If you are receiving intramuscular injections of medication, it is important that you receive them at the same time each month.

---

condition also should be assessed to plan appropriate nursing interventions. Schizophrenic patients may be unable to feed themselves. They often refuse to eat because of paranoid thoughts, or may exhibit bizarre eating habits. Daily functions such as bathing, showering, and dressing may be overwhelming tasks requiring assistance.

Reality should be presented when caring for the patient who is disoriented. The nurse can do this by pointing out what would be appropriate behavior, for example, "I'd like you to put your shoes on now." Recognizing the presence of hallucinations and delusions, but not reinforcing such behavior or thoughts, is an appropriate response when interacting with patients. The nurse should look for factors causing hallucinations and attempt to intervene before they occur. The delusional system should be ignored.

Safety measures may need to be incorporated to protect patients who display poor judgment, disorientation, destructive behavior, suicidal ideation, or agitation. Limit setting, acknowledging spatial territory (giving patients "room to breathe"), and providing protective safety measures are examples of such nursing interventions. Patients must be protected from themselves because they may injure themselves accidently, or may try to destroy themselves or attack other patients as a result of auditory hallucinations or paranoid ideations.

Efforts should be made to plan activities to improve the patient's self-concept. Sincere compliments should be given as often as possible, focusing on positive aspects of the person's personality or capabilities. Encourage participation in activities.

The nurse must observe for extrapyramidal side effects of psychotropic drugs and monitor the patient's willingness to take the drugs. Patients may refuse to take medication, pretend to take medication by palming it, or pretend to swallow the medication while retaining the pill in the mouth (only to get rid of it at the first possible moment). They may refuse to have blood drawn to monitor liver function or complete blood count. One patient on Clozaril refused weekly laboratory work to monitor new white blood cell count because she felt the laboratory technician was "draining her blood from her body." The patient finally allowed a nurse whom she trusted to draw the blood.

Examples of nursing diagnoses used while planning care of individuals with clinical symptoms of schizophrenia include *altered thought processes, *impaired verbal communication, *fear, *altered health maintenance, *ineffective individual coping, *noncompliance, *personal identity disturbance, *self-esteem disturbance, *sleep pattern disturbance, and *social isolation.

Nursing Care Plan 22–1 (on p. 420) shows a nursing diagnosis and goal-related nursing interventions for an individual with the DSM-IV diagnosis of schizophrenia.

✿ Summary

This chapter focused on the various theories regarding the development of schizophrenia. The latest research findings were described. Clinical symptoms of the five subclassifications or subtypes of schizophrenic disorder were listed. The positive and negative syndrome scale of schizophrenia was included. Transcultural considerations were addressed. Clinical examples were cited. Schizophrenic-like disorders, including schizoaffective disorder, schizophreniform disorder, brief psychotic disorder, and psychotic disorder due to a general medical condition, were described. Shared psychotic disorder was discussed in the previous chapter. Four treatment methods were discussed. Nursing diagnoses and interventions were included.

NANDA-approved nursing diagnosis.

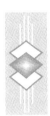

NURSING CARE PLAN 22-1
The Patient with Schizophrenia

Nursing Diagnosis: Agitation related to the presence of audiovisual hallucinations

Goal: Before discharge the patient will demonstrate control of behavior because of a decrease in or absence of audiovisual hallucinations.

Nursing Interventions	Outcome Criteria
	The patient will do the following:
Decrease environmental stimuli such as loud music or television shows, extremely bright colors, or flashing lights.	Verbalize feelings of agitation as they occur Identify stimuli that increase agitation
Present reality, for example: "The voices may be real to you but I don't hear anything."	Openly discuss presence of hallucinations with others
Attempt to identify precipitating factors by asking the patient what happened before the onset of the hallucination.	Describe thoughts and behavior prior to onset of hallucinations
Focus on the here-and-now by identifying underlying needs being met by the hallucinations.	Demonstrate insight regarding the purpose of hallucinations Demonstrate a decrease in agitation as insight regarding hallucinations improves
Medicate with prescribed antipsychotic agent.	Verbalize a decrease in or absence of audiovisual hallucinations when therapeutic level is reached
Educate regarding purpose of antipsychotic medication.	State the rationale for taking antipsychotic medication

Learning Activities

I. Clinical Activities
   A. Begin a relationship with a person experiencing schizophrenia.
   B. Identify any positive and negative symptoms that the patient exhibits.
   C. Identify examples of symptoms included in the terminology list in number III.
   D. List the therapies used and discuss the patient's responses.

E. Identify any antipsychotic drugs prescribed. State the rationale for their use; observe for side effects; evaluate effectiveness.

F. Identify nursing interventions used in caring for the patient.

II. Schizophrenia: Situations for Discussion

A. JW, 58 years old, has been admitted to the psychiatric unit and diagnosed as a schizophrenic, paranoid type. He blames his wife for his losing his job and states his employer "bugged" his telephone in the office. He confides in you that he "sees" Jesus frequently and that Jesus tells him everything is okay. JW keeps to himself and rarely shows any emotion.

　　1. Name the defense mechanisms that JW is using.

　　2. List the positive and negative symptoms present.

　　3. List the behaviors JW displays.

　　4. State the appropriate nursing interventions in response to this behavior.

B. MC has been admitted to the hospital with the diagnosis of schizophrenia, undifferentiated type. She is hostile, aggressive, and verbally abusive. She tells you she hears voices, acts inappropriately at times, and is regressive in her behavior. She tells you her "phillies have covered the thung."

　　1. Why is the patient diagnosed as undifferentiated schizophrenia?

　　2. List all symptoms, including positive and negative symptoms.

　　3. State the nursing problems presented by MC.

　　4. List the appropriate nursing interventions.

III. Terminology Related to Psychosis

The following is a list of terminology related to psychosis.

Apathy: Devoid of feeling, emotion, interest, or concern. A patient may show a lack of interest when visited by relatives.

Automatic obedience: An impaired thought process in which one does what one is told to do. The person responds to commands or suggestions in much the same way as a dog that has attended obedience school. The person does not appear to have a free will or to act independently.

Blocking: Sudden loss of thought content due to an anxiety-producing situation.

Clang association: A speech pattern characterized by the use of a series of sound-alike or rhyming words without regard to logic. May be used to compensate for defects in memory or communication. The sound of a word sets off a new train of thought.

Déjà vu (French for "already seen"): The sensation that a new situation has occurred previously

Depersonalization: Feelings of unreality or strangeness of self or the environment, a sense of not being oneself

Dissociation: A coping mechanism used to protect oneself from uncomfortable feelings by denying their existence

Echolalia: Repetition of another person's words or phrases (*e.g.*, a parrot mimicking a person's spoken word). Echolalia is seen in catatonic schizophrenia.

Echopraxia: Repetition or imitation of another person's movements (seen in catatonic schizophrenia)

Feelings of estrangement: The person feels detached or removed from people, the environment, or concepts.

Flight of ideas: Ideas or thoughts occur quickly and are so fragmentary that no single thought can be expressed clearly (*e.g.*, "I like money. Money is the root of all evil. Evil things have happened lately").

Folie à deux: Two closely related or associated persons, usually in the same family, share psychopathologic conditions that are nearly identical.

Ideas of reference: A person feels or believes that conversation and gestures occurring around the person have meaning intended especially for him or her (*e.g.*, a patient observing nurses giving report at the change of shift says, "They're plotting against me").

Neologisms: Coining or forming new words to express a complex idea

Word salad: Severe associative looseness, characterized by meaningless and incoherent mixtures of words and phrases (*e.g.*, "Sky is a blue rainbow my father's barrel").

IV. Independent Activities

Read the following for additional information on psychotic behavior:

A. H. Green, *I Never Promised You a Rose Garden*, 1964.

B. "Questions and Answers About Schizophrenia" in *Journal of Psychosocial Nursing and Mental Health Services*, August 1990.

Critical Thinking Questions

1. As you take the first bite of your burger in a fast-food restaurant, you notice a disheveled, dirty man in the booth across from you. He is talking to himself and gesturing wildly. Describe your thought process as you assess this man. What interventions, if any, would be appropriate?

2. Observe a psychiatric milieu unit. Discuss your findings: how is this unit organized, what are the characteristics of the environment, how does it feel?

3. Observe a client being treated with electroconvulsive therapy. How did you feel about what you observed? Discuss your thoughts and feelings with a classmate.

Self-Test

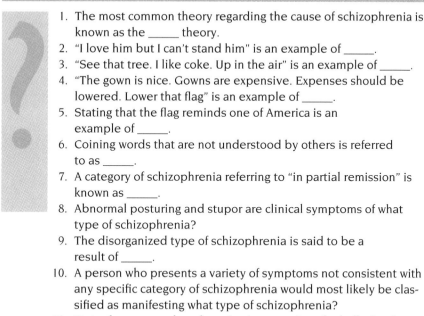

1. The most common theory regarding the cause of schizophrenia is known as the _____ theory.
2. "I love him but I can't stand him" is an example of _____.
3. "See that tree. I like coke. Up in the air" is an example of _____.
4. "The gown is nice. Gowns are expensive. Expenses should be lowered. Lower that flag" is an example of _____.
5. Stating that the flag reminds one of America is an example of _____.
6. Coining words that are not understood by others is referred to as _____.
7. A category of schizophrenia referring to "in partial remission" is known as _____.
8. Abnormal posturing and stupor are clinical symptoms of what type of schizophrenia?
9. The disorganized type of schizophrenia is said to be a result of _____.
10. A person who presents a variety of symptoms not consistent with any specific category of schizophrenia would most likely be classified as manifesting what type of schizophrenia?
11. State three examples of nursing interventions for hallucinations.
12. List three psychotropic drugs used to treat schizophrenia.
13. List three types of neuroimaging tests used to conduct research on schizophrenia.
14. Why is it important to monitor the white blood cell count of a patient receiving Clozaril?

SELECTED REFERENCES

Abrams, A. C. (1995). *Clinical drug therapy: Rationales for nursing practice* (4th ed.). Philadelphia: J. B. Lippincott.

American Psychiatric Association. (1994). *Diagnostic and statistical manual of mental disorders* (4th ed.). Washington, DC: American Psychiatric Press.

Andrews, M. M., & Boyle, J. S. (1995). *Transcultural concepts in nursing care* (2nd ed.). Philadelphia: J. B. Lippincott.

Bender, K. J. (1996, February). SDA antipsychotics show promise in phase III trials. *Psychiatric Times.*

Carpenito, L. J. (1995). *Nursing diagnosis: Application to clinical practice* (6th ed.). Philadelphia: J. B. Lippincott.

Dzurec, L. C. (1990, August). How do they see themselves? Self-perceptions and functioning for people with chronic schizophrenia. *Journal of Psychosocial Nursing and Mental Health Services.*

Holman, L., & Devous, M. D., Sr. (1992, October). Functional brain SPECT: The emergence of a powerful clinical method. *Journal of Nuclear Medicine.*

Iqbal, N., Schwartz, B. J., Cecil, A., Imran, Z., & Canal, C. (1993, March). Schizophrenia diagnosis. *Psychiatric Annals*.

Karch, A. M. (1997). *Lippincott's nursing drug guide*. Philadelphia: Lippincott–Raven Publishers.

Kaufmann, C. A., & Malaspina, D. (1993, March). Molecular genetics of schizophrenia. *Psychiatric Annals*.

Lego, S. (1996). *Psychiatric nursing: A comprehensive reference* (2nd ed.). Philadelphia: Lippincott–Raven Publishers.

Marder, S. R., & Van Putten, T. (1995). Antipsychotic medications. In A. F. Schatzberg & C. B. Nemeroff (Eds.). *The American Psychiatric Press textbook of psychopharmacology*. Washington, DC: American Psychiatric Press.

Pfefferbaum, A., Lim, K. O., et al. (1990). Brain magnetic resonance imaging: approaches for investigation schizophrenia. *Schizophrenia Bulletin, 16*.

Schultz, J. M., & Videbeck, S. D. (1994). *Manual of psychiatric nursing care plans* (4th ed.). Philadelphia: J. B. Lippincott.

Sharif, Z., Gewirtz, G., & Iqbal, N. (1993, March). Brain imaging in schizophrenia: A review. *Psychiatric Annals*.

Yaktin, U. S., & Laabban, S. (1992, June). Traumatic war stress and schizophrenia. *Journal of Psychosocial Nursing and Mental Health Services*.

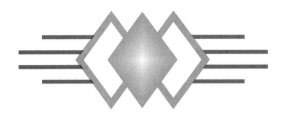

CHAPTER 23

IMPAIRED COGNITION: DELIRIUM, DEMENTIA, AMNESTIC, AND OTHER COGNITIVE DISORDERS

The death of the mind is the worst death imaginable, and for millions of Americans the slow death . . . creates a world of pain and suffering. The number of affected individuals signal the profound magnitude of the public health challenges to our society.

D. *Cohen*, *PhD*
Somebody Tell Me Who I Am, 1995

LEARNING OBJECTIVES

1 State the clinical features of

Delirium

Dementia

Amnestic disorder

2 Differentiate between dementia of the Alzheimer's type and vascular dementia.

3 Explain the purpose of the following assessment tools:

JOMAC

Mental Status Questionnaire

Rapid Disability Rating Scale

Brief Cognitive Rating Scale

Global Deterioration Scale

4 State the diagnostic tests used to identify the precipitating cause of a cognitive disorder.

5 Discuss the latest research findings related to cognitive disorders.

6 Cite short- and long-term nursing goals for a person with a cognitive disorder.

7 List nursing interventions for the following nursing diagnoses of a person with dementia:

Altered thought processes related to disorientation of person, place, and time

Risk for injury related to inability to ambulate independently

✿ Introduction

Acquired cognitive impairment is a broad general classification used to categorize disorders due to transient or permanent brain dysfunction caused by a disturbance of physiologic functioning of brain tissue. The DSM-IV has reclassified the disorders in this category. The term *organic mental disorder* is no longer used because it incorrectly implies that "nonorganic" mental disorders do not have a biologic basis.

The following disorders are discussed in this chapter: delirium, dementia, amnestic disorder, dementia due to other general medical conditions, and cognitive disorder not otherwise specified. Substance-related disorders are included in this classification but are discussed in separate chapters.

The differential diagnosis of dementia or delirium is based on the type of onset and course of symptoms. Mental processes, speech, behavior, and level of consciousness as well as presumed or established etiology are considered in determining a diagnosis.

Clinical Types of Cognitive Disorders

Delirium

Delirium is one of the most common and, by far, one of the most life-threatening psychiatric illnesses. Estimates vary from as low as 10% to 15% for patients on acute medical/surgical units to as high as 60% in postcardiotomy patients. High-risk populations include elderly patients, burn patients, patients with previous brain injury, as well as drug-dependent patients and those with human immunodeficiency virus (HIV) infection. In individuals older than 65 years of age who are hospitalized for a general medical condition, approximately 10% are reported to exhibit delirium on admission and another 10% to 15% may develop delirium while in the hospital.

Delirium is defined as a transient cognitive disorder, usually acute or subacute in onset, that presents as a reversible global dysfunction in cerebral metabolism. Various terms are used to identify delirium including ICU psychosis, encephalopathy, acute brain failure, and acute confusional state.

Clinical symptoms include a rapid onset (hours to days), in which symptoms may vary sharply in a short period of time. Judgment may be impaired. Affect or mood fluctuates. Memory is impaired, especially for recent events. Disorientation to person and place usually occurs. Language disturbances, referred to as dysnomia, or the inability to name objects, and dysgraphia, or the impaired ability to write, may occur. Speech may be incoherent, sparse, or fluent. Perceptual disturbances may include misinterpretations, illusions, or hallucinations. Thought process appears confused, with possible delusional content. Behavior exhibited may include agitation, restlessness, wandering, and disturbance in sleep–wake cycle. Asterixis, an abnormal movement in which the patient exhibits a peculiar flapping movement of hyperextended hands, is seen in various delirious states. Although the patient may perform poorly on mental status tests, cognitive ability generally improves when the patient recovers unless the delirium is superimposed on moderate to severe dementia. The prognosis includes a return to premorbid function if the cause is corrected in time.

The diagnosis of delirium due to a general medical condition is used when findings indicate that the cognitive disturbance is the direct physiologic consequence of a general medical condition such as urinary tract infection, respiratory tract infection, septicemia, or end-stage renal disease. Certain focal lesions of the right parietal lobe and occipital lobe also may cause delirium. Other causes can include metabolic disorders, fluid or electrolyte imbalances, hepatic disease,

⟡ CLINICAL EXAMPLE 23-1
Delirium Due to Urinary Tract Infection

LS, a 65-year-old retired mechanic, had just been transferred to a rehabilitation center from a local hospital after surgical repair of a fractured
hip. During hospitalization he had an indwelling Foley catheter in place.
The catheter was removed two days after surgery. On the fifth postoperative day, LS began to exhibit agitation and complained of seeing animals
in his room. He also expressed a concern that someone was going to hurt
him. He was oriented to person only. At night LS attempted to crawl out
of bed over the siderails. During the day he appeared to be aware of his
surroundings and was able to make his needs known. He had no recall of
the episodic confusion or disorientation he exhibited. The result of a urinalysis with culture and sensitivity revealed a urinary tract infection due
to *Escherichia coli*. LS was exhibiting clinical symptoms of delirium that
resolved after a 10-day course of treatment with Bactrim.

thiamine deficiency, postoperative states, hypertensive encephalopathy, and
sequelae of head injury.

Substance-induced delirium occurs within minutes to hours after taking relatively high doses of certain drugs and the delirium resolves as the substance is
discontinued or eliminated from the body. Various substances and medications
have been reported to cause delirium. They include anesthetics, analgesics,
antihistamines, anticonvulsants, antiasthmatics, antiparkinsonian drugs, corti-
costeroids, and muscle relaxants. Bactrim and Septra as well as nonsteroidal
anti-inflammatory drugs have been identified as causative factors of delirium in
the elderly.

Delirium due to multiple etiologies is a diagnosis used to alert clinicians to
the common situation in which the delirium has more than one etiology. Delirium not otherwise specified refers to a delirium that does not meet criteria for
any of the specific types of delirium. There is insufficient evidence to establish
a specific etiology.

Dementia

The annual incidence of newly diagnosed dementia rises from about 20 per
100,000 population at age 60 to 2,000 per 100,000 population at age 80 years.
Clinicians now estimate that about 50% of those persons aged 65 years and
older have "pure" Alzheimer's disease and about 15% have "pure" vascular
dementia. An overlap between these two dementias occurs in approximately
10% to 15% of patients. Between 5% and 10% of patients with dementia suffer
from diffuse Lewy body disease, and the remaining 10% of dementia cases rep-

resent progressive supranuclear palsy, Parkinson's dementia, and other, less common diagnoses (Geldmacher, 1996).

Dementia is a form of global or diffuse brain dysfunction that is characterized by a gradual, progressive, chronic deterioration of intellectual function. Judgment, orientation, memory, affect, emotional stability, cognition, and attention are affected either by a pattern of simple, gradual deterioration or by rapid, complicated deterioration. Impaired judgment, or the inability to make reasonable decisions, is one of the earliest signs of dementia and may occur in business dealings or social functions (*e.g.*, the person engages in a reckless business venture or displays a disregard for conventional rules of social conduct).

Disorientation to person, place, and time is one of the most common signs of brain dysfunction. The more extensive the dysfunction, the more severe the disorientation. A minimally impaired person may misjudge the date by weeks or months. Moderate impairment generally involves confusion about geographic location such as city or state as well as time, whereas severe impairment is demonstrated by disorientation with respect to time, place, and person. Short-term memory, attention, and concentration deficits are observable in this disorder because the person loses his or her train of thought, forgets what was said just a few minutes earlier, and may be unable to repeat the information just communicated.

Other characteristics or associated features include confabulation, perseveration, concrete thinking, and emotional lability. Confabulation is the filling in of memory gaps with false but sometimes plausible content to conceal the memory deficit. Perseveration is the inappropriate continuation or repetition of a behavior such as giving the same details over and over even when told one is doing so. Abstraction skills are impaired; therefore, the person tends to think in concrete terms. The tendency to manifest rapid, inappropriate, exaggerated mood swings often occurs, and marked anxiety or depression may be seen in mild cases.

Personality changes are often seen in persons with dementia. The normally active person may become withdrawn and apathetic when social involvement narrows.

Psychotic or behavioral disturbances include agitation, wandering, hallucinations, delusions, suspiciousness, reversal of sleep–wake pattern, inappropriate sexual behavior, hostility, aggressiveness, and combativeness.

Subtypes of Dementia

The DSM-IV lists 12 subtypes of dementia. They include

Dementia of the Alzheimer's type
Vascular dementia
Dementia due to HIV disease
Dementia due to head trauma

Dementia due to Parkinson's disease
Dementia due to Huntington's disease
Dementia due to Pick's disease
Dementia due to Creutzfeldt-Jakob disease
Dementia due to other general medical conditions
Substance-induced persisting dementia
Dementia due to multiple etiologies
Dementia not otherwise specified

Clinical symptoms of dementia of the Alzheimer's type and and vascular dementia are discussed because these two disorders comprise approximately 65% to 80% of all dementias.

Dementia of the Alzheimer's Type Alzheimer's disease is considered to be the fourth or fifth most common cause of death for people older than 65 years of age in the United States. It is not a natural course of aging. It is considered to be a silent epidemic characterized by the development of multiple cognitive deficits including memory impairment, aphasia (language disturbance), apraxia (impaired ability to carry out motor activities despite motor function), agnosia (failure to recognize or identify objects despite intact sensory function), and disturbance in executive functioning (*e.g.*, planning, organizing).

The course is characterized by gradual onset and the person is aware of the loss of mental abilities as they occur. If clinical symptoms appear before age 65 years, the diagnosis is dementia of the Alzheimer's type with early onset; after age 65, the coding is with late onset. Additional coding indicates with delirium, with delusions, with depressed mood, or uncomplicated. The specifier, with behavioral disturbance, is not coded but can be used to indicate clinically significant behavior such as wandering, throwing items, or combativeness.

As the dementia progresses, personality changes, paranoia, stooped gait, loss of voluntary functions, seizures, and violent behavior may occur. Death can result from neglect, malnutrition, dehydration, incorrect diagnosis, inappropriate treatment, or suicide.

Risk factors associated with the occurrence of Alzheimer's disease include advanced age, female gender, head trauma, low education, and family history of Down's syndrome (Cummings & Brentwood, 1995).

Stages of Dementia of the Alzheimer's Type Clinical symptoms of Alzheimer's disease were summarized earlier. Attempts to describe the progression of this disease have resulted in two frequently used classification systems. The first system groups clinical symptoms into three progressive stages described as mild, moderate, and severe in nature (Williams, 1986). The second system identifies

CLINICAL EXAMPLE 23-2
Dementia of the Alzheimer's Type, Stage 6

MM is an 80-year-old female patient admitted to the special care unit of a long-term care facility because her family is no longer able to meet her needs. During the assessment process, MM scored 8 of 30 points on the Folstein Mini Mental State Exam. Deficits were noted in the area of orientation, recall, inability to spell WORLD backwards, inability to write a complete sentence, and the inability to copy a diagram. MM also had difficulty performing activities of daily living while residing at home. She had become incontinent of bowel and bladder and was resistant to care provided by her family. MM had wandered outside at night and was returned home by the police. During the interview process, MM used confabulation during responses to questions about her husband, family, and past employment as an executive secretary. After the completion of a dementia workup, the diagnosis of Dementia of the Alzheimer's Type, Late Onset, Stage 6 was noted.

the seven stages of Alzheimer's disease according to functional consequences (Reisberg, 1986). For example, stage 3 lists functional manifestations of normal aging such as forgetting names and location of objects and exhibiting decreased ability to recall appointments. In comparison, stage 7 lists functional manifestations such as progressive loss of all verbal and psychomotor abilities in which the individual eventually requires total assistance in all activities. Knowledge of both classification systems is important when providing care for individuals with the diagnosis of Alzheimer's disease.

Research on Dementia of the Alzheimer's Type   The following articles have appeared recently in the newspapers and professional journals:

   "The Hunt for an Early Alzheimer's Disease Cure"
   "Alzheimer's Study Looks at Vessels into Brain"
   "Finns Find Genetic Links to Alzheimer's Disease"
   "Alzheimer's Disease: Clinical Drug Trials"
   "Future Research: New and Investigational Agents"

The contents of these articles reveal that neuroimaging has been used in the diagnostic evaluation of patients with memory and cognitive abnormalities. The predominant finding of bilateral posterior temporal and parietal perfusion defects in these patients is highly predictive of Alzheimer's disease (Holman & Devous, 1992).

It has also been hypothesized that beta amyloid is deposited in the blood vessels of the brain, causing the release of an often-toxic form of oxygen known as a free radical. These roaming radicals destroy the brain's nerve cells, resulting in development of the dementia of Alzheimer's disease (Ricks, 1996).

The administration of Tropicamide solution before an eye examination resulted in hypersensitivity in pupil dilation in individuals with Down's syndrome and Alzheimer's disease. This test has not been approved as a clinical diagnostic procedure (Scinto et al., 1994).

Several clinical drug trials are being conducted on patients with mild to moderate Alzheimer's disease. The drugs include calcium channel blockers, neuroplasticity-enhancing agents, antipsychotic agents, anxiolytics, estrogen, physostigmine, and prednisone (Cummings & Brentwood, 1995). Aricept (donezepil) was approved in November, 1996 by the Food and Drug Administration to treat early symptoms of Alzheimer's disease. Investigations will continue during the next two years to determine if Aricept can be used in the later stages of the disease. Ampakine CX-516 is an investigational drug that accelerates signals between brain cells and appears to improve memory significantly in healthy elderly men. Tests are inconclusive when used to treat individuals with the diagnosis of Alzheimer's disease.

Research continues to focus on the effect of acetylcholine in the brain, genetic transmission, toxic effect of high levels of aluminum in the brain, dysfunction of the immune system, and infectious agents or slow-acting viruses.

Three genes on three separate chromosomes (14, 19, 21) have now been linked to Alzheimer's disease. Researchers are working diligently to determine what these genes do and how their actions can be modified (Alzheimer's Association, 1995).

Vascular Dementia (Formerly Multi-Infarct Dementia) This DSM-IV diagnosis is used when focal neurologic signs and symptoms or laboratory evidence indicative of cerebrovascular disease are judged to be etiologically related to the disturbance. Memory impairment and cognitive disturbances are similar to those seen in dementia of the Alzheimer's type. The focal neurologic signs and symptoms include exaggeration of deep tendon reflexes, extensor plantar response, pseudobulbar palsy, gait abnormalities, or weakness of an extremity. Computed tomography (CT) scan usually reveals multiple infarcts involving cortex and underlying white matter. Anxiety, depression, socially inappropriate behavior, lack of inhibition, and increased agitation related to environmental stimulation may also be seen.

Coding is based on predominant features, such as with delirium, with delusions, with depressed mood, or uncomplicated. Behavioral disturbances may be specified as part of the diagnosis.

Dementia Due to Other General Medical Conditions This classification is used to diagnose dementia due to the medical conditions listed earlier under the subtypes of dementia (*e.g.*, HIV, traumatic brain injury, Parkinson's disease) as well as endocrine conditions, nutritional conditions, infectious conditions, structural lesions of the brain, and renal or hepatic dysfunction.

Identifying the specific type of dementia is important. For example, persons with Lewy body dementia may be misdiagnosed as having dementia of the Alzheimer's type. Often individuals with Lewy body dementia have extreme adverse reactions, such as stiff, rigid movements, or immobility, to drugs commonly used to treat behavioral problems associated with dementia. These adverse reactions can be serious and could jeopardize the person's health.

Amnestic Disorder

Three subtypes of amnestic disorder are described in the DSM-IV. They include amnestic disorder due to a general medical condition, substance-induced persisting amnestic disorder, and amnestic disorder not otherwise specified. Individuals with amnestic disorder are impaired in their ability to learn new information or are unable to recall previously learned information or past events.

An impairment in social or occupational functioning occurs and represents a significant decline from a previous level of functioning. If there is evidence from the history, physical examination, or laboratory findings that the disturbance is the direct physiologic consequence of a general medical condition, the diagnosis amnestic disorder due to (the specific medical condition) is listed. Examples include closed head trauma, penetrating missile wounds, surgical intervention, metabolic conditions, or seizures. The specifier "transient" is used if memory impairment lasts for one month or less. If the condition lasts for more than one month, the specifier "chronic" is used.

Substance-induced persisting amnestic disorder can occur in association with alcohol, sedatives, hypnotics, anxiolytics, and other or unknown substances. The diagnostic criteria are the same as listed for amnestic disorder due to a general medical condition.

Cognitive Disorder Not Otherwise Specified

This category is for disorders that are characterized by cognitive dysfunction presumed to be due to the direct physiologic effect of a general medical condition that do not meet criteria for any of the specific deliriums, dementias, or amnestic disorders already described in this classification.

Box 23-1 summarizes behavior due to central nervous system pathology.

BOX 23-1 Behavior Due to Central Nervous System Pathology

Frontal lobe:	Lack of attention, tenacity, or persistence
	Loss of emotional control, rage, violent behavior
	Changes in mood and personality, uncharacteristic behavior
	Expressive aphasia or dysphasia
Parietal lobe:	Neglect or inattention to left half of space resulting in possible self-injury or unintentional contact with others that could be viewed as aggressive behavior
Temporal lobe:	Inability to store or retrieve information
	Inability to comprehend speech due to loss of hearing or receptive aphasia
Occipital lobe:	Visual disturbances such as agnosia or the inability to recognize by sight
Limbic lobe:	Inability to feed self
	Decrease in socialization
	Lack of emotional expression or apathy
	Inability to learn or store information

Interventions consist of nonverbal communication; providing a safe, secure environment; and maintaining activities of daily living.

✦ Transcultural Considerations

Cultural and educational background should be taken into consideration when evaluating an individual's cognitive capacity. Individuals from various backgrounds may have difficulty answering questions in certain tests because they are unfamiliar with the general knowledge of other cultures or their cultures do not place an emphasis on information such as date of birth, state capitals, names of presidents, and so forth. The prevalence of different causes of dementia varies across cultural groups; for example, dementia secondary to nutritional deficiency or infections may occur with more frequency in countries where poverty is prevalent.

If an interpreter is used, it is imperative that the interpreter not provide additional information or elaborate on the patient's responses.

Assessment

Assessment of persons with impaired cognition is important in the early diagnostic phase. Various tools are used during the interview process to assess the
individual's cognitive status. The Folstein Mini Mental State Exam is discussed
in Chapter 5. Other assessment tools include the Brief Cognitive Rating Scale,
Global Deterioration Scale, Rapid Disability Rating Scale, Functional Assessment Staging Test (FAST; Table 23-1 on p. 436) and the Behavioral Syndromes Scale for Dementia. Judgment, orientation, memory, affect, and cognition (JOMAC) are evaluated in an attempt to differentiate among delirium,
dementia, and depression in the elderly.

The following aspects should be considered during the assessment process:

1. Intellectual ability, past and present
2. Changes in personality (*e.g.*, depression, irritability, loss of interest, and
   decrease or loss of interest in personal appearance)
3. Past and present health status
4. Any evidence of confabulation, negativistic behavior, perseveration, feign-
   ing deafness, projection, or rationalization for lack of appropriate response
5. Ability to provide self-care

A variety of diagnostic tests are used to identify the precipitating cause of
impaired cognition. After a complete history and physical examination, an electroencephalogram, electrocardiogram, CT scan or magnetic resonance imaging,
sedimentation rate, complete blood count, urinalysis, thyroid profile, liver profile, serum electrolytes, serology test, vitamin B_{12} level, and folic acid level are
included in the workup. Cerebrospinal fluid may be examined. A polypharmacy
review is conducted. An evaluation for depression is included. The patient may
be referred to a memory disorder clinic for this complete workup. Information
regarding past psychiatric history and toxin exposure is also obtained.

Social support is also assessed to determine which resources are needed and
whether they are available. For example, members of the family may benefit
from attending a support group, from reading educational material about
Alzheimer's disease and its related disorders, and from the caretaker teaching
checklist on page 437.

 Nursing Diagnoses and Interventions

Interventions include environmental modification to reduce agitation, allow
for wandering or pacing, avoid overstimulation, minimize confusion, prevent
falls, maintain dignity, and allow aging-in-place to occur. Most persons with
impaired cognition or the diagnosis of dementia are placed in long-term care
(*text continues on page 438*)

Stage	Characteristics	Clinical Diagnosis	Average Duration
1	No objective or subjective functional decrement	Normal adult	
2	Subjective deficit in word finding and/or recalling location of objects No objectively manifest functional deficits	Normal aged adult	
3	Deficits in demanding employment and social settings (*e.g.*, patient may begin to forget important appointments for the first time)	Compatible with incipient AD	7 yr
4	Deficits in performing complex tasks (*e.g.*, handling finances and marketing)	Mild AD	2 yr
5	Deficient performance in choosing proper clothing and independent community functioning	Moderate AD	18 mo
6a	Requires actual assistance in putting on clothing properly	Moderately severe AD	5 mo
6b	Requires assistance in bathing properly	Moderately severe AD	5 mo
6c	Requires assistance with the mechanics of toileting	Moderately severe AD	5 mo
6d	Urinary incontinence	Moderately severe AD	4 mo
6e	Fecal incontinence	Moderately severe AD	10 mo
7a	Speech ability limited to approximately six intelligible words a day	Severe AD	12 mo
7b	Intelligible vocabulary limited to a single word	Severe AD	18 mo
7c	Ambulatory ability lost	Severe AD	12 mo
7d	Ability to sit up lost	Severe AD	12 mo
7e	Ability to smile lost	Severe AD	18 mo
7f	Ability to hold up head lost	Severe AD	12 mo+

Reisberg, B. (1986, April). Dementia: A systematic approach to identifying reversible causes. *Geriatrics*. Reprinted with permission from *Geriatrics*, *41* (4). Copyright Advanstar Communications, Inc.

Dementia and Delirium

The following checklist has been developed to help you understand the difference between dementia, a gradual deterioration in a person's mental processes, and delirium, the acute deterioration in a person's mental processes. Reporting these changes to the patient's nurse or attending physician could enhance the individual's quality of life.

Symptoms	Dementia	Delirium
Judgment	Impaired	May be impaired
Mood	Fluctuates	Fluctuates
	Apathetic	
Memory	Impaired	Impaired
Cognition	Disordered reasoning	Disordered reasoning
Orientation	Disoriented	Disoriented
Thoughts	Confused	Confused
	Suspicious	Suspicious
		Incoherent
Perception	No change	Misinterpretations
		Visual hallucinations
Consciousness	Normal	Clouded
Speech	Sparse	Sparse or fluent
	Repetitive	
Behavior	Agitation	Agitation
	Wanders	Insomnia
		May wander
Mental status	Poor testing	Poor testing
	Progressively worsens	Improves when medically
	Inappropriate answers	stable
Activities of daily living	Deteriorate as dementia progresses	Usually remain stable unless medically unstable

Approximately 80% of persons who develop dementia of the Alzheimer's type or a related dementia exhibit behavioral disturbances as the dementia progresses. They may include agitation, suspiciousness, hallucinations, combativeness, sexually inappropriate behavior, impulsivity, wandering, or hoarding of items. Such behaviors are manageable and should be reported to the nurse or doctor.

facilities when they exhibit clinical symptoms similar to stage 6 of dementia of the Alzheimer's type.

Moyer (1995) addresses the issue of medication evaluation. The question is posited, "Whose quality of life will benefit by the use of medication?" A variety of medications may be used, depending on presenting symptoms, including antidepressants, anxiolytics, beta blockers, anticonvulsants, and neuroleptics (see Chapter 12).

A calm, supportive approach is necessary when handling the patient's emotional responses or defenses against the acknowledgment of intellectual deficits. Moyer (1995) lists the following programs to minimize behavioral problems, including catastrophic consequences. They include using creative reality by entering the world of the patient; using validation rather than reality orientation; using low-stimulation activities; focusing on former life-style and current capabilities; and providing for physical activities appropriate to the patient's age and physical capabilities.

Nursing goals may vary depending on the differential diagnosis of delirium, dementia, or amnestic disorder. Short-term goals include maintaining the patient's contact with reality, preventing injury, promoting adequate nutritional and fluid intake, promoting adequate sleep and rest, encouraging expression of feelings, and stimulating the memory through various activities.

Long-term goals focus on promoting optimal level of independence, decreasing socially inappropriate behavior, encouraging satisfactory social relationships, and assisting the patient to live in as nonrestrictive an environment as possible. The environment should allow the person the opportunity to adapt to impairments by doing things in less complex ways than in the past. Meeting basic needs becomes more demanding as physical deterioration occurs.

Remaining learning potential should be maximized while the person is made to feel comfortable both physically and emotionally. New material or devices to provide self-care should be introduced simply and gradually.

Delusional thought processes increase as the intellectual functioning deteriorates. Hallucinations may occur. Sudden deterioration may indicate a superimposed treatable disease.

Examples of common nursing diagnoses include *impaired verbal communication related to confusion, *risk for injury related to poor judgment, *self-care deficit, *altered thought processes related to lack of reality orientation, *sleep pattern disturbance due to wandering at night, and *impaired social interaction.

Nursing Care Plan 23-1 lists sample nursing diagnoses and goal-related nursing interventions for an individual with the DSM-IV diagnosis of dementia who is exhibiting *altered thought processes and who is having difficulty ambulating independently.

*NANDA-approved nursing diagnosis.

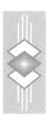

NURSING CARE PLAN 23-1
The Patient with Dementia

Nursing Diagnosis: *Altered thought processes as evidenced by disorientation to time and place

Goal: The patient will experience periods of orientation to reality.

Nursing Interventions	Outcome Criteria
	Within 24 to 48 hours of admission the patient will do the following:
Orient to person, place and time. Provide verbal reminders.	Verbalize forgetfulness
Address the patient by name.	Respond to name
Establish a set daily routine.	Respond to daily routine
Encourage the use of personal belongings or possessions.	Recognize personal belongings
Assign same staff to care for the patient whenever possible.	Recognize staff
Provide the patient with clear, simple, step-by-step directions.	Respond to directions by staff
Use supportive statements if fabricated stories are given in defense of memory loss.	Exhibit decreased use of confabulation

*NANDA-approved nursing diagnosis.

Nursing Diagnosis: *Risk for injury related to inability to ambulate independently

Goal: The patient will remain injury free during hospitalization.

Nursing Interventions	Outcome Criteria
	Within 24 to 48 hours of admission the patient will do the following:
Provide a safe environment by placing a call light in reach of patient.	Request assistance by using call light
Provide a walker, cane, or wheelchair as needed to encourage safe mobility.	Demonstrate compliance by using device provided to encourage safe mobility
Provide a gerichair with lap tray or seatbelt as needed if patient is disoriented and physically unable to ambulate independently.	Remain injury free

*NANDA-approved nursing diagnosis.

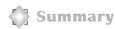 **Summary**

Cognitive disorders are due to transient or permanent brain dysfunction caused by a disturbance of physiologic functioning of brain tissue. This chapter focused on delirium, dementia, amnestic disorder, dementia due to other general medical conditions, and cognitive disorder not otherwise specified. Clinical symptoms of each disorder were described. The latest research findings were discussed. Transcultural considerations were addressed. Cognitive assessment tools were listed. Diagnostic tests used to identify the precipitating cause of impaired cognition were discussed. Nursing diagnoses and interventions for impaired cognition were cited, including short- and long-term goals. Examples of nursing diagnoses and nursing interventions were stated. Clinical examples of delirium and dementia were included.

Learning Activities

I. Clinical Activities
   A. Provide care for a patient with the diagnosis of impaired cognition such as delirium or dementia.
   B. List the clinical features or symptoms evident during hospitalization.
   C. State the diagnostic tests used to identify the cause of the disorder.
   D. Develop a nursing care plan for this assigned patient, focusing on sensorimotor deficits and behavioral symptoms.
II. Independent Activities
   A. Research literature on the following:
      1. Alzheimer's disease
      2. Amnestic disorder
      3. Vascular dementia
      4. Creutzfeldt-Jakob disease
   B. Compare the personality changes seen in these disorders.
   C. Discuss the impact of such illnesses on family members.
   D. Discuss the types of care available to persons with these chronic debilitating diseases.

Critical Thinking Questions

1. Attend a local support group for families of people with Alzheimer's disease What did you observe? What group techniques were employed by the group leader? What role can nursing play to help these families?
2. Your 75-year-old patient begins to exhibit signs of delirium after dark. He was alert and oriented when you admitted him yesterday. What data do you

need to collect? What can nurses do to attempt to prevent this common occurrence of delirium in elderly patients?

3. Observe a patient with stage 3 Alzheimer's and a patient with stage 6. What similarities and differences do you observe? How does nursing care differ for these two patients?

Self-Test

1. Differentiate among delirium, dementia, and amnestic disorder.
2. Differentiate between dementia of the Alzheimer's type and vascular dementia.
3. Discuss the most recent research finding regarding dementia of the Alzheimer's type.
4. Explain the importance of transcultural considerations during the assessment of patients with the diagnosis of dementia.
5. Explain the acronym JOMAC.
6. What are the diagnostic tests used to identify causative factors of cognitive disorders?
7. Name behavioral disturbances frequently seen in persons with cognitive disorders.
8. State four short-term nursing goals for patients with dementia.
9. List nursing interventions for
   Altered thought processes related to disorientation
   Risk for injury related to inability to ambulate independently

SELECTED REFERENCES

Allen, T. (1995, October). Alzheimer's disease: Lending a helping hand. *Advance for Nurse Practitioners*.

Allen, T. G. (1995, March). An overview of Parkinson's disease. *Advance for Nurse Practitioners*.

Alzheimer's Association. (1995, Fall). Research round-up: Discovery of early-onset gene makes headlines. *Advances in Alzheimer Research*.

American Psychiatric Association. (1994). *Diagnostic and statistical manual of mental disorders* (4th ed.). Washington, DC: American Psychiatric Press.

Batt, L. J. (1989, May). Managing delirium: Implications for geropsychiatric nurses. *Journal of Psychosocial Nursing and Mental Health Services*.

Carlson, D. L., Fleming, K. C., Smith, G. E., & Evans, J. M. (1995, November). Management of dementia-related behavioral disturbances: A nonpharmacologic approach. *Mayo Clinic Proceedings*.

Carpenito, L. J. (1995). *Nursing diagnosis: Application to clinical practice* (6th ed.). Philadelphia: J. B. Lippincott.

Cohen, D. (1995). Preface. In R. E. Cairl (Ed.). *Somebody tell me who I am*. St. Petersburg, FL: Caremor Publications.

Cummings, J., & Brentwood, V. A. M. C. (1995, November). Alzheimer's disease: A look at disease characteristics and etiology. *Current Approaches to Dementia.*

Foreman, M. D., & Zane, D. (1996, April). Nursing strategies for acute confusion in elders. *American Journal of Nursing.*

Geldmacher, D. S. (1996, February). Dementia: An overview of types. *Current Approaches to Dementia.*

Holman, L., & Devous, M. D. (1992, October). Functional brain SPECT: The emergence of a powerful clinic method. *Journal of Nuclear Medicine.*

Lego, S. (1996). *Psychiatric nursing: A comprehensive reference* (2nd ed.). Philadelphia: Lippincott–Raven Publishers.

Medina, J. (1996, February). Molecules of the mind: A real treatment for Alzheimer's? *Psychiatric Times.*

Moyer, D. M. (1995, November). Dementia care: The nurse practitioner's role. *Advance for Nurse Practitioners.*

Perlaky, D. (1994, January). A bearable solution: Responding creatively to dementia. *Nursing '94.*

Peskind, E. R., & Raskind, M. A. (1996). Cognitive disorders. In E. W. Busse & D. G. Blazer (Eds.). *The American Psychiatric Press textbook of geriatric psychiatry* (2nd ed.). Washington, DC: American Psychiatric Press.

Reisberg, B. (1986, April). Dementia: A systematic approach to identifying reversible causes. *Geriatrics.*

Ricks, D. (1996, March 14). Alzheimer's study looks at vessels into brain. *Orlando Sentinel.*

Scinto, L. F. M., Daffner, K. R., Dressler, D., et al. (1994, November 11). A potential non-invasive neurobiological test for Alzheimer's disease. *Science.*

Williams, L. (1986, February). Alzheimer's: The need for caring. *Journal of Gerontological Nursing.*

Yudofsky, S. C., Silver, J. M., & Hales, R. E. (1994). Treatment of aggressive disorders. In A. F. Schatzberg & C. B. Nemeroff (Eds.). *The American Psychiatric Press textbook of psychopharmacology.* Washington, DC: American Psychiatric Press.

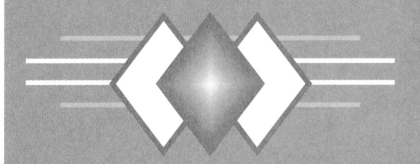

Special Populations in Psychiatric–Mental Health Nursing

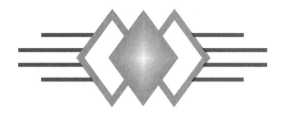

CHAPTER 24

Disorders of Infancy, Childhood, and Adolescence

Children Learn What They Live

If children live with criticism, they learn to condemn.
If children live with hostility, they learn to fight.
If children live with ridicule, they learn to be shy.
If children live with shame, they learn to feel guilty.
If children live with tolerance, they learn to be patient.
If children live with encouragement, they learn confidence.
If children live with praise, they learn to appreciate.
If children live with fairness, they learn justice.
If children live with security, they learn to have faith.
If children live with approval, they learn to like themselves.
If children live with acceptance and friendship, they learn to
find love in the world.

Dorothy Law Nolte

1 Discuss at least three causative factors pertaining to disorders of infancy, childhood, or adolescence.

2 Differentiate the four types of mental retardation.

3 Define the following disorders:

Conduct disorder

Adjustment disorder

Tourette's disorder

4 State the clinical symptoms of attention-deficit/hyperactivity disorder.

5 Describe the clinical symptoms of childhood depression.

6 Explain the dynamics of autistic behavior.

7 List nursing diagnoses associated with psychiatric disorders of infancy, childhood, and adolescence.

8 State nursing interventions for the following persons:

A depressed 12-year-old boy with suicidal ideation

A 7-year-old boy with attention-deficit/hyperactivity disorder

A 4-year-old girl with autistic behavior

 Introduction

This chapter focuses on disorders of infancy, childhood, or adolescence, which usually occur as a result of complex reactions during one's early developmental stages. The child's age, stage of personality development, motor and physical development, and ability to communicate are a few of the factors influencing such reactions. These factors are grouped into four main categories: constitutional factors, effects of physical disease or injury, temperamental factors, and environmental factors.

Constitutional factors are a result of genetic inheritance and the condition of the intrauterine environment during pregnancy. Genetic effects cause few psychiatric disorders in childhood; however, they can cause mental impairment or retardation, associated with Down's syndrome and phenylketonuria, for example. A decreased supply of oxygen and the presence of a disease such as syphilis create an adverse intrauterine environment that can affect the central nervous system (CNS) of the fetus. Fetal alcohol syndrome, which occurs in the pregnant woman who abuses alcohol; premature birth; and birth trauma are also causes of abnormal development, including mental impairment. Genetic counseling, good prenatal care, well equipped and competently staffed labor and delivery units, and the presence of neonatal intensive care units all help to decrease the onset of abnormal development, which may be accompanied by emotional disturbance or mental impairment.

Severe malnutrition, physical disease (*e.g.*, diabetes, rheumatoid arthritis, or congenital heart defect), brain damage due to infection or trauma, and injuries such as severe burns or traumatic amputation all may lead to the development of a psychiatric disorder.

A temperamental factor is described by *Webster's* as a "mode of emotional response," "disposition," or "excessive sensitiveness" exhibited by a person. Adverse or negative temperamental factors include withdrawal, slow or impaired adaptation to environmental change, unstable mood states, and exaggerated, intense reactions to an environmental stimulus. Heredity, interpersonal relationships, and the environment all influence one's temperament. Children with a positive temperament display a happy, contented mood, the ability to adapt readily, a positive approach to new situations, and a low-key or mild reaction to environmental stimuli. They are less apt to develop a behavior disorder than are children who exhibit adverse temperamental factors.

Environmental factors are considered to be the main cause of behavior disorders in children during early and middle childhood. Family, school, and neighborhood are considered functioning systems of the environment shaping the child's development. The family provides a protective training ground for the child as she or he learns to adapt, to live as a member of society, and to become independent. Any negative or maladaptive responses learned within one of the functioning systems can be extended to the other systems. For example, a child who uses the maladaptive behavior of a temper tantrum at home to get his or her way will probably attempt to use such behavior at school until limits are set.

Scapegoat is a term used to describe the role of a person within a family who is the recipient of angry, hostile, frustrated, or ambivalent emotions experienced by various family members. Such a person is singled out by family members who project their feelings onto her or him. As a result, the child may use acting-out behavior in an attempt to cope, to decrease anxiety, to receive love and attention, or to preserve self-esteem.

Placing too much responsibility on a child, making him or her a "little adult," creates an abnormal family role that can cause a behavior disorder. Such a child might be expected to babysit siblings, to help with adult tasks, or even to fulfill the role of an absent adult. The child does not have the opportunity to progress through the normal stages of growth and development.

A child whose mother is depressed or is experiencing severe emotional trauma is at risk because of the influence of a negative environment. Mental or physical abuse may occur in such a setting. The child receives little love and attention, if any, and lacks a model for close interpersonal relationship as he or she attempts to relate to others, develop trust, and gain independence.

Barker (1983) lists the characteristics of a school environment that influence the development of normal, positive behavior in children. The characteristics are summarized as follows:

1. An integration of the intellectually able and less able children provides for a well balanced classroom, encouraging normal growth and development.
2. Acknowledgment and praise by teachers promotes the development of a positive self-concept.
3. Encouragement of participation in running the school fosters responsibility.
4. Placing moderate emphasis on academic achievement permits the child to participate in a variety of activities and to develop a well rounded personality.
5. Good role modeling by teachers promotes positive behavior in children.
6. A comfortable, pleasant, and attractive environment is conducive to the development of mentally healthy persons.

Neighborhoods also can influence the development of behavior disorders. Poor socioeconomic conditions in crowded inner cities produce higher rates of psychiatric disorders in children than are seen in suburban areas. Delinquency, substance abuse, childhood depression, and antisocial personalities are just a few examples of disorders prevalent in such neighborhoods.

 Classification of Clinical Disorders

Disorders usually evident in infancy, childhood, or adolescence have been classified by the DSM-IV as follows:

1. Developmental disorders such as mental retardation
2. Learning disorders related to reading, writing, and mathematics
3. Motor skills disorders related to coordination
4. Communication disorders characterized by difficulties in speech or language
5. Pervasive developmental disorders characterized by severe deficits and pervasive impairment in multiple areas of development, such as social interaction and communication, and the presence of stereotyped behavior
6. Attention-deficit and disruptive behavior disorders characterized by prominent symptoms of inattention or hyperactivity–impulsivity
7. Feeding and eating disorders characterized by persistent disturbances in feeding and eating

8. Tic disorders characterized by vocal or motor tics
9. Elimination disorders focusing on the repeated passage of feces and urine into inappropriate places
10. Other disorders of infancy, childhood, and adolescence such as excessive anxiety, selective mutism, or repetitive nonfunctional motor behavior

Other categories discussed in this text are appropriate for children or adolescents, and age-specific features are included in each chapter. They include diagnoses such as affective disorders, personality disorders, organic mental disorders, and substance use disorders. Adjustment disorder, as well as the more frequently diagnosed childhood and adolescent disorders, will be presented in this chapter. Eating disorders are discussed in the following chapter.

Many texts present an excellent summary of psychological development, focusing on the developmental stage, motor and physical development, language or communication, cognitive behavior, interpersonal behavior, developmental crisis, and the most frequent disturbing behaviors in that particular developmental stage. The reader is referred to such texts on growth and development for additional information because it is important in the assessment and treatment of disorders affecting infants, children, and adolescents.

Mental Retardation

The last two decades have seen enormous changes taking place in services for children with learning difficulties such as mental retardation. The trend toward deinstitutionalization has made family and community support a central issue.

Mental retardation is described in the DSM-IV as the presence of a subaverage general intellectual functioning associated with or resulting in impairments in adaptive behavior. The onset occurs before age 18 years. Persons with mental impairment experience or exhibit significant limitations in at least two of the following skill areas: communication, self-care, home living, social/interpersonal skills, use of community resources, self-direction, functional academic skills, work, leisure, health, and safety.

Causative factors are numerous. They include defective genes, an abnormal number of chromosomes, malnutrition, radiation exposure, maternal infections, Rh incompatibility, syphilis, anoxia, birth injury, brain tumor, head trauma, early infant infections (*e.g.,* meningitis), and deprivation of normal growth and developmental experience (seen in children with a low socioeconomic status).

Mental retardation is classified by the intelligence quotient (IQ) scores and deficits in adaptation. Examples of standardized intelligence tests include the Wechsler Intelligence Scales for Children (Revised), Stanford-Binet, and Kaufman Assessment Battery for Children. Box 24-1 illustrates the categories of mild, moderate, severe, and profound mental retardation.

(*Text continues on p. 451*)

BOX 24-1 Categories of Mental Retardation

Subtype	IQ Level	Deficits	Comments
Mild	50 to 70	None in early childhood Difficulty adapting to school Achieve to sixth-grade level by late teens May need assistance when experiencing social or economic stress	85% of all persons with mental retardation Can achieve social and vocational skills for minimum self-support "Educable"—acquire academic skills up to approximately sixth-grade level
Moderate	35 to 55	Poor awareness of needs of others Need moderate supervision due to self-care deficit Usually do not progress beyond second-grade level Require supervision and guidance under mild social or economic stress	10% of all persons with mental retardation May profit from vocational training Can function in sheltered workshops as un-skilled or semiskilled persons "Trainable"
Severe	20 to 40	Poor motor development and minimal speech Unable to learn academic skills but may learn to talk and be trained in elementary hygiene skills or activities of daily living	3% to 4% of all persons with mental retardation Require complete supervision in a controlled environment May learn to perform simple work tasks
Profound	Below 20 or 25	Require total nursing care and highly struc-tured environment with supervision due to a self-care deficit Possess a minimal capacity for sensorimotor functioning	1% to 2% of all persons with mental retardation May learn some productive skills "Custodial"

⚙ CLINICAL EXAMPLE 24-1
Mental Retardation, Severe Level

MW, 21 years old, was born by a normal spontaneous vaginal delivery without any complications. Two months after birth, MW developed a temperature of 105°F and had a grand mal seizure. He was admitted to the neonatal intensive care unit with the diagnosis of fever of undetermined origin (FUO). Diagnostic tests revealed the presence of encephalitis. MW recovered but his parents were cautioned about the possibility of CNS damage because of the severity of his illness. During early childhood, ages one to five, MW was able to communicate with his parents to some extent but exhibited poor motor development. He was unable to learn basic skills such as reading, writing, and arithmetic, and it became evident that he needed supervision in a controlled environment. IQ testing revealed MW's IQ to be that of a person with severe retardation or mental impairment. At age 21 he continues to live at home with very supportive parents who have been able to teach him some self-care activities. He relates well to a pet cat, helps his mother with simple household chores, and helps his father with gardening and lawn care.

Various associated features of mental retardation include irritability, aggressiveness, temper tantrums, stereotyped repetitive movements, nail biting, and stuttering.

The prevalence rate of mental retardation has been estimated at approximately 1%. It occurs twice as frequently in male as in female children.

Attention-Deficit and Disruptive Behavior Disorders

Two commonly diagnosed disorders include attention-deficit/hyperactivity disorder and conduct disorder (childhood-onset type and adolescent-onset type). A summary of each follows.

Attention-Deficit/Hyperactivity Disorder (ADHD) According to the National Institute of Mental Health, this disorder affects approximately 3% to 5% of the nation's 63 million youngsters. On average, at least one child in every classroom in America needs help for this condition. In 1995, an estimated two million children, mostly boys, were diagnosed with this disorder, two and one-half times the number in 1990.

Characteristics of this disorder include a short attention span, impulsivity, and distractibility. Causative factors may include inherited temperament, in which the child displays symptoms since birth, cardiac abnormality, electrophysiologic abnormality of the cortex, stressful interpersonal family relationships, or an organic brain disorder.

⬚ CLINICAL EXAMPLE 24-2
Attention-Deficit/Hyperactivity Disorder

BS, aged six, diagnosed as having an attention-deficit/hyperactivity disorder, was interviewed by a clinical psychologist in the presence of several student nurses. When BS first entered the room he jumped up and down several times, giggled nervously, and then said "I'm sorry." The psychologist asked BS to sit still as he attempted to time the child's ability to remain immobile for a period of time. One minute seemed an eternity to BS, who insisted time was up in 15 seconds. When asked to draw a picture of the psychologist, BS was unable to sit still long enough to complete the drawing. He ran about the room investigating electrical outlets and various pieces of equipment in the room. After he knocked over a table lamp, BS repeatedly stated that he was sorry. As the psychologist asked him to participate in a ring-toss game, he stated "You go first, I always go last." He was unable to stand still as he awaited his turn.

The student nurses who observed BS's behavior stated they were exhausted after 30 minutes. "How do his parents keep up with him 24 hours a day?" "Does he ever unwind?" "Does he always break things?" and "Why does he say that he is sorry so often?" are just a few of the comments by the students. One student questioned how his behavior would affect other children when he played with them. Another student wanted to know how long BS would remain hyperactive. Postclinical conference discussion focused on assessment of BS's behavior and the development of a nursing care plan.

Clinical symptoms may include stubbornness, negativism, temper tantrums, obstinacy, inability to tolerate frustration, deficit in judgment, poor self-image, and aggressiveness. Symptoms may occur around age 3 but usually are not diagnosed until the child enters school, at which time academic and social functioning may be impaired.

The DSM-IV diagnostic criteria describe the child who has ADHD as follows:

1. Inattention resulting in failure to complete a task, failure to pay attention or listen, distractibility, inability to concentrate, and difficulty participating in play activity over a period of time
2. Impulsivity, since the child often acts before thinking, shifts frequently from one activity to another owing to a short attention span and inner "driven-ness," is unable to organize work, requires much supervision, disrupts class or groups by frequently speaking out of turn, and is unable to sit still and await his or her turn

3. Hyperactivity, demonstrated by fidgeting, being unable to sit still, running or climbing on things, moving about in sleep, and appearing to be in high gear all the time. The child's "motor," or inner drivenness, never "idles" or "stalls."
4. Onset before age seven years and lasting at least six months. The behavior is not caused by disorders such as schizophrenia, affective disorder, or severe or profound retardation.

Conduct Disorder Studies indicate that conduct disorders are the largest single group of psychiatric illnesses in adolescents. Conduct disorders affect approximately 6% to 16% of boys and 2% to 9% of girls younger than the age of 18 years. They usually occur just before, during, or immediately after puberty. Causes of such behavior may include

1. A poor parent–child interpersonal relationship
2. Lack of a father figure
3. Parental rejection
4. Lack of a secure, permanent family group as experienced by orphans or foster children during institutional living
5. Failure to bond during infancy
6. Incompatibility of the child's and parents' temperaments
7. Inconsistency in setting limits and disciplining a child by parents or authority figures
8. Large family size
9. Association with lower socioeconomic class children, including exposure to "delinquent groups"

Conduct disorders, as stated earlier, usually are seen during the developmental stages before, during, or just after the onset of puberty. Interpersonal behavior at this time includes developing peer relationships, participating in activities outside the family, lessening family ties, and exhibiting independence. If the child does not successfully complete these developmental stages of industry versus inferiority (ages six to puberty) and identity versus role confusion (puberty and adolescence) as described by Erikson (1964), the child may develop a sense of inferiority, may experience difficulty learning and working, and may fail to develop a sense of identity.

Symptoms may develop first within the family unit when the child attempts to cope with anxiety or resolve an inner conflict. Involvement in adolescent gangs also may precipitate the onset of antisocial behavior. In either case, there are usually unstable or poor interpersonal relationships within the family.

In general, such a disorder is seen more frequently in boys, is more common in children whose parents display antisocial behavior or alcohol dependence, and may occur in varying degrees of impairment from a mild to a severe form.

The DSM-IV states that the individual with a conduct disorder violates the basic rights of others or major age-appropriate societal norms or rules. Clinical symptoms include aggression to people and animals, destruction of property, deceitfulness or theft, and serious violations of rules. Clinical symptoms are present for 12 months and do not meet the criteria for antisocial personality if the person is 18 years of age or older. Various complications are listed as the result of conduct disorder. They include suspension from school, difficulty with the law, and phyical injury from accidents, fights, or other physical encounters. The specifiers mild, moderate, or severe are used to describe the number of conduct problems and the effect on others.

Tic Disorders

According to the DSM-IV, there are four disorders included in this classification. They include Tourette's disorder, chronic motor or vocal tic disorder, transient tic disorder, and tic disorder not otherwise specified.

A tic is a rapid, largely involuntary movement or noise. Tics are divided into motor tics, involving the rapid movement of a muscle, or vocal tics, which can range from a simple throat clearing to more complex vocalizations involving words or phrases. Tics are relatively common in childhood, with 5% to 24% of school-age children reporting past or present tics. In most cases, tics are mild and last less than one year, and in those cases the diagnosis is transient tic disorder. Chronic tic disorder refers to the presence of either motor tics or vocal tics, but not both. The tics occur many times a day nearly every day for more than a year. This disorder occurs before age 18 years.

Tourette's syndrome, or Gilles de la Tourette's syndrome, is described as a combination of motor tics and involuntary vocal and verbal utterances that often are obscene (coprolalia). Repeating one's own sounds or words (palilalia), repeating the last-heard sound, word, or phrase (echolalia), and imitation of someone else's movements (echokinesis) may be present. The tics occur many times a day nearly every day or intermittently throughout a period of more than one year. The onset is before age 18 years. This disorder can persist for a lifetime.

Although the etiology of tics is unknown, possible causes include stress, tension, brain damage, or a decreased production of the neurotransmitters serotonin and dopamine. Approximately 50% of patients with

Tourette's syndrome also have obsessions and complusions (obsessive–compulsive disorder).

Elimination Disorders

The two elimination disorders listed in the DSM-IV include enuresis and encopresis. Enuresis is the repeated urination, day or night, into bed or clothes at least twice a week for a period of at least three months. The presence of clinically significant distress or impairment in social, academic, occupational, or other important areas of functioning is also considered when using the diagnosis of enuresis, which usually begins by age five. Subtypes include nocturnal only, diurnal only, or nocturnal and diurnal. Causative factors may include regression, anxiety, adjustment reaction, or psychosis. A secondary emotional disorder may result from social ostracism by peers or familial attitude toward the child's behavior, such as anger, rejection, or punishment.

Encopresis, or fecal soiling, is the passage of feces into inappropriate places. The behavior may be involuntary or intentional. At least one event per month for a period of three months occurs before the diagnosis is given. Age of onset is at least four years or equivalent developmental level. Subtypes include with constipation, with overflow incontinence, and without constipation and overflow incontinence. In the absence of a physical disorder, the main causative factor is said to be a dysfunctional relationship between the child and parents, usually the mother. The child may be poorly cared for, under stress, experiencing increased anxiety, immature, regressed, or mentally retarded.

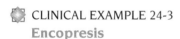 CLINICAL EXAMPLE 24-3
Encopresis

WJ, age four and a half, was completely toilet trained by age three. Her mother gave birth to a baby girl when WJ was four years old. Shortly after the birth of her sister, WJ began to have difficulty with retentive soiling. She refused to use the toilet when encouraged, only to be found later hiding behind a couch or drapes with soiled underwear. On one occasion, she disappeared from the living room while company was present and was later found in her bedroom closet grunting as though having a bowel movement. This behavior, which was quite frustrating to WJ's parents, continued for three months. At that time, WJ's mother consulted with the pediatrician. With his help, Mrs. J was able to tolerate her daughter's behavior. She continued to reassure WJ that she was loved and wanted by her parents. WJ's behavior eventually subsided as she was allowed to help care for her baby sister.

Other Disorders of Infancy, Childhood, or Adolescence

Five disorders are listed in the DSM-IV under this classification. They include separation anxiety disorder, selective mutism, reactive attachment disorder of infancy or early childhood, stereotypic movement disorder, and disorder of infancy, childhood, or adolescence not otherwise specified. Separation anxiety disorder is discussed.

Separation Anxiety Disorder This disorder may develop after some life stress. Onset may be as early as preschool age and may occur at any time before age 18 years. There may be periods of exacerbation and remission. It is characterized by excessive anxiety that is severe and persistent when the child is separated from the parent (usually the mother), a significant other, the home, or familiar surroundings. As the child grows older, he or she may refuse to travel independently from home, spend the night at a friend's house, attend camp, or go to school (school phobia). Psychophysiologic symptoms, such as headache, nausea, vomiting, and stomachache, are seen frequently when the child anticipates separation or when it actually occurs. The child may show a reluctance or refusal to go to sleep at night or to stay alone in the home, and may withdraw socially. The child may become housebound or incapacitated in the severe form of separation anxiety disorder owing to the presence of morbid fears of illness, injury, danger, or death. Duration of such a disturbance must be at least four weeks before a diagnosis is made.

Pervasive Developmental Disorders

Five disorders are included in this classification. They include autistic disorder, Rett's disorder, childhood disintegrative disorder, Asperger's disorder, and per-

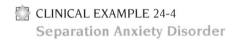

CLINICAL EXAMPLE 24-4
Separation Anxiety Disorder

CW, five years old, began to complain of a stomachache each morning as her mother prepared to go to work. The complaint had persisted for approximately a week when CW began to wander into her parents' bedroom each night after she had gone to bed. During the day the babysitter noticed that CW would follow her from room to room and refuse to play outside. The babysitter brought CW's behavior to the attention of her parents, who decided to consult the pediatrician. A diagnosis of separation anxiety disorder was made. Fortunately CW's behavior was identified early in its development, and she responded well to the pediatrician's suggestions for managing her anxiety.

vasive developmental disorder not otherwise specified. A summary of autistic disorder follows.

Autistic Disorder Sometimes referred to as early infantile autism, childhood autism, or Kanner's autism, this disorder is characterized by qualitative impairment in social interaction, qualitative impairments in communication, and restricted repetitive and stereotyped patterns of behavior, interests, and activities. Before age three years, the child exhibits delays or abnormal functioning in social interaction, language as used in social communication, or symbolic or imaginative play. Statistics reveal that as many as 4 of 10,000 children are afflicted.

Symptoms include the inability to establish a meaningful relationship owing to the lack of responsiveness to others; gross deficits in language development, including mutism, echolalia, and the inability to name objects; withdrawal, which may be mistaken for deafness; obsessive ritualistic behavior, such as rocking and spinning; obsessional attachments to particular objects; and anxiety or fear associated with harmless objects. Approximately 50% of autistic children have an IQ below 50.

Autistic children do not display an interest in or need for cuddling, touching, or hugging. They ignore people as if they were inanimate objects or not present in the environment. Their interest may focus on mechanical objects as they participate in ritualistic behavior at a basic sensorimotor level.

Language deficits may consist of pronominal reversal, or the use of the pronoun *you* when *I* should be used; immature grammar; echolalia; and the inability to name objects. An obsessive desire for sameness is usually present. The

---

❀ CLINICAL EXAMPLE 24-5
   Autistic Disorder

TJ, age 16, was diagnosed as being autistic at age 2. He lives at home with his parents and attends a school for developmentally disabled children. His ability to communicate verbally is restricted to his making guttural sounds at times. TJ requires constant supervision owing to masochistic behavior such as head banging and biting himself. Custodial care is also necessary to feed and toilet TJ. He has occasional outbursts in which he hits others and attempts to bite them. TJ responds to music, which seems to have a soothing effect on him, and he will stand on the basketball court for hours shooting baskets. Although he appears to be in his own world, TJ will unexpectedly respond to the voice of his classroom teacher by looking directly at her and nodding his head or making guttural sounds. His parents report that his conduct at home fluctuates from manageable behavior to hostile, aggressive outbursts, at which time he needs to be sedated.

child becomes resistant to change and is severely distressed if environmental change occurs.

Overactivity, distractibility, poor concentration, sudden unprovoked anger or fear, or aggressive outbursts also may occur. Autistic children do not experience delusions, hallucinations, incoherence, or looseness of association.

Intellectual functioning varies, because children who are autistic may function at a normal, high, or retarded level. Memory may be exceptional, as observed in the behavior of an autistic child who played several pieces of complicated classical music on the piano.

Adjustment Disorder

An adjustment disorder is a classification differentiated from other disorders in that the maladaptive reaction is in response to an identifiable event or situation that is stress producing and is not the result of or part of a mental disorder. The reaction usually occurs within three months after the onset of the stressor, manifests itself as impaired social or occupational functioning, and is exaggerated beyond the normal reaction to an identified stressor. Remission of the reaction usually occurs within six months as the stressor diminishes or disappears.

The DSM-IV lists six subtypes that describe an adjustment reaction. The behavioral manifestations that define the subtypes are as follows:

1. with depressed mood
2. with anxiety
3. with anxiety and depressed mood
4. with disturbance of conduct
5. with mixed disturbance of emotions and conduct
6. unspecified

The specifiers *acute* (less than six months) and *chronic* (six months or longer) may be used to indicate the persistence of symptoms. The criteria listed in the DSM-IV apply to children, adolescents, and adults.

Types of stressors considered include natural or man-made disasters; unwanted pregnancy; physical illness or injury; developmental stressors (*e.g.*, puberty, adolescence, or menopause); legal difficulties (*e.g.* being arrested or incarcerated); financial problems; living circumstances (*e.g.*, change in residence or immigration); occupation changes (*e.g.*, unemployment or retirement); conjugal stressors (*e.g.*, separation or death of a spouse); parenting (*e.g.*, becoming a parent); and interpersonal problems (*e.g.*, relating to one's friends, neighbors, or associates). A review of Erikson's eight developmental stages or Havinghurst's six periods of development is suggested to help one to identify anticipated transitions and resulting conflicts or stressors that can occur at various times in life, especially during childhood or adolescence.

Young children are considered quite vulnerable to stressors because of limited coping abilities and dependency on their environment. Vacationing with the family, starting school, or changing teachers are considered minimal-to-mild stressors, whereas the divorce of parents, hospitalization, the death of a peer, or a geographic move could be considered severe stressors. Examples of extreme stress in children include repeated physical or sexual abuse, or the death of a parent.

Adolescence has received attention as one of the most difficult adjustment periods. Breaking up with a steady significant other, being "cut" from a sport, experiencing the death of a peer, or leaving home for the first time are examples of stressors that may occur during adolescence, any of which may result in adjustment disorders. When the adolescent receives support during this developmental period, the likelihood of the onset of additional emotional disturbances is lessened.

Childhood Depression

The idea that children can develop conditions that are the same as the depressive disorders of adults has been controversial. The use of symptom-oriented, personal interviews with children has led to widespread recognition that disorders resembling adult depression can and do occur in childhood. In the DSM-IV, the criteria for prepubertal, adolescent, and adult depression are identical (Harrington, 1994). Epidemiologic surveys indicate a prevalence of depressive disorders among preadolescents in the range of 0.5% to 2.5%. Studies of adolescents have reported a higher prevalence, with current rates of 2.0% to 8.0% (Harrington, 1994). Some teenagers are simply unable to adjust to the rapid changes brought on by adolescence and become depressed. Suicide may occur as a result to end emotional pain. It is the third leading cause of death among people aged 15 to 24 years.

The following is a list of clinical symptoms usually present during childhood depression:

1. A pervasive sadness that is constantly present
2. Withdrawal
3. Irritable, negative behavior demonstrating the inability to have fun; destructive behavior

4. A poor or low self-esteem
5. Excessive guilt feelings, especially over minor incidents or situations that are not the person's fault
6. Disturbance in sleep (*e.g.*, insomnia, night terrors, or excessive napping)
7. Running-away behavior
8. A change in appetite (either decrease or lack of appetite, or overeating)
9. Somatic or physical complaints (*e.g.*, headaches, stomachaches, and earaches)
10. Difficulty in school (*e.g.*, inattention, school anxiety, or sudden change in performance, resulting in poor grades)
11. Preoccupation with death such as undue concern about the health of a parent, persistent thoughts related to the death of a pet, or suicidal thoughts

Causes of childhood depression are not cited specifically. Possible factors include poor or stressful environmental conditions, biochemical malfunction of the brain, or unusual sensitivity. Various theories also are discussed in the chapter on affective disorders, including precipitating events such as illness, trauma, or death of a loved one.

The following are warning signs of depression:

1. The child appears to be sad for at least one week.
2. The child refers to himself or herself as being unhappy.
3. She or he discusses suicide.
4. The child refuses to attend school.

❋ CLINICAL EXAMPLE 24-6
Childhood Depression

JK, a 13-year-old male athlete who was an excellent student, began doing poorly in class, skipping basketball practice, and staying out later than usual. His behavior resulted in arguments at home with his parents, especially his father, who attempted to discipline him. On one occasion, JK was caught smoking marijuana on the school grounds. JK's basketball coach, who had a good relationship with JK, asked him to stop by his office about two weeks after he began skipping practice. JK revealed to the coach that his parents were both very involved in their jobs and seemed to be too busy to enjoy family life. Everyone was going a separate way. JK was referred to the school counselor, who recognized the symptoms of depression.

If one or more of these warning signs is present, professional help should be sought.

 Transcultural Considerations

Intelligence testing should reflect adequate attention to ethnic or cultural background to avoid a misdiagnosis such as mental retardation. Cultural habits should be considered when assessing for feeding or eating disorders of infancy or early childhood. In some cultures, eating dirt, clay, or a nonnutritive substance is believed to be of value. Immigrant children may be diagnosed with a communication disorder because of refusal to speak to strangers or inability to speak the language of the host country. The diagnosis of conduct disorder may be given to a teenager who, in fact, is exhibiting a specific behavior necessary for survival. The environment, including social and economic context, should be assessed before making such a diagnosis.

 Research

Moon (1995) discusses the use of magnetic resonance imaging to detect biologic markers in children with ADHD. The findings indicate a lack of symmetry normally found in the anterior frontal lobe of the brain. There is also decreased volume in specific areas of the basal ganglia. Such findings constitute a biologic correlate of ADHD and may eventually lead researchers to the etiology and prevention of this disorder.

Kwasman, Tinsley, and Lepper (1995) conducted a study to evaluate pediatricians' knowledge and attitude regarding the diagnosis and treatment of attention-deficit disorder and ADHD. Results showed that attitudes toward treating patients with both disorders were mostly positive. Time required to care for these patients presented the biggest problem. Parents and children demonstrated a poor understanding of causes of the condition and treatment goals. Four needs were identified: greater improvement in teacher education and involvement, increases in availability of resources for parent education, more interdisciplinary contact, and better insurance coverage.

 Treatment

The following is a list of various methods used to treat infant, childhood, and adolescent disorders that require psychiatric help. Such disorders include depression, conduct disorders, pervasive developmental disorders, and adjustment disorders.

Individual psychotherapy
Family therapy or systems therapy
Group therapy
Play therapy
Behavioral therapy
Art therapy
Music therapy
Drug therapy or psychopharmacology
Hospitalization
Day hospitals or partial hospitalization programs
Alternative families

A brief summary of each therapy follows. (For more in-depth discussion, see Chapters 8, 10, 11, and 12.)

Individual Psychotherapy

Individual psychotherapy should include the following principles. These principles may serve as guidelines for a therapeutic nurse–patient relationship.

1. Accept the child but not necessarily the behavior. Remember that all behavior has meaning. The child may be acting-out to receive attention or love. Limit setting may be necessary to protect the patient or therapist.
2. Do not criticize the child.
3. Avoid discussing symptoms with the child unless the child refers to them.
4. Attempt to understand the child's feelings and point of view.

Individual psychotherapy may focus on specific problems, such as poor self-concept, feelings of depression, extreme dependency, or the inability to communicate.

Family Therapy (Systems Therapy)

The family is viewed as a biosocial subsystem that may be functional or dysfunctional (faultily integrated). Dysfunctional families may display poor interpersonal relationships, power struggles, extreme interdependency, or dis-integration. Disturbed behavior often is seen in children who become the focus of such family problems. Family therapists attempt to provide help for disturbed children and families as a whole. This may include altering the family situation rather than treating the child individually.

Group Therapy

Children and adolescents may be treated in groups. Peer relationships play an important part in group therapy because peers often help each other by exchanging information, identifying with the group, expressing feelings openly, and suggesting solutions to problems. Group therapy is used in the treatment of disorders such as substance abuse, oppositional disorders, depression, and anorexia nervosa, which is discussed in the next chapter.

Play Therapy

Play therapy usually is used with children between the ages of 3 and 12 years. The child is given the opportunity to act out feelings such as anger, hostility, frustration, and fear. Various toys, puppets, or materials such as crayons and fingerpaints may be used. A dollhouse and dolls can be used to simulate family, sibling, or peer relationships. For example, a young girl may play with a doll and punish it or refer to it as a "bad girl," treating the doll the way she is treated by her parents. Watching a child at play allows the care-giver the opportunity to learn about a child's real and imaginary emotional life.

Behavioral Therapy

Behavioral therapy attempts to alter a person's behavior and modify or remove symptoms such as temper tantrums or bedwetting. It often is used with hyperactive children to reduce the activity and to organize play. This is done by altering the circumstances before or after a particular behavior by using learning theory.

Operant conditioning, or behavior modification, is a second type of behavioral therapy used to modify behavior through manipulation. The person is given a reward or positive reinforcement for desired behavior, and negative reinforcement for undesired behavior. This type of therapy is used in the treatment of anorexia nervosa, delinquent behavior, enuresis, mental retardation, and several other disorders or problems.

Art and Music Therapy

Therapies involving art or music allow the child to express herself or himself in these disciplines and can be effective with those who have difficulty communicating with others. For example, a seven-year-old depressed child was able to draw a picture of his fear of death after separation from his father, who was hospitalized for treatment of Hodgkin's disease. He had overheard family conversation regarding the seriousness of his father's condition and feared that his father would never return home.

Drug Therapy (Psychopharmacology)

Drugs are used to control hyperactivity or attention-deficit disorder, depression, anxiety, and epilepsy.

Hyperactivity may be treated with a CNS stimulant such as methylphenidate hydrochloride (Ritalin), dextroamphetamine sulfate (Dexedrine), or magnesium pemoline (Cylert) to prevent flooding of the cerebral cortex by a stream of impulses.

Antidepressant agents may include Tofranil, Elavil, Pamelor, Desyrel, Prozac, and Wellbutrin. Plasma levels may be monitored. Anxiolytics such as Klonopin, Xanax, Ativan, Valium, Buspar, and Librium have proven to be effective. A combination of these drug classifications may be used if the patient exhibits clinical symptoms of both depression and anxiety. Lithium is used to treat bipolar disorder.

Neuroleptic agents such as Clozaril, Thorazine, Mellaril, Prolixin, Moban, and Trilafon are used to treat disorders such as autism, pervasive developmental disorder, schizophrenia, and Tourette's syndrome. Orap is a new medication used to treat Tourette's syndrome by controlling vocal outbursts and reducing the frequency and severity of tics.

Hypnotics such as Noctec and Triclos are prescribed for anxiety and sleep disturbances. These agents are used as an adjunctive, symptomatic treatment to alleviate distress.

Anticonvulsants may be used to treat challenging behaviors such as autism, conduct disorders, and agitation secondary to organic changes. Tegretol, Dilantin, Mysoline, or Depakote require the monitoring of serum blood levels as well as liver enzymes.

The U.S. Food and Drug Administration recently approved Adderall for the treatment of ADHD. It is intended for use in children 3 years of age and older (Pharmaceutical Update, 1996).

Hospitalization

Hospitalization of children or adolescents serves various purposes, for example, removing the child from a dysfunctional environment; treating severely disturbed behavior (*e.g.*, psychosis) in a controlled setting; providing protective care for suicidal, destructive, aggressive, or hyperactive behavior; or treating severe anxiety disorders.

Day Hospitals (Partial Hospitalization Programs)

Treatment in a day hospital setting provides a therapeutic milieu for children. It serves as an extended outpatient clinic during the day, yet allows children to return home to their families evenings, nights, and weekends. It is quite useful in the care of emotionally disturbed children, providing observation, treatment, and care. Classrooms or special education programs are structured so that the child is able to continue his or her education while receiving psychiatric care.

Alternative Families

Runaways, delinquents, and disturbed children often benefit from placement in the homes of alternative families. Children's services, group homes, and foster homes may provide much-needed physical and emotional care.

Assessment

The assessment of a young person is complicated by the interaction of psycho-pathology with the child's environment and with developmental processes. An interview with at least one parent or adult caretaker is essential. Information from teachers is desirable. Standardized rating scales are useful. A recent med-ical history and physical examination are necessary, with laboratory testing as indicated. Psychoeducational testing is used when the student's school functioning is impaired (Dulcan, Bregman, Weller, & Weller, 1995).

Children suspected of having autism or a related developmental disorder are evaluated by a treatment team consisting of a developmental specialist, pedia-trician or neurologist, psychologist, speech–language pathologist, and physician or occupational therapist (Church, 1996).

Roye (1995) describes the HEADSS (W) assessment tool for obtaining a psychosocial history from teens. The acronym stands for home, education, activities, drug use and abuse, sexual behaviors, suicidal thoughts, and depres-sion and weight.

Nursing Interventions

The nurse may participate in several of the treatment modalities described pre-viously. Ground rules for establishing a therapeutic relationship with children or adolescents are summarized as follows:

1. Accept a child or adolescent as an equal when able, keeping in mind the person's age.
2. Do not use baby talk or substandard English, or talk down while communi-cating with the child or adolescent. Listen to the emotions expressed and encourage verbalization of feelings.
3. Do not force yourself on the patient or push him or her to confide in you.
4. Accept the person but discuss any undesirable behavior. Ignoring behavior such as tics also may be acceptable. Each behavior needs to be evaluated to decide the appropriate approach.
5. Be a good role model.

Another suggestion is to watch one's body language or nonverbal commu-nication. Children and adolescents are quite observant of what adults say and how they communicate feelings both verbally and nonverbally. They should know that adults have good and bad days that can affect their interpersonal rela-tionships, especially in the area of communication.

The following rules for parents to live by were written by boys in a reform school for delinquent behavior.

1. Don't lose control in stressful situations because children are great imitators of parental behavior.
2. Don't use alcohol or pills as a crutch. Your behavior tells children it's okay to do the same.
3. Be a strict and consistent disciplinarian. Call a bluff. Don't compromise. Such an attitude denotes love and provides security. Children don't always want what they ask for; they just test parents.
4. Set a good spiritual example. Children need to know that a supreme being exists.
5. Don't try to imitate your children by dressing, talking, or acting younger. Children need good role models, not parents who try to be peers.
6. Be honest and give a few compliments if they are deserved.

Such suggestions can also apply to nurses who work with children and adolescents in the psychiatric setting.

Other aspects of nursing interventions include (1) helping the child to master developmental tasks to overcome regressive, slow, or impaired developmental behavior; (2) establishing a method of communication with persons who have difficulty communicating, such as the withdrawn, disoriented, mute, hostile, preoccupied, or autistic child; (3) identifying stimuli that might foster abusive, destructive, or otherwise negative behavior; and (4) allowing time for the person to respond to therapeutic interventions.

Nurses should be aware of their own reactions to patients' behaviors. If unable to handle feelings or behaviors, they should seek assistance from peers or supervisory personnel. They also should respect the child's spatial territory and not invade her or his privacy. Therapeutic touch is used only after exploring the person's feelings about being touched (*e.g.*, a battered or abused child would probably withdraw and resist touch).

Nursing personnel may plan activities appropriate for the child's developmental level and age. They should consider the child's energy level and need to calm down after an activity.

Specific nursing interventions are discussed here for the following disorders of infancy, childhood, and adolescence: mental retardation, ADHD, conduct disorder, autistic disorder and childhood and adolescent depression. Examples of nursing diagnoses and nursing interventions are included at the end of this chapter.

Mental Retardation

As stated previously, persons with mental retardation may be educable or trainable, or require custodial care. Such persons may have dual diagnoses of mental retardation and mental illness, as well as a physical disability or limitation.

The nurse working in an institutional setting is challenged to provide environmental stimulation as well as to meet the needs of the child emotionally and physically because persons with mental retardation do not always communicate physical symptoms. Helping the child to master the activities of daily living may be a slow process involving behavioral therapy. Protective care may be necessary if the person is epileptic, prone to acting-out behavior, disoriented, or masochistic (head banging or biting self). The administration of anticonvulsant and psychotropic drugs is also the responsibility of the nurse.

Education of the family is an important factor not to be overlooked because many persons who are mentally retarded attend an institution during the week but go home for weekend or holiday visits. Others attend a day hospital, special school, or sheltered workshop, and return home at night as well as weekends. The nurse is the patient's advocate, both in the institutional setting and when relating to the family. Identifying the family's ability to cope and continue with the therapy at home is important to promote progress as well as to minimize the stress that can occur when changing environments.

Attention-Deficit/Hyperactivity Disorder

The main treatment for ADHD is to change the environment so that the child is able to alter or improve his or her reaction to the environment. Environmental stimuli are kept at a minimum while the child is medicated with CNS stimulants (e.g., Ritalin, Cylert, Dexedrine, or Benzedrine) that have a paradoxical effect that prevents flooding of the cerebral cortex by impulses (this in effect slows the child down). Other medication used in the treatment include tricyclic antidepressants, alpha-adrenergic stimulating agents such as Clonidine, and beta-blockers such as Inderal to decrease aggressive behavior (Dulcan, Bregman, Weller, & Weller, 1995).

The role of the nurse is to identify, reduce, or eliminate such stimuli as well as to administer the medication. The nurse may also work with the family or teachers to plan a firm, consistent, predictable environment. Limits and standards must be set while employing behavior therapy. The symptoms usually subside at puberty.

Conduct Disorder

The suggestions by delinquents listed earlier serve as a basic list of approaches when dealing with conduct disorders. Stated positively, they are included in the following list of interventions:

1. Establish trust by being honest.
2. Maintain control by setting limits for manipulative, acting-out behavior.
3. Be consistent with limit setting.
4. Respect the person's age and maintain an adult–child or adult–adult relationship, whichever is appropriate.
5. Establish realistic expectations. Discuss such expectations with the person and encourage verbalization of feelings.

Autistic Disorder

Autism is very difficult to treat because it is considered the most irreversible childhood disorder. The nurse is challenged as she or he assesses the child and

1. Helps the child establish a meaningful interpersonal relationship
2. Develops an effective way to communicate
3. Provides a safe, consistent environment to prevent self-destructive behavior
4. Allows time for the patient to develop tolerance for physical closeness
5. Encourages the child to participate in self-care
6. Administers medication for symptomatic relief (*e.g.*, Haldol)
7. Helps the child's family to handle difficult behavior effectively by employing behavioral therapy

Kaufman's (1975) article on autism describes a long-term, deeply committed, two-phase program for his son, Raun. The first phase was to motivate Raun to explore the world outside himself. The second phase focused on a program of instruction to master developmental tasks. In 3 months, he accomplished 14 months of development. Not all autistic children make such progress, but Raun's story is encouraging.

Childhood and Adolescent Depression

Childhood and adolescent depression can go unrecognized or untreated, resulting in a chronic or severe form of depression, possibly leading to suicide. The nurse needs to be aware of the differences between childhood or adolescent depression and adult depression if effective nursing intervention is to be provided. A comparison of the depressions is given in Table 24-1.

The nurse's role is to assist the depressed child or adolescent in verbalizing feelings such as suicidal ideation or anger, in developing a positive self-image, and in developing independence. The nurse also educates the patient regarding prescribed psychotropic drugs and discusses the importance of compliance. Participation in therapies such as individual, family, or peer group counseling is encouraged. Providing parents with the teaching checklist on disorders of childhood and adolescence may also be helpful. (Other nursing interventions are discussed in Chapter 19.)

The following are examples of nursing diagnoses frequently used when developing a care plan for children and adolescents who exhibit emotional or behavioral problems. They include *anxiety, *body image disturbance, *impaired verbal communication, *ineffective individual coping, depression, loneliness, manipulation, altered impulse control, *impaired social interaction, disturbance in self-concept, and *sleep pattern disturbance.

Nursing Care Plan 24-1 (on p. 470) lists an example of a nursing diagnosis and goal-related nursing interventions for a child with the DSM-IV diagnosis of anxiety.

* NANDA-approved nursing diagnosis.

TABLE 24-1 CHARACTERISTICS OF CHILDHOOD/ADOLESCENT AND ADULT DEPRESSION

Childhood/Adolescent Depression	Adult Depression
Constant depression, involving every aspect of one's world	Depression usually improves during the day.
It can paralyze emotional growth and social development.	Worse in the early morning hours
Anger or hostility leads to aggressive behavior.	Not normally aggressive
Reality testing reinforces feelings of depression.	Reality testing allows the adult an opportunity to examine objectively feelings and events regarding depression.
Higher percentage of suicidal ideation than observed in adults	
Does not recognize need for help	Usually recognizes need and seeks help

PARENT TEACHING CHECKLIST

Disorders of Childhood and Adolescence

The following checklist has been developed to reinforce the parent's knowledge about _____. Please inform the nurse if you are uncertain about any of the items listed below.

✔ Clinical symptoms my child may experience include:
✔ The reasons my child may exhibit a change in clinical symptoms include:
✔ Interventions that may stabilize my child's clinical symptoms include:
✔ Support persons I may contact:
✔ The name of the medication my child is taking is:
✔ Instructions regarding this medication
  ▪ Take this medication as directed by the doctor
  ▪ Do not give your child over-the-counter medication without informing the nurse or doctor
  ▪ Usual side effects include:
  ▪ Report any unusual side effects promptly
  ▪ Do not discontinue giving your child medication without first consulting your child's nurse or doctor

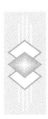

NURSING CARE PLAN 24-1
The Child with Anxiety

Nursing Diagnosis: *Sleep pattern disturbance related to change in environment (relocation)

Goal: The patient will establish regular hours for sleeping.

Nursing Interventions	Outcome Criteria
	Before discharge the patient will do the following:
Provide for quiet, relaxing activities before the hour of sleep.	Demonstrate compliance by participating in quiet structured activities before sleep
Assign a staff person to stay with the child to discuss fears or homesickness.	Verbalize feelings of fear or loneliness as they occur
Provide reassurance. Establish a bedtime routine. Provide a night light.	Verbalize feelings of security prior to falling asleep

*NANDA-approved nursing diagnosis.

 ## Summary

This chapter focused on the disorders of infancy, childhood, and adolescence. Factors influencing the onset of such disorders were discussed. These include constitutional, temperamental, and environmental factors, as well as the effects of physical disease or injury. Diagnostic criteria, etiology, treatment, and nursing interventions were described for each of the following subclassifications: mental retardation; ADHD; conduct disorder; anxiety disorders; tic disorders; disorders with physical manifestations, such as enuresis and encopresis; pervasive developmental disorders, such as autistic disorder; separation anxiety disorder; adjustment disorder; and childhood depression. Clinical examples of severe mental retardation, ADHD, separation anxiety disorder, encopresis, autism, and childhood depression were given. Transcultural considerations and research related to the disorders of childhood and adolescence were discussed. A brief summary of treatment regimens focused on individual psychotherapy, as well as family, group, play, behavioral, art, music, and drug therapy. Hospitalization, day hospitals or partial hospitalization programs, and alternative families were also presented. Nursing assessment and interventions were discussed.

Examples of nursing diagnoses related to children and adolescents with emotional or behavioral disturbances were cited. An example of nursing interventions and outcome criteria related to childhood anxiety was included.

Learning Activities

I. Clinical Activities
- A. Care for a patient exhibiting a disorder of infancy, childhood, or adolescence.
  1. Identify the developmental level of the patient. State the tasks appropriate for the developmental level and identify those tasks uncompleted. State nursing interventions to facilitate completing such tasks.
  2. Assess the patient's ability to relate to others. Consider peers, family, and members of the health team. In what manner does the patient communicate?
  3. Review the patient's treatment plan. Is it appropriate? If not, what changes or additions would you make?
- B. Care for a patient with an adjustment disorder.
  1. Identify the source(s) and duration of stressor(s) experienced by the patient.
  2. Assess the patient's past and present coping mechanisms.
  3. Identify positive coping mechanisms and situational supports.
  4. Develop short-term goals appropriate for this patient.
  5. State nursing diagnoses and interventions based on the patient's behavioral symptoms.
  6. Discuss those stressors and appropriate supportive nursing interventions during clinical conference.
- C. Identify in your clinical facility a list of agencies available as support systems to persons who exhibit symptoms of adjustment disorders.

II. Independent Activities
- A. Identify facilities in your community that provide care for infants, children, or adolescents with psychiatric disorders. Consider hospitals, foster homes, children's services, and rehabilitative services.
- B. Investigate the role of the school psychologist in the diagnosis and care of a child with a behavioral disorder.
- C. Contact a local law enforcement agency and obtain information regarding the various types of disturbed or disturbing children or adolescents who are brought to their attention. What options are available when handling such people?

Critical Thinking Questions

1. Watch a current movie about gangs. Can you identify characters in the movie with conduct or attention-deficit/hyperactivity disorders? What causative factors would you identify if one of these characters were your client?
2. A friend comes to you for advice. Her five-year-old son has been wetting the bed every night for the past several months. She is at her "wit's end" and says she "can't understand why he keeps doing this—after all, he's been toilet trained for two and one half years." Identify some common causes for this type of behavior regression. What questions would you ask your friend? What interventions would be appropriate?
3. Read several articles or chapters about family systems therapy. What principles can you apply with any family you assess and work with?

Self-Test

1. List three causes of disorders in childhood.
2. State four behaviors that could be warning signs of depression.
3. Discuss the purpose of play therapy and when it would be an appropriate nursing intervention.
4. Describe autism.
5. List two nursing interventions to help a child relate to an adult.
6. Differentiate between adolescent and adult depression.
7. State three nursing interventions for adolescent depression.
8. List three ways in which a family may promote a positive interpersonal relationship with a disturbed adolescent.
9. State four nursing interventions appropriate for increasing an adolescent's self-esteem.
10. State the characteristics of an adjustment disorder.
11. Describe behavioral manifestations that may occur during an adjustment disorder.
12. State stressors in each of the following developmental levels that may occur during an adjustment disorder:
    Childhood
    Adolescence
13. Define the following terms:
    Tics
    Selective mutism
    Encopresis
    Enuresis
    Pervasive developmental disorder

14. List five symptoms of attention-deficit/hyperactivity disorder.
15. State nursing interventions for each of the symptoms listed in the previous question.
16. Differentiate the levels of mental retardation.
17. List five causes of conduct disorder.
18. Give a brief explanation of the following therapies as they apply to children and adolescents:

    Individual psychotherapy

    Group psychotherapy

    Art therapy

    Music therapy

    Drug therapy

19. Discuss the rationale for the following environmental changes for children and adolescents:

    Hospitalization

    Day hospital

    Alternative families

SELECTED REFERENCES

American Psychiatric Association. (1994). *Diagnostic and statistical manual of mental disorders* (4th ed.). Washington, DC: American Psychiatric Press.

Barker, P. (1983). *Basic child psychiatry* (4th ed.). Baltimore: University Park Press.

Barlow, D. J. (1989, January). Therapeutic holding: Effective intervention with the aggressive child. *Journal of Psychosocial Nursing and Mental Health Services.*

Carpenito, L. M. (1995). *Nursing diagnosis: Application to clinical practice* (6th ed.). Philadelphia: J. B. Lippincott.

Carrey, N. J., & Adams, L. (1992, May). How to deal with sexual-acting out on the child psychiatric inpatient ward. *Journal of Psychosocial Nursing and Mental Health Services.*

Church, C. C. (1996, February). Unlocking the mystery: An overview of autism in children. *Advance for Nurse Practitioners.*

Dulcan, M. K., Bregman, J. D., Weller, E. B., & Weller, R. A. (1995). Treatment of childhood and adolescent disorders. In A. F. Schatzberg & C. B. Nemeroff (Eds.). *The American Psychiatric Press textbook of psychopharmacology.* Washington, DC: American Psychiatric Press.

Erikson, E. (1964). *Childhood and society* (rev. ed.). New York: W. W. Norton.

George, M. S. (1993, September). Obsessive–compulsive disorder and Tourette syndrome. *Clinical Advances in the Treatment of Psychiatric Disorders.*

Gerchufsky, M. (1996, February). Helping families cope with ADHD. *Advance for Nurse Practitioners.*

Hahn, M. C. (1996, February). Talking to teens: What clinicians need to know. *Advance for Nurse Practitioners.*

Harrington, R. (1994). Affective disorders. In M. Rutter, E. Taylor, & L. Hersov (Eds.). *Child and adolescent psychiatry: Modern approaches* (3rd ed.). Oxford: Blackwell Scientific Publications.

Johnson, B. S. (1995). *Child, adolescent, and family psychiatric nursing.* Philadelphia: Lippincott–Raven Publishers.

Kaufman, B. (1975, February). Reaching the "unreachable" child. *New York Magazine.*

Kwasman, A., Tinsley, B. J., & Lepper, H. S. (1995, November). Pediatricians' knowledge and attitudes concerning diagnosis and treatment of attention deficit hyperactivity disorders. *Archives of Pediatrics and Adolescent Medicine.*

Moon, M. A. (1995, December). MRI reveals biologic marker of ADHD children. *Clinical Psychiatry News.*

Pharmaceutical Update. (1996, July). New option for ADHD. *Advance for Nurse Practitioners.*

Popper, C. W., & Frazier, S. H. (Eds). (1990, Spring). *Journal of Child and Adolescent Psychopharmacology.* New York: M. A. Liebert, Inc.

Rosner, T. A., & Pollice, S. A. (1991, January). Tourette's syndrome. *Journal of Psychosocial Nursing and Mental Health Nursing.*

Roye, C. G. (1995, December). CE credit: Breaking through to the adolescent patient. *American Journal of Nursing.*

Rutter, M., Taylor, E., & Hersov, L. (1994). *Child and adolescent psychiatry: Modern approaches* (3rd ed.). Oxford: Blackwell Scientific Publications.

Schultz, J. M., & Videbeck, S. D. (1994). *Manual of psychiatric nursing care plans* (4th ed.). Philadelphia: J. B. Lippincott.

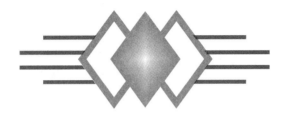

CHAPTER 25

EATING DISORDERS

To be nobody but myself—in a world which is doing its best . . . to make you everybody else—means to fight the hardest battle which any human being can fight, and never stop fighting.

e. e. cummings

1 Define the terms *anorexia nervosa* and *bulimia nervosa*.

2 Explain why simple obesity is not categorized as an eating disorder.

3 Cite at least five factors that may contribute to the development of an eating disorder.

4 Explain the rationale for medical evaluation and treatment of individuals with eating disorders.

5 State the criteria for inpatient treatment.

6 Discuss the rationale for using antidepressant agents in the treatment of anorexia nervosa or bulimia nervosa.

7 State at least three nursing diagnoses most frequently identified in the treatment of eating disorders.

8 Describe nursing interventions used in planning care for individuals exhibiting clinical symptoms of eating disorders.

Introduction

According to the DSM-IV, eating disorders are characterized by severe disturbances in eating behavior. Two specific diagnoses are included: anorexia nervosa and bulimia nervosa. Simple obesity is considered to be a general medical condition and does not appear in the DSM-IV because it has not been established that it is consistently associated with a psychological or behavioral syndrome.

Anorexia Nervosa

Anorexia nervosa, a condition that is seen mainly in young women, has become increasingly prevalent. Although most anorectics are teenaged girls or women who usually are bright achievers, males also suffer from this disorder. Characterized by an aversion to food, it may result in death owing to serious malnutrition. The age of onset is usually late adolescence; however, diagnosis has been made in young girls, 8 to 11 years of age, as well as women over age 30. According to statistics provided by Herzog (1988),

1. Of all anorectics, 90% to 95% are female.
2. Of diagnosed anorectics, 10% to 20% die. Half of these deaths are due to suicide.

3. Anorexia occurs mainly in upper middle-class families; however, victims may be from any socioeconomic group.
4. Usually the youngest daughter of several children is afflicted.

Some factors that may contribute to the development of this disease include disturbed self-image, parent–child conflicts, past and present experiences resulting in feelings of dependency and helplessness, the adolescent's desire to return to the alleged comfort and safety of childhood, or a stressful life situation. Starvation is an attention-getting device that permits the anorectic patient full control of her body, allows her to remain in or revert to a prepubertal state, and is considered manipulative behavior.

The DSM-IV states that the anorectic has an intense fear of becoming obese although weight loss occurs. Even when emaciated, the person insists that she is fat, displaying a distortion of body image. A weight loss of at least 15% of the original body weight is seen, as well as the refusal to maintain at least minimal body weight for age and height. In postmenarcheal females, at least three consecutive menstrual cycles are absent before the diagnosis is considered. No known physical illness or disease is responsible for the weight loss. Two subtypes are used to describe anorectic behavior: restricting type (does not regularly engage in binge-eating or purging behavior) and binge-eating/purging type.

Various methods are used to lose weight. They include induced vomiting, laxatives, enemas, diuretics, diet pills, excessive exercise, binging and purging, stimulants, or refusal to eat. Deceitful behavior may prevail as the anorectic patient disposes of food she is supposed to eat. The following symptoms occur as the disorder progresses. Not all persons who are anorectic exhibit all the symptoms listed.

1. Dry, flaky, or cracked skin
2. Brittle hair and nails, hair beginning to fall out
3. Amenorrhea or menstrual irregularity
4. Constipation
5. Hypothermia
6. Decreased pulse, blood pressure, and basal metabolic rate
7. Skeletal appearance
8. Presence of lanugo (downy-soft body hair seen in newborn infants)
9. Intense fear of becoming obese
10. Distorted body image as patient continues to see self as fat
11. Loss of appetite
12. Dehydration, malnutrition, and electrolyte imbalance, which can result in death
13. A total lack of concern about symptoms

The preanorectic person is generally considered to be a "model child and student" who is meek, compliant, perfectionistic, and an overachiever. She usually is overly sensitive, fears independence and sexual relationships, has a low self-concept, and is resistant to growing up and maturing.

As the eating disorder progresses, the anorectic person presents behaviors such as manipulation, stubbornness, hostility, and deceitfulness. Defense mechanisms used are denial, displacement, projection, rationalization, regression, isolation, and intellectualization.

Warning signs that should alert parents, teachers, or others to the possibility of anorexia include

1. Drastic weight loss in the presence of unusual eating habits, such as fasting, binging, or refusal to eat except tiny portions
2. Obsession with neatness or personal appearance, including frequent mirror gazing. The person constantly checks her appearance, fearing unattractiveness and obesity.
3. Hostility and the desire to control others
4. Calorie counting, dieting, and excessive exercise or hyperactivity
5. Weighing oneself several times daily
6. Depressed mood
7. Amenorrhea or irregular menses
8. Wearing loose-fitting clothing to hide her physical appearance as it changes
9. Denying hunger

Living in an environment that is overprotective, rigid, or lacking in conflict resolution, the anorectic achieves secondary gains such as love and undue attention because she is considered to be a special or unique person.

Bulimia Nervosa

Episodic binge eating with a rapid consumption of a large amount of food in under two hours is classified as bulimia. The person is aware that the behavior is abnormal, fears the inability to stop eating voluntarily, is self-critical, and may experience depression after each episode.

According to the DSM-IV criteria, the person with bulimia nervosa consumes high-calorie, easily ingested food, eats inconspicuously, and terminates binging or gorging by self-induced vomiting, going to sleep, or engaging in social activities. The person may stop eating because of abdominal pain. Repeated attempts are made to lose weight by fasting or dieting; by abusing laxatives, enemas, or diuretics; by self-induced vomiting; or by abusing over-the-counter weight control medications. Weight fluctuation is seen owing to alternating

CLINICAL EXAMPLE 25-1
Anorexia Nervosa

MJ, 19 years old, was a sophomore in college when her psychology professor noted a change in classroom behavior as well as a sudden weight loss. When questioned about her behavior, MJ told the professor that she was losing weight to compete for a position on the track team, although she was unable to give him a specific goal regarding her desired weight. She began to wear clothing that was loose fitting and would refer to herself as overweight although others commented on her thinness. MJ's meek compliant behavior changed to that of a deceitful, hostile, and manipulative person. She isolated herself at mealtime and engaged in various exercises after eating. At times she would eat large amounts of food and then induce vomiting. A close friend observed MJ taking large amounts of over-the-counter diet pills as well as laxatives. In an effort to continue her weight loss, MJ would set her alarm so that she could exercise during the night and also awaken for early morning jogging. She became obsessed with exercising. Her physical appearance deteriorated as her hair began to fall out, her skin became quite dry, and acne developed. MJ also complained of being chilly all the time and wore layered clothing. During track practice, MJ became light-headed, felt irregular heart beats, perspired profusely, and experienced severe fatigue. The track coach took her to the college health clinic to be examined by the physician. Physical examination revealed poor skin turgor, as well as other symptoms of dehydration. The physician also suspected a potassium and protein deficit, although MJ denied any eating problems. Her weight was approximately 15 pounds under the desired weight for her height and body build. She had lost 25 pounds in a four-month period and experienced amenorrhea for three months. The college physician recommended that MJ see the school counselor regarding her concern about weight loss.

dieting or fasting and binging. Such behavior occurs on an average of at least twice a week for three months before the diagnosis is given. Subtypes include purging type (regularly engages in self-induced vomiting or the misuse of laxatives, diuretics, or enemas) and nonpurging type (uses inappropriate compensatory behaviors such as fasting or excessive exercise).

The onset of bulimia nervosa occurs in adolescence or early adult life. Many adolescents feel insecure about their physical shape and size in a society that places value on external appearance and nurturing. Parents and family members also wield a great deal of influence during the development of the adolescent's self-concept and perceptions of the world.

Certain traits are found among individuals who view themselves as unlovable, inadequate, and unworthy. The desire to please becomes very powerful as the adolescent strives to be perfect, thin, loved, and accepted. The psychiatric implications are significant because approximately 50% of those patients with bulimia nervosa also experience depression and require antidepressant medication. Substance abuse is commonly seen. Bulimia nervosa may develop into a chronic disorder and occur intermittently over several years.

Serious medical complications that may occur because of alternating binging and purging include

1. Chronic inflammation of the lining of the esophagus
2. Rupture of the esophagus
3. Dilatation of the stomach
4. Rupture of the stomach
5. Electrolyte imbalance or abnormalities, leading to arrhythmias of the heart and metabolic alkalosis
6. Heart problems, irreversible congestive heart failure, and death due to abuse of Ipecac syrup
7. Chronic enlargement of the parotid gland
8. Dehydration
9. Irritable bowel syndrome or abnormal dilatation of the colon
10. Rectal prolapse or abscess
11. Rupture of the diaphragm, with entrance of the abdominal contents into the chest cavity
12. Dental erosion
13. Chronic edema
14. Fungal infections of the vagina or rectum

The prevalence of this disorder among adolescent and young adult women is approximately 1% to 3%. The age of onset is usually between 17 and 25 years (American Psychiatric Association, 1994).

Obesity

Although obesity is not defined as a DSM-IV disorder, individuals exhibiting clinical symptoms of obesity and coexisting diagnoses such as anxiety or depression have been treated in the psychiatric setting. Such individuals frequently refer to themselves as bulimics who do not purge, and give a history of repeated attempts to lose or stabilize their weight. They usually respond to and benefit from treatment modalities similar to those used by individuals with bulimia nervosa.

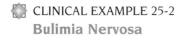 CLINICAL EXAMPLE 25-2
Bulimia Nervosa

LR, a 21-year-old secretary, was seen in the emergency room of a local community hospital with complaints of weakness, rapid pulse, dizziness, and difficulty swallowing. A physical assessment disclosed symptoms of dehydration, with a possible electrolyte imbalance. On being questioned further, LR confided to the physician that she was concerned about her weight and had tried various measures to control her appetite. She found herself craving sweets and other high-calorie foods. When such feelings occurred she would devour "everything in sight" that was easily ingested, eating for one to two hours at times. Her grocery and restaurant bills were quite high, over $150.00 per week, because of such cravings. After such binging episodes, LR would induce vomiting to avoid weight gain. She stated that she felt "out of control" and anxious when she binged. Her main fear was that of becoming fat, and when she vomited she was able to relieve herself of guilt feelings due to overeating. Recent publicity about anorexia and bulimia had caused her to seek help for physical symptoms that had been present for several weeks. LR agreed to a complete physical examination and referral to a counselor who had experience working with bulimic patients.

Conant (1996) describes obesity as a physical condition resulting from a medical condition, diet, side effect of medications such as steroids, or compulsive eating that is psychogenic in origin. Developmental obesity begins in childhood with overeating, and reactive obesity occurs in later life, when compulsive eating is used to cope with stress.

Rohland (1996) addresses obesity in childhood. Approximately 20% of children 6 to 17 years of age weigh 20% more than their ideal body weight. The social stigma of being overweight can have long-term, devastating effects on self-esteem because obese children are often teased and rejected by their peers. In August, 1996 a 12-year-old-boy in central Florida hanged himself the morning that school was to start. The parents stated that he had tried all summer to lose weight before he was scheduled to enter middle school. His pediatrician stated that the boy's body frame was large and, genetically, he was predisposed to developing faster than his peers. Bailey (1994) states that obesity in children is usually caused by a combination of excessive caloric intake and insufficient exercise; however, it is also a feature of various congenital and acquired syndromes such as Down's, Klinefelter's, and Prader-Willi.

Agras (1995) addresses the diagnosis of binge-eating disorder. The principal features include binge-eating at least twice a week for six months, causing marked distress, and not occurring during the course of bulimia nervosa. There is a substantial overlap between this proposed disorder and obesity. Because of insufficient information, this diagnosis was not officially included in the DSM-IV. It is hoped that research will help to determine the possible utility of this proposed category.

 ## Transcultural Considerations

Eating disorders are most commonly seen in industrialized societies where food is abundant and attractiveness is equated with being thin. They occur in the United States, Canada, Europe, Australia, Japan, New Zealand, and South Africa. Individuals who immigrate from other cultures may develop the disorder as thin-body ideals are assimilated.

 ## Medical Evaluation and Treatment of Anorexia and Bulimia

Medical assessment must begin with a physical examination. Medical complications, as stated earlier, can be serious and potentially life threatening. Profound emaciation is often the most striking feature of individuals with anorexia nervosa. The presence of physical signs may serve as a clue in making the diagnosis of bulimia nervosa in persons reluctant to disclose binge and purge behaviors. A dental examination should be included in the initial medical evaluation.

An electrocardiogram (EKG) should be done on all individuals to detect the presence of arrhythmias and other changes reflective of electrolyte imbalance. Laboratory tests may also reveal abnormal laboratory values such as severe leukopenia, low fasting blood sugar, elevation of serum enzymes and amylose levels, variance in blood urea nitrogen values, carotenemia, and elevation of serum cholesterol levels.

Endocrine assessments may reveal a decrease in urinary secretion and plasma levels of gonadotropins in anorexia nervosa. Other abnormalities may include elevated levels of growth hormone, hypothyroidism, and incomplete suppression of cortisol.

Abnormal electroencephalogram (EEG) tracings have been described in both anorexia nervosa and bulimia. It is also important to screen for abuse of alcohol, drugs, and Ipecac in bulimics to prevent the occurrence of a medical emergency due to irreversible cardiomyopathy.

The inpatient treatment of eating disorders is highly problematic because individuals often deny the illness, evade therapeutic treatment, and engender negative reactions in health care professionals. A variety of treatment approaches are available. They include individual, cognitive, psychoeducational, group, and family therapy as well as self-help groups. Criteria for inpatient treatment are listed in Box 25-1 (American Psychiatric Association, 1989).

Effective treatment programs use behavioral methods to treat anorexia nervosa. The mere act of hospitalization incorporates a behavioral contingency. One goal of such methods is to help the anorectic person to alter inappropriate eating habits and gain weight. For example, privileges are earned if weight is gained, and they are taken away if weight is lost. Anorectic patients can be quite manipulative as they attempt to divert attention from their eating habits, which may include eating slowly, hiding food, or giving food to other persons. They need to be supervised on a one-to-one basis to discourage such manipulative ploys.

The use of psychotropic drugs has been effective; however, administering antidepressant drugs before weight restoration may be hazardous in individuals with a low serum potassium level or history of cardiac arrhythmias. Trial doses of antidepressant drugs such as Elavil may be tried once anorectic behavior is stable. Periactin may be prescribed to increase the person's appetite. Luvox or Anafranil may be used to reduce obsessive–compulsive traits. Far more success has been demonstrated in the pharmacologic treatment of bulimic disorder than of anorexia. Individuals who exhibit clinical symptoms of bulimia may respond well to Prozac, Zoloft, Desyrel, lithium carbonate, Norpramin, Pamelor, or Elavil. Such medication is also effective in treating concomitant depression (Agras, 1995; Pope & Hudson, 1989). Other related disorders include phobias, substance abuse, impulse control disorder, and borderline personality disorder. Agras (1995) discusses pharmacologic treatment of concomitant disorders.

Outpatient treatment, designed to meet the needs of the individual with an eating disorder, may require a team approach. Members would include a medical physician or internist, psychiatrist, nutritionist, and group or family therapist. If

BOX 25-1 Criteria for Hospitalization

1. Low weight or failure to maintain outpatient weight contract
2. Metabolic abnormalities, especially hypokalemic alkalosis
3. Depressed mood; suicidal ideation or plan
4. Severe binging and purging
5. Psychosis
6. Family crisis
7. Nonsupportive environment
8. Failure to respond to outpatient treatment

the individual remains at home, the approach usually used is to ignore eating habits as well as self-induced vomiting, purging, or excessive exercising. Such avoidance reduces the possibility of manipulation or confrontation when the individual is indecisive, ambivalent, or hostile.

❖ Nursing Assessment and Interventions

"Clients may not eat for a number of reasons, both physiologic and psychologic. A client may refuse to eat, be uninterested in eating, or be unaware of the need or desire to eat. A client may be experiencing physical problems that interfere with appetite or that make it difficult for the client to eat" (Schultz & Videbeck, 1994).

It is imperative that the nurse use an assessment tool to determine whether a psychiatric problem may underlie the individual's inability or refusal to eat. Conant (1996) presents an assessment guide for eating disorders that focuses on weight, eating habits or pattern, level or type of activities, family relationships, and physical signs and symptoms. Sample questions include "Do you often feel fat?", "Do you induce vomiting after you have eaten?", "Do you exercise?", "How do members of your family express anger?", and "Do you use laxatives or diuretics to lose weight?"

Some individuals exhibit bulimarectic behavior in which they alternate between periods of excessive and minimal food intake. The chance of successful treatment is better if the patient maintains a body weight greater than 90 pounds. That weight appears to be a critical turning point in the patient's response to therapy. As stated earlier, if the patient is in no physical distress, outpatient therapy may be employed. If an underlying depression exists, protective care may be necessary.

The nurse plays an important role in the care of individuals with eating disorders. The nurse needs to adjust readily to mood swings and changes of behavior. This is done effectively by

1. Being matter-of-fact, friendly, and casual if the patient is withdrawn or sullen
2. Setting limits to avoid manipulative behavior
3. Remaining uninvolved when the patient is indecisive or ambivalent
4. Avoiding confrontation when the patient exhibits hostility or anger
5. Stating that eating three nutritional meals a day is necessary to maintain a healthy body
6. Avoiding long discussions or explanations about food or the body
7. Approaching the person with positive expectations in spite of negative behavior
8. Allowing the patient to maintain some control, for example, in decision making

━━━━━━━━━━━━━━━ PATIENT TEACHING CHECKLIST ━━━━━━━━━━━━━━━
Eating Disorder

The following checklist has been developed to reinforce your knowledge about eating disorders. Please inform the nurse if you are uncertain about any of the items listed below.

✔ Clinical symptoms I may experience include:
✔ The reasons I binge and purge or avoid eating include:
✔ Interventions I have learned to control this behavior are:
✔ Support persons I may contact include:
✔ The name of the medication I am taking is:
✔ Instructions regarding this medication
   ▪ Take this medication as directed by your doctor
   ▪ Do not drink alcohol while taking this medication
   ▪ Do not take any over-the-counter medication without informing your nurse or doctor
   ▪ Usual side effects include:
   ▪ Report any unusual side effects promptly
   ▪ Antidepressant agents usually reach therapeutic levels within two to three weeks
   ▪ Anxiolytic agents are usually fast acting because onset occurs within 30 minutes
   ▪ Dosage adjustment may be necessary
   ▪ Do not discontinue taking this medication without first consulting your nurse or doctor

Other nursing interventions may include providing the patient with a teaching checklist, monitoring intake and output, weighing the patient weekly, setting activity limits, and inserting a nasogastric tube or administering intravenous therapy if the physical condition warrants such care.

As denoted previously, short-term goals and interventions focus on stabilization of medical problems and restoration of normal nutritional status. Long-term goals and interventions focus on the development of improved self-esteem, positive coping skills, and healthy relationships.

Nursing diagnoses frequently used when planning nursing care include *ineffective denial, *self-esteem disturbance, *noncompliance with treatment plan, *ineffective family coping, *fatigue, *fluid volume deficit, and *risk for violence: self-directed or directed at others. Nursing Care Plan 25-1 summarizes nursing diagnoses and goal-related nursing interventions for a patient with a DSM-IV diagnosis of anorexia nervosa.

*NANDA-approved nursing diagnosis.

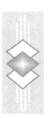

NURSING CARE PLAN 25-1
The Patient with Anorexia Nervosa

Nursing Diagnosis #1: *Altered nutrition (less than body requirements) related to self-induced vomiting after eating

Goal: Patient will avoid use of self-induced vomiting as a coping behavior.

Nursing Interventions	Outcome Criteria
	Within 24 to 48 hours the patient will do the following:
Educate patient on how self-induced vomiting is used to cope with feelings.	Demonstrate insight regarding relationship between feelings and binge–purge behavior
Encourage patient to discuss negative feelings that precipitate self-induced vomiting.	Verbalize feelings, including urge to vomit
Give positive reinforcement for appropriate expression of feelings.	Verbalize feelings appropriate to situations
Restrict use of bathroom for one to two hours after eating to prevent vomiting or disposal of concealed food.	Demonstrate compliance by not vomiting or disposing of concealed food after meals

Nursing Diagnosis #2: *Noncompliance related to depression as evidenced by presence of low self-esteem, blunted affect, poor eye contact, and isolation

Goal: Patient will demonstrate compliance.

Nursing Interventions	Outcome Criteria
	Within 24 to 48 hours the patient will begin to do the following:
Explain rationale for treatment modalities.	Demonstrate an understanding of prescribed treatment modalities
Assess causative or contributing factors.	Identify causative or contributing factors
Reduce or eliminate causative factors if possible.	Exhibit improvement in self-esteem, affect, eye contact, and socialization
Reinforce importance of adhering to prescribed regimen.	Demonstrate compliance with prescribed regimen

*NANDA-approved nursing diagnosis.

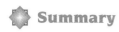 **Summary**

This chapter focused on contributing factors and characteristics of anorexia nervosa, bulimia nervosa, and obesity. Statistics regarding the frequency of eating disorders were cited. Clinical examples of anorexia nervosa and bulimia nervosa were presented. Transcultural considerations were discussed. The rationale for medical evaluation was stated. Criteria for inpatient treatment were listed. Treatment modalities, including the use of psychotropic drugs, were described. Nursing assessment, diagnoses, and appropriate interventions were discussed. A brief sample care plan focusing on altered nutrition (less than body requirements) and noncompliance related to depression was presented.

Learning Activities

I. Clinical Activities
   A. Care for a patient exhibiting clinical symptoms of an eating disorder.
      1. Assess for the presence of anxiety or depression.
      2. Identify the source(s) and duration of stressor(s) experienced by the patient.
      3. Assess present coping skills.
      4. Review the patient's treatment plan. Is it appropriate? If not, what changes or additions would you make?
   B. Identify a list of agencies available as support systems to persons who exhibit clinical symptoms of eating disorders.
II. Independent Activities
   A. Identify facilities in your community that provide support groups for persons with eating disorders.
   B. Contact the mental health association in your community. Obtain samples of educational material used to educate adolescents regarding eating disorders. Critique the accuracy of the information provided.

Critical Thinking Questions

1. While performing an admission health assessment on a 21-year-old woman admitted for a breast biopsy, you find the following: dry, flaky skin, brittle nails and hair, low blood pressure, slow pulse, and very visible bony prominences. Your questions uncover amenorrhea and a distorted body image. What nursing interventions are appropriate?
2. Contact a nurse practitioner at a local college health center. What materials about eating disorders does she have available for students? Ask the nurse practitioner to discuss her view of her role in caring for this population.

3. Search the literature for a body image assessment tool developed by a nurse. Administer the tool to classmates who appear thin, average, and overweight. What are your findings?

Self-Test

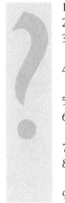

1. Define anorexia nervosa.
2. State five clinical symptoms of anorexia nervosa.
3. List a nursing intervention for each of the symptoms stated in the previous item.
4. Discuss the rationale for using behavior modification when caring for an anorectic patient.
5. Define bulimia nervosa.
6. State at least five medical complications that may occur because of binging and purging behavior.
7. Compare obesity to bulimia nervosa.
8. Explain the rationale for medical evaluation and treatment of eating disorders.
9. Cite the criteria for inpatient treatment of individuals with clinical symptoms of eating disorders.
10. Discuss the rationale for using antidepressant medication.
11. State three nursing diagnoses and interventions frequently used when planning nursing care for individuals with the diagnosis of bulimia nervosa.

SELECTED REFERENCES

Agras, W. S. (1995). Treatment of eating disorders. In A. F. Schatzberg & C. B. Nemeroff (Eds.). *The American Psychiatric Press textbook of psychopharmacology.* Washington, DC: American Psychiatric Press.

American Anorexia/Bulimia Association, 133 Cedar Lane, Teaneck, NJ 07666.

American Psychiatric Association. (1989). *Treatments of psychiatric disorders: A task force report of the American Psychiatric Association.* Washington, DC: Author.

American Psychiatric Association. (1994). *Diagnostic and statistical manual of mental disorders* (4th ed.). Washington, DC: Author.

Bailey, A. (1994). Physical examination and medical investigations. In M. Rutter, E. Taylor, & L. Hersov (Eds.). *Child and adolescent psychiatry* (3rd ed.). Cambridge, MA: Blackwell Scientific Publications.

Bates, B. (1995, December). Bulimia nervosa linked to history of sexual assault and rape. *Clinical Psychiatry News.*

Bender, K. J. (1996, February). Reconsidering anorectics: Dexfenfluramine recommended for obesity, without DEA controls. *Psychiatric Times.*

Bruch, H. (1973). *Eating disorders: Obesity, anorexia nervosa and the person within.* New York: Basic Books.

Carley, J., & Rooda, L. (1995, September). Profile of a support group: Help for eating disorders. *Advance for Nurse Practitioners.*

Carpenito, L. J. (1995). *Nursing diagnosis: Application to clinical practice* (6th ed.). Philadelphia: J. B. Lippincott.

Conant, M. (1996). The client with an eating disorder. In S. Lego (Ed.). *Psychiatric nursing: A comprehensive reference* (2nd ed.). Philadelphia: Lippincott–Raven Publishers.

Herzog, D. (1988). Eating disorders. In *The new Harvard guide to psychiatry.* Boston: Harvard University Press.

Hofland, S. L., & Dardis, P. O. (1992, February). Bulimia nervosa: Associated physical problems. *Journal of Psychosocial Nursing and Mental Health Services.*

Kolody, B., & Sallis, J. F. (1995, February). A prospective study of ponderosity, body image, self-concept, and psychological variables in children. *Journal of Developmental and Behavioral Pediatrics.*

McKenna, M. S. (1989, September). Assessment of the eating disordered patient. *Psychiatric Annals.*

Pope, H. G., & Hudson, J. I. (1989, September). Pharmacologic treatment of bulimia nervosa: Research findings and practical suggestions. *Psychiatric Annals.*

Rohland, P. (1996, June). The battle of the bulge. *Advance for Nurse Practitioners.*

Schultz, J. M., & Videbeck, S. D. (1994). *Manual of psychiatric nursing care plans* (4th ed.). Philadelphia: J. B. Lippincott.

Staples, N. R., & Schwartz, M. (1990, February). Anorexia nervosa support group: Providing transitional support. *Journal of Psychosocial Nursing and Mental Health Services.*

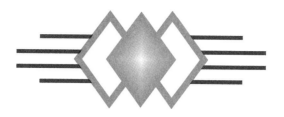

CHAPTER 26

INEFFECTIVE INDIVIDUAL COPING: ALCOHOLISM

> **Twelve Steps to Destruction**
>
> 1. I stated that I could hold my liquor and was master of my own life.
> 2. Came to believe I was sane and rational in every respect.
> 3. Decided to run my own life and be fantastic in all my undertakings.
> 4. Made a thorough and searching inventory of my fellow man and found him lacking.
> 5. Admitted to no one including God and myself that there was anything wrong with me.
> 6. Sought through alcohol to avoid all my responsibilities and to escape from the realities of life.
> 7. Continued to get drunk in an attempt to remove these shortcomings.
> 8. Made a list of all persons that had harmed me, whether imaginary or real, and swore to get even.

9. Got revenge whenever possible, except when to do so might further injure me.
10. Continued to find fault with the world and the people in it and when I was right promptly admitted it.
11. Sought through lying, cheating, and stealing to improve myself materially at the expense of my fellow man, asking only for the means to get drunk or stay high.
12. Having a complete mental, moral, physical and financial breakdown as the result of these steps, I endeavored to drag those around me down to my level and practiced these insanities in all my affairs.

Alcoholics Anonymous

LEARNING OBJECTIVES

1 Define alcoholism.

2 Differentiate between alcohol abuse and dependence.

3 State the more common physiologic effects of alcoholism.

4 Describe the more common psychological consequences of misuse of alcohol.

5 Compare and contrast the drinking habits of adolescents and adults.

6 Discuss the treatment of alcoholism.

7 Differentiate between the stages of alcohol withdrawal.

8 Develop a nursing care plan for a patient undergoing withdrawal due to alcoholism.

9 State the purpose of

AA

Al-Ateen

Al-Anon

Halfway houses

Introduction

The statistics on alcoholism's prevalence and impact can be startling. The National Institute of Mental Health noted in 1990 that approximately 5.1 million Americans abused alcohol. The latest statistics estimate that 18 million individuals are heavy drinkers and approximately 10 million of this number are alcoholics (Riggin, 1996). Other statistics indicate that 30% of all patients seen in acute care settings are alcoholic. As many as 36% of emergency department visits and 40% of admissions to medical–surgical units are prompted by alcohol-related problems. Alcoholism is responsible for up to 20% of acute care hospitalizations of elders (Antai-Otong, 1995).

In the United States, the high rate of alcohol involvement in fatal injuries has been well documented. Alcohol has been found in the blood of approximately 40% to 60% of motor vehicle accident victims, 32% to 46% of homicide victims, 20% to 50% of suicides, 25% to 50% of drowning victims, and 40% to 64% of fire and burn fatalities (Guohua, Smith, & Baker, 1994).

Abuse of alcohol is a major health problem for older children and adolescents. Unintentional injuries are the leading cause of death for adolescents, and approximately 40% of these injuries are related to alcohol use (U. S. Public Health Service, 1994).

The exact number of elderly Americans who abuse alcohol is not known. According to research conducted over the past decade, approximately 10% of all elderly patients treated in geriatric mental health facilities may have this problem (Daniels, 1996).

According to statistics quoted in the DSM-IV, as many as 90% of adults in the United States have had some experience with alcohol, and a substantial number (60% of men and 30% of women) have had one or more alcohol-related adverse life events.

Alcoholism is responsible for dysfunctional marital and family relationships, divorce, desertion, child abuse, displaced children, and impoverished families. Alcohol-related medical problems include cirrhosis, pancreatitis, chronic gastritis, blood dyscrasias, cardiac arrhythmia, and cerebral degeneration or dementia. Furthermore, fetal alcohol syndrome is one of the leading causes of birth defects in the United States.

 Etiology

According to the National Council on Alcoholism, the alcoholic is powerless to stop the drinking that seriously alters her or his normal living pattern. Alcoholics Anonymous describes alcoholism as a physical condition associated with a mental obsession. It is considered to be one part physical, one part psychological, one part sociologic, and one part alcohol.

Why do persons who, for example, are unable to cope with environmental pressures, have an unhappy childhood, or are emotionally unstable, become alcoholics? Various theories have been stated, but none has been accepted as being a complete explanation. Biologic theories propose that some individuals have a predisposition to alcoholism. Psychological theories focus on the "alcoholic personality." Early childhood rejection, overprotection, or undue responsibility can produce a dependent personality. Behavioral theorists believe alcoholism is the result of the positive effect of mood alterations that are experienced while drinking.

The following causative factors of alcohol abuse in teenagers have been discussed in literature:

1. Alcohol is the drug of choice among most adults. It is legal, and it is socially acceptable.
2. Advertising campaigns are aimed at youth with "soda pop wine" advertisements. Over 100 million dollars are spent yearly in such advertisement.
3. Parents indirectly sanction the use of alcohol by telling teenagers alcoholic beverages are okay but "don't touch any of those dangerous drugs like marijuana."
4. Teenagers possess more leisure time and money, and experience less parental or community supervision, especially at weekend parties.

Attempts have been made to describe the alcoholic personality. Common characteristics include the presence of increased anxiety or depression, social, or sexual inadequacy, increased social pressures, a desire to lower one's inhibitions, or self-destructive tendencies. The alcoholic personality may exhibit dependency needs or avoid any type of dependent behavior in an attempt to exhibit typical masculine characteristics. Alcohol meets the hidden dependency needs of such a person.

Alcohol consumption early in life may lead to a high tolerance of alcohol and lead to pattern drinking over a period of years. Later in life (*i.e.*, over age 50), such tolerance decreases and problem drinking occurs. The National Council on Alcoholism lists *13 Steps to Alcoholism* (1975). They are presented here.

Step 1 The person has begun to drink alcoholic beverages. Social drinking occurs in moderation as one drinks a cocktail, a few beers, or a glass of wine occasionally. No particular drinking pattern is established.

Step 2 The person is experiencing blackouts. Drinking results in inebriation with some regularity, although the person feels he or she can stop at will. During these drinking episodes the person gets "tight," gets "high," or feels good, and does not remember getting intoxicated or what was said or done afterwards. The person is experiencing amnesia or loss of memory.

Step 3 Liquor becomes very important. The person stops sipping and begins gulping alcoholic beverages. Sneaking drinks may become an established behavior. The person is reluctant to discuss how important liquor has become in his or her life. Chances of becoming an alcoholic at this step are very high if drinking does not slow down or stop.

Step 4 The person consistently drinks too much. This behavior occurs approximately two years after the first blackout. At this point the person cannot control the amount she or he drinks on any given occasion, although the person is not driven to drink. The person can control when he or she will drink again. During this period of drinking, the person may become extravagant with money because liquor has helped overcome a feeling of inferiority. This step is referred to as the basic or crucial phase of alcoholism. At this point the person can stop drinking, but if he or she begins to make excuses to self or anyone else, it is usually too late to stop drinking. These four steps are referred to as the early "danger signs" of alcoholism.

Step 5 The person makes excuses for drinking. "It's only beer. It relaxes me and helps me unwind," "I drive better after a few drinks," "I'm just celebrating my new promotion at work," or "It's rude to refuse a drink from the host" are a few examples of excuses made for excessive drinking. The person believes that he or she can handle drinking. Guilt feelings are experienced, and the person becomes defensive, building a repertoire of alibis, excuses, or falsehoods to rationalize behavior.

Step 6 The person wants alcohol available at all times (especially a morning drink or "eye-opener"). Drinking is a source of energy, strength, or motivation for the day and serves a "medicinal" purpose. It also eases the person's conscience, lifts the ego, and reinforces denial about abusing alcohol.

Step 7 The person drinks alone. Solitary drinking occurs because the person prefers to drink alone any time of day without listening to critical remarks of others who feel she or he drinks too much, or the person lives in a fantasy world while drinking, distorting reality. Drinking has now become an escape from reality.

Step 8 The person becomes antisocial while drinking. Solitary drinking can cause the person to become destructive or violent in behavior while the desire to cause damage becomes intense. Such destructive feelings may be directed toward self or others. Alcoholism causes the person to lose inhibitions and results in the loss of control or the ability to judge conduct. The person may react as a child or animal to meet immediate wants or needs. Realization of such behavior results in feelings of inadequacy and incompetency. The solution to such feelings is to drink more. The person is now experiencing the middle stages of alcoholism. The alcoholic pattern is set, and the person will follow it *unless* intervention occurs (*e.g.*, counseling or attending an alcoholic treatment program).

Step 9 The person experiences benders. This step begins the acute stage of compulsive drinking. The person is a true alcoholic with uncontrollable behavior. This usually occurs one to three years after morning drinking began. A bender is described as a period of days during which the person drinks continuously and helplessly with one goal in mind: to get drunk. The person no longer can control when she or he drinks. No thought is given to family, friends, job, food, or shelter.

Step 10 The person experiences a deep sense of remorse and resentment. During sober moments deep remorse is felt for uncontrollable actions and behavior. As guilt feelings become unbearable, the person drinks more and begins to blame others. The world is against him or her.

Step 11 The person experiences intense anxiety. Physical deterioration shows as hands tremble, steps are shaky, and nerves are jumpy. The person is experiencing "the shakes." Alcohol is the only thing that calms the person, so she or he guards the supply.

Step 12 The person realizes that liquor controls her or him. This realization generally occurs after the person has delirium tremens (DTs) or has talked with someone whose opinion he or she values, for example, a member of the clergy or psychiatrist.

Step 13 The person may get help or give in to alcoholism. If the person refuses to admit the truth to himself or herself, the alcoholism is incurable. Severe deterioration of health, family, work, and other relationships have occurred by now. The person may have lost job, home, and family. The last five steps are considered to be the late stages of alcoholism and are referred to as compulsive drinking. Death is inevitable unless some form of intervention occurs.

 ## Diagnostic Criteria for Alcohol Dependence and Abuse

This diagnostic class includes the alcohol use disorders: alcohol dependence and alcohol abuse. Alcohol-induced disorders are also discussed in the DSM-IV. They include alcohol intoxication, withdrawal, intoxication with delirium, and withdrawal delirium. Dementia, amnestic disorder, psychotic disorder with delusions or hallucinations, mood disorder, anxiety disorder, sexual dysfunction, and sleep disorder may also be alcohol induced.

The DSM-IV states that alcohol dependence and abuse share features with those of sedatives, hypnotics, and anxiolytics. The essential feature of dependence is a cluster of cognitive, behavioral, and physiologic symptoms indicating that the individual continues use of the substance (alcohol) despite critical substance-related problems. The symptoms of dependence are similar for most substances. There is a maladaptive pattern of substance use resulting in distress as the individual experiences a cluster of three or more of seven stated symptoms during a 12-month period:

1. Tolerance, which is defined as a need for markedly increased amounts of alcohol to achieve desired effect or a markedly diminished effect with continued use of the same amount of alcohol.
2. Withdrawal symptoms or the continued use of alcohol to relieve or avoid withdrawal symptoms.
3. Intake of alcohol is in larger amounts or over a longer period of time than was intended.
4. Persistent desire or unsuccessful efforts to cut down or control use of alcohol.
5. A significant amount of time is spent in activities necessary to obtain alcohol, drink alcohol, or recover from its effects.
6. Social, occupational, or recreational activities are given up or reduced because of drinking alcohol.
7. Drinking alcohol is continued despite knowledge of having a persistent or recurrent physical or psychological problem that is likely to have been caused or exacerbated by alcohol.

Specifiers during diagnosis include with physiologic dependence (evidence of tolerance or withdrawal) or without physiologic dependence (no evidence of withdrawal or tolerance).

The criteria for alcohol abuse do not include tolerance, withdrawal, or a pattern of compulsive use. The individual exhibits one or more of the following symptoms within a 12-month period:

1. Recurrent drinking of alcohol resulting in a failure to fulfill major role obligations at work, school, or home
2. Recurrent drinking in situations in which it is physically hazardous
3. Recurrent alcohol-related legal problems
4. Continued use despite having persistent or recurrent social or interpersonal problems caused by alcoholism

As stated earlier, the differentiation between dependence and abuse applies to 11 classes of drugs listed in the DSM-IV. Other substance-related disorders are discussed in Chapter 27.

Effects of Alcohol

Table 26-1 shows a comparison of the blood-alcohol level, approximate amount of beverage for each level, effects of alcohol, and the amount of time it takes alcohol to leave the body (Walker, 1982; Liska, 1981; and Altrocchi, 1980).

Physiologic effects of alcoholism are numerous. Most texts list the effects according to the system involved. The more common effects seen include

1. Gastrointestinal tract complications, such as acute gastritis, pancreatitis, hepatitis, cirrhosis of the liver, esophageal varices, hemorrhoids, and ascites.
2. Cardiovascular system complications, such as portal hypertension, weakened heart muscle, and heart failure. Broken blood vessels in the upper cheeks close to the nose and bloodshot eyes are not uncommon.
3. Respiratory tract complications include respiratory depression and a depressed cough reflex because of the sedative effect of alcohol. The alcoholic person is susceptible to pneumonia and other respiratory infections.
4. Reproductive system complications include prostatitis, interference with voiding, and release of sexual inhibitions. Fetal alcohol syndrome during pregnancy results in abnormalities in the newborn such as heart defects, abnormally shaped heads and limbs, genital defects, and mental retardation.
5. Central nervous system depression, resulting in peripheral neuropathy, interference with nerve conduction, gait changes, and nerve palsies, is frequently seen.

The alcoholic usually has a poor nutritional status, including deficiencies of vitamins A, D, and K. Anemia, an increased susceptibility to infection, bruising tendencies, and bleeding tendencies occur as a result of a decrease in red and white blood cells and abnormal bone marrow functioning.

Two central nervous system disorders associated with the chronic use of alcohol are Korsakoff's psychosis and Wernicke's encephalopathy. *Korsakoff's psychosis*, a form of amnesia often seen in chronic alcoholics, is characterized by a loss of short-term memory and the inability to learn new skills. Clinical symptoms also include disorientation and the use of confabulation. Degenerative changes in the thalamus occur because of a deficiency of B complex vitamins, especially thiamine and B_{12}. *Wernicke's encephalopathy* is an inflammatory, hemorrhagic, degenerative condition of the brain caused by a thiamine deficiency, usually in association with chronic alcoholism. Lesions occur in the

TABLE 26-1 BLOOD-ALCOHOL LEVELS

Blood-Alcohol Level (%)	Approximate Amount of Beverage	Effects of Alcohol	Time Needed for Alcohol to Leave the Body
0.03	1 cocktail, 1 bottle beer, or 5½ oz wine	Slight tension Euphoria Feeling of superiority	2 hr
0.06	2 cocktails, 3 bottles beer, or 11 oz wine	Feeling of warmth and relaxation Decreased mental efficiency Loss of normal inhibitions Loss of some motor coordination	4 hr
0.09	3 cocktails, 5 bottles beer, or 16½ oz wine	Talkative Clumsy Exaggerated behavior	6 hr
0.10	3 to 5 cocktails, 6 to 7 bottles beer, or 20 to 22 oz wine	Legally drunk in most states Impaired motor, mental, and speech activity Decreased feelings of guilt	6 hr

(continued)

499

TABLE 26-1 BLOOD-ALCOHOL LEVELS (Continued)

Blood-Alcohol Level (%)	Approximate Amount of Beverage	Effects of Alcohol	Time Needed for Alcohol to Leave the Body
0.15	5 to 7 cocktails or 26 to 27 oz wine	Gross intoxication Slurred speech Impaired motor coordination	10 hr
0.20	8 cocktails	Angers easily Motor abilities severely impaired Blackout level Unable to recall events	At least 10 or more hrs
0.30	10 cocktails	Stupor likely; possible aggressive behavior Death may occur owing to deep anesthetic effect or paralysis of the respiratory center.	
0.40	13 cocktails	Coma leading to death	
0.60	20 cocktails	Severely impaired breathing and heart rate Death will probably occur	

hypothalamus, mammillary bodies, and tissues surrounding ventricles and aqueducts. Clinical symptoms include double vision, involuntary and rapid eye movements, lack of muscular coordination, and decreased mental function, which may be mild or severe.

The reader is referred to the DSM-IV to obtain information on the 12 alcohol-induced disorders mentioned earlier in the text.

Transcultural Considerations

Andrews and Boyle (1995) discuss the use and abuse of alcohol by adolescents. It is noted that most teenagers have their first alcoholic drink between the ages of 12 and 15 years. Alcohol may serve as an informal rite of passage from childhood to adulthood for African-American teens. Studies indicate that alcohol use among white and Native American males is relatively high compared with consumption by blacks and Asian-American teens. The reason for drinking cited by white, black, and Hispanic adolescents was to relax. Indochinese youths drink to forget.

Carpenito (1995) summarizes drinking habits of various cultures. It is considered to be the number-one health problem in the black community, the primary factor being unemployment. Irish Americans exhibit the highest or near-highest amount of alcohol consumption because of a need for reassurance, to escape psychological burdens, and to repress sexuality and aggression. Mexican Americans celebrate life while drinking alcohol. The very high percentage of alcoholism among Native Americans is, in part, a result of an increased sensitivity to alcohol.

As noted in the DSM-IV, there are wide cultural variations in attitudes toward alcohol consumption, patterns of use, and accessibility of alcohol. Some groups forbid the use of alcohol, whereas drinking alcohol may be widely accepted in other cultures. Such factors must be considered during the assessment process.

Assessment

Two screening tests are frequently used during the assessment process: the Michigan Alcohol Screening Test (MAST) and the CAGE Screening Test for Alcoholism (Boxes 26-1 and 26-2).

Five or more points on the MAST indicates the presence of alcoholism. Four points suggests a potential problem with alcohol. Three or fewer points indicate the individual does not have a problem with alcohol.

A positive response to one question in the CAGE questionnaire indicates the individual has a potential problem with alcoholism. Two affirmative responses correctly identifies 75% of persons with an alcohol problem.

BOX 26-1	Michigan Alcohol Screening Test (MAST)

Points	Questions
(0)	1. Do you enjoy a drink now and then?
(2)	2. Do you feel you are a normal drinker?*
(2)	3. Have you ever awakened the morning after some drinking the night before and found that you could not remember a part of the evening before?
(1)	4. Does your spouse (or parents) ever worry or complain about your drinking?
(2)	5. Can you stop drinking without a struggle after one or two drinks?*
(1)	6. Do you ever feel bad about your drinking?
(2)	7. Do friends and relatives think you are a normal drinker?*
(0)	8. Do you ever try to limit your drinking to certain times of the day or to certain places?
(2)	9. Are you always able to stop drinking when you want to?*
(4)†	10. Have you ever attended a meeting of Alcoholics Anonymous (AA)?
(1)	11. Have you gotten into fights when drinking?
(2)	12. Has drinking ever created problems with you and your spouse?
(2)	13. Has your spouse (or other family member) ever gone to anyone for help about your drinking?
(2)	14. Have you ever lost friends or girl- or boyfriends because of drinking?
(2)	15. Have you ever gotten into trouble at work because of drinking?
(2)	16. Have you ever lost a job because of drinking?
(2)	17. Have you ever neglected your obligations, your family, or your work for two or more days because you were drinking?
(1)	18. Do you ever drink before noon?
(2)	19. Have you ever been told you have liver trouble? Cirrhosis?
(2)	20. Have you ever had delirium tremens (DTs), severe shaking, heard voices, or seen things that were not there after heavy drinking?
(4)	21. Have you ever gone to anyone for help about your drinking?
(4)	22. Have you ever been in a hospital because of drinking?
(0)	23. a. Have you ever been a patient in a psychiatric hospital or on a psychiatric ward of a general hospital?

BOX 26-1 Michigan Alcohol Screening Test (MAST) (Continued)

(2)†	b. Was drinking part of the problem that resulted in hospitalization?
(0)	24. a. Have you ever been seen at a psychiatric or mental health clinic, or gone to any doctor, social worker, or clergyman for help with an emotional problem?
(2)†	b. Was drinking part of the problem?
(2)	25. Have you ever been arrested, even for a few hours, because of drunk behavior?
(2)	26. Have you ever been arrested for drunk driving after drinking?

*Negative responses are indicative of alcoholism.

†Positive response would be diagnostic of alcoholism.

A total of 4 or more points is presumptive evidence of alcoholism, while a 5-point total would make it extremely unlikely that the individual was not alcoholic. However, a positive response to 10, 23, or 24 would be diagnostic; a positive response indicates alcoholism.

From Gallant, D. S. (1982). *Alcohol and drug abuse curriculum guide for psychiatric faculty* (pp. 53–54). Rockville, MD: National Institute on Alcohol Abuse and Alcoholism.

The nurse uses the interview process to obtain additional data from the patient, including the patient's interpretation of the drinking problem and attitude toward control of the problem. Information regarding the person's level of sensorium and general physical condition is pertinent. Is the patient inebriated, undergoing withdrawal, dehydrated, malnourished, or in any physical distress? Information regarding available support systems is also important at this time.

BOX 26-2 CAGE Screening Test for Alcoholism

1. Have you ever felt you ought to **C**ut down on your drinking?
2. Have people **A**nnoyed you by criticizing your drinking?
3. Have you ever felt bad or **G**uilty about your drinking?
4. Have you ever had a drink first thing in the morning to steady your nerves or get rid of a hangover (**E**ye-opener)?

From Ewing, J. A. (1984). Detecting alcoholism: The CAGE questionnaire. *Journal of the American Medical Association, 252,* 1905–1907.

Riggin (1996) mentions two frequently used assessment instruments in clinical settings with individuals who have a problem with alcohol dependence or abuse: the Diagnostic Interview Schedule (DIS), which contains an alcohol dependence subscale, and the Addiction Severity Index (ASI), designed to assess alcohol and drug use as well as the medical, psychological, and legal complications of use within the family, employment, and social settings.

Diagnostic laboratory tests include liver function tests and the mean corpuscular volume, which, when elevated, are indicators of heavy alcohol use. Other tests may be ordered depending on the physical condition of the patient or complaints verbalized during the assessment process (*e.g.*, blood alcohol level or urine screen for alcohol).

A neurologic evaluation may be requested as well as a psychiatric consult to rule out coexisting psychiatric disorders such as depression, delirium, dementia, or anxiety.

 ## Treatment Including Nursing Interventions

"Few, if any patient groups present . . . with treatment options as puzzling as do alcoholics. The settings in which such patients are treated vary greatly, as do the professional backgrounds of the care givers" (American Psychiatric Association, 1989, p. 1063).

It has been estimated that approximately 25% of individuals entering an alcoholic treatment program have a major preexisting psychiatric disorder such as schizophrenia or affective disorder. In such instances, the individual is given a dual disorder diagnosis, and treatment also focuses on the psychiatric disorder. Eighteen million U.S. alcoholics cannot be ignored. The pain of their alcoholism must be treated. The three general steps in the difficult treatment of alcoholism according to Liska (1981) are

1. Managing acute episodes of intoxication to save life and to overcome the immediate effects of excess alcohol
2. Correcting the chronic health problems associated with alcoholism
3. Changing the long-term behavior of alcoholic persons so that destructive drinking habits are not continued

A chronic state of intoxication requires a "drying-out" period, such as withdrawal or detoxification, before treatment can begin. During withdrawal, various symptoms may develop within 12 to 48 hours after abrupt cessation of alcoholic intake. Some patients may experience withdrawal symptoms three to four days after they quit drinking. Such symptoms may last 48 hours or longer.

The first stage of withdrawal, also referred to as the tremulous stage or the shakes, is characterized by psychomotor hyperactivity with tremors, headache, elevated blood pressure, nausea, loss of appetite, nervousness, flushed face, and agitation. This stage can last 36 hours to several days and may progress to the second stage of acute hallucinosis. During this second stage, the person experiences the symptoms of stage one as well as visual, auditory, or tactile hallucinations. Such hallucinations usually disappear in a day or two, but may last several months. The most severe stage, stage three or the DTs, occurs within one to seven days after the person's last drink and may last up to 72 hours. Relapses can occur. Symptoms include tremors; hallucinations; disorientation in person, time, and place; elevated temperature; profuse diaphoresis; severe agitation; tachycardia; delirium; and convulsions, or grand mal seizures.

Treatment protocols vary during the withdrawal or detoxification period according to the physiologic status of the patient. For example, if liver enzymes are elevated or liver damage is suspected, benzodiazepine therapy is considered to be a safe and effective protocol. There is a 5% risk of mortality in patients with severe alcohol withdrawal symptoms. Patients who have medically complicated or severe alcoholic withdrawal must be treated in a hospital as they may require intravenous barbiturates to control extreme agitation. Risperdal or Haldol may be necessary to control symptoms of delirium. Close observation may

CLINICAL EXAMPLE 26-1
Chronic Alcoholism

AK, a 54-year-old accountant, was admitted to the general hospital with symptoms of acute abdominal pain, hematemesis, and generalized edema. A thorough physical evaluation, including a neurologic examination, revealed peripheral neuropathy, an enlarged liver, hemorrhoids, ascites, and several ecchymotic areas in his upper and lower extremities. During the admitting interview, AK admitted to drinking "a six-pack or two" of beer nightly to relax after a stressful day at work. He further stated he had been drinking "on and off since his early 20s" but was always "able to handle his drinking." When asked whether he felt his drinking was affecting his health, AK stated that he did not think he was an alcoholic, just a "social drinker." Further testing revealed that AK was malnourished and anemic, and had portal hypertension from cirrhosis of the liver. When AK's attending physician suggested that he seek counseling or the support of a group such as Alcoholics Anonymous, AK denied that he had a serious drinking problem. Approximately six months after his discharge from the hospital, AK was readmitted with the diagnosis of hepatic coma due to chronic alcoholism. He died the following day.

be required because these agents tend to reduce seizure threshold, potentiate orthostatic hypotension and sedation, and produce anticholinergic adverse effects (Antai-Otong, 1995).

Patients may require fluid and electrolyte replacement because of severe dehydration and malnourishment. Cardiac status may need to be monitored. Laboratory tests may need to be repeated because of abnormal values. Computed tomography scan and electroencephalography may be ordered to rule out metabolic encephalopathy or coexisting neurologic disorders.

An example of a nursing diagnosis and goal-related nursing interventions for the patient undergoing symptoms of alcohol withdrawal is given in Nursing Care Plan 26-1.

Once the patient has undergone withdrawal or detoxification, he or she must learn to "stay dry in a drinking world." This is not an easy task because recovery is a long-term or lifelong struggle. Sobriety is maintained on a day-to-day basis and depends on the client's ability to recognize and change those living patterns that trigger drinking behavior. Treatment and rehabilitation often break down once the patient returns to the outside world, in which alcohol is a major part of the life-style.

During hospitalization, after withdrawal, the individualized care plan should focus on the following goals:

1. Increasing factual knowledge about alcoholism
2. Fostering interdependence on people, rather than dependence on alcohol
3. Encouraging the person to participate in self-determination by identifying personal strengths
4. Encouraging the patient to reestablish broken relationships
5. Encouraging the alcoholic patient to accept her or his own humanity
6. Allowing the person to grieve over the loss of alcohol
7. Fostering change in or modification of the person's life-style, which has contributed to drinking
8. Encouraging development of alternative approaches to coping with stressors

Various types of supportive care are available to the alcoholic person to assist her or him in meeting the goals just described. They include individual or group psychotherapy, family therapy, aversion therapy, Alcoholics Anonymous (AA), halfway houses, and industrial programs. Individual psychotherapy generally approaches the use of alcohol as a method of defending oneself from stress, frustration, or guilt feelings, and explores the patient's use of denial, hostility, and feelings of depression. Group therapy is a more effective type of support for the alcoholic patient, providing the opportunity for human interaction and discussion of commonly shared problems. Providing the patient with the teaching

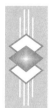

NURSING CARE PLAN 26-1

The Patient Experiencing Alcohol Withdrawal Symptoms

Nursing Diagnosis: *Sensory perceptual alterations: visual hallucinations and illusions secondary to alcohol withdrawal

Goal: The patient will demonstrate absence of visual hallucinations and illusions by the end of the withdrawal period.

Nursing Interventions	Outcome Criteria
	Within 24 to 48 hours the patient will begin to do the following:
Provide a calm, quiet, protective environment, avoiding loud noises, abrupt movements, and dimly lit rooms because shadows increase the likelihood of visual hallucinations and illusions, and may increase the patient's fears.	Verbalize feeling safe and comfortable in the present environment
Display a calm, empathetic, and pleasant attitude. Be readily available when the patient's behavior indicates a need for support.	Describe the presence of any visual hallucinations or illusions she or he experiences
Reinforce reality by referring to the patient's actual surroundings during conversation.	Demonstrate orientation to person, place, and time
Reassure the patient that hallucinations will cease once withdrawal is completed.	Verbalize insight into the cause of hallucinations and illusions
Administer prescribed anticonvulsant or sedative medication when necessary. Explain rationale for medication.	Demonstrate an understanding of the rationale for the use of specified medication during the withdrawal process

*NANDA-approved nursing diagnosis.

checklist (on p.508) will help the nurse assess the patient's knowledge of his or her disease as well as the supportive care available.

Family therapy serves many purposes, such as understanding the alcoholic's ability to arouse anger or provoke loss of temper and to create anxiety within the family unit. Helping the family to gain knowledge about alcoholism and put the knowledge into effect may also occur during family therapy, because problem-solving guidance and direction are available.

The concept of codependency, or living in the shadow of another person's chemical dependency, is usually addressed in family or marital therapy. The codependent becomes so involved with the family member's drinking problem that the codependent's needs and desires are ignored. As a result, the codependent

═══════════ PATIENT TEACHING CHECKLIST ═══════════
Alcoholism

The following checklist has been developed to reinforce your knowledge about alcoholism. Please inform the nurse if you are uncertain about any of the items listed below.

✔ The reasons I may desire to drink alcohol include:
✔ Coping skills I have developed to avoid drinking alcohol include:
✔ The role of a sponsor is:
✔ Other support persons I may contact include:
✔ Adequate nutrition is necessary because:
✔ Laboratory tests may be ordered because:
✔ The name of the medication I am taking is:
✔ Instructions regarding this medication
  ▪ Take this medication as directed by your doctor
  ▪ Do not drink alcohol while taking this medication
  ▪ Do not take any over-the-counter medication without informing your nurse or doctor
  ▪ Side effects or adverse reactions may occur if alcohol is consumed while taking this medication
  ▪ Report any side effects promptly
  ▪ Do not discontinue taking this medication without first consulting your nurse or doctor

may allow abusive behavior to continue even when it is dangerous. Codependent behavior impedes recovery.

Aversion therapy consists of giving a drug such as emetine and then following it with alcohol. Nausea and vomiting are induced by the emetine, causing an aversion to alcohol based on the reflex association between alcohol and vomiting. Disulfiram (Antabuse) interferes with the breakdown of alcohol, causing an accumulation of acetaldehyde, a by-product of alcohol, in the body. The person who takes Antabuse and drinks alcohol experiences severe nausea and vomiting, hypotension, headaches, rapid pulse and respirations, flushed face, and bloodshot eyes. This reaction lasts as long as there is alcohol in the blood. Persons with serious heart disease, diabetes, epilepsy, liver impairment, or mental illness should not take Antabuse.

Naltrexone (ReVia) is a new drug recently approved for use in the treatment of alcoholism. It is considered to be approximately 50% effective in reducing craving and blocking the reinforcing effects of alcohol. It is contraindicated in patients with hepatitis or liver failure and those who have recently taken opioid drugs. Additional research is indicated to determine long-term effects of the drug.

Alcoholics Anonymous is a self-help group that emphasizes both group and individual treatment approaches. Meetings are devoted to testimonials and discussions of the problems that arise from drinking alcohol. Through mutual help and reassurance, the alcoholic gains a new sense of confidence and more successful coping abilities. AA promotes maturity as its members assume increasingly greater responsibility. It also helps members to gain a new self-concept and willingness to accept assistance.

Halfway houses provide group living in a structured environment for recovering alcoholic patients who need a "home away from home" or who have no home. Comprehensive industrial programs for alcoholic employees have been developed in an effort to save corporations an estimated 10 billion dollars per year. Employee assistance programs include in-house alcohol counseling and AA programs.

Other services available to families of alcoholics include Al-Anon family groups and Al-Ateen. Al-Anon family groups help members to understand and assist the alcoholic person, whereas Al-Ateen tries to help children understand their parents' drinking problems and find mutual support in a group situation. The young members learn that their situations are not unique, and they cease to feel alone.

✿ Summary

Alcoholism, a major health problem in the United States, affects approximately 18 million people and is considered by AA to be a physical condition with a mental obsession. The etiology of alcoholism was described. The *13 Steps to Alcoholism*, by the National Council on Alcoholism, were discussed, citing the early danger signs of alcoholism, the middle stages of alcoholism, and the late stages of alcoholism, or compulsive drinking. The DSM-IV diagnostic criteria for alcohol dependence and abuse were listed. The more common physiologic and behavioral effects of alcoholism were stated. The symptoms of withdrawal or detoxification after alcohol intoxication were described by stages: 1) the first stage, also referred to as the tremulous stage; 2) the second stage, characterized by hallucinations; and 3) the third stage, also known as delirium tremens or DTs. Transcultural considerations were discussed. Screening tests frequently used during the assessment process were described. The role of the nurse during withdrawal or detoxification was explained. Treatment protocols were stated. Nursing interventions were listed, focusing of goals, supportive care for the individual as well as the family, and aversion therapy. The concept of codependency was explained. A clinical example of chronic alcoholism was given. An example of nursing diagnosis and goal-related nursing interventions for the patient experiencing alcohol withdrawal symptoms was cited.

Learning Activities

I. Clinical Activities
   A. Care for a patient with the diagnosis of alcohol dependence or abuse.
   B. Describe the patient's symptoms.
   C. Does the patient exhibit any insight into his or her problem?
   D. Does the patient express a desire to be helped?
   E. Develop a nursing care plan for this patient.
   F. Discuss supportive care for the patient after discharge.
II. Independent Activities
   A. Attend an AA meeting or visit a local chapter of Al-Ateen.
   B. Obtain information about the presence or absence of industrial alcohol programs in your community.
   C. Review the *13 Steps to Alcoholism* by the National Council on Alcoholism. Discuss appropriate nursing interventions for each step to impede progress toward compulsive drinking.

Critical Thinking Questions

1. Prepare a genogram of an alcoholic's family. What patterns do you find? What conclusions can you make about alcoholism as a disease?
2. Attend an AA, Al-Anon or Al-Ateen meeting in your community. What kinds of appropriate and inappropriate coping skills did you see? What kinds of group tasks did you observe?
3. Many alcoholics are admitted to clinical facilities for medical problems, where their alcoholism goes unnoticed. Using what you know about patient assessment and alcoholism, how might you reword questions or gather information to uncover alcoholism?

Self-Test

1. State the diagnostic criteria for
      Alcohol abuse
      Alcohol dependence
2. Explain the causative factors of alcohol abuse in teenagers.
3. Describe the following:
      The early stages of alcoholism
      The middle stages of alcoholism
      The late stages of alcoholism
4. State the blood-alcohol level with which one is considered legally drunk in most states.

5. List the more common physiologic effects of alcoholism in the
   Gastrointestinal tract
   Cardiovascular system
   Respiratory tract
   Reproductive system
   Central nervous system
6. Describe the nutritional status of a chronic alcoholic.
7. State behavioral patterns generally seen during alcoholism.
8. Describe the stages of alcohol withdrawal or detoxification.
9. Discuss supportive care available to alcoholics.
10. Differentiate between aversion therapy and Antabuse therapy.
11. Explain the rationale for the use of the following tests:
    MAST
    CAGE

SELECTED REFERENCES

Altrocchi, J. (1980). *Abnormal behavior*. New York: Harcourt Brace Jovanovich.

American Psychiatric Association. (1994). *Diagnostic and statistical manual of mental disorders* (4th ed.). Washington, DC: Author.

American Psychiatric Association. (1989). *Treatment of psychiatric disorders: A task force report of the American Psychiatric Association*. Washington, DC: Author.

Andrews, M. M., & Boyle, J. S. (1995). *Transcultural concepts in nursing care* (2nd ed.). Philadelphia: J. B. Lippincott.

Antai-Otong, D. (1995, August). Helping the alcoholic patient recover. *American Journal of Nursing*.

Carpenito, L. J. (1995). *Nursing diagnosis: Application to clinical practice* (6th ed.). Philadelphia: J. B. Lippincott.

Daniels, J. L. (1996, August). Chemical dependence in the elderly. *Advance for Nurse Practitioners*.

Gerchufsky, M. (1996, November). Alcoholism: Making screening part of your routine. *Advance for Nurse Practitioners*.

Guohua, L., Smith, G. S., & Baker, S. P. (1994, September). Drinking behavior in relation to cause of death among U.S. adults. *American Journal of Public Health*.

Jellinek, E. M. (1960). *The disease concept of alcoholism*. New Haven, CT: Hills-House Press.

Liska, K. (1981). *Drugs and the human body: With implications for society*. New York: Macmillian.

Merrill, M., Kraft, P. G., Gordon, M., Holmes, M., & Walker, B. (1990). *Chemically dependent older adults: How do we treat them?* Center City, MN: Hazelden Foundation.

National Council on Alcoholism. (1975). *13 steps to alcoholism: Which steps are you on?* New York: Author.

O'Neil, A. (1995, September). Identifying alcohol dependence in women. *Advance for Nurse Practitioners*.

Riggin, O. Z. (1996). The client who is addicted to alcohol. In S. Lego (Ed.). *Psychiatric nursing: A comprehensive reference* (2nd ed.). Philadelphia: Lippincott–Raven Publishers.

Schultz, J. M., & Videbeck, S. D. (1994). *Manual of psychiatric nursing care plans* (4th ed.). Philadelphia: J. B. Lippincott.

U. S. Public Health Service. (1994, September). Alcohol and other drug abuse in adolescents. *American Family Physician*.

Walker, J. I. (1982). *Everybody's guide to emotional well-being*. San Francisco: Harbor Publishing.

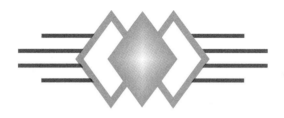

CHAPTER 27

INEFFECTIVE INDIVIDUAL COPING: PSYCHOACTIVE SUBSTANCE ABUSE

A ddiction is a person problem, not a chemical problem . . . use is determined by the experience the drug creates for the user.

American Psychiatric Association,
Treatments of Psychiatric Disorders, 1989

1   Discuss the causative factors associated with psychoactive substance abuse and dependence.

2   Define the following terminology:

Addiction

Psychological dependence

Tolerance

Physical dependence

3   Discuss why individuals abuse or become dependent on sedatives, narcotics, amphetamines, cannabis or marijuana, hallucinogens, inhalants, or nicotine.

4   Describe the common medical problems associated with psychoactive substance abuse.

5   Discuss treatment measures, including nursing interventions, for acute drug intoxication and detoxification.

6   State examples of nursing diagnoses related to individuals who exhibit clinical symptoms of psychoactive substance abuse or dependence.

7   List services available to persons who abuse drugs.

8   Develop a nursing care plan, including short- and long-term goals, for an individual experiencing withdrawal because of substance abuse.

✿ Introduction

According to the 1990 statistics provided by the National Institute of Mental Health, approximately 2.4 million citizens of the United States (1.3% of the population) admitted to abusing psychoactive drugs. In 1987, the American Nurses Association estimated that 6% to 8% of nurses used alcohol or other drugs to an extent sufficient to impair their professional performance. In 1995, the Institute of Medicine estimated that 5.5 million Americans required treatment for substance abuse.

The use of drugs, as noted, has increased in recent years. About 33% of the U.S. population, 70.4 million Americans, have experimented with illegal drugs. Among the most frequently abused drugs are marijuana and cocaine. Marijuana is often used in combination with other addictive substances, such as alcohol or nicotine. Cocaine is consistently used by approximately 6 million Americans

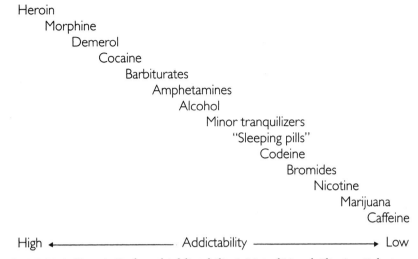

FIGURE 27-1 Mann's "Index of Addictability": List of Mood-Altering Substances Arranged According to the Potential Each Has for Causing Addiction

(Pfizer, Inc., 1996). According to articles published by the news media, heroin has begun to make a comeback in a more pure form, putting users at risk for medical complications and death due to overdose.

Figure 27-1 represents a list of mood-changers categorized by George Mann, M.D., of The Johnson Institute in Minneapolis, Minnesota, and referred to as "The Index of Addictability." It indicates the higher degrees of addictability from top to bottom (*i.e.*, heroin at the top has a high potential for addiction, whereas caffeine at the bottom has a low potential for addiction).

◈ Etiology of Drug Abuse or Dependence

Five theories regarding the etiology of psychoactive substance abuse or dependence are described in *Treatments of Psychiatric Disorders* (American Psychiatric Association, 1989). They focus on immature or deficient personalities, disruptive environment, adaptive difficulties, peer pressure, and inability to cope with stress or tension. Information cited in literature also states that sociologic factors, personality type, and availability of drugs contribute to psychoactive substance abuse or dependence. A discussion of each of these factors follows:

1. *Sociologic factors.* The whole socializing process of adolescence seems to contribute to drug abuse. Peers and their values are particularly strong influences. Experimentation, curiosity, rebellion, and boredom are just a few reasons

cited by adolescents when asked why they use or abuse drugs. Pot (marijuana) parties make marijuana readily accessible to adolescents. Marijuana, cocaine, and heroin frequently are dispensed at adult social gatherings.

2. *Personality type.* Although a particular addictive personality has not been identified, many theorists consider drug abusers to be fixed at an oral or infantile level of development. Such a person searches for immediate gratification of needs or ways to escape tension, and turns to drugs to experience feelings of euphoria or oblivion. Characteristics frequently seen in persons who abuse drugs include low self-esteem, feelings of dependency, low tolerance for frustration and anxiety, antisocial behavior, and fear. Theorists are not certain whether these characteristics were present before the addictive behavior or whether the characteristics are a result of substance abuse.

3. *Availability of drugs.* Over-the-counter drugs; prescriptions readily obtained for sleeplessness, nervousness, anxiety, and pain relief; and medication offered on an as-needed basis during hospitalization—all are factors that make drug abuse easy. For example, EW, a 52-year-old executive, was admitted to the general hospital with symptoms of peptic ulcer disease. During the initial intake interview, the nurse asked EW to list any medication he was taking. She was surprised to find that he was taking Librax, Valium, Seconal, and Percocet. EW had seen three different doctors before being hospitalized and was given the prescriptions to treat symptoms of a peptic ulcer, hiatal hernia, acute low back pain, and insomnia. None of the physicians questioned EW about previous prescriptions, and he did not volunteer any information because he was "afraid the doctors wouldn't give me medication for my abdominal and low back pain and sleeplessness."

 ## Classification of Substance Use Disorders

Various terms are used to describe persons who use and abuse drugs, although the DSM-IV clearly refers to substance abuse and substance dependence (described in Chapter 26). *Addiction* is a term used to define a state of chronic or recurrent intoxication and is characterized by psychological and physical dependence, and tolerance. Psychological dependence or habituation implies an emotional dependence on a drug, or desire or compulsion to continue taking a drug. Tolerance refers to the person's ability to obtain a desired effect from a specific dose of a drug. For example, as a person develops a tolerance for 10 mg of Valium, she or he increases the dose to 15 mg or 20 mg to obtain the effects originally experienced when taking 10 mg of Valium. Physical dependence is manifested by the appearance of withdrawal symptoms after the person stops taking a specific drug.

Ten classes of substances are associated with both abuse and dependence: nicotine; caffeine; sedatives, hypnotics, or anxiolytics; opioids; amphetamines or similarly acting sympathomimetics; cannabis; cocaine; hallucinogens; inhalants;

and phencyclidine. A diagnosis of multiple substance or polysubstance abuse occurs when people mix drugs and alcohol. The severity of psychoactive substance dependence is classified according to the following criteria: mild, moderate, severe, in partial remission, or in full remission.

This chapter focuses on disorders related to the use of sedatives, hypnotics, anxiolytics, opioids, amphetamines, and cannabis (marijuana). The diagnostic criteria for substance dependence and substance abuse were presented in the previous chapter, which focused on alcoholism. A summary of other categories such as hallucinogens, inhalants, and nicotine is included.

Sedative-, Hypnotic-, or Anxiolytic-related Disorders

Substances included in this category are benzodiazepines, carbamates, barbiturates, barbiturate-like hypnotics, all prescription sleeping medications, and all anxiolytic medications except the nonbenzodiazepine antianxiety agents, such as BusPar. The ingestion of these drugs in high doses can be lethal, especially when mixed with alcohol.

The DSM-IV describes the subclassifications of dependence, abuse, intoxication, withdrawal, intoxication delirium, withdrawal delirium, persisting dementia, persisting amnestic disorder, psychotic disorder with delusions or hallucinations, mood or anxiety disorder, sexual dysfunction, or sleep disorder induced by sedatives, hypnotics or anxiolytics. Specifiers include with physiologic dependence or without physiologic dependence.

These drugs are used to relax the central nervous system or slow down body processes. They temporarily ease tension and induce sleep. Medically, they may be used in the treatment of hypertension, peptic ulcers, or epilepsy; as a relaxant before and during surgery; and as a sedative for use in mental and physical illness.

Normal effects of these drugs include a decrease in cardiac and respiratory rate; a lowered blood pressure; and a mild depressant action on nerves, skeletal muscles, and the heart. Overdoses may include symptoms such as slurred speech, drowsiness, drunken appearance, staggering gait, quick temper, quarrelsome disposition, and death. Street names include "libs," "blues," "rainbows," "yellowjackets," and "downers."

Barbiturates are the leading cause of accidental poisoning, as well as a primary method of committing suicide. Barbiturate dependency is one of the most difficult disorders to cure. Withdrawal can cause severe discomfort, accompanied by tonic–clonic convulsions, mental confusion, psychotic delirium, hallucinations, fever, exhaustion, and death.

Opioid-related Disorders

According to the DSM-IV, the opioids include natural opioids such as morphine, semisynthetics such as heroin, and synthetics with morphine-like action such as codeine or methadone. Medications such as Talwin and

Buprenex that have both opiate agonist and antagonist effects are also included in this classification.

Opiates are narcotic drugs that relieve pain, often induce sleep, suppress coughing, and alleviate pain. People abuse opiates by taking them orally, inhaling them, or injecting them into their veins in an attempt to help relieve withdrawal symptoms, for "kicks," or to "feel good." The user becomes passive and listless as the opiates depress the respiratory center of the brain, causing shallow respirations. The person also experiences reduced feelings of hunger, thirst, pain, and sexual desire. As the effects of the drug wear off, the abuser, who becomes physically and emotionally addicted by requiring increasingly larger dosages, suffers withdrawal symptoms unless another dose of the drug is taken.

Opiates, also referred to as "white stuff," "hard stuff," and "junk," are considered to be the most addictive drugs. Acute overdose is identified by symptoms of decreased, slow respirations; constricted pupils; and a rapid, weak pulse.

Opiate withdrawal symptoms begin within 12 to 16 hours after the last dose and are characterized by watery eyes, rhinitis, yawning, sneezing, and diaphoresis. Other symptoms include dilated pupils, restlessness and tremors, goose bumps, irritability, loss of appetite, muscle cramps, nausea and vomiting, and diarrhea. Symptoms subside within 5 to 10 days if no treatment occurs.

Methadone is used to decrease the severity of withdrawal and as a maintenance narcotic by transferring the person's addiction to methadone, which allows him or her to function better in society. The cure rate among opiate addicts is extremely low, and overdose can be lethal. Experts state that it takes up to five years to cure an opiate addict.

Subclassifications of this disorder include dependence, abuse, intoxication, withdrawal, intoxication delirium, psychotic disorder with delusions or hallucinations, mood disorder, sexual dysfunction, and sleep disorder. The specifiers, with or without physiologic dependence, are used further to describe the disorder.

Amphetamine-related Disorders

Medical indications for the use of amphetamines or amphetamine-like substances include attention deficit disorder with hyperactivity, narcolepsy, weight reduction, and treatment-resistant depression. Dexedrine, Benzedrine, Ritalin, Cylert, and Preludin are examples of such drugs.

Amphetamines (pep pills) are drugs that directly stimulate the central nervous system and create a feeling of alertness and self-confidence in the user. They are also referred to by drug abusers as "wake-ups," "speed," "eye-openers," "copilots," "truck drivers," "uppers," or "bennies."

These drugs are often abused by oral ingestion, injection into veins, smoking, or inhaling increased dosages to obtain an exaggerated effect of the stimulating action. People also take these drugs for kicks, for thrills, or to combat boredom; to stay awake or to allow greater physical effort; or to counteract the effects of alcohol and barbiturates. They are considered to be dangerous because they can drive a user to do things beyond his or her physical limits; they can cause mental fatigue, dizziness, and feelings of fear and confusion; and sudden withdrawal can lead to depression and suicide. The heart and circulatory system also may be damaged as a result of overproduction of adrenalin.

Effects of stimulants on the body include increased heart rate, elevated blood pressure, excitability, tremors of the hands, increased talkativeness, profuse diaphoresis, dry mouth, abnormal heart rhythms, headaches, pallor, diarrhea, and unclear speech. The abuser can develop a psychological dependence on stimulants and may experience delusions, auditory and visual hallucinations, or a drug psychosis that resembles schizophrenia.

Subclassifications of this disorder are the same as those listed for opioid-related disorders. Amphetamine-induced anxiety disorder may also occur.

Cannabis-related Disorders

Marijuana is the most widely used illegal drug. It is often used in combination with other addictive substances such as alcohol or nicotine. Most users in the 18- to 25-year age range are male. Many people who try marijuana go on to use it extensively, and many of those people eventually use other drugs, such as cocaine (Pfizer, Inc., 1996).

Marijuana is a common plant with the biologic name of *Cannabis sativa*. It can act as a stimulant or depressant and is often considered to be a mild hallucinogen with some sedative properties. Researchers are studying its possible antiemetic effect on persons with AIDS and those receiving chemotherapy. Its use as an anticonvulsant or antidepressant is also being researched. Studies have indicated that it may lower pressure in the eyeball, making it effective in the treatment of glaucoma.

Persons who abuse marijuana usually smoke it in a pipe or as a rolled cigarette ("joint") but also may take it orally as capsules or tablets, on sugar cubes, or in food. Holders ("roach clips") are used to get the last puffs from marijuana butts once they become too short to handle with fingers. Slang names for marijuana include pot, herb, grass, weed, smoke, and Mary Jane.

Marijuana acts quickly, in about 15 minutes, once it enters the bloodstream, and the effects last approximately two to four hours. It affects a person's mood, thinking, behavior, and judgment in different ways, and in large doses it may cause hallucinations. General physiologic symptoms include increased appetite, lowered body temperature, depression, drowsiness, unsteady gait, inability to think clearly, excitement, reduced coordination and reflexes, and impaired judgment. Users of large amounts may feel suicidal or have delusions of invulnerability, causing them to take chances.

Although marijuana is not physically addicting, it may lead to psychological dependence, thereby retarding personality growth and adjustment to adulthood. Its use also can expose the user to those using and pushing stronger drugs.

Reasons for using marijuana include "getting high," "escape," "to have greater personal insights," "make life more meaningful," and "expanding one's mind."

The following differential diagnoses are included in the DSM-IV: cannabis dependence, abuse, intoxication, intoxication with delirium, cannabis-induced psychotic disorder with delusions or hallucinations, and cannabis-induced anxiety disorder.

Other Classifications of Drugs

Other categories of frequently abused substances are hallucinogens, phencyclidine hydrochloride (PCP), inhalants, caffeine, and nicotine. Hallucinogens and PCP are associated only with abuse because physiologic dependence has not been demonstrated. They are referred to as "mind benders" or psychedelic drugs, affecting the mind and causing changes in perception and consciousness. Examples include lysergic acid diethylamide (LSD), mescaline, dimethyl-tryptamine (DMT), 2,5 dimethoxy-4-methylamphetamine (STP), and psilocybin. Similar to marijuana, but stronger in effect on the body, hallucinogens are dangerous because they can lead to panic, paranoia, flashbacks, or death. Physiologic symptoms can include an increased pulse rate, blood pressure, and temperature; dilated pupils; tremors of hands and feet; cold, sweaty palms; flushed face or pallor; irregular respirations; and nausea. Effects on the central nervous system include an increased distortion of senses, loss of the ability to separate fact from fantasy, loss of sense of time, ambivalence, and the inability to reason logically.

Hallucinogens are quite unpredictable. One experience ("trip") with them may be good but the next may be disastrous. The daughter of television personality Art Linkletter leaped from her apartment in a suicidal panic brought on by LSD. Diane had an exciting career, loving family, good health, and no material worries. According to her father, no explanation could be found for her tragic death except the fact that she had taken LSD.

PCP, commonly known as "angel dust," is an extremely dangerous hallucinogen. Originally used as a surgical anesthetic, PCP was found to cause extreme agitation, stupor, hallucinations, and psychosis. Persons who experience PCP intoxication have enormous strength, experience unbelievably paranoid reactions, and literally do not know pain. They may become violent, destructive, and confused after one dose. Medical complications of PCP include vomiting, seizures, and extremely high blood pressure.

Inhalants are any chemicals that give off fumes or vapors and, when inhaled, produce symptoms similar to intoxication. The person who inhales or sniffs such substances may become confused or excited, or experience hallucinations. After such a "high," the person may experience a loss of coordination, a distorted perception of reality, and hallucinations and convulsions.

Dangers of inhaling gasoline, glue, or paint thinners include temporary blindness and damage to the lungs, brain, and liver. Deaths have occurred as a result of suffocation caused by placing a plastic bag, moistened cloth, or plastic container against one's face. Commonly abused inhalants include glue, gasoline, lighter fluid, paint thinner, varnish, shellac, nail polish remover, and aerosol-packaged products.

Caffeine is available in a variety of sources such as coffee, soda, tea, over-the-counter analgesics and cold remedies, stimulants, and weight-loss aids. Some individuals display clinical symptoms of dependence, tolerance, and withdrawal when consuming large amounts of caffeine. These symptoms include restlessness, nervousness, excitement, insomnia, flushed face, diuresis, gastrointestinal disturbance, muscle twitching, rambling flow of thought or speech, tachycardia or arrhythmia, periods of inexhaustibility, and psychomotor agitation.

Nicotine, the active ingredient in tobacco, is a stimulant that elevates one's blood pressure and increases one's heartbeat. Tar, found in the smoke, contains many carcinogens. Long-term effects of tobacco dependence include emphysema, chronic bronchitis, coronary heart disease, and a variety of cancers.

Approximately 28% of adult women and 30% of adult men smoke cigarettes for stimulation, to relax or feel better, or from habit. Regular smokers become psychologically dependent on cigarettes and find it difficult to stop smoking. Tobacco dependence usually begins in late adolescence or by early adult life and may result in tobacco withdrawal when the person attempts to stop smoking. Symptoms of withdrawal include a craving for tobacco, irritability, difficulty concentrating, restlessness, anxiety, headache, drowsiness, and gastrointestinal disturbances.

Riggin (1996) discusses the abuse of designer drugs and steroids. Designer drugs are manufactured in clandestine laboratories and are then made available on the street. They are described as potent reinforcers and addictive, usually taken intravenously or snorted. Steroids are abused by athletes and adolescent men to enhance masculine appearance or by both men and women to maximize physical development. Adverse behavioral effects as well as medical complications may result.

Medical Treatment of Psychoactive Substance Abuse

Several medical problems are associated with substance abuse. They include

1. Malnutrition with vitamin deficiencies
2. Fluid and electrolyte imbalance
3. Constipation

4. Amenorrhea
5. Respiratory infections
6. Skin abscesses
7. Cellulitis
8. Dental caries and loss of teeth
9. Impotence
10. Hepatic dysfunction
11. Bacterial endocarditis
12. Thrombophlebitis
13. Pulmonary embolism
14. Seizures

Treatment measures for various types of substance use disorders focus on medical care of acute intoxication, chronic intoxication, detoxification, and withdrawal as well as prevention of medical complications.

Medical treatment protocols vary; however, the generic treatment includes a physical examination, use of diagnostic aids such as blood or urine drug levels, a neurologic evaluation when indicated, and use of medication to avoid seizures or hypertensive crisis. If delirium occurs, low dosages of phenothiazines may be used. Gastric lavage may be necessary. Ascorbic acid may be given to enhance excretion of the drug through acidification of the urine. Diazepam may be used to decrease anxiety, to reduce the possibility of seizures, or to provide skeletal muscle relaxation (Bernstein, 1988).

Detoxification is not necessary when treating persons who abuse marijuana, amphetamines, or cocaine. Individuals who abuse hallucinogens may require three months of neuroleptic maintenance therapy to avoid the risk of recurrent symptoms. Methadone or clonidine is used to detoxify individuals who abuse opiates and synthetics. Abrupt discontinuation of sedatives may be fatal owing to status epilepticus, hyperthermia, or possible intravascular coagulation disorder. Detoxification uses gradually diminishing dosage of drugs such as phenobarbital based on a phenobarbital tolerance test. Long-term use of low doses of sedatives may produce discomfort when drug use is stopped. Patients require careful observation, but may not require detoxification (Bernstein, 1988).

The following treatment principles of substance abuse should be considered by health care professionals when providing initial care:

1. Treat a patient symptomatically if the drug is unidentifiable.
2. Do not accept at face value what a patient tells you if clinical symptoms are contrary.
3. Use pharmacologic antagonists sparingly.

4. Intoxicated persons should not be sent to jail or left unobserved or unattended.
5. Do not administer phenothiazines if a seizure disorder or respiratory distress is suspected.
6. Gastric lavage should not be performed if the patient has ingested petroleum products and is alert.
7. Do not use gastric lavage if the patient appears psychotic and if a drug such as LSD or mescaline has been ingested approximately two hours or more before admission.

Services available for individuals who require treatment for substance abuse include

Individual psychotherapy
Group therapy
Family therapy
Encounter groups
Parent support groups
Recreational therapy
Occupational therapy
Short-term residential rehabilitation (3 months)
Longer-term therapeutic community (6 to 18 months)
Day treatment center
Reentry programs
Outpatient and aftercare treatment

 Assessment

The individual who abuses substances presents a variety of challenges because of fear, dependency needs, feelings of insecurity, low self-esteem, the inability to cope, a low tolerance for frustration or anxiety, rebellion, or boredom. Persons who self-prescribe medication frequently do not admit readily to substance abuse. Defense mechanisms such as rationalization, projection, and repression commonly are used by persons who abuse substances.

During the assessment process, which may occur in the emergency room, general hospital, psychiatric unit, or drug treatment center, questions should be directed toward identifying the name of drug(s) used, amount and frequency of use, duration of use, and route of administration. Assessment should also focus on history of suicidal ideation or attempts; withdrawal symptoms, including hallucinations, confusion, tremors, seizures, and the like; longest drug-free period; and desire for treatment.

It is imperative that the nurse be able to recognize symptoms of drug over-dose or drug withdrawal during the assessment process. Each drug reacts differently and is identified in part by behavioral and physical manifestations. Assessment measures therefore should focus on obtaining baseline data and monitoring vital signs; observing for signs of central nervous system depression, such as irregular respirations or lowered blood pressure; recognizing signs of impending seizures or coma; assessing the person for cuts, bruises, infection, or needle tracks; assessing general nutritional status; determining the patient's level of sensorium; listening to physiologic complaints; and observing behavioral symptoms. If it is a crisis situation, data collection focuses on whatever is essential for immediate care. In a less acute situation, information gathering provides the basis for developing a care plan.

 ## Nursing Diagnoses and Interventions

Common nursing diagnoses frequently used to plan care for individuals exhibiting symptoms of psychoactive substance abuse include *risk for injury, depression, *anxiety, *sleep pattern disturbance, *altered nutrition, possible *fluid volume deficit, *altered health maintenance, *noncompliance, *ineffective individual coping, and *risk for violence.

Attitudes of nursing personnel can influence the quality of care given to persons who abuse drugs. Nurses may view patients who overdose on drugs with disapproval, intolerance, moralistic condemnation, or anger, or they may not display any emotional reaction. They need to display an accepting, nonjudgmental attitude while coping with various behaviors such as manipulation, noncompliance, aggression, or hostility. Nursing personnel need to be aware of the various signs and symptoms of abused drugs if they are to administer appropriate nursing care.

Nursing interventions also include providing medical relief for symptoms such as nausea, vomiting, skin bruises, fluid and electrolyte imbalance, and withdrawal symptoms. Patient education can be presented once the individual's condition stabilizes.

Schultz and Dark (1990) list several goals for persons during drug withdrawal. Summarized, the goals state the patient will

1. Remain drug free
2. Verbalize decreased feelings of fear and anxiety
3. Experience a safe environment

*NANDA-approved nursing diagnosis.

4. Experience minimal discomfort during the withdrawal process
5. Demonstrate decreased clinical symptoms of confusion, delusions, or environmental misperceptions
6. Demonstrate compliance

Long-term or discharge goals cited by Schultz and Dark indicate the individual will

1. Continue to abstain from the use of chemicals
2. Agree to participate in a chemical dependency treatment program
3. Demonstrate knowledge of prevention of human immunodeficiency virus transmission
4. Continue to maintain an optimum level of health
5. Demonstrate insight regarding illness and knowledge of recovery process

Nursing Care Plan 27-1 describes a nursing diagnosis and goal-related nursing interventions for an individual diagnosed with multiple substance abuse.

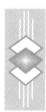

NURSING CARE PLAN 27-1
The Patient with Multiple Substance Abuse

Nursing Diagnosis: *Ineffective individual coping related to multiple substance abuse

Goal: Before discharge, the patient will state alternative coping skills or strategies to avoid the use of drugs.

Nursing Interventions	Outcome Criteria
	Within 48 to 72 hours the patient will be able to do the following:
Establish rapport	Demonstrate trust
Initiate one-to-one relationship	Respond appropriately to questions
	Express feelings openly
Assist patient in identifying positive coping skills	Identify stressors contributing to substance abuse
	Explore alternative coping skills to deal with identified stressors
Teach problem-solving and decision-making skills	Demonstrate knowledge of problem solving and decision making

*NANDA-approved nursing diagnosis.

Summary

The problem of drug abuse has become a national crisis in the United States. Frequently abused drugs include marijuana, sedatives, hypnotics, amphetamines, barbiturates, and cocaine. Several causes of drug abuse or dependence were cited, including sociologic factors, personality type, and the availability of drugs. The DSM-IV classifications of drugs associated with both abuse and dependence were discussed, including anxiolytics; sedatives or hypnotics; opiates or narcotics; amphetamines and related stimulants; cannabis or marijuana; hallucinogens; PCP; inhalants; and nicotine. Reasons for use of drugs, routes of administration, symptoms of physical or psychological dependence, effects of the drugs on the body, and examples of street names were given. Common medical problems associated with drug abuse were stated. Treatment measures were explained. Treatment principles were listed, as well as services for persons who require treatment for substance abuse. Attitudes of persons caring for people who abuse drugs were explored. Assessment measures, nursing diagnoses, and nursing interventions were discussed. Goals for persons during withdrawal, as well as recovery from drug addiction, were listed.

Learning Activities

I. Clinical Activities
   A. Care for a patient with a history of substance abuse or dependence.
   B. Evaluate the patient's treatment plan.
   C. Does the patient display insight into the problem?
   D. Does the patient express the desire to be helped?
   E. Is the patient cooperative?
   F. Should the patient be in another hospital or treatment program?
   G. Are the patient's plans for the future realistic?
   H. Discuss supportive care for the patient after discharge.
II. Independent Activities
   A. Discuss how the following possible symptoms may be related to substance abuse:
      1. Change in school or work attendance or performance
      2. Alteration of personal appearance
      3. Sudden mood or attitude changes
      4. Withdrawal from family contacts
      5. Withdrawal from responsibility
      6. Unusual patterns of behavior
      7. Unresponsiveness to environmental stimuli
   B. Research your local newspaper for a week, paying specific attention to articles on substance abuse.
      1. What drugs are frequently listed, if any?

2. What age group of people is involved?

3. Describe the circumstances in the articles pertaining to substance abuse (*e.g.*, a crime, abuse, auto accident).

C. Contact your state's board of professional regulation to ascertain what program(s) are available for impaired nurses.

Critical Thinking Questions

1. Professional nurses are not exempt from substance abuse; in fact, many communities have support groups for recovering nurses. Research the available services for impaired nurses at your hospital and in the community. Explore the behaviors and personality traits of the impaired nurse. What assessment parameters might assist the profession quickly to identify and help these nurses?

2. One only needs to turn on a television or read a newspaper to realize that drug abuse is a major social, economic, and political problem in this country. What actions might a community mental health nurse take to create an awareness among children in her community? What actions might a hospital-based nurse take?

3. While removing your patient's basin from his bedside cabinet, you notice a packet of pills in the far corner of the cabinet. What should you do?

Self-Test

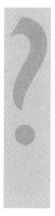

1. Describe the "Index of Addictability."
2. Describe how the following contribute to drug abuse or dependence:
   Sociologic factors
   Personality type
3. Define tolerance.
4. Match the following:

   (1) Amphetamines   (a) Can be a stimulant or depressant; mild hallucinogen

   (2) Opioids   (b) Fumes or vapors producing mild intoxication

   (3) Cannabis   (c) Relaxes central nervous system and slows down the body processes

   (4) Inhalants   (d) Narcotic drugs to relieve pain or induce sleep

   (5) Barbiturates   (e) Stimulates the central nervous system

5. State the more common medical problems of substance abuse.
6. List supportive care available to persons who abuse drugs.
7. Discuss short-term goals during drug withdrawal.
8. State the long-term or discharge goals for the patient.

SELECTED REFERENCES

Allen, K. M. (1996). *Nursing care of the addicted client*. Philadelphia: Lippincott–Raven Publishers.

American Psychiatric Association. (1994). *Diagnostic and statistical manual of mental disorders* (4th ed.). Washington, DC: Author.

American Psychiatric Association. (1989). *Treatments of psychiatric disorders: A task force report of the American Psychiatric Association*. Washington, DC: American Psychiatric Press.

Bernstein, J. G. (1988). *Handbook of drug therapy in psychiatry* (2nd ed.). Littleton, CT: PSG Publishing.

Carpenito, L. J. (1995). *Nursing diagnosis: Application to clinical practice* (6th ed.). Philadelphia: J. B. Lippincott.

Compton, P. (1989, March). Drug use: A self-care deficit. *Journal of Psychosocial Nursing and Mental Health Services*.

Hughes, T. L., & Smith, L. L. (1994, September). Is your colleague chemically dependent? *American Journal of Nursing*.

Jeffries, K. (1988, January). Abuse: A nurse's journey out of a nightmare. *Journal of Christian Nursing*.

McCaffery, M., & Ferrell, B. R. (1994, August). Understanding opioids & addiction. *Nursing '94*.

McCormick, M. (1989). *Designer drug abuse*. New York: Watts, Franklin.

Navarra, T. (1995, January). Enabling behavior: The tender trap. *American Journal of Nursing*.

Pfizer, Inc. (1996, March/April). Understanding psychiatric disorders: What is substance abuse? *Clinical Advances in the Treatment of Psychiatric Disorders*.

Riggin, O. Z. (1996). The client who is abusing substances other than alcohol. In S. Lego (Ed.). *Psychiatric nursing: A comprehensive reference* (2nd ed.). Philadelphia: Lippincott–Raven Publishers.

Schultz, J., & Dark, S. (1990). *Manual of psychiatric nursing care plans* (3rd ed.). Boston: Little, Brown.

Schultz, J. M., & Videbeck, S. D. (1994). *Manual of psychiatric nursing care plans* (4th ed.). Philadelphia: J. B. Lippincott.

Shame and addiction (video). Santa Barbara, CA: FMS Productions.

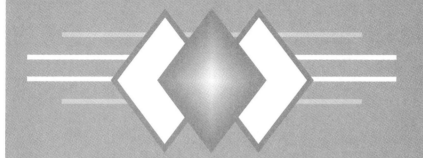

Relational
Problems

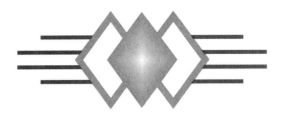

CHAPTER 28

CHILD ABUSE AND NEGLECT

1   Identify risk factors that create an environment for abuse of a child to occur.

2   Differentiate between child abuse and neglect.

3   State at least three possible causative factors in child neglect.

4   Describe the three categories of childhood sexual abuse.

5   State at least five common physical findings indicating physical abuse of a child.

6   Discuss the multidisciplinary treatment approach to child abuse.

7   List community support services available to help prevent the repetition of abuse.

8   Discuss the steps in reporting child abuse or neglect.

9   Develop a nursing care plan for a victim of child abuse.

Introduction

The DSM-IV lists relational problems as a category to describe patterns of interaction between or among members of a relational unit that are associated with clinically significant impairment in functioning. The problems are included because they are frequently a focus of clinical attention identified by health professionals.

Child abuse has become increasingly frequent since the onset of the industrial revolution. Terms used to describe child abuse include *battered child syndrome* and *nonaccidental injury to children*. Barker (1983) states that the cause of child abuse is complex and can occur at three levels: (1) in the home, where the abusers are parents or parent substitutes; (2) in the institutional setting, such as day-care centers, child-care agencies, schools, welfare departments, correctional settings, and residential centers; and (3) in society, which allows children to live in poverty or be denied the basic necessities of life.

Every day, more than three children die in the United States as the result of abuse or neglect. Clinicians who routinely provide care for children will see an average of four to six victims of abuse and neglect each year. More than 2.4 million cases of suspected child abuse and neglect are reported yearly to state child protective services agencies in the United States (Berkowitz, 1992).

Defining Child Abuse and Neglect

Numerous factors are involved in defining child abuse and neglect. They include cultural and ethnic backgrounds, attitudes concerning parenting, social factors, and environmental or circumstantial factors. Abuse is considered an act of commission in which intentional physical, mental, or emotional harm is inflicted on a child by a parent or other person. It may include repeated injuries or unexplained cuts, bruises, fractures, burns, or scars; harsh punishment; or sexual abuse or exploitation. Abuse is not to be confused with discipline. Discipline is a purposeful action to restrain or correct a child's behavior. It is done to teach, not punish, and it is not designed to hurt the child or result in injury. Neglect is an act of omission and refers to a parent's or other person's failure to (1) meet a dependent's basic needs such as proper food, clothing, shelter, medical care, schooling, or attention; (2) provide safe living conditions; (3) provide physical or emotional care; or (4) provide supervision, thus leaving the child unattended or abandoning him or her.

Causes of Abuse and Neglect: Risk Factors

Anyone can neglect or abuse a child under certain circumstances, such as stress due to illness, marital problems, financial difficulties, or parent–child conflict. Parents or other persons may lose control of their feelings of anger or frustration and direct such feelings toward a child.

Three elements that generally create the environment for an incident of abuse to occur include the abuser, the abused, and a crisis. The abuser is usually a parent or caretaker. Many abusers have a history of having been brought up in very strict families and being abused themselves. Abusive parents usually are young; pick a mate who is indifferent, passive, or of little help to them; keep to themselves; and move from place to place. In general, they display a poor self-concept, immaturity, fear of authority, lack of skills to meet their own emotional needs, belief in harsh physical discipline, fear of spoiling a child, poor impulse control, and unreasonable expectations for a child. The mate, who usually knows about the abuse, either ignores it or may even participate in it. The abused or neglected child victim is usually younger than six years of age, is more vulnerable to abuse than others, and may have a physical or mental handicap. Emotionally disturbed, temperamental, hyperactive, or adopted children also demonstrate a higher incidence of abuse. The child may irritate the parent to the point of loss of control or may provoke abuse while attempting to get attention. A crisis (*e.g.*, loss of job, divorce, illness, or death in the family) is usually the precipitating factor that sets the abusive parent in motion. The parent overreacts because he or she is unable to cope with numerous or complex stressors, becomes frustrated and anxious, and suddenly loses control, abusing the child.

Other Characteristics of Potentially Abusive or Neglectful Parents

Characteristics of potentially abusive or neglectful parents are warning signals but do not mean that abuse or neglect will inevitably occur. They are often present in high-risk families and may be noticeable before the birth of a child. Such characteristics (described following), displayed for a short period of time, may indicate the result of anxiety in a new mother or father; however, if they persist, the parent should seek help.

The profile of abusive or neglectful parents of a soon-to-be born or newborn child include

1. Denial of a pregnancy by a mother who has made no plans for the birth of the child and refuses to talk about the pregnancy
2. Depression during pregnancy
3. Fear of delivery
4. Lack of support from husband or family
5. Undue concern about the unborn child's sex and how well it will perform
6. Fear that the child will be one of too many children
7. Giving birth to an unwanted child
8. Resentment toward the child by a jealous parent
9. Indifference or a negative attitude toward the child by the parent after delivery
10. Inability to tolerate the child's crying, viewing child as being too demanding

There are no physical characteristics that automatically identify the potential child abuser. The person may be rich or poor, of any racial origin, male or female, and living in a rural area, the suburbs, or a city.

Transcultural Considerations

Family income, ethnicity, region of residence, and type of metropolitan area are all associated with risk of victimization, according to a national survey (Finkelhor & Leatherman, 1994). Hispanic and black children, those living in Mountain and Pacific states, and those from large cities were at greater risk for victimization. Black youths had elevated rates for sexual assault and kidnapping, whereas low-income children had high rates of family assault and general violence. Approximately 6.2 million youths participated in this national survey.

Skuse and Bentovim (1994) believe cross-cultural variability in child-rearing beliefs and behavior is so great that it would be difficult, although probably not impossible, to define a framework of acceptable child-rearing practices that would be universally applicable.

Areas of Child Abuse or Neglect

Maltreatment of children usually falls into the following general areas: (1) physical abuse, (2) neglect, (3) emotional maltreatment, and (4) sexual abuse.

Physical, behavioral, and environmental indicators often afford clues to a child's needs and treatment by parents. They are discussed in reference to each of the four general areas of maltreatment.

Physical Abuse

The most common physical indicators seen in child abuse are bruises in which there is no breakage of the skin. They are usually seen on the posterior side of the body or on the face, in unusual patterns or clusters, and in various stages of healing, making it difficult to determine the exact age of a bruise. Burns are also frequently seen and usually are due to immersion in hot water, contact with cigarettes, tying with a rope, or the application of a hot iron. Areas of the body where burns are seen include the buttocks, palms of hands, soles of feet, wrists, ankles, or genitals. Lacerations, abrasions, welts, and scars may be noted on the lips, eyes, face, and external genitalia. Other physical indicators include missing or loosened teeth; skeletal injuries such as fractured bones, epiphyseal separation, or stiff, swollen, enlarged joints; head injuries; and internal injuries. Such physical injuries should be considered with respect to the child's medical history, developmental ability to injure self, and behavioral indicators.

Behavioral indicators of physical abuse depend on the age at which the child is abused, as well as the frequency and the severity of abuse. The behavioral profile of a physically abused child includes

1. Fear of parents as well as fear of physical contact with adults
2. Extremes in behavior such as passivity or aggressiveness, or crying very often or very seldom
3. Sudden onset of regressive behavior such as thumb sucking, enuresis, or encopresis
4. Learning problems that cannot be diagnosed
5. Truancy from school or tardiness
6. Fatigue causing the child to sleep in class
7. Inappropriate dress to hide burns, bruises, or other marks of abuse
8. Inappropriate dress, resulting in frostbite or illness due to exposure to inclement weather

9. Overly compliant to avoid confrontation
10. Sporadic temper tantrums
11. Hurting other children
12. Demanding behavior

If such behaviors are present in a child, she or he should be observed for physical injuries.

Münchausen syndrome by proxy is now a well known phenomenon in which the parent, almost invariably the mother, fabricates illness in her child or children and presents the problem to doctors. The child is usually persistently brought for medical examinations, yet acute symptoms and the signs of illness cease when the child is separated from the parent, who denies having any knowledge of the etiology of the disorder. Comorbidity is a major problem because it is highly likely that the child will have more than one fabricated illness. Failure to thrive and nonaccidental injuries are also commonly associated. Forms of fabricated illnesses include poisonings, seizures, apparent bleeding from a variety of orifices, skin rashes, and pyrexia (Skuse & Bentovim, 1994).

The "shaken baby syndrome" is a sometimes fatal form of abuse that typically occurs when an adult loses control and violently shakes a child who has been crying incessantly. The physical findings usually include major head injury. Bruising occurs from being grabbed firmly. Physical findings may include subdural hematoma, cerebral edema, or retinal hemorrhage (Brasseur, 1995).

Environmental indicators of increased likelihood for physical abuse in children include severe parental problems such as drug addiction, alcoholism, and mental illness; family crisis; and geographic or social isolation of the family.

Child Abuse: Examples Parents of an eight-month-old girl hired two babysitters, ages 14 and 12 years, to watch their daughter while they celebrated their wedding anniversary. The young sitters physically abused the child by tossing her back and forth in a game of catch and suspended her from a ceiling light fixture, allowing her to fall on the floor. She sustained several internal injuries and was hospitalized in serious condition. The babysitters were charged with delinquency, and the parents were found guilty of child abuse and neglect by placing her in the care of two minors.

In another case of child abuse, a man was accused of beating his girlfriend's five-year-old daughter severely enough to cause permanent brain damage. The child was beaten with a stick and forced to drink dishwashing liquid because she was "too sassy." After the beating, the child was kept on the floor of the apartment because she appeared to be unconscious at times. The mother force-fed her daughter oatmeal and bananas in an effort to revive her. Two days later the child was taken to the hospital and was found to have burn marks on her buttocks, a head injury, and bruises on her body. The mother was charged with child abuse, and the boyfriend was sentenced to 15 years in prison for aggravated child abuse.

Neglect

As stated earlier, neglect is an act of omission and includes abandonment; lack of adequate supervision; and failure to meet the child's basic human needs of shelter, adequate nutrition, good hygiene, adequate clothing, and proper medical or dental care. Financial status, cultural values, and parental capacity should be considered before a parent or adult is accused of neglecting a child.

Behavioral indicators of neglect commonly seen include failure to thrive; learning difficulties due to poor attention span; inability to concentrate, or autistic behavior; use of drugs or alcohol; delinquency; and sexual misconduct.

Neglected children may live in an environment characterized by poverty, come from a large family with marital conflict, lack material resources, or experience indifferent parental attitudes.

Characteristics of neglectful parents include lack of understanding of the child's physical and emotional needs, lack of interest in the child's activities, poor parenting skills, and poor personal hygiene.

Child Neglect: Examples   A fundamentalist mother and father denied medical care to their infant son, resulting in the child's death due to suffocation from pneumonia. The parents, who were convicted of reckless homicide and child neglect, were sentenced to five years in prison.

A second case of child neglect occurred when a young, divorced, working mother entrusted the care of her one- and two-year-old children to her eight-year-old daughter while she worked as a waitress from approximately 7:00 P.M. to midnight. Before she left for work each evening, she locked the younger children in their bedrooms and instructed the older daughter to stay indoors and "keep an eye on the children." One evening a fire began on the second floor of the apartment, killing the two younger children by smoke inhalation. The eight-year-old was able to escape the fire. The mother told the authorities she made minimum wage and was unable to afford to pay a babysitter, so she worked at night while her older daughter was home.

Emotional Maltreatment (Abuse or Neglect)

Emotional maltreatment or psychological abuse may consist of verbal assaults or threats that provoke fear; poor communication that may send double messages; and blaming, confusing, or demeaning messages. Inappropriate discipline, immature parenting, continuous friction or conflict in the home, rejecting parents, discriminatory treatment of the children in the family, and abuse of drugs or alcohol are examples of environmental indicators or pathologic, destructive parenting patterns. Such parents may tell the child that she or he is unwanted, unloved, or unworthy of care. The child may become the scapegoat of the family, that is, accused of causing family problems. "If it weren't for your bad habits, Daddy wouldn't leave us!," "It's all your fault we don't have enough money. You're sick all the time," and "The family got along fine until you started to act so selfish." The child often develops a low self-concept as he or she hears such negative comments and may exhibit behavioral indicators such as

1. Stuttering
2. Enuresis or encopresis
3. Delinquency, truancy, or other disciplinary problems
4. Hypochondriasis
5. Autism or failure to thrive
6. Overeating
7. Childhood depression
8. Suicide attempts

Emotional neglect occurs when parents or other adults responsible for the child fail to provide an emotional climate that fosters feelings of love, belonging, recognition, and an enhanced self-esteem. Examples of emotional neglect include ignoring the child, providing minimal human contact, and failing to provide opportunities to foster growth and development.

Emotional Maltreatment and Sexual Abuse: Example Two brothers, ages five and seven years, were found on several occasions acting as if they were dogs. Their mother stated they would walk and eat like dogs as well as bark and carry objects in their mouths. At times they would drop their heads in their cereal or soup bowls and lap their food like a dog. They had to be reminded continually that they were little boys. When questioned by the police, the young boys stated that their father hooked them to a chain and harness and told them to act like dogs. Their father and other men also performed sexual acts on the boys. The father was sentenced to two years imprisonment.

Sexual Abuse

Sexual abuse is not easy to identify because the physical signs of abuse usually are not seen outside a clinical or medical setting. The child victim is usually reluctant to share information about the abuse because the child fears she or he may alienate or anger the person who provides food, shelter, and a family bond.

Estimates of childhood sexual abuse in the United States range from 100,000 to 500,000 cases per year. An estimated one half of sexually abused children are between 6 and 12 years of age (Gibbons & Vincent, 1994).

Episodes of childhood sexual abuse are classified as acute, subacute, or non-acute. Acute episodes include cases of sexual abuse that have occurred within the previous 72 hours of examination by a clinician. Evidence of moderate to severe injury such as vaginal bleeding or genital lacerations may be present. Subacute episodes involve sexual abuse cases that have occurred more than 72 hours before an examination by a clinician. Symptoms such as minor abrasions or dysuria may be present. Nonacute abuse cases occur more than 72 hours before a clinician's examination. There are no significant injuries or symptoms.

Three terms are frequently used to describe sexual abuse of children: sexual misuse, rape, and incest. Sexual misuse of a child is defined as sexual activity that is inappropriate because of the child's age, development, and role within the family unit. Examples of sexual misuse of a child include fondling, genital manipulation, voyeurism, or exhibitionism.

Rape refers to actual penetration of an orifice of a child's body during sexual activity. Oral penetration is the most frequent type of penetration experienced by very young children.

Incest, or sexual intercourse between family members who are so closely related as to be legally prohibited from marrying one another because of consanguinity, is usually a well guarded secret. Approximately 100,000 cases of incest occur each year, but fewer than 25% are reported, according to the American Psychological Association and the National Center on Child Abuse and Neglect. Victims of incest are usually very young. The average age of an incest victim is 11 years, although most child victims experience their first incestuous encounter between the ages of 5 and 8 years.

Physical indicators of sexual abuse that may be present during an examination include

1. Itching, pain, bruises, or bleeding in the external genitalia, vagina, or anal area
2. Edema of the cervix, vulva, or perineum
3. Torn, stained, or bloody undergarments
4. Stretched hymen at a very young age
5. Presence of semen or of a sexually transmitted disease
6. Pregnancy in an older child
7. Bladder infections

Behavioral indicators or characteristics exhibited by a sexually abused child are quite numerous. The more commonly seen behaviors include

1. Difficulty in walking or sitting
2. Reluctance to participate in recreational or physical activities
3. Poor peer relationships
4. Delinquency, truancy, acting-out, or runaway behavior
5. Preoccupation with sexual organs of self or others (occurs with younger children)

6. Sexual promiscuity or prostitution in older children
7. Change in sleeping patterns, nightmares, or sudden fear of falling asleep
8. Bed wetting or thumb sucking (inappropriate to age)
9. Use of drugs and alcohol
10. Confiding in a friend, a teacher, or the authorities

Environmental indicators or elements common in cases of child sexual abuse are as follows:

1. Overcrowding in the home
2. Prolonged absence of a parent
3. Social or geographic isolation of a family
4. Intergenerational pattern of incest
5. Alcoholism
6. Extremely protective attitude toward the child by a jealous parent who refuses to allow the child to have any social contact, distrusts the child, and accuses the child of sexual promiscuity
7. Marital difficulties
8. Personality disorders in the parents
9. Lack of knowledge of childhood developmental issues

Sexual Abuse: Examples A six-year-old girl, daughter of a well liked and respected member of the community, was forced by her father to have oral sex with him when her mother was away at club meetings. The sexual encounters lasted only a few months but had a profound effect on the young girl, whose parents divorced when she was 14. She loved her father but also hated him and swore that she would never tell anyone about the incest. A few years after she married, her deteriorating sexual relationship with her husband prompted her to admit the incest and to seek therapy.

Another case of sexual abuse involved several children in an unlicensed babysitting service. The owner was arrested for charges of violating his probation from a previous child molestation conviction, filming infants and toddlers during incidents of child abuse, and having oral sex with some of the children under his care. One child was found to have gonorrhea of the throat.

Multidisciplinary Treatment

Treatment of victims of child abuse or neglect is considered to be a multidisciplinary process, frequently beginning with crisis intervention. Members of the treatment team may include doctors, nurses, psychologists, psychiatrists, social workers, teachers, and law enforcement officers. Once child abuse is established, the child welfare agency is responsible for the child's immedi-ate welfare and decides whether to remove the child from his or her natural environment by placing the child in a hospital or foster home. A social worker from the child welfare agency usually investigates the family and recommends whether psychiatric treatment is needed for the child, family, or both. Barker (1983) recommends that a nonpunitive, empathetic approach be used when the parents or responsible adults are questioned about the child's abuse. The helping person or interviewer should not become overinvolved or display anger toward them because such approaches negate the development of a therapeutic relationship. He also recommends temporary removal of abused children from their natural environment, depending on the details of the abuse, during psychiatric evaluation and treatment of the child. Child abuse may result in a serious injury, permanent brain or other physical damage, growth failure, personality or behavioral problems, intellectual retardation, or death.

Support services available in the community to help prevent the repetition of abuse may include the following:

1. Visiting or public health nurses
2. Protective services for children
3. Emergency shelter for children
4. Day-care centers or nurseries
5. Self-help groups such as Parents Anonymous
6. Telephone hot lines
7. Homemaker services
8. Financial assistance such as local welfare department
9. Employment counseling
10. Parent education classes
11. Foster home care
12. Transportation services
13. Counseling
14. Assertiveness training

Nursing Care of Abused Children

Nursing personnel generally respond to child abuse with feelings of shock, anger, rage, or revulsion. People who have abused children anticipate such responses from helping persons and authority figures, thus resisting efforts to involve them in therapy. If the nurse displays negative responses such as frustration, hope-lessness, sadness, or sympathy, she is unable to be objective and to plan compe-tent nursing interventions. Nurses should realize that abusive parents as well as abused children have severe, unmet dependency needs; nurses should accept abusive parents as worthwhile people.

Parents of physically abused children brought to emergency room settings usually give a predictable history of the child's injuries, namely, falling out of bed, against a piece of furniture or household appliance, or down a flight of stairs. They are usually inconsistent in giving details that are nearly always incompatible with the child's injuries. The child may appear guarded or afraid of any physical contact with the examiner or parents while receiving treatment. Victims of sexual abuse usually try to protect the offender and may act in a pseudoadult manner.

Assessment

The assessment process includes a thorough physical and x-ray examination, including inspection of the genitals and anus. Play therapy and art therapy also serve as assessment tools when child abuse is suspected. A mature, patient, empathetic approach should be used, while focusing on physical, behavioral, and environmental indicators of abuse as well as family dynamics. Evidence of malnutrition, dehydration, old fractures, bruises, internal injuries, or intracranial hemorrhage may be present. The child's behavioral characteristics may include withdrawal, low self-esteem, oppositional behavior, compulsive behavior, hypervigilance, or an increased awareness of the environment, and a fearful attitude toward the parents.

The results of the assessment process should be well documented, with particular emphasis on the child's physical status, emotional status, developmental level or stage, interpersonal skills, and behavioral response to the family. Photographs should be taken before medical treatment to document the initial appearance of the injuries.

Nursing Diagnosis

Once the data are analyzed, nursing diagnoses are formulated. Examples of nursing diagnoses commonly seen in victims of child abuse or neglect include *anxiety, *powerlessness, guilt, *altered comfort due to pain from physical abuse, *impaired verbal communication owing to the psychological barrier of fear, *ineffective individual coping because of delayed developmental growth,

*NANDA-approved nursing diagnosis.

self-concept disturbance and potential for less than adequate nutritional requirements due to parental neglect.

Intervention

Nursing intervention may occur in a variety of settings such as in the school, by the school nurse; the home, by the public health nurse; the hospital, by the emergency room or staff nurse; or the doctor's office, by the office nurse.

The hardest task for the nurse is to develop a trusting relationship with the abused child and family. Immediate care should focus on meeting physical and emotional needs to promote homeostasis and comfort, and to reduce fear. Once these needs are met, problems such as impaired verbal communication, ineffective individual coping, ineffective family coping, and disturbance in self-concept can be addressed. Ideally, during this time, intervention also may focus on treating the family as a unit to facilitate a healthy, safe environment for the child later.

Prevention of Child Abuse and Neglect

The nurse may help prevent child abuse by recognizing early signs of abuse, supporting and working for legislation to interrupt the child abuse syndrome, promoting educational courses on family interpersonal relationships and child raising practices, promoting community awareness programs, participating in continuing educational courses, and participating in nursing research of child abuse and effective treatment measures.

In most states, certain professional people are required by law to report suspected child abuse, neglect, or sexual abuse. Even if the law does not require nurses to report such a case, they have an ethical obligation to protect a child from harm. It is not the intent of the law to remove a child from his or her home unless the child is in danger. Parents are not punished unless undue harm has occurred. In most situations, the family is helped so that the parents and child can stay together. Directions on how to report child abuse follow. Such a report may be made by telephone, in person, or in writing to the children's services board of a local welfare department or to the local police department. The nurse should state the following information:

1. Name and address of the suspected victim
2. Child's age
3. Name and address of the child's parent or caretaker
4. Name of the person suspected of abusing or neglecting the child

5. Why abuse or neglect is suspected
6. Any other helpful information
7. Nurse's name, if she or he wishes (Some states require a signature.)

The case will be investigated whether the reporter remains anonymous or gives a name.

 ## Summary

Child abuse can occur at three levels: in the home, in institutional settings, and in society. This chapter discussed the factors contributing to child abuse and neglect; defined abuse, discipline, and neglect; and listed the three elements necessary for abuse to occur. Characteristics of potentially abusive or neglectful parents were stated. The four areas of child abuse or neglect were described and examples of each were given. They include physical abuse, neglect, emotional maltreatment, and sexual abuse. Physical, behavioral, and environmental indicators of child abuse were explored. The multidisciplinary treatment approach was explained, and support services available to abusive families were listed. Nursing care of abused children focused on the nurse's response to an abused child, the assessment process, and prevention of abuse. Information on how to report child abuse was detailed.

Learning Activities

I. Clinical Activities
   A. Care for a victim of physical abuse, neglect, emotional maltreatment, or sexual abuse if possible.
   B. Assess the victim's physical, behavioral, and environmental stressors.
   C. Develop a nursing care plan, stating appropriate diagnoses and interventions.
II. Independent Activities
   A. Obtain data from the local child welfare agency regarding its role and function in child abuse.
   B. Investigate the law on reporting child abuse in the state in which you reside.

Critical Thinking Questions

1. Child abuse and neglect is epidemic in the United States. What might be the role and responsibility of nursing in responding to this crisis?
2. Explore your feelings about child abuse. How might you cope with meeting the parents of a child you are caring for whom you suspect is being abused?

Self-Test

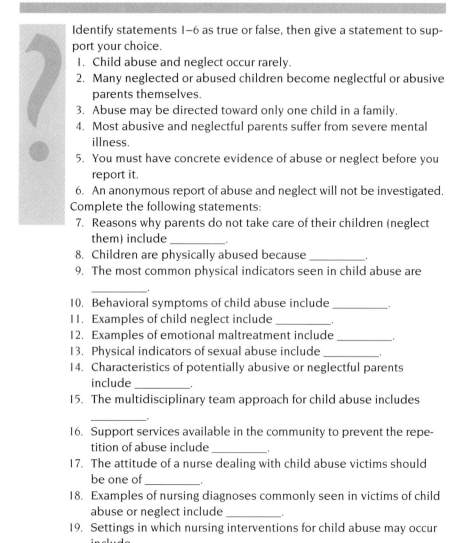

Identify statements 1–6 as true or false, then give a statement to support your choice.

1. Child abuse and neglect occur rarely.
2. Many neglected or abused children become neglectful or abusive parents themselves.
3. Abuse may be directed toward only one child in a family.
4. Most abusive and neglectful parents suffer from severe mental illness.
5. You must have concrete evidence of abuse or neglect before you report it.
6. An anonymous report of abuse and neglect will not be investigated.

Complete the following statements:

7. Reasons why parents do not take care of their children (neglect them) include _____.
8. Children are physically abused because _____.
9. The most common physical indicators seen in child abuse are _____.
10. Behavioral symptoms of child abuse include _____.
11. Examples of child neglect include _____.
12. Examples of emotional maltreatment include _____.
13. Physical indicators of sexual abuse include _____.
14. Characteristics of potentially abusive or neglectful parents include _____.
15. The multidisciplinary team approach for child abuse includes _____.
16. Support services available in the community to prevent the repetition of abuse include _____.
17. The attitude of a nurse dealing with child abuse victims should be one of _____.
18. Examples of nursing diagnoses commonly seen in victims of child abuse or neglect include _____.
19. Settings in which nursing interventions for child abuse may occur include _____.
20. Examples of prevention of child abuse include _____.

SELECTED REFERENCES

American Psychiatric Association. (1994). *Diagnostic and statistical manual of mental disorders* (4th ed.). Washington, DC: Author.

Barker, P. (1983). *Basic child psychiatry* (4th ed.). Baltimore: University Park Press.

Berkowitz, C. D. (1992, January). Child sexual abuse. *Pediatric Review.*

Bowers, J. J. (1992, June). Therapy through art: Facilitating treatment of sexual abuse. *Journal of Psychosocial Nursing and Mental Health Services.*

Brasseur, J. W. (1995, July/August). Child abuse: Identification and intervention. *Clinician Reviews.*

Carpenito, L. J. (1995). *Nursing diagnosis: Application to clinical practice* (6th ed.). Philadelphia: J. B. Lippincott.

Elvik, S. L. (1995, September). Sexual abuse of the developmentally disabled: Recognizing the signs. *Advance for Nurse Practitioners.*

Finkelhor, D., & Leatherman, J. D. (1994, October). Children as victims of violence: A national survey. *Pediatrics.*

Gibbons, M., & Vincent, E. C. (1994, January). Childhood sexual abuse. *American Family Physician.*

Greenfeld, M. (1990, July). Disclosing incest: The relationships that make it possible. *Journal of Psychosocial Nursing and Mental Health Service.*

Kestenbaum, C. J. (1994, November). *Play therapy with young children: Practical strategies.* Presentation at 7th Annual U. S. Psychiatric & Mental Health Congress, Washington, DC.

Murphy, J. L. (1993, October). An overview for school nursing professionals: Child sexual abuse. *Journal of School Nursing.*

Polk-Walker, G. C. (1990, November). What really happened? Incidence and factor assessment of abused children and adolescents. *Journal of Psychosocial Nursing and Mental Health Services.*

Schultz, J. M., & Videbeck, S. D. (1994). *Manual of psychiatric nursing care plans* (4th ed.). Philadelphia: J. B. Lippincott.

Skuse, D., & Bentovim, A. (1994). Physical and emotional maltreatment. In M. Rutter, E. Taylor, & L. Hersov (Eds.). *Child and adolescent psychiatry* (3rd. ed.). London: Blackwell Scientific Publications.

Whitfield, C. L. (1989). *Healing the child within: Discovery and recovery for adult children of dysfunctional families.* Deerfield Beach, FL: Health Communications.

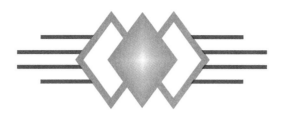

CHAPTER 29

THE ABUSED ADULT
WITHIN THE FAMILY UNIT

A 1994 U.S. Justice Department study showed that 13,000 acts of violence were committed against women at work by their husbands or boyfriends. Nationwide, domestic violence takes its toll on businesses as well as the victims. As much as $10 billion is spent on health care each year treating victims of domestic violence.

U. S. *Justice Department*, 1994

1 Describe causative factors related to abusive behavior.

2 Describe the dynamics of spouse abuse.

3 Explain how elderly persons are abused.

4 Discuss the assessment process of a physically abused person.

5 Describe emotional reactions of individuals who are victims of abuse.

6 List nursing diagnoses frequently used in developing a care plan for a victim of violent behavior.

7 Cite nursing interventions for the following nursing diagnoses of a physically abused person:

   Disturbance in self-concept

   Anxiety due to a physical assault

   Ineffective family coping because of abusive behavior by a spouse

 Introduction

Domestic violence, or abuse within the family unit, is a common occurrence in today's society. A domestic violence victim suffers emotional, psychological, and physical abuse, all of which can result in a variety of health problems. Because of the number of individuals affected, it is essential that health care professionals are taught to recognize and accurately interpret behaviors associated with domestic violence.

National statistics indicate that a woman is battered every 15 seconds in the United States. On a national scope, abuse of women cannot be predicted by demographic features related to age, ethnicity, race, religious denomination, education, socioeconomic status, or class (Makar, 1996).

Family or domestic violence is defined as any act carried out with the intention of, or perceived intention of, physically or psychologically hurting another person. It includes individuals who are emotionally involved, usually spouses or intimate partners, but may also involve children, siblings, and the elderly. Child abuse and neglect were discussed in the previous chapter.

It has been estimated that as many as 25% of women are abused by their partners and 52% of women who are murdered die at the hands of their own partners. As high as 35% of women who seek emergency room treatment have been battered, but only 5% to 10% of these women are identified as victims of domestic violence (Loring & Smith, 1994).

It has also been estimated that approximately one to two million elderly experience some form of mistreatment each year, including physical abuse, verbal abuse, neglect, and material or financial exploitation (Lachs & Pillemer, 1995).

Theories Regarding Abusive Behavior

Physical abuse involves a willful, nonaccidental attempt to injure a person by way of a direct, overtly aggressive attack. Examples of abuse include throwing objects at a family member, threatening to injure, or physically beating the individual. *Men usually push, shove, grab, slap, hit repeatedly, torture, or threaten with a lethal object. Women hit with or throw objects, use fists, kick, bite, or scratch.

Various theories describe the causative factors for abusive behavior toward spouses and elderly parents. The following is a summary of commonly cited theories:

1. The abuser is deprived of nurturing and mothering as a child; therefore, he is unable to nurture others as an adult. Such a person may be a victim of physical or sexual abuse and unable to trust others.
2. The abuser may have a history of antisocial behavior, including drug and alcohol abuse, and is unable to control impulsive behavior owing to frustration or anxiety. Persons often act more violently when they are under the influence of alcohol or drugs.
3. Specific behaviors learned during various developmental stages become part of a person's interactions with spouse and family. For example, a child who lives in an environment in which spouse or parental abuse occurs probably will believe that abuse is normal unless intervention occurs to prohibit such behavior.
4. Poor socioeconomic conditions resulting in increased stress, anxiety, or frustration may precipitate abusive behavior within the family unit.
5. Poor communication skills may result in the use of verbal or physical abuse.
6. Abusive behavior may increase after the death of a significant family member, the loss of a job, a geographic move, the onset of physical or mental illness, a developmental change, or a family change such as pregnancy or the birth of a child.

*Although men are also victims of abuse, victims most commonly are women. In this chapter, the portrayed victims are female.

Abuse by Spouse or Significant Other

The profile of the abused person includes a history of being raised in insecure living conditions, having been abused as a child, and getting married when a teenager. Abused women often exhibit a pattern of learned helplessness as well as characteristics of low self-esteem and shame. They may hold religious or cultural beliefs about the traditional gender roles of men and women.

Spouse abuse takes many forms. In the Duluth, Minnesota, Domestic Abuse Intervention Project (1985), a power and control wheel was developed to serve as a teaching model for counseling groups of batterers. Eight forms of abuse are defined. They include

1. Anger and intimidation in which the individual uses looks, actions, expressions, or a loud voice to intimidate a partner psychologically
2. Isolation or restriction of a partner's freedom by controlling or limiting what she does, who she sees, what she reads, and where she goes
3. Threats and psychological abuse in which the partner may experience humiliation, or fear financial or emotional harm such as blackmail
4. Physical abuse in which the individual attempts physically to hurt or scare the partner
5. Abusing traditional male role as head of household by treating partner as a servant
6. Economic abuse by attempting to make one's partner dependent for money and survival
7. Emotional abuse by making negative statements about one's partner, which results in low self-esteem or self-concept
8. Sexual abuse by compelling one's partner to have sex or perform sexual acts involuntarily

Professional staff, who have worked with and studied men who batter, have made the following observations. Battering men usually have a low self-esteem. They believe that a man should be the head of the household and have the final say in the family decisions. Because of insecurities and fears, the batterers experience extreme jealousy. Growing up in violent homes, they have not developed positive ways to communicate feelings and needs or the ability to compromise. They typically blame everyone and everything but themselves for their actions. Because they do not want to face the seriousness of their behavior and its consequences, denial is a common defense mechanism used by batterers.

Dynamics of Physical Spouse Abuse

Walker (1984) describes three phases of the pattern of spouse abuse: the tension-building phase, the acute beating phase, and the loving phase. Spouse abuse usually occurs as a result of the inability to cope with an increase in daily stressors. During the tension-building phase, disagreements may occur between a couple as the battered person is unable to assert herself and withdraws rather than attempting to display any anger verbally or nonverbally. The spouse becomes possessive, jealous, and fearful as he senses the partner's anger, causing emotional distancing to occur. Such nonassertiveness on the part of the battered person is rationalized by the spouse as acceptance and permission to vent tensions. Minor physical abusive incidents may cause the battered person to cope with abuse by somatizing while the spouse attempts to reduce tension by taking drugs or drinking alcohol, which further decreases inhibitions and precipitates abusive episodes.

During the acute battering phase, the spouse loses control of behavior because of blind rage. The battered person also loses control and is unable to stop the physical abusiveness experienced. Both persons are in a state of shock immediately after the incident. The spouse is unable to recall his behavior; the battered person depersonalizes during the abusive incident and is able to recall in detail what occurred. As both calm down, the spouse may exhibit feelings of remorse, beg forgiveness, promise not to abuse in the future, and state that he

 CLINICAL EXAMPLE 29-1
Family Violence Due to Spouse Abuse

JW, a 43-year-old housewife, was beaten, bruised, and afraid. She stood in her bedroom pointing a pistol at her angry, abusive husband. Both her eyes were swollen, choke marks were on her neck, and bruises were evident on several areas of her body. She killed her husband with the pistol. When questioned by police, she stated that he was totally out of control after drinking beer. His blood alcohol level was 0.236 (A person is considered legally intoxicated if the level is above 0.10.) JW described her husband as a hard worker and good father who was a loving person when he was sober but a totally different person when he was intoxicated. He had beaten her on several occasions in the past six months but never to the point of choking and punching her. In the past, JW's husband would wake up in the morning after physically abusing her and ask "Did I do that?" He would promise such behavior "wouldn't happen again" and she would believe him.

cannot live without the battered partner. During this loving phase, the abused person believes her spouse's promises and forgives him because she then feels less helpless. Such behavior on her part is interpreted by the spouse as an act of love and acceptance. She usually does not take assertive action to stop the abuse because she believes her husband will change; is afraid of more violence; lacks self-confidence; feels trapped; feels guilty, ashamed, embarrassed, helpless, or powerless; is dependent emotionally and financially on her spouse; feels that her child or children need their father; or rationalizes that life is "not so bad."

 ## Abuse of the Elderly

Elder abuse is considered to be a widespread problem. The typical victim is female, 75 years of age or older, dependent on the abuser for basic needs, and mentally or physically impaired. Causative factors eliciting abusive behavior include severe physical or mental disabilities, financial dependency, personality conflicts, societal attitudes toward aging (*e.g.*, considering the elderly person to be a burden), and frustration while caring for an impaired elderly person. Many times, elderly persons are expected to meet the needs of their grown children. These family members may become abusive if the elderly parent is unable to communicate clearly with them or meet their emotional needs.

The abuse of elderly persons can occur in a variety of settings, such as nursing homes, general hospitals, retirement centers, their own homes, or the homes of adults who care for them. Many states have adopted laws similar to child abuse laws to prevent the abuse of the elderly.

Forms and examples of abuse of the elderly are listed in Box 29-1.

Elderly persons may not report abusive behavior because of fear of retaliation by the abuser, fear of rejection, a low self-esteem (whereby they feel they deserve such treatment), loyalty to caretakers, or lack of contact with helping persons.

 ## Assessment of Abused or Assaulted Persons

Clinical assessment by the nurse and attending physician is done to determine if the abused or assaulted victim is in any physical or life-threatening danger due to injuries requiring emergency medical care. The battered person may present multiple bruises or injuries, somatic complaints or symptoms associated with trauma that may not be observable, or characteristic behavioral reactions such as acute anxiety reaction, depression, or suicidal ideation. Determining the

BOX 29-1 Forms of Elder Abuse

Forms	Examples
Physical	Direct beating, slapping, or kicking
	Lack of or withholding food or medical care
	Lack of supervision
	Overmedication
	Withholding life-sustaining medication
Psychological	Verbal assault or threats
	Intentional isolation of the elderly by refusing to transport the person who is unable to leave home unattended.
Violation of rights	Placing the elderly person in a nursing home against his or her wishes when the person is not dangerous to self or others
Material abuse or financial ex- ploitation	Misuse of money or property by children or legal guardians
	Stealing of social security checks, credit cards, property
Neglect	Failure to give medication, food, or personal care; withholding aids such as hearing aids, dentures, or eyeglasses
Other	Allowing the elder to live in unsanitary conditions

emotional status of the victim is imperative. Obtaining a medical history is also important to acquire additional clues to battering and to make a tentative medical, psychological, and nursing diagnosis. The person may describe a history of multiple injuries, psychiatric problems, medical problems, or self-abusive behavior (*e.g.*, alcohol abuse, drug abuse, or suicidal gestures).

Interview questions directed at possible battered persons should be carried out in a supportive and sensitive manner. Inquiries focus on any suspicious-looking injuries; how the injuries occurred; whether the battered person is living with the abuser; the victim's emotional response to the abuser; a safe place for the victim and any children to go such as a shelter; and whether the victim wants to press charges.

Campbell (1986) developed a Danger Assessment Instrument for assessing the potential for homicide. The questions denote risk factors that have been statistically associated with homicides of abused women. They focus on the frequesncy of abuse, type of abuse, presence of lethal weapons in the home, forced sex, use of drugs or alcohol, jealous behavior or violence toward family members by the abuser, and suicidal ideation verbalized by the abused.

Grant (1996) refers to the Migrant Clinicians Network Domestic Violence Assessment Form developed by McFarlane for use in a migrant health center setting. Four questions are posed:

1. Within the last year, have you been hit, slapped, kicked, or otherwise physically hurt by someone? (The perpetrator is then identified, the frequency of abuse noted, and the area of injury is noted on a body map.)
2. If pregnant, since the pregnancy began, have you been hit, slapped, kicked, or otherwise physically hurt by someone? (The frequency of abuse is noted and the area of injury is noted on a body map.)
3. Within the last year, has anyone forced you to have sexual activities? (The perpetrator is then identified and the frequency of abuse is noted.)
4. Are you afraid of your partner or anyone you identified?

During the assessment process, colored photographs are taken to complement the data noted on the body map. Laboratory and diagnostic tests as well x-rays may be ordered. Figure 29-1, the Abuse Assessment Screen, is a similar form developed by the Nursing Research Consortium on Violence and Abuse.

 ## Nursing Interventions

The physician's primary concerns center on immediate care of physical injuries, prevention or alleviation of psychological damage, and proper medical examination.

The nurse's role is to give emergency medical care and to plan appropriate interventions because an acute anxiety reaction may occur after abuse. Crisis intervention skills are used to reduce anxiety and provide supportive care. It is important that arrangements are made for someone to stay with the battered or abused person. If an in-depth formal interview is necessary, the assault victim is informed of her rights and arrangements are made for the story to be told in detail only once so that the victim does not have to relive the incident psychologically by unnecessary repetition.

Other initial nursing interventions after abuse include providing privacy and respecting the right to confidentiality, displaying a nonjudgmental attitude, encouraging verbalization of feelings and thoughts about the assault, explaining the examination process, and assisting with an examination.

1. Have you *ever* been emotionally or physically abused
   by your partner or someone important to you?   Yes ☐ No ☐

2. **WITHIN THE LAST YEAR,**
   have you been hit, slapped, kicked, or otherwise
   physically hurt by someone?   Yes ☐ No ☐

   If YES, by whom? _____
   Total number of times _____

3. Since you've been pregnant, were you hit, slapped,
   kicked, or otherwise physically hurt by someone?   Yes ☐ No ☐

   If YES, by whom? _____
   Total number of times _____

**MARK THE AREA OF INJURY ON THE BODY MAP. SCORE
EACH INCIDENT ACCORDING TO THE FOLLOWING SCALE:**

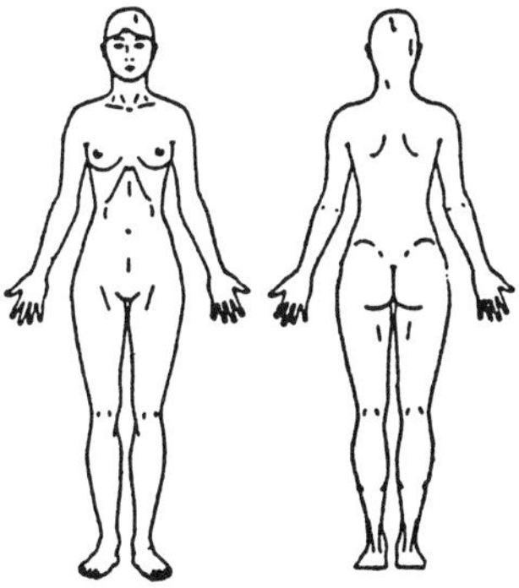

SCORE

1= **Threats of abuse including
   use of a weapon**   _____

2= **Slapping, pushing; no injuries
   and/or lasting pain**   _____

3= **Punching, kicking, bruises,
   cuts and/or continuing pain**   _____

4= **Beating up, severe contusions,
   burns, broken bones**   _____

5= **Head injury, internal injury,
   permanent injury**   _____

6= **Use of weapon; wound
   from weapon**   _____

If any of the descriptions for the higher number apply, use the higher number.

4. **WITHIN THE LAST YEAR,**
   has anyone forced you to have sexual activities?   Yes ☐ No ☐

   If YES, who? _____
   Total number of times _____

5. Are you afraid of your partner or anyone you
   listed above?   Yes ☐ No ☐

Source: Developed by the Nursing Research Consortium on Violence and Abuse.
Readers are encouraged to reproduce and use this assessment tool.

FIGURE 29-1 Abuse Assessment Screen

BOX 29-2 Action Plan to Avert Violence

1. Develop an emergency kit containing money, car keys, medical records, medical cards, important phone numbers, clothing, and copies of pertinent papers to validate identity and eligibility for assistance.
2. Secure access to emergency transportation.
3. Identify a safe place to go.
4. Pack clothing for children.
5. List information about partner's place of employment, including name, address of company, and employer's name.

After the person has been examined and crisis intervention has been used, the abused person may benefit from one or more of the following therapeutic interventions: (1) individual psychotherapy; (2) family or couple therapy; (3) group psychotherapy; (4) temporary emergency housing, such as a shelter for battered persons, hospital, boarding house, or community church facility; (5) emergency financial assistance for food, shelter, or clothing; (6) vocational counseling; (7) legal counseling; and (8) referral to a crisis hotline, self-help group, or social worker. Medication may be prescribed for symptoms of depression, anxiety, insomnia, or agitation, or for the presence of nightmares.

If the abused individual prefers to return home, an action plan is developed in the event that violence recurs. Box 29-2 lists the concrete steps necessary to provide a safe environment.

Older adults may benefit from additional services such as alternative housing, nursing care by the visiting nurse or public health nurse, food from Meals on Wheels, assistance from a visiting homemaker program, visits by persons involved in a foster grandparent program, and transportation for the elderly provided by community organizations.

Nursing Care Plan 29-1 lists examples of nursing diagnoses and goal-related nursing interventions for the abused person.

Summary

Abusive or battering behavior can result in feelings of fear, embarrassment, and humiliation, thus making it one of the most underreported crimes. This chapter discussed physical, psychological, economic, social, and sexual abuse. Theories regarding abusive behavior were summarized. The profile of a victim of spouse abuse was described. The dynamics of physical spouse abuse were explained, followed by an example of family violence due to spouse abuse. Abuse of the elderly person was discussed. Examples of each form were cited. Assessment of abused or assaulted persons was described, including the use of the Danger Assessment Instrument, the Migrant Clinicians Network Domestic Violence Assessment Form, and the Abuse Assessment Screen. Nursing interventions were cited, including the development of an action plan to avert violence. Examples of nursing diagnoses and goal-related nursing interventions were given, focusing on disturbance in self-concept because of severe trauma of physical abuse; anxiety due to actual threat to biologic integrity; and ineffective family coping because of family conflict.

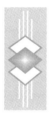

NURSING CARE PLAN 29-1
The Abused Person

Nursing Diagnosis: Disturbance in self-concept related to severe trauma as a result of physical abuse

Goal: The patient will understand the dynamics of low self-concept secondary to physical abuse.

Nursing Interventions	Outcome Criteria
	The patient will do the following:
Establish trust and rapport by encouraging expression of feelings, avoiding negative criticism or judgmental comments, and providing a safe, protective environment.	Verbalize trust Describe feelings
Display acceptance.	Feel accepted
Help patient to identify present strengths and coping skills by using crisis intervention technique.	State present strengths and coping skills
Explain dynamics of abuse.	Verbalize understanding of dynamics of abuse Acknowledge she is not responsible for the abuse she experienced

(continued)

Nursing Diagnosis: *Anxiety related to actual threat to biologic integrity (physical assault)

Goal: The patient will experience less anxiety.

Nursing Interventions	Outcome Criteria
	The patient will do the following:
Identify level of anxiety.	Identify symptoms of anxiety
Decrease environmental stimulation.	Identify stressors or behavior that precipitates symptoms of anxiety
Support present coping mechanisms.	Identify positive coping mechanisms that decrease anxiety
Explore alternative coping mechanisms such as relaxation techniques.	Verbalize a decrease in symptoms of anxiety when using alternative coping mechanisms such as relaxation techniques
Administer prescribed medication as ordered.	Verbalize understanding of actions of antianxiety agents
Educate regarding use of antianxiety agents.	

Nursing Diagnosis: *Ineffective family coping because of family conflict related to violence

Goal: Family will avoid the use of violence by using family discussions to resolve conflict.

Nursing Interventions	Outcome Criteria
	The family members will do the following:
Explore communication skills within the family unit.	Communicate more directly
Teach positive communication skills.	Actively listen to each other
Encourage a realistic perception of the situation.	Verbalize an understanding of misperception
Encourage expression of feelings.	Verbalize feelings without fear of reprisal Verbalize anger in a socially acceptable manner
Encourage family discussion.	Use family discussions to resolve conflict

*NANDA-approved nursing diagnosis.

Learning Activities

I. Clinical Activities
  A. If possible, spend a day of observation in a shelter for abused persons or in an emergency room of a large metropolitan hospital.
  B. Discuss the support systems made available to abused persons at this shelter or in the emergency room.
II. Independent Activities
  A. Obtain a list of community agencies available to abused persons.
  B. Discuss the services provided by each agency.
  C. Contact the National Clearinghouse on Domestic Violence, P.O. Box 2309, Rockville, MD 20852, for additional information on family violence.
  D. Review the daily newspaper for a week and collect data on the types of domestic or family violence reported. Discuss the reported intervention for each case of abuse. Was it appropriate?

Critical Thinking Questions

1. Spend a day at a local women's shelter. Explore your feelings about spouse abuse. What do these women have in common with you? How are they different?
2. Interview a local police officer to ascertain how a domestic violence case is handled. Ascertain his or her understanding of interpersonal dynamics. How does the officer perceive the effectiveness of our legal system in such cases? What role can nursing play?
3. As you perform a physical assessment on 78-year-old Mr. Brass, you notice bruises and tender areas on his upper arms and back. When you question him, he becomes agitated and tells you not to bother about them. You suspect elder abuse. What do you do?

Self-Test

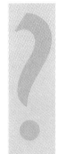

1. Describe abusive or battering behavior.
2. Give examples of
     Psychological abuse
     Social abuse
     Sexual abuse
3. Describe the personality of an abusive person.
4. State the dynamics of spouse abuse.
5. State why an abused spouse may not take assertive action to stop abuse.
6. State why elderly persons may be abused.

7. Cite examples of abuse of elderly persons.
8. State the rationale for clinical assessment of abused or assaulted victims.
9. List nursing interventions for an individual who has experienced severe trauma as a result of spouse abuse.
10. List nursing interventions for an elderly patient who is experiencing anxiety related to an actual threat to biologic integrity.

SELECTED REFERENCES

Berrios, D. C., & Grady, D. (1991). Domestic violence risk factors and outcomes. *Western Journal of Medicine*.

Burgess, A. W., Hartman, C. R., & Grant, C. A. (1991, December). Drawing a connection from victim to victimizer. *Journal of Psychosocial Nursing and Mental Health Services*.

Campbell, J. (1986, August). Nursing assessment for risk of homicide in battered women. *Advances in Nursing Science*.

Carpenito, L. J. (1995). *Nursing diagnosis: Application to clinical practice* (6th ed.). Philadelphia: J. B. Lippincott.

Chez, N. (1994, July). Helping the victim of domestic violence. *American Journal of Nursing*.

Grant, C. A. (1996). The client who has been battered. In S. Lego (Ed.). *Psychiatric nursing: A comprehensive reference* (2nd ed.). Philadelphia: Lippincott–Raven Publishers.

Hinojosa, I. C., & Meagher, T. F. (1996, November). Taking control of violence in the workplace. *Advance for Nurse Practitioners*.

Lachs, M. S., & Pillemer, K. (1995, February). Abuse and neglect of elderly persons. *New England Journal of Medicine*.

Loring, M. T., & Smith, R. W. (1994, March). Health care barriers and interventions for battered women. *Public Health Reports*.

Makar, M. C. (1996). "When violence hits home." Continuing education for Florida nurses. *Continuing Medical Education Resource*.

McFarlane, J., Christoffel, K., Batemen, L., Miller, V., & Bullock, L. (1991, August). Assessing for abuse: Self-report versus nurse interview. *Public Health Nursing*.

Quillian, J. P. (1996, April). Screening for spousal or partner abuse in a community health setting. *Journal of the Academy of Nurse Practitioners*.

Walker, L. (1987, July). Identifying the wife at risk of battering. *Medical Aspects of Human Sexuality*.

Walker, L. E. (1984). *The battered woman syndrome*. New York: Springer Publishing.

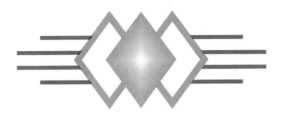

CHAPTER 30

RAPE AND SEXUAL ASSAULT

C hildhood sexual abuse is a significant issue for many adults who receive psychotherapy or other nursing services. Whereas only a small portion of adults who were sexually abused as children manifest severe psychopathology, there are several long-term psychological and behavioral effects that are believed to be related to childhood sexual abuse.

Draucker, 1996

Introduction

Sexual harassment has received extensive publicity within the past four or five years. One much publicized case included attorney Anita Hill, who accused Supreme Court nominee Clarence Thomas of sexually harassing her while they were working together. A second case involved Republican Senator Bob Packwood of Oregon, who allegedly harassed dozens of female employees and associates.

Petrocelli and Repa (1992) define sexual harassment as any unwelcome sexual advance or conduct on the job that creates an intimidating or offensive working environment. Sexual harassment may range from sexual innuendo to coerced sexual relations. Both men and women may be victimized. Davidhizar and Giger (1995) cite various court cases.

Rape is considered to be a universal crime against women: a violent sexual act committed against a woman's will and involving the threat or use of force.

Three essential elements are necessary to define rape legally: (1) the use of force, threat, intimidation, or duress; (2) vaginal, oral, or anal penetration; and (3) nonconsent by the victim. Rape statutes vary from state to state, and in some states a wife may charge her husband with rape. Attempted rape is defined as an assault on a woman in which oral, vaginal, or anal penetration is intended but does not occur. Statutory rape is the act of sexual intercourse with a girl younger than the age of consent (usually 16 years) *with* her consent.

Incest, as described in the chapter on child abuse, is also classified as sexual assault and can occur at any age. Unfortunately, adult survivors of incest do not always seek help at the time of sexual assault, and they may experience clinical symptoms of rape trauma syndrome described in this chapter.

Motives for Rape or Sexual Assault

There is no typical rape victim profile. Every woman is a potential victim regardless of age, race, or socioeconomic status. Men who commit rape are from all walks of life and ethnic backgrounds; often from single-parent homes; young, usually younger than age 25 years; and often married, leading otherwise normal sex lives. Persons at high risk as rape victims include single females between the ages 11 and 25 years who are African American and come from a low socioeconomic background. Although most victims are women, men also experience sexual assaults.*

Elvik (1995) addresses sexual abuse of the developmentally disabled. Individuals with mild developmental delays usually want to be accepted and to fit in with a "normal" society. Such a person may also exhibit some degree of impulsivity or gregariousness that could put him or her at risk for sexual abuse.

Several patterns of rape or sexual assault have been described by theorists according to the motive involved: (1) anger rape, (2) power rape, (3) sadistic rape, and (4) impulsive or opportunistic rape. In the first pattern, anger rape, sex is used as a means of expressing rage, hatred, and contempt toward the victim. The rapist exhibits physical brutality by beating, kicking, or choking while he views the victim as a symbol of those women who wronged him at some point in life. Power rape is generally committed by persons with low self-esteem and a history of poor relationships with women, and is done in an attempt to prove manhood, competency, and strength. The offender forces the victim to become weak, helpless, and submissive, the exact qualities he despises in himself. Sadistic rape occurs because the person feels a need to inflict pain and torment on his victim to achieve sexual satisfaction. He misinterprets the victim's emotional anguish as sexual excitation rather than a refusal of his advances. Bizarre ritualistic behavior may occur during a sadistic rape. Impulsive, opportunistic rape may occur in conjunction with another antisocial act, such as a robbery. A person who is so antisocial takes what he wants whenever he desires it; rape therefore becomes a form of stealing.

Sexual attacks are considered to be one of the following: (1) blitz rape, in which an unexpected surprise attack occurs in the absence of prior interaction with the victim; (2) confidence rape, in which the offender and victim have had a prior interaction; (3) marked victim rape, in which the offender assaults a woman he has been acquainted with in some way; (4) accessory-to-sex rape, which refers to a vulnerable victim's inability to give consent (as in the case of a person who is mentally retarded); and (5) date rape, which refers to the exploitation of an individual's friendliness or behavior during a date.

*Although men can also be victims of sexual assault, victims are most commonly women. In this chapter, the portrayed victims of rape and sexual assault are female.

Emotional Reactions to Rape and Sexual Assault

Rape trauma syndrome is a diagnosis used to describe the result of being raped, including an acute phase of disorganization and a longer phase of reorganization in a victim's life. The DSM-IV recognizes the reaction to rape as a post-traumatic stress disorder. The acute phase of rape trauma occurs when the victim is disrupted by the crisis and displays emotional reactions of anger, guilt, embarrassment, humiliation, denial, shock, disbelief, or fear of death; multiple physical or somatic complaints; or a wish for revenge. After a period of several weeks, the acute-phase reactions give way to deeper, more long-term feelings or reorganization that cause the victim to change daily life patterns, experience recurring dreams and nightmares, seek support from friends and family, initiate or refuse counseling, or develop irrational fears (phobias). One or more of six major phobic reactions may occur: (1) fear of being indoors if the rape occurred in the home; (2) fear of the outdoors if the victim was sexually assaulted outside the home; (3) fear of crowds; (4) fear of being alone; (5) fear of people around the victim while the person engages in daily activities; and (6) fear of sexual activity if the person had no prior sexual experience. Long-term reactions to rape and sexual assault may take several years to resolve, especially if the person goes through legal court action. During this time, the victim may move into a new residence, change the telephone number, change jobs, or move to a new state. If the victim is married, severe marital conflict may occur.

A maladaptive stress reaction referred to as "silent rape syndrome" may occur. The victim fails to disclose information about the rape to anyone, is unable to resolve feelings about the sexual assault, experiences increased anxiety, and may develop a sudden phobic reaction. Behavioral changes may include depression, suicidal behavior, somatization, and acting-out (*e.g.*, alcohol or drug abuse or sexual promiscuity).

 ## Assessment of Victims of Rape or Sexual Assault

Assessment by the nurse, attending physician, or other health care professional is done to determine if any physical or life-threatening danger exists. Emergency medical care may be given while the assessment process occurs if multiple bruises or injuries are present. The abused person may have somatic complaints or symptoms associated with trauma that are not readily observable.

Characteristic behavioral reactions that may be identified during a psychological assessment include an acute anxiety reaction, depression, or suicidal ideation. Other assessment data that should be collected if the patient can be questioned are a history of the rape or attempted rape; legal information, including the names of persons who have been notified, such as the police; what evidence has been preserved; and support persons or systems available to the abused person.

If the victim gives consent and is able to tolerate the procedure, usually a gynecologic examination, pregnancy test if indicated, and laboratory tests are performed after a rape situation. The date of the victim's last menstrual period should be obtained.

Evidence the nurse should be aware of includes the presence of semen, stains, fiber, or hair on clothing or the body; fingernail scrapings; and pieces of torn clothing. If the victim has any of these in her possession or on her body, the evidence or specimens must be saved to be analyzed and documented, according to hospital protocol.

Grant (1996) presents guidelines for interviewing rape victims in crisis. Specific information focuses on demographic data, crisis status, type of assault, services needed or requested, and leading questions to consider. Available services usually include medical, police/legal, shelter, transportation, and counseling. Questions to consider during the interview include "Does she feel the rape was her fault?", "Does she believe in the myths about rape?", and "Which ones and what are their impact on her?". The more common myths and facts about rape are presented in Table 30-1 (on p. 566).

Emotional responses by the victim to rape or sexual assault vary according to the person's developmental level; therefore, the nurse needs to be familiar with developmental stages of the life cycle. Foley (1984) gives excellent examples of reactions to rape according to developmental levels from childhood to older adulthood. Reactions cited include preoccupation with wrong or bad acts during childhood (4–7 years); misperception of rape as a sexual act during latency (7 years to puberty); confusion over normal sexual behavior and concern about pregnancy or venereal disease as an adolescent (puberty to 18 years); concern over credibility, life-style, morality, and character as a young adult (18–24 years); concern over how rape will affect family and life-style during adulthood (25–45 years); and concern over physical safety, fear of death, reputation, and respectability as an older adult (45 years and older).

During the initial assessment process, the nurse may experience strong reactions to the sexual assault, including conflict over who is to blame; anxiety about the possibility of becoming a sexual assault victim herself; anger and

TABLE 30-1 RAPE: MYTHS AND FACTS	
Myth	Fact
Attractive women provoke men into raping them.	Between 70% and 80% of all rapes are violent, planned aggressive acts not based on physical attractiveness or age. Statistics show rape victims range in age from approximately 3 months to over 90 years.
If a woman struggles, rape can be avoided; no woman can be raped against her will.	Rapists frequently overpower smaller and physically weaker women and carry weapons to harm, mutilate, or kill their victims. Counterattack by the victim may cause more injury to occur.
Only women with bad reputations or who are friendly to strangers outside their homes are raped.	All women are potential sexual assault victims. The rapist's desire is control, not sex. Approximately one third to one half of all rapes occur in a victim's home. Rapists include husbands, ex-husbands, neighbors, lovers, and boyfriends.
Women "cry rape" to get revenge.	Rape is an underreported crime owing to feelings of guilt. Approximately 2% of all reported rape cases are false.
Most sexual assaults involve African-American men raping white women.	The rapist and victim tend to be of the same race (intraracial) in most cases of sexual assault.

hostility toward the victim, the rapist, and society for allowing such an act to occur; or a desire to learn more about rape to resolve personal feelings.

Identification of the victim's response to the assault as acute stress reaction, maladaptive stress reaction, or reorganization stress reaction is important because not all rapes are reported immediately after the assault occurs.

 Nursing Intervention

The physician's primary concerns center on immediate care of physical injuries, prevention or alleviation of psychological trauma, and referral for gynecologic, medical, or psychological follow-up. Documentation of the patient's physical and emotional status, and any evidence, including stained clothing, fingernail scrapings, and mouth or anal smears containing semen, are important. Prevention of venereal disease and pregnancy also are concerns of the attending physician. The victim has the right to request medical treatment only and to refuse examination for the collection of legal evidence, so that a consent for examination and treatment is necessary *before* the examination.

The nurse's role is to plan appropriate interventions to help the victim recover from the physical, emotional, social, or sexual disruption that she is experiencing. During the acute stress reaction phase of rape, the nurse uses crisis intervention skills to reduce anxiety and to provide supportive care. It is imperative that arrangements be made for a nurse to stay with the victim. She should be calm and supportive, listen carefully to what the victim has to say, encourage the victim to speak distinctly and clearly when describing the rape incident, and reassure her that the information given will be confidential and handled discreetly. The victim should be treated with respect and dignity while receiving care.

Other interventions after abuse or during the acute stress reaction include providing privacy; displaying a nonjudgmental attitude; explaining the examination process; and, if rape occurred, assisting with a rape examination according to hospital protocol. When preparing the victim for a physical and gynecologic examination, the nurse should find out if the patient has ever been examined. She should arrange for physical comfort by providing, for example, drinks of water to relieve thirst and a place to wash after the initial examination has been completed. It is not unusual for the victim to feel dirty or contaminated.

Treatment of maladaptive stress reactions after rape should include a psychiatric referral once the rape has been discovered to help with the victim's unresolved feelings and reactions resulting in increased psychological distress.

During the reorganization phase of the rape syndrome, nursing interventions vary according to individual needs of the victim, generally focusing on (1) providing a community resource list for medical and legal assistance; (2) providing written information about examinations, test results, or medications for the person to refer to once the state of anxiety decreases following delayed treatment; (3) documenting conversations and observations for possible legal action; and (4) arranging for follow-up medical care and counseling until the patient has recovered.

Patient education includes stating the rationale for medication (*e.g.*, penicillin as a prophylaxis for infection or venereal disease, and the "morning-after pill" to prevent pregnancy). Tranquilizers or antianxiety agents may be prescribed. Emphasis should be placed on follow-up appointments to repeat serology, cultures, and pregnancy tests, as well as to provide counseling services as necessary. Concerns immediately after treatment include safety, transportation home, and attendance or absence from work or school.

Emergency room personnel should ask the victim for permission to provide a crisis center with her telephone number, with the understanding that a follow-up person will take the initiative in contacting the victim. The establishment of ongoing support systems is important if the person is to resolve an abuse or rape experience. Such support systems include crisis hot lines, self-help groups, counseling, or shelters if the person requests a protective environment.

Walter (1992) addresses the topic of elderly survivors of incest and their need for nursing interventions as they review the life process. The lack of research regarding the impact of incest survival on older adults may, in part, be due to the relative unavailability of the elderly, disinterest in older adults, or the stigma associated with this type of victimization. Geriatric assessment forms may ask for information regarding elder abuse but do not assess for a past history of incest or sexual abuse. Many survivors exhibit symptoms of depression or anxiety. Once an elderly person is identified as a survivor of incest, goals for nursing care should include improving coping skills and increasing self-esteem. The individual should be encouraged to ventilate emotions and supportive measures such as individual therapy should be provided.

Davis (1990) discusses survival skills for victims of childhood sexual abuse. It is realistic to experience emotional and practical upheaval, which stirs up old feelings of terror, powerlessness, rage, and grief. The feelings may be strong enough to precipitate a crisis during the delayed recovery phase.

The survival protocol includes listing the names and telephone numbers of people to contact in an emergency; recognizing signs and symptoms of anxiety or panic attacks; listing effective coping skills to decrease anxiety; listing a suicide prevention plan; and obtaining a survivor sponsor to provide encouragement as well as a positive attitude.

Nursing Care Plan 30-1 lists nursing diagnoses and goal-related nursing interventions for the victim of rape.

Summary

This chapter focused on sexual harassment, sexual assault, and rape. Definitions of each were given. Motives for rape or sexual assault were described. Emotional reactions were described, with emphasis on the rape trauma syndrome. "Silent rape syndrome" was defined. The assessment process was explained, including physical, psychological, and behavioral assessment. Rape myths and facts were stated. Medical and nursing interventions were listed for both phases of the rape trauma syndrome and for maladaptive stress reactions after rape. Nursing care and survival skills for victims of childhood sexual abuse were discussed. Examples of nursing diagnoses and nursing interventions were given.

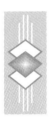

NURSING CARE PLAN 30-1
The Victim of Rape

Nursing Diagnosis: Acute phase of *rape trauma syndrome, as evidenced by feelings of guilt, fear, and anger

Goal: The patient will share feelings about traumatic incident with staff.

Nursing Interventions	Outcome Criteria
	During hospitalization the patient will do the following:
Establish trust.	Verbalize feeling of trust toward staff and feel secure in present environment
Maintain a nonjudgmental attitude. Convey acceptance.	Verbalize a feeling of acceptance in the presence of staff and peers
Provide crisis counseling.	Demonstrate an understanding of rationale for crisis intervention
	Describe feelings related to traumatic experience

Nursing Diagnosis: *Situational low self-esteem as evidenced by statements of negative feelings about self

Goal: Before discharge, the patient will demonstrate increased feelings of self-worth.

Nursing Interventions	Outcome Criteria
	During hospitalization the patient will do the following:
Encourage patient to express feelings about the way she views herself.	Describe feelings related to self-worth
Clarify any misconceptions the person has about care-givers.	Demonstrate ability to accept explanations without doubt or mistrust
Avoid negative criticism. Provide positive feedback.	Accept positive feedback
Assist in identifying positive aspects of self.	Identify at least two positive attributes about self

*NANDA-approved nursing diagnosis.

Learning Activities

I. Clinical Activities
   A. Spend a day in the emergency room of your clinical facility if possible, and obtain information regarding their rape treatment protocol. Share this information in postclinical conference.
   B. Identify support systems made available to rape victims *while* they are receiving treatment in the facility.
II. Independent Activities
   A. List measures suggested for preventing rape relevant to
      1. Environmental protection
      2. Physical protection
      3. Self-protection as an attack occurs
   B. Read the following for professional growth:
      1. *The Courage to Heal* by E. Bass & L. Davis
      2. *Sexual Harassment Today* by R. Davidhizar & J. N. Giger

Critical Thinking Questions

1. You have been asked to speak to a high school class about date rape. How would you go about preparing this presentation? What would you say?
2. Attend a local hearing of a rape case. What did you observe? How was the case handled?
3. Interview a layperson who has been trained as a rape counselor. How does her focus differ from a nursing focus? What can you teach each other about the care of a rape survivor?

Self-Test

1. List the three essential elements necessary legally to define rape.
2. State the motives for rape or sexual assault.
3. Differentiate between blitz and confidence rape.
4. Explain the phases of rape trauma syndrome.
5. Describe maladaptive stress reaction to rape.
6. Discuss the following myths about rape:
   Attractive women provoke men into raping them.
   Women "cry rape" to get revenge.
   Women can avoid rape by struggling with the rapist.

SELECTED REFERENCES

American Psychiatric Association. (1994). *Diagnostic and statistical manual of mental disorders* (4th ed.). Washington, DC: Author.

Bass, E., & Davis, L. (1988). *The courage to heal: A guide for women survivors of child sexual abuse.* New York: Harper & Row.

Carpenito, L. J. (1995). *Nursing diagnosis: Application to clinical practice* (6th ed.). Philadelphia: J. B. Lippincott.

Curry, J. (1993, January). Rape treatment models studied at Medical College Hospital of Pennsylvania. *Nursing Spectrum.*

Davidhizar, R., & Giger, J. N. (1995, December). Sexual harassment today: Workplace policy is the best form of prevention. *Advance for Nurse Practitioners.*

Davis, L. (1990). *The courage to heal workbook: For women and men survivors of child sexual abuse.* New York: Harper & Row.

Draucker, C. B. (1996). The client who was sexually abused. In S. Lego (Ed.). *Psychiatric nursing: A comprehensive reference* (2nd ed.). Philadelphia: Lippincott–Raven Publishers.

Elvik, S. L. (1995, September). Sexual abuse of the developmentally disabled. *Advance for Nurse Practitioners.*

Foley, T. S. (1984). The client who has been raped. In S. Lego (Ed.). *The American handbook of psychiatric nursing.* Philadelphia: J. B. Lippincott.

Grant, C. S. (1996). The client who has been raped. In S. Lego (Ed.). *Psychiatric nursing: A comprehensive reference* (2nd ed.). Philadelphia: Lippincott–Raven Publishers.

Greenfeld, M. (1990, July). Disclosing incest: The relationships that make it possible. *Journal of Psychosocial Nursing and Mental Health Services.*

McFarlane, J., Greenberg, L., Weltge, A., & Watson, M. (1995, October). Identification of abuse in emergency departments: Effectiveness of a two-question screening tool. *Journal of Emergency Nursing.*

Petrocelli, W., & Repa, B. (1992). *Sexual harassment on the job.* Berkeley, CA: Nolo Press.

Pohl, J. D. (1992). The theory of revictimization and suggestions for treatment. *Highland Highlights.*

Walter, K. (1992, January). That was then: Elderly survivors of incest. *Journal of Psychosocial Nursing and Mental Health Services.*

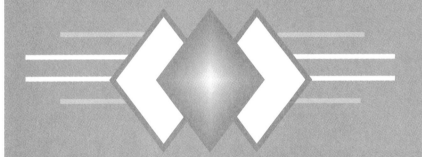

Populations with Special Needs

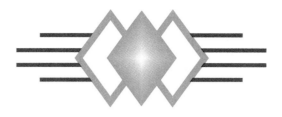

CHAPTER 31

COPING WITH ACQUIRED IMMUNODEFICIENCY SYNDROME (AIDS)

T he far-reaching consequences of infection with human immunodeficiency virus (HIV) have spurred an ever-growing data base of knowledge that changes rapidly from one month to the next. The problems associated with providing the necessary care for persons with HIV infection or AIDS are significant. Perhaps with continued education and constant awareness that this crisis will abate only with the preparation of health care providers and the public at large, we will be able to survive as a society.

J. C. Norman, 1996

LEARNING OBJECTIVES

1 Describe the acquired immunodeficiency syndrome.

2 Discuss the psychological effects of AIDS.

3 Define the effects of AIDS on the family.

4 Discuss the goals of psychotherapy with AIDS patients.

5 Outline the types of treatments available.

6 Discuss nursing interventions for AIDS patients who are
   experiencing anticipatory grief
   experiencing fear related to biologic changes

 Overview of AIDS

Acquired immunodeficiency syndrome (AIDS) is a life-threatening disease. AIDS is now the leading cause of death among U.S. men between the ages of 25 and 44 years. It is the fourth leading cause of death among U.S. women between the ages of 25 and 44 years. At this time, 18 million persons worldwide are human immunodeficiency virus (HIV) positive and, of these, more than three million are women of childbearing years. Worldwide, one million people have AIDS (Centers for Disease Control Semiannual HIV/AIDS Surveillance Report, June, 1996).

Recent statistics also revealed that of all AIDS cases reported, 10% have involved individuals 50 years of age or older, and about 3% have been among persons over 60 years old. Primary risk groups include gay men, injecting drug users, and sexually active heterosexuals.

Extensive research has led to the discovery of the virus that is believed to cause AIDS and AIDS-related complex (ARC). The virus was originally named HTLV-III (human T-cell lymphotropic virus), then renamed human immunodeficiency virus (HIV). The time period between exposure to the virus and diagnosis of the illness is between six months and five years, although some people may carry the virus without showing symptoms of the disease for an indefinite period of time. The AIDS virus is carried in the blood and blood-related products, especially semen, and is primarily contagious through intimate sexual contact or through the sharing of needles by IV drug users.

The AIDS virus attacks an individual's immune system and emerges in the form of 1 of 12 secondary infectious diseases or 2 types of malignant cancer. The two most common diseases of AIDS patients are *Pneumocystis carinii* pneumonia and Kaposi's sarcoma, a rare form of skin cancer. All of the AIDS diseases have extremely painful, debilitating, and devastating physical and psychological effects. The physical symptoms may include nausea and vomiting, constant fever, chronic headaches, diarrhea, painful mouth infections, hypotension, liver and kidney failure, central nervous system dysfunction with psychomotor retardation, severe respiratory distress, and incontinence. Persons with ARC most commonly experience fever, weight loss, debilitating fatigue, night sweats, and pain. One third to one half of these individuals will go on to develop the AIDS infection, whereas the others will show no progression of the disease. Additional information pertaining to the medical aspect of AIDS and its impact on health care providers can be obtained in various medical–surgical nursing textbooks.

Psychological Effects of AIDS

AIDS is frequently described as a tragic and complex phenomenon that provokes shattering emotional and psychological reactions in all who are involved with the illness. AIDS connects medicine and psychiatry to a greater degree than any other major illness. Forstein (1984) describes three population groups that can be delineated in discussing the psychological impacts of AIDS.

1. Clients with the disease and their sexual partners
2. Individuals at high risk for AIDS based on epidemiologic data
3. Individuals not specifically at risk but who are aware of and affected by the presence of AIDS within society

The overall psychosocial impact of AIDS is significantly affected by the fact that each of the identified risk groups, especially homosexual men, has a minority status within the American culture. Collins (1983) and others demand that the emotional impact of AIDS be discussed within the context of the preexisting socially condoned antipathy toward homosexual and bisexual men.

The most serious psychological problems occur for those clients who actually have the disease. Most people with AIDS are relatively young. Most of these persons have previously been healthy and have not had experience with a major medical illness. The confirmation of this diagnosis can be catastrophic for the client, eliciting a series of emotional and social reactions. These reactions include a loss of self-esteem, fear of the loss of physical attractiveness and rapid changes in body image, feelings of isolation and stigmatization, an overwhelming sense of hopelessness and helplessness, and a loss of control over their lives.

Nichols has described a four-stage reaction process similar to the pattern designated by Kübler-Ross in dying patients (Kübler-Ross, 1969; Nichols, 1983). The initial stage consists of shock, numbness, and disbelief. The severity of the psychological reaction may depend on existing support systems for the individual. During this period, patients report sleep problems and an experience of depersonalization and derealization. For some, the acknowledgment of the AIDS diagnosis causes severe emotional paralysis or regression.

The second stage is denial, and the person may attempt to ignore the diagnosis of AIDS. Although it may serve a necessary psychic function, this denial can cause the patient to engage in behaviors that are both self-destructive and potentially very dangerous to others. Some patients begin to plunge into complete isolation, avoiding human contact as much as possible.

The third stage is when the individual begins to ask the question "Why did I get AIDS?" Expressions of guilt and anger are frequent as the patient seeks to understand the reason for his or her illness. Homosexual or bisexual men may experience feelings of homophobia and believe that God is punishing them for their homosexual preference.

The final stage of resolution and acceptance depends on the individual's personality and ego integration and may be signified by the acceptance of the illness and its limitations, a sense of peace and dignity, and a preparation for dying. As the debilitating symptoms progress, other patients may become increasingly despondent and depressed, stop eating, express suicidal ideations, and develop almost psychotic fixations and obsessions with their illness. A significant and growing number of AIDS patients make successful suicide attempts.

In addition, emotional crises are caused by the person's increasing isolation as he or she attempts to cope with the nearly universal stigma faced on a daily basis. AIDS patients experience rejection from all parts of society, including families, friends, lovers, social agencies, landlords, and health care workers. For many, this constant rejection causes a reliving of the "coming-out process," with a heightening of the associated anxiety, guilt, and internalized self-hatred. The fear of spreading AIDS to others causes further isolation and abandonment at a time when there is an ever-greater need for physical and emotional support. Patients with AIDS may respond with intense anger and hostility as their conditions deteriorate and they confront the other everyday realities of this illness: loss of job and home; forced changes in life-style; the perceived lack of response by the medical community; and the often crippling expense associated with the illness.

An even larger group of homosexual men suffer from ARC or test positive for the HIV infection but have not yet developed any of the physical signs or symptoms. Individuals in these two groups also experience severe psychological stress. The issues involve

1. Preoccupation with shifting and frightening physical symptoms
2. Initial confrontation with societal stigmas
3. Overwhelming anxiety at developing a painful and debilitating terminal illness
4. Poor social and occupational functioning

5. Chronic fatigue
6. The inability to predict or control the onset of this life-threatening process

These persons are often referred to as the *gray zone* (Morin, Charles, Malyan, 1984) and are at risk for development of an anxiety disorder, a major depression, a dysthymic disorder, or in some cases a psychosis.

The family of an AIDS patient also experiences severe psychological stress and trauma. The issue of the individual's sexuality and life-style, often something of which the family had not been aware, creates an additional crisis at a time when they are confronted with the knowledge that their son or daughter (or sibling) has a terminal illness. The pressure on the family system causes members to respond with quiet anger, confusion, and possible rejection of the AIDS patient and his or her whole life-style. Families may blame the patient's lover for the condition but simultaneously find themselves forced to include the lover in their grief and in their attempts to cope with the illness. Coleman (1988) describes the diagnosis of AIDS as creating a further challenge to the fragile balance of roles within the family system. An adult child who has been functioning independently for many years must now rely again on parental support to meet daily self-care needs. Parents are confronted with a change in their new retired life-style as the dying child comes home to live. Families also are forced to assume financial responsibility, which can further magnify their anger, guilt, and frustration. Some families are able to achieve resolution of their own painful psychological conflicts and provide the necessary physical and emotional support to the AIDS patient. However, a significant number of families become fixed in their rejection, grief, and anger and are never able to resolve the distance and estrangement from the family member with AIDS.

In response to this familial abandonment, the individual with AIDS often develops an alternative family that assumes the support and care-taker role. This new family may include a gay partner and close gay and straight friends who significantly alter their life-style to care for the patient. These friends experience the same sense of loss, isolation, and bereavement as the more traditional family but are denied the customary social support systems and public recognition for their role.

 Transcultural Considerations

Andrews and Boyle (1995) discuss the HIV/AIDS pandemic. Heterosexual intercourse has become the dominant mode of transmission in North America, Australia, Asia, and Northern Europe. Nearly 90% of the projected HIV infections and AIDS cases for this decade will occur in less-developed countries.

CLINICAL EXAMPLE 31-1
Acquired Immunodeficiency Syndrome

GD, age 38, a single white man, has been seeing a psychiatrist weekly for eight months with the complaints of anxiety, mood swings, sleep disturbances, angry outbursts, and increasing social and occupational dysfunction. GD is a banker with a master's degree in business adminis-tration. He is a member of the Jaycees, an active member of his church, and the captain of his bank's softball team. He grew up in Ohio and remains close to his parents and younger brothers. A gourmet cook, GD had planned to retire early and travel around the world. He is a homo-sexual and was diagnosed with AIDS five months before beginning indi-vidual therapy. The goals of ongoing individual or group psychotherapy with GD or other people with AIDS include the following:

1. Assisting the individual to verbalize anger, guilt, and fears and to face fears of disfigurement, loss of control, and death
2. Restructuring or enabling the person to accept his illness and to find new meaning in life while adapting to the limitations of his illness
3. Assisting the person to cope with the condemnation and rejection from society, family, friends, and health care workers
4. Evaluating the appropriateness of a therapeutic dose of a psycho-pharmacologic agent
5. Maintaining continuing communication among all involved social and medical agencies and providers
6. Resolving multiple and complex financial and legal concerns
7. Assisting the individual to face death while maintaining respect and dignity

Norman (1996) discusses the problems of homophobia and stigmatization of men having sex with men (MSM) in ethnic communities of color as well as in the society at large. Social and emotional isolation, disapproval, prejudice, judgments of shame and immorality, and even violence may occur. Attitudes of various ethnic communities may be influenced by organized religion, concep-tualizations of MSM, and the value placed on civil liberties. Dual standards for men and women extend to cultural attitudes toward monogamy, expression of sexuality, talking about sexuality, condom use, who may initiate sexual inter-course, and reproduction.

According to the statistics released by the Centers for Disease Control in 1994, the largest number of AIDS cases occurred in the white population, fol-lowed by African Americans, Hispanics, Asians or Pacific Islanders, American Indians or Alaska Natives, and people of unknown race or ethnicity.

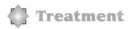 **Treatment**

Various DSM-IV diagnoses may be used during the treatment of persons who are HIV positive or are known to have AIDS: depression, anxiety, relational problems, sleep disorders, or dementia due to HIV disease. Providing the appropriate treatment to meet the complex needs of the AIDS patient involves the utilization and coordination of multiple resources. The primary therapeutic goal is to assist the individual to gain control over his or her life for as long as possible. Psychiatric intervention, as outlined in the clinical example, may be appropriate with intensive individual or group therapy and with referral to the appropriate community agencies. Most communities have now established full-service agencies made up of volunteers from the community and health professionals who work together to provide support and education to individuals with AIDS and their families. The types of comprehensive services provided include

1. A 24-hour hotline
2. A buddy system
3. People-with-AIDS support group
4. Social service advocacy
5. Financial and legal counseling
6. Crisis intervention
7. Religious support
8. Referrals
9. Printed materials
10. Emergency assistance fund
11. Professional education
12. Disability applications and assistance

Support groups have become the key element in the provision of treatment. These groups, established by community and gay-oriented organizations to respond to this health crisis and to lessen the isolation of people with AIDS, involve a unique variety of concerned volunteers. Through use of the buddy system, and with the assistance of trained professionals, these specialized groups provide emotional and physical support, assistance with daily chores, legal and financial planning, and advocacy with the appropriate social and government agencies. Lawyers can minimize some of the emotional trauma by assisting the individual to make crucial decisions regarding hospital visitation rights, treatment options, power of attorney, and disposition of property. Hirsch and Enlow (1985) describe the benefit of helping the person with AIDS to retain legal and personal control over his or her life for as long as possible.

Many hospitals have responded to the demand for treatment by providing a special care unit within the hospital. These units are specifically designed to address the particular medical and psychological needs of the AIDS patient. They are staffed by health care professionals and gay volunteer counselors who have been trained in the techniques of working with the terminally ill patient.

 ## Nursing Intervention

Regan-Kubinski and Sharts-Engel (1992) discuss the prevalence of HIV infection in the female population. The assessment of negative emotional responses, anxiety, and uncertainty about the future is addressed, with emphasis on augmenting the individual's motivation to cope with physical symptoms, and, eventually, to prepare for death with dignity.

Whipple and Scura (1996) discuss HIV infection in older adults. Many clinicians do not consider older adults to be at risk because of society's stereotype of older people as sexually inactive. Older adults may be reluctant to speak frankly about their sexual orientation. AIDS dementia complex may be confused with other dementias that occur in the elderly. Cognitive impairment may be attributed to the aging process. Because clinicians do not consider older adults to be at risk for HIV/AIDS, failure to assess or diagnose this disorder denies the patient proper treatment and care.

Ferri (1995) states that HIV infection within the adolescent community does not get the attention it deserves because of time constraints, uneasiness about HIV/AIDS issues, and lack of understanding about adolescent development. Making decisions about disclosure is difficult for teens, who may lack certain social experiences and skills. They fear the loss of friends, family, and other supports.

Lego (1996) discusses clinical phenomena that occur in the early and middle phases of HIV/AIDS. During the early phase, the emphasis is on stages of the grief process, fear of incapacitation due to physical and mental deterioration as well as deformity and pain, shame, and suicidal thoughts. Several phenomena are identified during the middle phase. They include loss of control, helplessness and vulnerability, passivity and victimization, severe reduction in self-esteem, sense of isolation, guilt, anger, depression, paranoia, fear of violence, sense of betrayal, alcohol or substance abuse, somatic preoccupation, and projective identification. Nursing interventions are listed for each of the clinical phenomena. During the late phase, death is relatively near. The individual may exhibit clinical symptoms of dementia, personality changes, or acute psychotic reaction. Various psychoactive drugs may be used to reduce anxiety, stabilize depression, or minimize psychotic symptoms.

The nurse is an integral member of the multidisciplinary team that provides comprehensive care to AIDS patients and their families. The use of the team approach to manage care is beneficial and supportive to both the patient and staff. The role of nursing in the terminal phase of this illness is a critical one. Nurses must continually help the health care team, family, and significant others to focus on the patients' desires.

Caring for patients with AIDS is an extremely challenging assignment; it is important first of all for the nurse, as well as all members of the team, to be aware of their own feelings, fears, and lack of education about AIDS. Hospital administrators have continually reported that the incurable and epidemic nature of AIDS causes considerable stress for all hospital personnel, particularly nurses (Shohen, 1988). Nurses must also be cognizant of their own possible negative feelings about these patients and examine how their feelings might interfere with their ability to provide high-quality, comprehensive nursing care to AIDS patients and their families. To assist with this exploration, the nurse manager, with support from social workers, chaplains, and counselors, should help establish a support group for the nurses. Such a group provides regular opportunities for nurses to verbalize their own feelings about the stress of caring for these very difficult patients, to complain about the inadequate community support and resources, to vent their own fears about possibly acquiring the HIV infection through an accidental needle stick, and to grieve together over the continuing deaths of these young AIDS patients. Nursing Care Plan 31-1 (on p. 584) lists examples of nursing diagnoses and goal-related nursing interventions for individuals with AIDS.

Summary

A description of the disease called acquired immunodeficiency syndrome (AIDS) was presented along with the physical symptoms of the illness. The psychological effects of AIDS were discussed, with concentration on three population groups: clients with the disease, individuals at high risk for AIDS, and individuals aware of and affected by the disease. The stages of emotional response to the AIDS diagnosis and illness were discussed. The psychological and physical risks and complications of AIDS-related complex (ARC) were also reviewed. The often complex response of the family system to this critical illness was described as well as the vital caretaking role of the alternative family. A clinical example described a young male client with AIDS and outlined the goals of individual or group psychotherapy with AIDS patients. The remaining sections discussed the complex treatment needs of people with AIDS and the use and coordination of multiple community resources and support groups. The chapter conclusion focused on the nursing interventions and the unique role of the nurse as a key member of the multidisciplinary health care team.

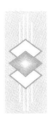

NURSING CARE PLAN 31-1
The Patient with AIDS

Nursing Diagnosis: *Fear related to biologic changes from disabling illness (AIDS)

Goal: During hospitalization the patient will verbalize a decreased fear of biologic changes related to AIDS.

Nursing Interventions	Outcome Criteria
	During hospitalization the patient will do the following:
Develop trust by conveying respect, acceptance, and concern.	Verbalize decreased feelings of being overwhelmed
Encourage patient to verbalize feelings and fears.	Describe fears related to illness
Use physical contact (touch arm, hold hand) if appropriate as a means to offer comfort.	Verbalize feelings of comfort with staff and present environment
Educate about clinical course of illness focusing on the here and now.	Demonstrate an understanding of present physical status
	Verbalize decreased fear

Nursing Diagnosis: *Anticipatory grieving related to progression of illness

Goal: The patient will progress through the grieving process.

Nursing Interventions	Outcome Criteria
	During hospitalization the patient will do the following:
Encourage patient to share concerns about illness.	Discuss concerns openly
Educate regarding the grief process.	Demonstrate an understanding of the grief process
Assist in identifying present stage of grief process.	Identify present stage of grief process
Promote grief work with each stage (*e.g.*, denial, anger, depression).	Express feelings even if painful or uncomfortable through talking, writing, drawing, etc.
Refer patient to spiritual resource person if the need is identified.	Indicate whether spiritual counseling is desired

*NANDA-approved nursing diagnosis.

Learning Activities

I. Clinical Activities
  A. Care for a patient with AIDS.
  B. Describe the emotional reactions exhibited by the patient.
  C. Identify which stage of the grieving process the patient is experiencing.
  D. If possible, develop a relationship with the patient's family or support system and identify their psychological needs.
  E. Discuss the community resources and support systems available to persons with AIDS.
II. Independent Activities
  A. Obtain a list of community resources and agencies available to persons with AIDS.
  B. Contact your local health department to receive information about the incidence and treatment of AIDS in your specific community.
  C. Initiate a group discussion with other students regarding how you and others feel about the AIDS dilemma.

Critical Thinking Questions

1. Review nursing history to learn about other epidemics to which nurses have responded. How are the social, economic, and political conditions surrounding those epidemics similar to conditions surrounding the AIDS epidemic? How are the conditions different?
2. Considering developmental, social, and psychological issues, what would you tell a group of sexually active teenagers about AIDS?
3. Nurses in the forefront of providing care for patients with AIDS in the home and hospice environments are seldom recognized by the media. What strategies would you use to create media interest in this remarkable work?

Self-Test

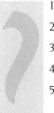

1. Define the acquired immunodeficiency syndrome.
2. Describe the psychological effects of AIDS.
3. Explain the role of the family when caring for an AIDS patient.
4. List four goals of psychotherapy with the AIDS patient.
5. List five resources available for assisting the patient and family in coping with AIDS.
6. What are the key nursing interventions for assisting an AIDS patient?

SELECTED REFERENCES

American Psychiatric Association. (1994). *Diagnostic and statistical manual of mental disorders* (4th ed.). Washington, DC: Author.

Andrews, M. M., & Boyle, J. S. (1995). *Transcultural concepts in nursing care* (2nd ed.). Philadelphia: J. B. Lippincott.

Bassetti, M. (1996, November). Primary care strategies for AIDS prevention. *Advance for Nurse Practitioners.*

Centers for Disease Control. (1996, June). Semiannual HIV/AIDS surveillance report. In *Continuing education for Florida nurses, 1996.* Sacramento, CA: Continuing Medical Education Resource.

Coleman, D. (1988). Nursing care of the AIDS patient. In *AIDS: A health care management response.* Rockville, MD: Aspen.

Collins, G. (1983, May 30). Facing the emotional anguish of AIDS. *The New York Times.*

Ferri, R. S. (1995, July). HIV and adolescents: A primary care perspective. *Advance for Nurse Practitioners.*

Forstein, M. (1984, March). The psychosocial impact of the acquired immunodeficiency syndrome. *Seminars in Oncology.*

Gerchufsky, M. (1995, March). "Waste anything but time." *Advance for Nurse Practitioners.*

Grant, I. (1996, June). HIV and dementia. *Current Approaches to Dementia: Caring for the Older Adult.*

Hirsch, D., & Enlow, R. (Annual 1985). *The effects of the acquired immune deficiency syndrome on gay lifestyle and the gay individual.* New York: New York Academy of Science.

Kübler-Ross, E. (1969). *On death and dying.* London: Macmillan.

Lego, S. (1996). *Psychiatric nursing: A comprehensive reference* (2nd ed.). Philadelphia: Lippincott–Raven Publishers.

Morin, S., Charles, K., & Malyan, A. (1984, November). The psychological impact of AIDS on gay men. *American Psychologist.*

Nichols, S. (1983). Psychiatric aspects of AIDS. *Psychosomatics, 24.*

Norman, J. C. (1996). Essentials of nursing management: HIV-AIDS. *Continuing Medical Education Resource.*

Regan-Kubinski, M. J., & Sharts-Engel, N. (1992, February). The HIV-infected woman: Illness cognition assessment. *Journal of Psychosocial Nursing and Mental Health Services.*

Shohen, S. (1988). Public relations issues. In *AIDS: A health care management response.* Rockville, MD: Aspen.

Whipple, B., & Scura, K. W. (1996, February). The overlooked epidemic: HIV in older adults. *American Journal of Nursing.*

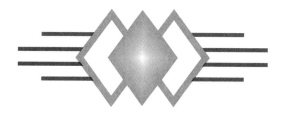

CHAPTER 32

PSYCHOSOCIAL ASPECTS OF AGING

P sychiatric syndromes—rather than discrete disorders—are more realistic as diagnostic entities in geriatric psychiatry. The most common of these syndromes are memory loss, depression, anxiety, suspicions and agitation, sleep disorders, and hypochondriasis.

Blazer, 1994

1 Define the term *aging*.

2 Describe factors that affect the aging process.

3 State Duvall's developmental tasks of aging.

4 List the eight categories of mental disturbances in older adults.

5 Differentiate between dementia, depression, and delirium in the elderly.

6 Define failure to thrive.

7 Identify elements of a comprehensive assessment of geropsychiatric patients.

8 Discuss the importance of obtaining family input during the assessment process.

9 State the rationale for prescribing low doses of psychoactive drugs for geriatric patients.

10 State nursing diagnoses commonly used when planning care for elderly persons with mental health problems.

11 Plan nursing interventions for elderly persons who demonstrate needs for

    Psychological safety and security

    Loving and belonging

    Self-esteem

    Self-actualization

Introduction

Various statistics have been published regarding the elderly population (ages 65 years and older). According to Taeuber (1993), 6% of the world's population is 65 years of age or older. The elderly represent 12% or 31.1 million of the U.S. population. Of these, approximately 18 million were ages 65 to 74, 10 million were ages 75 to 84, and 3 million were age 85 years or older. By the year 2020, approximately 52 million persons will be 65 years of age or older.

The prevalence of psychiatric symptoms in community populations of older adults is discussed by Blazer (1996). They are listed as follows:

15% Depression
14% Hypochondriasis

17% Suspiciousness
4% Persecutory ideation
14% Difficulty falling asleep
34% Unable to stay asleep
31% Sleepy all day
2% Generalized anxiety

This chapter focuses on the psychosocial aspects of aging. Common emotional, behavioral, and cognitive disorders are briefly discussed. The reader is referred to specific chapters in the text for additional information regarding psychiatric disorders experienced by the elderly.

Theories About Aging

Wantz and Gay (1981) describe two aging theories, (1) cellular theory and (2) genetic theory. The cellular theory lists three possible causes of aging: an accumulation of insufficient proteins within the cells that causes cellular aging, an accumulation of defective cells with impaired cellular functions, and an accumulation of harmful wastes and by-products in the body that affects the cells (metabolic waste product theory). According to the genetic theory, longevity, or one's life span, is determined at conception because genetic factors may cause cellular irregularities and mutations to occur. These irregularities and mutations, as well as one's environment and any disease processes, can influence the aging process. Genetic factors are discussed in the next section.

Havinghurst (1968) also discusses two theories of aging, (1) the activity theory and (2) the disengagement theory. The activity theory states that older persons experience the same psychological and social needs as when they were younger. The disengagement theory states that older persons and society initiate a decrease in social interaction and activity. Older persons accept and may even desire this interrupted relationship to occur as they become increasingly self-centered.

Ebersole and Hess (1985) categorize the theories of aging as evolutionary, biologic, psychological and sociologic. Evolutionary theorists view old age as an addendum to the life of sexual maturation and propagation (Ebersole). The theories of biologic and physiological aging are concerned with cellular changes. They include damage theory, program theory, and popular theory. The psychological and sociologic theories are based on developmental stages and tasks throughout one's life span. Certain psychological growth mechanisms are ascribed to various ages. Examples can be found in the works of Jung, Piaget, Erikson, Clayton, Butler, Neugarten, and Lowenthal.

Nurses caring for aging persons should be aware of these theories as they plan nursing interventions for patients.

Factors Influencing the Aging Process

Busse (1996) states that aging usually refers to the adverse effects of the passage of time but can also refer to the positive processes of maturation or acquiring a desirable quality. The multiple processes of decline associated with growing old are separated into primary and secondary aging. Primary aging is intrinsic and is determined by inherent or hereditary influences. Secondary aging refers to extrinsic changes (defects and disabilities) caused by hostile factors in the environment, including trauma and acquired disease.

Intrinsic factors include biologic and physiologic components such as sex, race, intelligence, familial longevity patterns, and genetic diseases. According to statistics, women live longer than men by approximately seven years. Factors assumed to contribute to this longevity of women over men include endocrine metabolism before menopause that provides protection against circulatory or cardiovascular diseases, higher activity level, less stress from occupation, better weight control, and less use of tobacco. Although the life expectancy for whites is approximately five years more than for all other races, the death rate for whites older than age 75 years is higher than for all other races. Persons with a higher level of intelligence appear to live longer than persons with lower levels of intelligence. This fact may be due, in part, to the lifestyle selected by persons with higher intelligence quotients (IQs). Such persons may remain physically active by participating in events that promote physical, mental, and social well-being. Persons with type A personality seldom relax or enjoy themselves because of a drive-to-succeed quality. They are prime candidates for heart attacks. The type B personality is an easygoing individual who takes life in stride.

Personality also influences the adoption of abusive behaviors, such as overeating, tobacco dependence, and alcohol abuse. These abuses definitely impair one's physical health and shorten one's life span. Familial longevity patterns are indicators of a person's potential life span. A 45-year-old man from a family with a record of long-lived great-grandparents, grandparents, and parents probably will live longer than a man of the same age whose family history includes heart attacks by his father and grandfather at middle age. Genetic disease may cause a person to experience a short life span; for example, persons with Down's syndrome, cystic fibrosis, or Tay-Sachs disease have shortened life spans. Although people have minimal if any control over these intrinsic factors influencing the aging process, a high quality of life possibly could promote one's sense of physical, mental, and social well-being.

Extrinsic components or factors of aging can be controlled to some degree by the person. Examples of these environmental factors include employment, economic level, education, health practices and related diseases, and societal attitude. Income, economic level, and educational level definitely determine how one lives. Health care may not be sought because of high medical–surgical costs, lack of insurance, or ignorance about contributing factors to or symptoms of various diseases. People who eat inadequate diets, have poor living conditions, ignore or minimize health problems, or experience financial stress are definitely at risk for a shortened life span. Substance abuse and poor diets are seen in all age groups. These practices have a negative effect on health and have proven to contribute to earlier deaths. Societal attitudes affect persons psychologically and definitely have an impact on the aging process. Most persons seek the approval of society and will behave the way they think society expects them to behave. Such thinking could lead to a lifestyle that is detrimental to one's health. Older adults should seek intellectual, emotional, and physical stimulation to maintain an optimal level of health and longevity.

Myths About Aging

A local hospital recently published a pamphlet entitled *On Center*. The topic was "Growing Older: Adding Life to Your Years." Five myths about aging were presented. They are included in Box 32-1 (on p. 592).

Developmental Tasks of Aging

In addition to various factors that influence aging, consider how aging can affect one's psychosocial needs. Statistics quoted by Ebersole and Hess (1985) reveal that approximately 5% of older persons are institutionalized for health or emotional problems. The larger percentage of aging adults live in central parts of cities or in rural locations. Statistics released in 1986 by the American Association of Retired Persons showed that Florida, California, and New York contained approximately 35% of the elderly population. These statistics may be relatively higher at this time.

Duvall (1977) lists developmental tasks of the elderly that influence their emotional needs. They are summarized in the following sections.

Establishing Satisfactory Living Arrangements

Many factors influence this developmental task. Is the person single, widowed, divorced, or married? Does the elderly person have an incapacitating illness or handicap? Does the person require assistance or supervision with the activities of daily living (ADLs)? Are the grocery store, pharmacy, doctor's office, and church located close by or within walking distance? Is the person able to stay in her or his own home or does the person need to be relocated? These are just a

BOX 32-1 Myths About Aging

Myth: Growing old means growing set in your ways.
Fact: The American Association of Retired Persons counts over 2 million computer users among its 33 million members. They track finances, keep in touch with grandchildren, produce memoirs, and research family trees.
Myth: Growing old means growing senile.
Fact: Today's seniors are well educated about the importance of health care, exercise, and nutrition and they are embracing life-styles that significantly combat physical and mental inactivity.
Myth: Growing old means a growing gap between the old and the young.
Fact: Since the early 1990s, grandparents have provided sole care for close to 1 million children younger than age 15 and 708,000 younger than age 5 years. With grandparents raising their children's children, the intergenerational gap may be a thing of the past.
Myth: Growing old means a growing dependency on medical care and drugs.
Fact: Research confirms active, involved seniors remain healthy, both physically and mentally. They are learning to become active patients, seeking prompt, effective medical attention.
Myth: Growing old means growing invisible.
Fact: The masters of art, literature, and science have shaped the world, often making their best contributions in their senior years. In 1990, 15.4 million persons age 55 years and older were in the work force. Older workers are among the most productive employees of all.

few questions that the family and the aging person consider when satisfactory living arrangements are made. Loneliness, anxiety, or depression, as well as other emotional reactions, may occur if these needs are not met.

Adjusting to Retirement Income

Not all people are fortunate enough to have a savings account and receive social security, retirement benefits, or some other form of supplemental income. Retirement may be a time planned for relaxation and leisure activities or may pose a financial crisis. Adjusting one's standard of living to a reduced income can be quite stressful for the elderly when the cost of living continues to rise.

Establishing Comfortable Routines

Retirement, which provides a person with newfound leisure time, allows one to establish a comfortable routine such as going on a last-minute trip, participating in a weekly bowling league during the day, doing volunteer work, or developing new hobbies. Retirement may be stressful for the "workaholic," or type A personality, who needs to be busy all the time. "All my husband does is get in my way. He's always underfoot like a little puppy dog. I wish he was still working"; "I thought we'd do things together such as golf, bowl, or play bridge. He's not interested in doing anything"; and "I don't enjoy life any more. There's nothing to look forward to now that I am retired" are just a few comments by persons having difficulty adjusting to new routines during retirement. On the positive side, the following comment was made by a senior citizen thoroughly enjoying retirement: "I don't know how I managed to work before. I don't have enough time in the day to do everything."

Maintaining Love, Sex, and Marital Relationships

"Most older people want—and are able to lead—an active, satisfying sex life. . . . When problems occur they should not be viewed as inevitable, but rather as the result of the disease, disability, drug reactions, or emotional upset—and as requiring medical care" (National Institute on Aging, 1981). Walker (1982) states, "The notion that old age will be sexless has been proven false in study after study. Provided that they are healthy, elderly people are capable of an active sex life into their 80s and 90s. Sexual performance may be slowed somewhat with aging, but sexual pleasure and capacity remain intact" (p. 171). Sexual problems can arise in later years from physiologic changes, fear of impotence, fear of a heart attack because of physical exertion, or boredom. An older widowed man is able to establish a new marital relationship more readily than a woman because of the availability of women in his age group or younger. Older women are frowned on if they marry a man much younger.

Keeping Active and Involved

Special characteristics that demonstrate the ability of the elderly to keep active have been identified by Butler and Lewis (1982). These characteristics include the desire to leave a legacy, the desire to share knowledge and experience with younger generations, the ability to demonstrate an increased emotional investment in the environment, a sense of immediacy or "here and now" owing to the decreased number of years left, the ability to experience an entire life cycle, increased creativity and curiosity, and a satisfaction with life. Physical illness may prevent a person from being active and becoming involved with others. The theory of disengagement also offers an explanation for the aging person's lessened activity and interaction with society. Active senior citizens may participate in various volunteer employment programs such as Retired Senior Volunteer Program (RSVP), Service Core of Retired Executives (SCORE), Volunteers in Service to America (VISTA), Peace Corps, Foster Grandparents Programs, and Senior Opportunities and Service programs (SOS).

Staying in Touch with Other Family Members

"I cry inside every day. Each time they come to visit me, I beseech them to take me home. . . . All I want . . . is to hold my daughter's hand and be surrounded by those people and things I love." This statement was made by a 94-year-old woman placed in a nursing home by her family.

The following poem appeared in a local newspaper along with a drawing of a forlorn-looking elderly woman sitting alone in her home:

> Next year.
>   They said they'll
> come down for Christmas
>   next year.
> Excuses again.
>   It's warm today.
> Too warm for Christmas anyway.
>   I don't think I can wait
> another year.
>
>   *Larry Moore, 1983*

This verse depicts the loneliness experienced by many elderly people, especially at holidays, anniversary dates, and birthdays, because they do not have family or a substitute support system.

Loneliness can lead to depression and thoughts of suicide. The elderly are considered to account for approximately 25% of suicides reported yearly. Persons who meet the developmental tasks of maintaining love, sex, and marital relationships, as well as keeping active and involved, probably would be able to cope with separation from family members more readily than those who choose to disengage themselves from society.

Sustaining and Maintaining Physical and Mental Health

It is not easy to experience a slowing of one's mental and physical reactions and be unable to do anything about it, or to look on as younger people perform one's job and assume one's role. Various emotional and behavioral reactions occur as one undergoes the physiologic changes of the aging process. These reactions include anxiety, frustration, fear, depression, intolerance, stubbornness, loneliness, decreased independence, decreased productivity, low self-esteem, and numerous somatic complaints (also referred to as hypochondriasis).

Imagine what your own emotional or behavioral reactions would be to the following physical impairments: loss of hearing or sight, inability to speak because of a stroke, inability to perform ADLs because of a paralyzed left side or disorientation, and incontinency of urine or stool from loss of bladder or bowel control. Loss is a predominant theme in characterizing the emotional experiences of older people. The aged person fears loss of control over daily routines, loss of identity, confinement (*e.g.*, placement in a nursing home or hospital), social isolation because of failing health, and death (20% to 25% of the elderly occupy nursing homes when they die).

Finding Meaning in Life

"Listen to the aged. They will teach you. They are a distinguished faculty who teach not from books but from long experience in living" (Burnside, 1975, p. 1800). The elderly reminisce frequently as they adapt to the aging process. They are eager to talk about days gone by. Schrock (1980) refers to Roger C. Peck's concept of ego transcendence versus ego preoccupation in her discussion of the elderly person's outlook on life. *Ego transcendence* describes a positive approach to find meaning in life as aging persons talk about past life experiences and realize that they have the wisdom and knowledge to serve as resource persons. They are willing to share themselves with others, remain active, and look to the future. Persons exhibiting *ego preoccupation* resign themselves to the aging process, become inactive, feel they have no future, and wait to die. They do not feel their lives have any significant meaning to themselves or others.

Neugarten (in Schrock, 1980) discusses five components of measuring the elderly's satisfaction with life: (1) zest versus apathy, (2) resolution and fortitude versus passivity, (3) congruence between desired and achieved goals, (4) self-concept, and (5) mood tone. Table 32-1 provides a comparison of ego transcendence and ego preoccupation using Neugarten's five components of life satisfaction, which is a helpful tool to use in the nursing assessment of aging persons.

TABLE 32-1 NEUGARTEN'S FIVE COMPONENTS OF LIFE	
Ego Transcendence	Ego Preoccupation
Zest Enthusiastic and personally involved in activities around him or her.	*Apathy* Bored, lacks energy and interest in others and activities around him or her.
Resolution and fortitude Assumes an active responsibility for one's life and actions. Maslow describes this self-actualized person as realistic; accepting of others; spontaneous in actions; displaying a need for privacy, autonomy, and independence; democratic; and humorous (Schrock, 1980).	*Passivity* Does not assume an active responsibility for one's life and actions. Remains inactive and passive, allowing things to happen.
Goal congruence (has achieved goals) Satisfied with the way goals have been met. Feels successful as a person.	*Goal incongruence (has not achieved goals)* Regrets actions taken to achieve goals. Dissatisfied with the way life is treating her or him.
Positive self-concept Likes one's physical appearance and cares about how one presents self to others. Feels competent. Is able to socialize with others without feeling like a "third party."	*Negative self-concept* Does not place much emphasis or concern on physical appearance. Feels incompetent. Is unable to relate to others socially without feeling as if he or she is imposing.
Positive mood tone Has the ability to appreciate life, displays a sense of humor, is optimistic and happy.	*Negative mood tone* Is unable to appreciate life; displays a pessimistic attitude; may be irritable, bitter, or gloomy in emotional reactions.

 ## Emotional Reactions or Behaviors

Emotional problems of the elderly have been classified from minor mental problems to the development of major psychotic disorders such as late-life schizophrena. Eight patterns of behavior or mental disturbance due to psychiatric disorders have been identified. They include

1. Aggressive, assaultive, hostile behavior
2. Anxious, agitated, restless, hyperactive behavior

3. Elation, rapid speech, decrease in ability to eat or sleep
4. Depression combined with paranoid ideation
5. Withdrawn, negativistic, mute condition
6. Delusions of persecution or grandiosity
7. Hallucinations
8. Simple deterioration displaying regression, confusion, and disorientation

A nonspecific condition often seen in the elderly is referred to as failure to thrive. This syndrome includes unexplained weight loss, deterioration in mental status and funtional ability, and social isolation. The more common emotional reactions, cognitive changes, and behavioral disturbances that occur in the elderly are discussed in this chapter. They include anxiety, loneliness, guilt, depression, somatic complaints, paranoid reactions, dementia, pseudodementia, and delirium.

Anxiety

Loss of mental acuity, admission to a nursing home, loss of a spouse, emergency surgery, confinement to bed because of a physical illness, and the diagnosis of a terminal illness are but a few causes of anxiety during old age. Aged persons may not be accustomed to expressing their feelings openly. Pent-up feelings, concerns, or reactions to loss may manifest themselves as numerous physical or somatic complaints, insomnia, restlessness, fatigue, hostility, dependency, and isolation (see Chapter 16 for additional information).

Loneliness

Loneliness is considered to be the "reactive response to separation from persons and things in which one has invested oneself and one's energy" (Burnside, 1981, p. 66). Burnside lists five causes of loneliness in the elderly:

1. *Death of a spouse, relative, or friend.*
2. *Loss of a pet.* Some elderly persons relate to pets as though they were people, and the death of a long-time pet can be very traumatic.
3. *The inability to communicate in the English language.* People feel isolated and lonely if they are in a foreign environment or are unable to understand what is being said.
4. *Pain.* People often complain of loneliness when pain occurs during the late evening or early morning hours because no one is around to provide comfort.
5. *Certain times of the day or night.* Changes in living habits due to institutionalization in a nursing home may cause loneliness because the elderly are no longer able to perform daily or nightly rituals. Daily activities generally provide some stimulation for the elderly, whereas quiet evenings can seem quite long, especially if no relatives or friends visit.

Guilt

As the elderly experience the life-review process, reminiscing about the past, guilt feelings may emerge from past conflicts or regrets. For example, an elderly man revealed guilt feelings about not lending his son-in-law and daughter money several years ago when they were in a financial bind. At the time of the request, the man felt that the couple should be able to support themselves. "Young people don't appreciate things given to them on a silver platter. They need to work for what they get. Then they'll take care of it" were his words of advice at the time they asked for help. He went on to state that they had plenty of money now, but "money doesn't keep one company." Guilt feelings may also occur when one considers past grudges, actions taken against others, outliving others, or unemployment or retirement.

Late-life Depressions

Depression can occur at any time during the life span but appears to increase in degree and frequency during old age. Although loss is the most common causative factor, unresolved grief, anger, loneliness, declining health, and guilt can result in feelings of mild to severe depression. Medications taken by the elderly also may precipitate or enhance a depressive reaction. As stated earlier, 25% of all suicides committed yearly are by persons 65 years of age or older. Elderly persons most at risk are white men older than age 85 years, isolated elderly persons, older persons experiencing increased dependency and changes in body function, and those persons with the diagnosis of a terminal illness. DSM-IV diagnoses frequently used to describe depression in older adults include dysthymia, major depression, bereavement, and adjustment disorder with depressed mood. (See Chapters 19 and 20 for additional information.)

Somatic Complaints

Hypochondriasis, or preoccupation with one's physical and emotional health resulting in bodily or somatic complaints, is common in the elderly patient. The aging person is rechanneling stress and anxiety into bodily concerns as he or she assumes the "sick" role described earlier in this text. Support, concern, and interest conveyed to the patient serve as secondary gains, reinforcing a sense of control. The care-giver should assess all complaints thoroughly and matter-of-factly, avoiding stereotyping the person as a "chronic complainer." Common somatic complaints include insomnia, anorexia, and pain. (See Chapter 17 for additional information about anxiety-related disorders such as somatic complaints.)

Paranoid Reactions

Loss of sight or hearing, sensory deprivation, or physical impairments often contribute to suspiciousness in elderly persons. Aging persons may feel others are talking about them or conspiring against them. Medication such as diazepam (Valium) or a strange environment also may contribute to confusion and suspicious behavior among the elderly. (See Chapter 21 for additional information.)

Dementia (Senility) or Cognitive Dysfunction

Dementia is described as impaired memory from a physical cause. The person forgets recent events more readily than past events, as well as names, telephone numbers, and conversations. Attempts to compensate for memory loss include social withdrawal, keeping lists, and confabulation, or the fabrication of material to fill gaps in stories in response to questions about situations or events one is unable to recall. As mental deterioration or cognitive dysfunction occurs, personality and behavioral changes are seen, including angry accusations, suspiciousness, vulgar language, poor personal hygiene, disregard for rules and regulations, and vague, incomprehensible speech.

The causative factor in 50% to 60% of all senile persons is an irreversible deterioration of the brain, termed Alzheimer's disease. Other factors include a series of ministrokes due to high blood pressure, chronic substance abuse, neurologic diseases, brain tumors, and metabolic diseases. (See Chapter 23 for additional information.)

Table 32-2 is a comparison of characteristics distinguishing pseudodementia from dementia.

Zung (1980) differentiates between dementia and depression. The individual with the diagnosis of dementia exhibits clinical symptoms including labile emotion; decreased attention span; decreased memory for recent events; confabulation; repetition of the same statements (perseveration); impaired intellect; disorientation to time and place; poor judgment; deterioration in personal hygiene; loss of bladder and bowel control; vague somatic complaints; visual hallucinations and delusions; and neurologic symptoms of dysphasia, apraxia, and agnosia.

TABLE 32-2 PSEUDODEMENTIA AND DEMENTIA

Pseudodementia	Dementia
Rapid onset	Insidious indeterminant onset
Symptoms of short duration	Symptoms of long duration
Depressed mood	Mood and behavior fluctuate
Patient replies "don't know"	Patient gives "near-miss" answers
Patient focuses on disabilities	Patient conceals disabilities
Fluctuation in level of cognitive impairment	Level of cognitive impairment relatively stable

In contrast, the depressed individual's affect is not influenced by suggestion. There is difficulty in concentration with impaired learning of new knowledge; a decrease in attention span; and a decrease in recent memory. The depressed individual can complete serial 7s. Confusion, if present, is not as profound as in dementia. Judgment may be poor. Common somatic complaints include insomnia, decrease in appetite, weight loss, decreased libido, low energy, and constipation. Psychotic depression including clinical symptoms of auditory hallucinations and delusions may occur. No neurologic symptoms are present.

Delirium

Delirium is characterized by a disturbance of consciousness and impairment of attention that fluctuates during the course of the day. It is usually due to disturbance of brain physiology by a medical disorder or ingested substance, and is one of the most common psychiatric diagnoses in the elderly population.

Delirium is particularly important to identify because it is assumed to be a reversible disorder, although it may persist for months in hospitalized medical or surgical patients. Peskind and Raskind (1996) and Jung and Grossberg (1993) discuss common causes of delirium in the elderly. They are classified as systemic illness, metabolic disorders, neurologic disorders, pharmacologic adverse effects, and miscellaneous causes.

Common clinical symptoms frequently seen include hallucinations, illusions, delusions, agitation, disorientation, memory impairment, anxiety, and abnormal vital signs. (See Chapter 23 for additional information.)

 ## Transcultural Considerations

McKenna (1995) discusses transcultural perspectives in the nursing care of the elderly by stating that culture defines who is old. Culture also establishes rituals for identifying the elderly, sets socially acceptable roles and expectations for behavior in the elderly, and influences attitudes toward the aged (p. 228).

Aging is viewed as a positive experience by those persons who achieve integrity. Older persons find meaning in their lives by sharing their traditions and values with others. It is imperative that the nurse consider the elderly patient's perspective on aging in at least three general areas:

1. How the person perceives health and illness
2. What expectations the person has of care
3. How nursing can support culturally determined patterns of dealing with health and coping with illness

Transcultural considerations were discussed in various chapters, including those on nursing assessment of psychiatric patients, therapeutic interventions, theories of personality development, emotional responses to illness and hospitalization, and loss and grief. The reader is directed to these chapters for additional information regarding the psychosocial aspects of aging in culturally diverse societies.

Assessment and Nursing Diagnosis

It has been said that what looks like chronic organic mental syndrome may actually be clinical symptoms of congestive heart failure, pneumonia, or some other medical disorder. The assessment of elderly patients is multifaceted, focusing on the collection of demographic data, the interview process, and review of medical records.

Brummel-Smith (1986) discusses interviewing the older adult patient. The physical setting may be a decisive factor in making an interview or assessment effective. Adequate lighting is necessary because of possible reduced visual acuity. The interviewer should speak clearly and distinctly, facing the patient. It is important that the nurse introduce himself or herself initially and establish how the patient prefers to be addressed (surname or first name). If dentures are worn, they should be in place to avoid embarrassment or impaired communication. Questions that are open-ended allow the patient to respond without difficulty or fear of giving incorrect responses that could result in institutionalization or hospitalization. Older adults may initially be resistant to or resent questions regarding personal problems. Patients with memory impairment may "reminisce" because they cannot converse in the here-and-now. Therefore, it is important to consider whether a family member or health care surrogate should be interviewed to validate data or obtain additional information as needed.

Biologic aspects as well as social, economic, environmental, and spiritual factors must be considered. Laboratory screening tests include, but are not limited to the following:

Complete blood count
Blood glucose
Blood urea nitrogen
Blood creatinine
Serum electrolytes
Liver profile
Thyroid profile
Serology

Vitamin B_{12} and folic acid
Urinalysis
Electrocardiogram
Chest x-ray
Computed tomography scan with and without contrast
Magnetic resonance imaging
Electroencephalogram

Lee (1996) addresses the importance of understanding physiologic changes in the elderly. Health problems and polypharmacy can put patients at risk for adverse drug reactions. Hepatic and renal impairment dictate which symptoms. The psychiatric nurse must be aware of drugs that impair absorption, which drugs require sufficient serum protein levels for binding, and which drugs have prolonged half-lives that cause unwanted sedation.

Various assessment tools used to determine DSM-IV clinical diagnoses have been discussed or referred to throughout the text. They include Geriatric Depression Scale, Beck's Depression Scale, Mini-Mental State Exam, Short Portable Mental Status Questionnaire, Global Deterioration Rating Scale, Brief Cognitive Rating Scale, Rapid Disability Rating Scale, and Yale-Brown Obsessive Compulsive Scale. Box 32-2 contains an example of a form used during the assessment of geriatric patients who present with emotional or behavioral disturbances.

Examples of nursing diagnoses most frequently seen in the elderly community include agitation, anger, *anxiety, *ineffective individual coping, situational crises, depression, *fear, *dysfunctional grieving, *noncompliance, *altered thought processes, *sleep pattern disturbance, and *risk for self-directed violence. Brief nursing care plans addressing most of these nursing diagnoses are available for review in other chapters of the text.

Nursing Interventions

Gerontologic nursing is described as the process of assessing the health care needs of older people, planning and implementing health care to meet these needs, and evaluating the effectiveness of such care. Emphasis is placed on maximizing the older person's independence in the ADLs; preventing illness or disability; promoting, maintaining, and restoring health; or maintaining life in dignity and comfort until death ensues.

Geropsychiatric nursing interventions focus on Maslow's (1968) theory of motivation, in which he identified five levels of basic human needs, which are

*NANDA-approved nursing diagnosis.

BOX 32-2 Geropsychiatric Assessment

Name:
Date of Birth:
Sex:
Marital Status:
Religion:
Medical Diagnosis:
Medications (Include start dates, dosage adjustments, and medications
     previously taken):
Allergies:
Laboratory Findings (Include dates obtained):
Neurologic Findings (Include tests performed):
Presenting Symptoms:
     Mental Status:
     Functional Status:
     Behavioral Assessment:
History of Previous Psychiatric Treatment:
Support Systems (Include social functioning, financial resources, and
     family dynamics):
Family Input:

---

listed in Chapter 13. Using Maslow's concept enables the care-giver to meet more than just survival needs, a condition that occurs too frequently in nursing care.

The following are statements about the aging process that may be helpful as one plans nursing care to meet the psychological or emotional needs of elderly patients, whether they are seen as outpatients or inpatients:

1. People who suffer great difficulty in the process of aging have been somewhat emotionally frail all their lives. Such frailty may be due to unmet needs
   of psychological safety and security. Nursing care should be planned to meet
   these needs by
       Minimizing the amount of change to which the person is exposed
       Determining the person's previous life-style and encouraging the con-
           tinuance of that life-style as much as possible
       Explaining new routines, medications, or treatments
       Introducing change gradually
       Including the person in decision making
       Encouraging relocated, hospitalized, or institutionalized patients or
           family members to bring familiar items from home

2. Older persons have a need for love and belonging as well as a need to maintain their status in society. As they become older, it may be increasingly difficult for them to remain active or make contributions to society. If they feel unwanted, they may resort to telling stories about earlier achievements. Nursing interventions to meet the need for love and belongingness include

   Encouraging expression of affection, touch, and human sexuality

   Permitting the person to select a roommate when appropriate

   Providing opportunities to form new friendships and relationships with persons of varying ages

   Permitting flexible visiting hours with family or friends

   Providing privacy when desired

   Encouraging expression of feelings such as loneliness and the need to be loved

3. Irritating behavior usually is related to the elderly person's frustration, fear, or awareness of limitations rather than a physiologic deficit or the actual issue at hand. The older person needs to feel a sense of self-worth, to take pride in her or his abilities and accomplishments, and to be respected by others. Nursing interventions are planned to restore, preserve, and protect the elderly person's self-esteem by

   Encouraging participation in decision making pertaining to ADLs

   Identifying strengths to promote self-confidence and independence

   Encouraging the person to take pride in personal appearance

   Communicating clearly with the elderly person at an adult level

   Occasionally seeking the older person's advice

   Listening thoughtfully as the person reminisces about life experiences

4. Self-actualization of self-fulfillment occur only after the lower needs of survival, safety and security, love and belonging, and a positive sense of self-esteem have been met. Peck's concept of ego transcendence, discussed earlier in this chapter, describes the self-actualized person. Nursing interventions to promote self-fulfillment in the elderly include

   Promoting decision making and independence. The elderly person is encouraged to take responsibility for actions.

   Encouraging participation in activities or the development of hobbies to promote socialization, productivity, and creativity, as well as fostering a sense of accomplishment.

   Encouraging the person to be a resource person as well as a teacher of skills or crafts to younger generations. Such activities serve a useful purpose and earn the elderly person recognition.

   Working with the elderly person to meet the developmental task of dying

As aging persons prepare to meet the fourth task, they experience a life-review process in which they attempt to put their life in order. They reflect on what life means and on the finiteness of life. They may read philosophy, study religion, or discuss their accomplishments and failures. Discussing the accomplishments of elderly persons enhances their self-respect and prestige.

The following comments were made by student nurses who cared for residents of a nursing home during their geriatric nursing clinical rotation. They were asked to assess their assigned patients' needs as well as degree of independence. The comments address the needs just discussed.

> The first day I walked into Mrs. K's room she was responsive to questions but volunteered no information on her own. The second day I asked her if she remembered me and she stated "Yes, you are the one who made me laugh." . . . She responded to the radio and talked about different programs. I think she might have enjoyed my reading to her. . . . She definitely wanted to maintain her independence.
>
> My patients taught me to live today to the best of my ability, accept where I am in life, do the best I can at all times, and don't worry about tomorrow. . . . I tried to give them a little extra attention and let them know they were special, worthwhile people.
>
> Mrs. D. made a lot of progress while I cared for her. She attended activities, began talking more, enjoyed going outside, and would tell me her likes and dislikes. A person working with the elderly has to be a very patient and caring individual.
>
> BC showed me a positive outlook on life. She appeared happy that she had fulfilled all her goals and was satisfied with the way the years have gone by. She said she had her memories and that's what she treasured most. . . . Working with the elderly taught me something important. . . . We must realize that every elderly person was once a young person who had ambitions, dreams, and goals. . . . We need to take care of their emotional as well as physical needs.

The time to prepare people for the adjustment to growing older is during the middle years. Emphasis should be placed on the development of new interests, hobbies, and friendships that will assist them in filling extra hours available due to retirement, widowhood, or an illness. This primary prevention can be done by nurses assisting persons in the community, working with family members, or caring for patients in acute care settings.

 ## Summary

This chapter focused on the psychosocial aspects of aging by defining aging, briefly stating the theories of aging, and listing intrinsic and extrinsic factors influencing the aging process. Duvall's eight developmental tasks of aging and the impact on one's emotional needs were discussed. They include establishing satisfactory living arrangements; adjusting to retirement income, establishing comfortable routines; maintaining love, sex, and marital relationships; keeping active and involved; staying in touch with other family members; sustaining and maintaining physical and mental health; and finding meaning in life. Common emotional reactions or behaviors, such as anxiety, loneliness, guilt, depression, somatic complaints, paranoid reactions, dementia, and delirium were explained. A comparison of pseudodementia, depression, and dementia was given. Transcultural perspectives in the nursing care of the elderly were addressed. The multifaceted assessment process was explained. Examples of nursing diagnoses most frequently seen in the elderly community were cited. Nursing interventions were discussed, focusing on the need for psychological safety and security, love and belonging, self-esteem, and self-actualization.

Learning Activities

I. Clinical Activities
   A. Care for an elderly patient.
      1. Identify any unmet developmental tasks as described by Duvall.
      2. State identified emotional needs of the patient.
      3. Plan nursing interventions for unmet needs and tasks.
   B. Assess the patient's satisfaction with his or her life. Does the patient appear to be ego transcendent or ego preoccupied? Why?
   C. Obtain a copy of the Mini-Mental State Exam, Global Deterioration Rating Scale, Geriatric Depression Scale, or Beck's Depression Scale for discussion in clinical postconference.
II. Independent Activities
   A. Research the community to identify volunteer employment programs for the elderly.
   B. Contact a local senior citizen's club. What activities are available to members of the community? Are special discount rates for dining, attending movies, bowling, and other activities available to senior citizens?

Critical Thinking Questions

1. Visit a local retirement community. Interview several people about what it is like to get older and how they cope. What conclusions can you draw about coping skills and healthy aging?
2. How do you feel about growing older?
3. Using Peck's concept of ego transcendence, how might an elderly person help you and your classmates understand aging?

Self-Test

1. Define the aging process.
2. List the intrinsic factors that influence aging.
3. Describe the extrinsic factors that influence aging.
4. Compare the cellular and genetic theories of aging.
5. Describe Duvall's eight developmental tasks of the elderly.
6. State the components of ego transcendence.
7. List causative factors of the following emotional reactions or behaviors in the elderly person:
   Anxiety
   Loneliness
   Guilt
   Depression
   Somatic complaints
   Paranoid reactions
   Dementia or cognitive dysfunction
8. List the five levels of basic human needs identified by Maslow.
9. List at least two nursing interventions for each of the needs listed in question no. 8 in relation to elderly persons.
10. Explain why elderly patients may experience adverse side effects while taking psychotropic medication.
11. Define failure to thrive.
12. Differentiate between delirium and dementia.
13. Describe the data obtained during a geropsychiatric assessment.

SELECTED REFERENCES

American Psychiatric Association. (1991). *Comprehensive review of geriatric psychiatry.* Washington, DC: American Psychiatric Press.

Blazer, D. G. (1996). Epidemiology of psychiatric disorders in late life. In E. W. Busse & D. G. Blazer (Eds.). *Textbook of geriatric psychiatry* (2nd ed.). Washington, DC: American Psychiatric Press.

Blazer, D. G. (1994). Geriatric psychiatry. In R. E. Hales, S. C. Yudofsky, & J. A. Talbott (Eds.). *The American Psychiatric Press textbook of psychiatry* (2nd ed.). Washington, DC: American Psychiatric Press.

Brummel-Smith, K. (1986F). Interviewing the older adult. In A. J. Enelow & S. N. Swisher (Eds.). *Interviewing and patient care.* New York: Oxford University Press.

Burnside, I. (1975, November). Listen to the aged. *American Journal of Nursing.*

Burnside, I. (1981). *Nursing and the aged* (2nd ed.). New York: McGraw-Hill.

Busse, E. W. (1996). The myth, history, and science of aging. In E. W. Busse & D. G. Blazer (Eds.). *Textbook of geriatric psychiatry* (2nd ed.). Washington, DC: American Psychiatric Press.

Buntinx, F., Kester, A., Bergers, J., & Knottnerus, J. A. (1996, May). Is depression in elderly people followed by dementia? A retrospective cohort study based in general practice. *Age and Aging.*

Butler, R., & Lewis, M. (1982). *Aging and mental health: Positive psychosocial and biomedical approaches* (3rd ed). St. Louis: C. V. Mosby.

Dubin, S. (1996, May). Geriatric assessment. *American Journal of Nursing.*

Duvall, E. M. (1977). *Marriage and family development* (5th ed.). Philadelphia: J. B. Lippincott.

Ebersole, P., & Hess, P. (1985). *Toward healthy aging: Human needs and nursing response* (2nd ed.). St. Louis: C. V. Mosby.

Feinberg, M. (1997, January). Self-medication in the elderly: Principles for preventing complications. *Advance for Nurse Practitioners.*

Hall, P. (1996, October). Providing psychosocial support. *American Journal of Nursing.*

Havinghurst, R. J. (1968, August). Personality and patterns of aging. *Gerontologist.*

Jung, R. J., & Grossberg, G. T. (1993, July/August). Diagnosis and treatment of psychiatric disorders in the nursing home. *Nursing Home Medicine.*

Kimball, M. J., & Williams-Burgess, C. (1995, April). Failure to thrive: The silent epidemic of the elderly. *Archives of Psychiatric Nursing.*

Lee, M. L. (1996, July). Drugs and the elderly: Do you know the risks? *American Journal of Nursing.*

Leininger, M. (1995). *Transcultural nursing concepts, theories, research, and practice.* New York: McGraw-Hill.

Maslow, A. H. (1968). *Toward a psychology of being.* New York: D. Van Nostrand.

McKenna, M. A. (1995). Transcultural perspectives in the nursing care of the elderly. In M. M. Andrews & J. S. Boyle (Eds.). *Transcultural concepts in nursing care* (2nd ed.). Philadelphia: J. B. Lippincott.

National Institute on Aging. (1981, October). *Age page: Sexuality in later life.* Washington, DC: U.S. Department of Health and Human Services.

Peskind, E. R., & Raskind, M. A. (1996). Cognitive disorders. In E. W. Busse & D. G. Blazer (Eds.). *Textbook of geriatric psychiatry* (2nd ed.). Washington, DC: American Psychiatric Press.

Schrock, M. M. (1980). *Holistic assessment of the healthy aged.* New York: John Wiley & Sons.

Taeuber, C. M. (1993f). *Sixty-five plus in America.* Malta: United Nations International Institute on Aging.

Valente, S. M. (1994, December). Recognizing depression in the elderly. *American Journal of Nursing.*

Walker, J. I. (1982). *Everybody's guide to emotional well-being.* San Francisco: Harbor Publishing.

Wantz, M., & Gay, J. (1981). *The aging process: A health perspective.* Cambridge: Winthrop Publishers.

Zung, W. W. K. (1980). Affective disorders. In E. W. Busse (Ed.). *Handbook of geriatric psychiatry.* New York: Van Nostrand Reinhold.

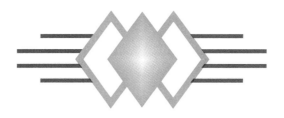

CHAPTER 33

PSYCHIATRIC PATIENTS WITH MEDICAL PROBLEMS/SYNDROMES

P hysical illness is highly prevalent among psychiatric patients. Individuals exhibiting emotional or psychiatric difficulties in the general hospital setting may require the use of psychotropic medication and adjunctive therapy to stabilize their conditions. These individuals would be better served by a unit that offers integrated care.

Fogel, 1989

1 Describe the rationale for the use of a med/psych unit.

2 List examples of admission criteria for a med/psych unit.

3 Give examples of medically ill patients admitted to a med/psych unit.

4 Discuss the symptoms and treatment of neuroleptic malignant syndrome.

5 State the qualifications of a nurse working on a med/psych unit.

6 Discuss the type of therapies available to patients with concurrent medical and psychiatric disorders.

❁ Admission Criteria

Admission to a med/psych unit is governed by diagnostic-related groupings (DRGs) and DSM-IV criteria. There are two types of such units. The first type (DRG-driven) states that the psychiatric patient with a medical problem must be discharged as soon as the medical disorder has stabilized. For example, if a person is admitted with unstable diabetes and has bipolar disorder, the DRG criteria for diabetes dictate the patient's length of stay on the unit. The second type (DSM-IV–driven) states that the person must have an unstable psychiatric disorder that adversely affects the medical condition, thus requiring hospitalization to treat both conditions. The psychiatric or psychological factors may influence the course of the general medical condition, may interfere with treatment of the general medical condition, or may constitute an additional health risk for the individual. The factors may precipitate or exacerbate symptoms of a general medical condition by eliciting stress-related physiologic responses (e.g., causing bronchospasm in individuals with asthma). Discharge occurs when both the psychiatric and physiologic disorders are stabilized.

Specific admission criteria may differ, also. One such unit states that a patient would be admitted if he or she is not actively suicidal, homicidal, or at risk for elopement; whereas a second unit admits actively suicidal patients.

Prescribing psychotropic medications in medically ill patients requires careful risk–benefit assessment (Stoudemire, Moran, & Fogel, 1995). Examples of medical conditions that may be seen on a med/psych unit include pseudoparkinsonism, lithium toxicity, seizure disorder, closed head injury, renal failure, metastatic carcinoma, and benign prostatic hypertrophy. Individuals with sleep disorders or those persons who need medical clearance for electroconvulsive therapy (ECT) may also be admitted to a med/psych unit.

Neuroleptic Malignant Syndrome

Neuroleptic malignant syndrome (NMS) is an uncommon, potentially fatal complication of neuroleptic treatment (less than 0.9%). It is characterized by the following clinical symptoms that can occur within 24 to 72 hours of administration of the first dose of medication:

1. Hyperpyrexia
2. Severe parkinsonism with muscle rigidity, catatonic appearance, or tremors
3. Elevated creatinine phosphokinase (CPK) blood levels
4. Elevated white blood count
5. Periods of altered consciousness manifested by dazed mutism, agitation, confusion, or comatose appearance alternating with periods of alertness
6. Elevated pulse
7. Hypertension with elevated diastolic pressure
8. Elevated liver enzymes
9. Profuse diaphoresis
10. Myoglobin in plasma
11. Difficulty swallowing and speaking
12. Excessive salivation

Symptoms persist for 5 to 10 days or longer in patients receiving oral short-acting antipsychotics and for 20 to 30 days or longer after fluphenazine (Prolixin) injections. Antipsychotic drugs that have caused the occurrence of NMS include Stelazine, Thorazine, Navane, Prolixin, Prolixin Depot, Haldol, and Mellaril (Maxmen, 1991; Stoudemire et al., 1995).

Care must be taken to consider all of the clinical symptoms in diagnosing NMS and not rely on two or three symptoms. For example, elevated CPKs can be seen in patients receiving intramuscular injections. Patients on neuroleptics frequently have difficulty swallowing and may exhibit excessive salivation. It is important to have a neurologic evaluation of the patient with suspected NMS. Psychological/emotional needs are also assessed while hospitalized on the unit.

Treatment is symptomatic to reduce fever and decrease elevated blood pressure. Careful monitoring and titration of medication is required as the syndrome can recur after the neuroleptic has been stopped (Masters & Spitler, 1986). Bromocriptine mesylate (Parlodel), a dopamine agonist, and dantrolene sodium (Dantrium), a peripheral muscle relaxant, have been used alone and together to treat NMS.

Neuroleptic malignant syndrome may develop after the removal of antiparkinsonian agents. The risk of recurrence on reexposure to neuroleptics may be minimized by delaying rechallenge by two weeks post-NMS and by using an alternative neuroleptic. ECT may be given to manage acute psychotic symptoms during NMS. Clozapine may be used if the patient is unable to tolerate other neuroleptics (Stoudemire et al., 1995).

 ## Staff Development

"As in all med/psych units, the quality of the nurses and their ability to deliver integrated care is a critical factor determining the program's success. Nurses must be cross-trained to perform both medical and psychiatric nursing" (Bruns & Stoudemire, 1990).

Because the concept of medical psychiatry is relatively new, there is little in the way of integration in training. Historically, psychiatric nurses have performed psychiatric nursing duties, and medical/surgical nurses have taken care of medical/surgical patients. Therefore, staff development focuses on both aspects of nursing care. Psychiatric nurses, who are trained to care for the mentally/emotionally ill, may need to be reeducated with courses including review of intravenous therapy, tracheotomy care, Foley catheterization, oxygen administration, interpretation of laboratory values, understanding of radiographic findings, electrocardiogram readings, and arterial blood gas results. Medical/surgical or intensive care nurses, who are already well versed in the above procedures, may need courses pertaining to psychiatric nursing. Included in such courses are sessions on the developmental and psychosocial needs of the elderly, neuropsychological assessment, communication skills, psychopharmacologic drug reactions and interactions, ECT, behavior modification, and the medical and psychiatric dynamics in the care of patients with dementia.

 ## Role of the Multidisciplinary Treatment Team

The core of the treatment team is the nursing staff, who function as a primary care model. Nurses use their professional skills to develop a nursing care plan that promotes holistic health care. Because of coexisting psychiatric and medical disorders, a variety of nursing diagnoses may be used.

The following are examples of nursing diagnoses used in the med/psych setting:

1. *Self-care deficit: poor grooming habits related to decreased interest in appearance, inability to make decisions, and feelings of worthlessness
2. *Ineffective individual coping: anger related to internal conflicts (guilt, low self-esteem) and feelings of rejection

*NANDA-approved nursing diagnosis.

3. *Impaired social interactions related to alienation from others due to constant complaining, ruminations, or loss of pleasure from relationship
4. *Ineffective individual coping: excessive physical complaints (without organic etiology) related to inability to express emotional needs directly
5. *Social isolation related to inability to initiate activities secondary to low energy levels
6. *Dysfunctional grieving: pathologic pattern related to unresolved grief secondary to prolonged denial and repression

Included on the treatment team is a psychiatric social worker whose duties are to assist in defining the patient's aftercare needs and in determining placement requirements. Another member of the team is the recreational therapist/adjunctive therapist. This member focuses on each patient's capabilities and cognitive skills. The therapist's assessment and input are useful in completing the plan of treatment. The head of the treatment team is the unit psychiatrist. He or she meets once a week with the team and other psychiatrists to assess each patient's progress and establish new goals. If the patient or family members are able to attend the meeting, they are encouraged to actively participate in setting goals.

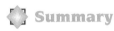 Summary

This chapter focused on the admission criteria, staff development, and the role of the multidisciplinary staff on a med/psych unit. Examples of concurrent medical problems, including NMS, were given. Nursing diagnoses used in the med/psych setting were cited.

Learning Activities

I. Clinical Activities
   A. Assess the patients on your assigned unit regarding the presence of a physical illness concurrent with a psychiatric disorder.
   B. Using the admission criteria in this chapter, identify those patients who would benefit from treatment on a med/psych unit.
II. Independent Activities
   A. Read "Neuroleptic Malignant Syndrome: Recognizing the Unrecognized Killer" by Hooper, Herren, and Goldwasser.
   B. Compare the clinical symptoms of the three case studies.
   C. Develop a plan of care for each. Refer to Carpenito (1995, p. 1046) for interventions related to NMS.

*NANDA-approved nursing diagnosis.

Critical Thinking Questions

1. Health care reform is exploring ways to cut costs. Develop a case to support the cost effectiveness of a med/psych unit.
2. Discuss with the members of a multidisciplinary team how they approach the patient. What are their priorities? What conflicts might occur if differences aren't appreciated?
3. What difficulties might you anticipate in staff nurses who work on a med/psych unit?

Self-Test

1. Describe the following aspects of a med/psych unit:
   Admission criteria
   Examples of diagnoses meeting admission criteria
   The role of the nurse
   Therapies available on the unit

2. Explain neuroleptic malignant syndrome.

3. State the medical treatment of neuroleptic malignant syndrome.

SELECTED REFERENCES

American Psychiatric Association. (1994). *Diagnostic and statistical manual of mental disorders* (4th ed.). Washington, DC: Author.

Blair, D. T., & Dauner, A. (1993, February). Neuroleptic malignant syndrome: Liability in nursing practice. *Journal of Psychosocial Nursing and Mental Health Services.*

Bruns, W., & Stoudemire, A. (1990, December). Development of a medical–psychiatric program within the private sector. *General Hospital Psychiatry.*

Carpenito, L. J. (1995). *Nursing diagnosis: Application to clinical practice* (6th ed.). Philadelphia: J. B. Lippincott.

Cowart, T., & Stoudemire, A. (1989, November). Nursing staff development and facility design for medical–psychiatry units. *General Hospital Psychiatry.*

Fogel, B. S. (1989, November). Med–psych units. *General Hospital Psychiatry.*

Fulop, G., & Strain, J. J. (1991, April). Diagnosis and treatment of psychiatric disorders in medically ill inpatients. *Hospital and Community Psychiatry.*

Hooper, J. F., Herren, C. K., & Goldwasser, H. (1989, July). Neuroleptic malignant syndrome: Recognizing an unrecognized killer. *Journal of Psychosocial Nursing and Mental Health Services.*

Lazarus, A., Mann, S. C., & Caroff, S. N. (1989). *The neuroleptic malignant syndrome and related conditions.* Washington, DC: American Psychiatric Press.

Masters, J. C., & Spitler, R. (1986, September). Neuroleptic malignant syndrome. *Journal of Psychosocial Nursing and Mental Health Services.*

Maxmen, J. S. (1991). *Psychotropic drugs fast facts.* New York: W. W. Norton.

Smith, R. G. (1991, June). *Somatization disorder in the medical setting.* Washington, DC: American Psychiatric Press.

Stoudemire, A., & Fogel, B. S. (1987). *Principles of medical psychiatry.* Orlando, FL: Grune and Stratton.

Stoudemire, A., Moran, M. G., & Fogel, B. S. (1995). Psychopharmacology in the medically ill patient. In A. F. Schatzberg & C. B. Nemeroff (Eds.). *American Psychiatric Press textbook of psychopharmacology.* Washington, DC: American Psychiatric Press.

Young, L. S., & Harsch, H. H. (1989, November). Length of stay on a psychiatry–medicine unit. *General Hospital Psychiatry.*

APPENDIX A

NURSING ASSESSMENT
OF THE ADULT/ADOLESCENT

TO BE COMPLETED WITHIN 8 HOURS OF ADMISSION

I. NAME: _____

DATE _____ TIME _____ UNIT _____

INFORMANT: _____

DATE OF BIRTH: _____ SEX: ____ RELIGION: _____ MARITAL STATUS: ☐ S ☐ M ☐ W ☐ D

OCCUPATION: _____ EDUCATION: _____ LANGUAGES: _____

NEXT OF KIN: _____ RELATIONSHIP: _____ PHONE NO: _____

ADDRESS OF NEXT OF KIN: _____

FAMILY OR REFERRING PHYSICIAN: _____

LEGAL STATUS:
☐ Voluntary BA40
☐ Treatment Form BA42
☐ Right to Release BA51
☐ Emergency Admission BA52B
☐ Involuntary Placement BA32
☐ Notice of Right to Petition BA36
☐ Exparte Court Order BA3001

PREVIOUS ADMISSION TO UNIVERSITY BEHAVIORAL CENTER?
☐ YES ☐ NO

BODY IDENTIFICATION MARKS.
(DRAW ALL SCARS, BRUISES, TATTOOS, ETC.)

PROSTHESIS: _____

DENTURES: _____

GLASSES: _____

CONTACT LENSES: _____

GLASS EYE: _____

LIMBS: _____

HEARING AID: _____

HAIRPIECE: _____

OTHER: _____

What is the reason you are coming into the hospital? (Describe the precipitating events, stress, etc.) _____

What problems are you having that you would like help with? _____

UNIVERSITY BEHAVIORAL CENTER
ORLANDO, FLORIDA

PATIENT ID

617

II. DAILY LIVING SITUATION

A. How do you spend your time each weekday and weekend? (*i.e.*, occupation, recreational activity, school, interests, hobbies, etc.) _____

_____

_____

_____

B. Where and with whom do you live? _____

_____

_____

C. What are your responsibilities at home? Has your performance changed at home or work? _____

_____

_____

D. What problems are there in your home? With whom? What would you like to be different at home?

_____

_____

_____

_____

_____

III. INDIVIDUAL MENTAL STATUS

A. Do you have thoughts that trouble you? _____

_____

B. Do you hear voices or see things that other people don't see or hear? (If so, describe them.)_____

_____

_____

C. What kind of future do you see for yourself? _____

_____

_____

D. What do you see as your strengths? _____

_____

Weaknesses? _____

E. (1) Have you ever thought of hurting yourself? Describe incident. _____

_____

_____

(2) Have you ever tried to hurt yourself? Describe incident. _____

_____

_____

F. (1) Have you ever thought of hurting someone else? Describe incident. _____

_____

_____

_____

F. (2) Have you ever attempted to hurt someone else? Describe incident. _____
_____

G. Describe your friendships. How do you relate to others? _____
_____

H. Have you noticed any changes in your sexual interest/functioning? _____
_____

IV. SCHOOL BEHAVIORS (For Adolescents)
1. Present grade in school _____
2. Number of days absent from school _____ Reasons _____
_____

3. Grade Point Average _____
4. Hx of fights at school _____
_____

5. Do you attend any special classes at school (ED or LD)? _____
_____

6. Do you consider yourself a follower or a leader? _____
7. In what extracurricular activities do you participate? _____
_____

8. What is your favorite class? _____
9. What is your relationship like with your teacher? _____
10. Have you run away from school or home? _____
11. Do you date? _____
12. Are you sexually active? _____
13. What birth control measures are you currently using? _____
14. Any Hx of sexually transmitted disorders (*e.g.* Gonorrhea, Syphilis, Herpes, AIDS)? _____

V. SUBSTANCE USE ASSESSMENT
A. Do you use any of the following? (Review and complete the chart below.)

SUBSTANCE	YES	NO	NAME	AMOUNT & FREQUENCY	DURATION	ROUTE
Coffee, Tea, Cola						
Tobacco						
Tranquilizers						
Barbiturates (downers)						
Stimulants (uppers & diet pills)						
Sleeping Pills						
Antidepressants						
Lithium						
Anticonvulsants						
Over-the-counter drugs (i.e., Aspirin, laxatives)						

SUBSTANCE	YES	NO	NAME	AMOUNT & FREQUENCY	DURATION	ROUTE
Alcohol						
Marijuana/Hashish						
PCP						
LSD, Hallucinogens						
Heroin						
Cocaine						
Methadone						
Glue, Aerosols						
Other						

    B. Please list date and name of chemical(s) last used _____

    C. Precipitating event (if any) _____

    D. Have you ever had blackouts? _____ Last episode _____

    E. Amount of drugs per week _____

    F. Have you ever tried to withdraw? _____

    G. What happened? (Check for hallucinations, confusion, tremors, seizures, D.T.'s etc.) _____

    H. Longest drug-free period over past 5 years _____

    I. How long have you been abusing? _____

    J. Ever treated for addiction? (Where, when, how long) _____

       Was treatment completed? _____

    K. What was successful about treatment? _____

       Ever on antabuse? _____ Any adverse reaction? _____ Helpful? _____

    L. Attend(ed) ☐ AA ☐ NA ☐ EA ☐ Alanon ☐ Alateen ☐ Other _____

       How often and how long? _____ Continued in followup (aftercare)? _____

       If no, why discontinued? _____

    M. Drug Screen: ☐ URINE ☐ SERUM: _____
                                  DATE

VI. PHYSICAL DATA

    A. Have you been sick for physical or mental health reasons? If so, were you hospitalized? _____

    B. Are you taking any prescribed medications (including birth control pills)? List name and dosage.

    C. Did you bring any of your medication to the hospital? ☐ YES ☐ NO

       Location in hospital? _____ Sent home _____

    D. Do you have any allergies? (specify drugs, food, environment and reaction) _____

E. Are you having problems with elimination? (bowel movements, urination)

_____

F. Do you require any assistance with your daily activities? (bathing, feeding self, ambulating independently) If so, explain. _____

_____

G. Tell me about your sleeping pattern. (number of hours, naps, changes in pattern, insomnia, nightmares) _____

_____

H. Tell me about your nutrition habits. (dietary restrictions, food, preferences, recent weight changes)

_____

_____

I. Is there anything else you would like to tell me that would help us in planning your treatment?

_____

_____

J. Vital Signs: Blood Pressure–Sitting _____ Standing _____

Temperature _____ Pulse _____ Respiration _____

K. Physical Characteristics:

Height _____ Weight _____ Eye Color _____ Hair Color _____

L. Family Medical History   ☐ Diabetes   ☐ Alcohol   ☐ Heart Disease

   ☐ Kidney Disease   ☐ Hypertension   ☐ Drugs   ☐ Arthritis   ☐ Stroke

   ☐ Epilepsy   ☐ Cancer   ☐ Mental Illness   ☐ T.B.   ☐ Other _____

M. Have you ever been pregnant?_____ ☐ para ☐ gravida

L.M.P. _____

NURSING INTERVIEW completed by: _____ ____/____/____

                                              Signature   Date

Doctor Notified: _____ _____

                                                                    TIME

VII. GENERAL DESCRIPTION OF PATIENT

1. Appearance:

    a. Facial expressions:

    ☐ Angry ☐ Cheerful ☐ Disinterested
    ☐ Blank ☐ Frowning ☐ Dissatisfied
    ☐ Happy ☐ Haggard ☐ Questioning
    ☐ Worn ☐ Smiling ☐ Bewildered
    ☐ Sad ☐ Tearful ☐ Interested

    b. Eyes:

    ☐ Open ☐ Sparkling ☐ Staring
    ☐ Closed ☐ Darting ☐ Fixed
    ☐ Pupils Dilated

    c. Complexion:

    ☐ Healthy ☐ Sallow ☐ Pasty
    ☐ Ruddy ☐ Other _____

    d. Grooming and dress:

    1. Clothing:

        ☐ Clean ☐ Soiled
        ☐ Ragged ☐ Wrinkled
        ☐ Pressed ☐ Burned

    2. Shoes:

        ☐ Shined ☐ Worn
        ☐ Scuffed

    3. Stockings:

        ☐ YES ☐ NO

    4. Socks:

        ☐ YES ☐ NO

    e. Body Language:

    1. Posture:

        ☐ Erect ☐ Sagging

    2. Movement:

        ☐ Normal ☐ Relaxed
        ☐ Slow ☐ Coordinated
        ☐ Fast ☐ Hyperactive

	HEAD	FACE	TORSO	EXTREMITIES
Trembling	☐	☐	☐	☐
Twitching	☐	☐	☐	☐
Spasms	☐	☐	☐	☐
Rocking	☐	☐	☐	☐
Immobile	☐	☐	☐	☐
Rigid	☐	☐	☐	☐
Tics	☐	☐	☐	☐

2. Behavior:

    ☐ Shy ☐ Oriented ☐ Impatient
    ☐ Bold ☐ Restless ☐ Attentive
    ☐ Aloof ☐ Euphoric ☐ Suspicious
    ☐ Bossy ☐ Sarcastic ☐ Ritualistic
    ☐ Alert ☐ Withdrawn ☐ Distrustful
    ☐ Labile ☐ Demanding ☐ Uninhibited
    ☐ Fearful ☐ Confident ☐ Distorted
    ☐ Playful ☐ Apathetic ☐ Apprehensive
    ☐ Confused ☐ Irritable ☐ Antagonistic
    ☐ Agitated ☐ Impulsive ☐ Distractible
    ☐ Critical ☐ Seductive

3. Communication:

    a. Tone: ☐ Soft ☐ Average
    ☐ Loud ☐ Clipped
    ☐ Whispering

    b. Speech difficulties: ☐ Language barrier
    ☐ Lisping ☐ Stuttering ☐ Other _____

    c. Flow of speech:

    ☐ Talkative ☐ Repetitious ☐ Guarded
    ☐ Average ☐ Relevant ☐ Constant Flow
    ☐ Hesitant ☐ Irrelevant ☐ Gregarious,
    ☐ Mumbles ☐ Mute   initiating
    ☐ Monosyllables ☐ Quiet,
                      noninitiating

4. Perception and Thinking:

    a. Intellectual functioning

    1. Impaired memory:

        ☐ YES ☐ NO
        ☐ Recent ☐ Remote

    2. Impaired judgment:

        ☐ YES ☐ NO

    3. Brief attention span:

        ☐ YES ☐ NO

    4. Lacks ability to concentrate:

        ☐ YES ☐ NO

    5. Misinterprets: ☐ YES ☐ NO

    6. Logical: ☐ YES ☐ NO

5. Self-evaluation:

    a. How do you see yourself?

    ☐ Polite ☐ Loving ☐ Honest
    ☐ Unkind ☐ Selfish ☐ Friendly
    ☐ Likable ☐ Reliable ☐ Cautious
    ☐ Dependent ☐ Easygoing ☐ Trustworthy
    ☐ Independent ☐ Considerate ☐ Short-tempered

    b. What is your usual mood? Has it changed? How?

    _____

VIII. MISCELLANEOUS CHECKLIST

    A. Patient given handbook: ☐ YES   ☐ NO

    B. Unit rules explained by staff: ☐ YES   ☐ NO

    C. Luggage and purse search completed: ☐ YES   ☐ NO

    D. Body search completed: ☐ YES   ☐ NO

    E. Valuables list completed: ☐ YES   ☐ NO

    F. Clothes list completed: ☐ YES   ☐ NO

    G. Summary and Recommendations:

_____ R.N.

APPENDIX B

DSM-IV CLASSIFICATION—
AXIS I AND II CATEGORIES
AND CODES

The official coding system in use in the United States is the International Classification of Diseases, Ninth Revision, Clinical Modification (ICD-9-CM). Most DSM-IV disorders have a numerical ICD-9-CM code that precedes the name of the disorder in each classification. The names of some disorders are followed by alternative terms enclosed in parentheses, which, in most cases, were the DSM-III-R names for the disorders.

An ellipsis (. . .) is used in the names of certain disorders to indicate that the name of a specific mental disorder or general medical condition should be inserted when recording the name (*e.g.*, 293.0 Delirium Due to Hypothyroidism).

An "x" appearing in a diagnostic code indicates that a specific code number is required.

If criteria are currently met, one of the following severity specifiers may be noted after the diagnosis:

Mild
Moderate
Severe

If criteria are no longer met, one of the following specifiers may be noted:

In Partial Remission
In Full Remission
Prior History

NOS = Not Otherwise Specified.

✦ Disorders Usually First Diagnosed in Infancy, Childhood, or Adolescence

Mental Retardation

Note: *These are coded on Axis II.*

317	Mild Mental Retardation
318.0	Moderate Mental Retardation
318.1	Severe Mental Retardation
318.2	Profound Mental Retardation
319	Mental Retardation, Severity Unspecified

Learning Disorders

315.00	Reading Disorder
315.1	Mathematics Disorder
315.2	Disorder of Written Expression
315.9	Learning Disorder NOS

Motor Skills Disorder

315.4	Developmental Coordination Disorder

Communication Disorders

315.31	Expressive Language Disorder
315.32	Mixed Receptive-Expressive Language Disorder
315.39	Phonological Disorder
307.0	Stuttering
307.9	Communication Disorder NOS

Pervasive Developmental Disorders

299.00	Autistic Disorder
299.80	Rett's Disorder
299.10	Childhood Disintegrative Disorder
299.80	Asperger's Disorder
299.80	Pervasive Developmental Disorder NOS

Attention-deficit and Disruptive Behavior Disorders

314.xx	Attention-Deficit/Hyperactivity Disorder
.01	Combined Type
.00	Predominantly Inattentive Type
.01	Predominantly Hyperactive-Impulsive Type
314.9	Attention-Deficit/Hyperactivity Disorder NOS
312.xx	Conduct Disorder (former code: 312.8)
.81	Childhood-Onset Type

.82 Adolescent-Onset Type
.89 Unspecified Onset

Feeding and Eating Disorders of Infancy or Early Childhood

307.52 Pica
307.53 Rumination Disorder
307.59 Feeding Disorder of Infancy or Early Childhood

Tic Disorders

307.23 Tourette's Disorder
307.22 Chronic Motor or Vocal Tic Disorder
307.21 Transient Tic Disorder
   Specify if: Single Episode/Recurrent
307.20 Tic Disorder NOS

Elimination Disorders

___.___ Encopresis
787.6   With Constipation and Overflow Incontinence
307.7   Without Constipation and Overflow Incontinence
307.6 Enuresis (Not Due to a General Medical Condition)
   Specify type: Nocturnal Only/Diurnal Only/Nocturnal and Diurnal

Other Disorders of Infancy, Childhood, or Adolescence

309.21 Separation Anxiety Disorder
   Specify if: Early Onset
313.23 Selective Mutism
313.89 Reactive Attachment Disorder of Infancy or Early Childhood
   Specify type: Inhibited Type/Disinhibited Type
307.3 Stereotypic Movement Disorder
   Specify if: With Self-Injurious Behavior
313.9 Disorder of Infancy, Childhood, or Adolescence NOS

❖ Delirium, Dementia, and Amnestic and Other Cognitive Disorders

Delirium

293.0 Delirium Due to . . . [*Indicate the General Medical Condition*]
___.___ Substance Intoxication Delirium (*refer to Substance-Related Disorders for substance-specific codes*)

___.___ Substance Withdrawal Delirium (*refer to Substance-Related Disorders for substance-specific codes*)

___.___ Delirium Due to Multiple Etiologies (*code each of the specific etiologies*)

780.09 Delirium NOS

Dementia

290.xx Dementia of the Alzheimer's Type, With Early Onset (*also code 331.0 Alzheimer's disease on Axis III*)

   .10   Uncomplicated

   .11   With Delirium

   .12   With Delusions

   .13   With Depressed Mood

        Specify if: With Behavioral Disturbance

290.xx Dementia of the Alzheimer's Type, With Late Onset (*also code 331.0 Alzheimer's disease on Axis III*)

   .0   Uncomplicated

   .3   With Delirium

   .20   With Delusions

   .21   With Depressed Mood

        Specify if: With Behavioral Disturbance

290.xx Vascular Dementia

   .40   Uncomplicated

   .41   With Delirium

   .42   With Delusions

   .43   With Depressed Mood

        Specify if: With Behavioral Disturbance

294.1 Dementia Due to HIV Disease (*also code 043.1 HIV infection affecting central nervous system on Axis III*)

294.1 Dementia Due to Head Trauma (*also code 854.00 head injury on Axis III*)

294.1 Dementia Due to Parkinson's Disease (*also code 332.0 Parkinson's disease on Axis III*)

294.1 Dementia Due to Huntington's Disease (*also code 333.4 Huntington's disease on Axis III*)

290.10 Dementia Due to Pick's Disease (*also code 331.1 Pick's disease on Axis III*)

290.10 Dementia Due to Creutzfeldt-Jakob Disease (*also code 046.1 Creutzfeldt-Jakob disease on Axis III*)

294.1 Dementia Due to . . . [Indicate the General Medical Condition not listed above] (*also code the general medical condition on Axis III*)

___.___ Substance-Induced Persisting Dementia (*refer to Substance-Related Disorders for substance-specific codes*)

_____.__ Dementia Due to Multiple Etiologies *(code each of the specific etiologies)*

294.8 Dementia NOS

Amnestic Disorders

294.0 Amnestic Disorder Due to . . . *[Indicate the General Medical Condition]*
Specify if: Transient/Chronic

_____.__ Substance-Induced Persisting Amnestic Disorder *(refer to Substance-Related Disorders for substance-specific codes)*

294.8 Amnestic Disorder NOS

Other Cognitive Disorders

294.9 Cognitive Disorder NOS

◈ Mental Disorders Due to a General Medical Condition not Elsewhere Classified

293.89 Catatonic Disorder Due to . . . *[Indicate the General Medical Condition]*

310.1 Personality Change Due to . . . *[Indicate the General Medical Condition]*
Specify type: Labile Type/Disinhibited Type/Aggressive Type/Apathetic Type/Paranoid Type/Other Type/Combined Type/Unspecified Type

293.9 Mental Disorder NOS Due to . . . *[Indicate the General Medical Condition]*

◈ Substance-related Disorders

[a]The following specifiers may be applied to Substance Dependence:
With Physiological Dependence/Without Physiological Dependence
Early Full Remission/Early Partial Remission
Sustained Full Remission/Sustained Partial Remission
On Agonist Therapy/In a Controlled Environment
The following specifiers apply to Substance-Induced Disorders as noted:
[I]With Onset During Intoxication/[W]With Onset During Withdrawal

Alcohol-related Disorders
Alcohol Use Disorders

303.90 Alcohol Dependence[a]

305.00 Alcohol Abuse

Alcohol-induced Disorders

303.00   Alcohol Intoxication
291.81   Alcohol Withdrawal
            Specify if: With Perceptual Disturbances
291.0   Alcohol Intoxication Delirium
291.0   Alcohol Withdrawal Delirium
291.2   Alcohol-Induced Persisting Dementia
291.1   Alcohol-Induced Persisting Amnestic Disorder
291.x   Alcohol-Induced Psychotic Disorder
    .5   With Delusions[I,W]
    .3   With Hallucinations[I,W]
291.89   Alcohol-Induced Mood Disorder[I,W]
291.89   Alcohol-Induced Anxiety Disorder[I,W]
291.89   Alcohol-Induced Sexual Dysfunction[I]
291.89   Alcohol-Induced Sleep Disorder[I,W]
291.9   Alcohol-Related Disorder NOS

Amphetamine (or Amphetamine-like)–related Disorders

Amphetamine Use Disorders

304.40   Amphetamine Dependence[a]
305.70   Amphetamine Abuse

Amphetamine-induced Disorders

292.89   Amphetamine Intoxication
            Specify if: With Perceptual Disturbances
292.0   Amphetamine Withdrawal
292.81   Amphetamine Intoxication Delirium
292.xx   Amphetamine-Induced Psychotic Disorder
    .11   With Delusions[I]
    .12   With Hallucinations[I]
292.84   Amphetamine-Induced Mood Disorder[I,W]
292.89   Amphetamine-Induced Anxiety Disorder[I]
292.89   Amphetamine-Induced Sexual Dysfunction[I]
292.89   Amphetamine-Induced Sleep Disorder[I,W]
292.9   Amphetamine-Related Disorder NOS

Caffeine-related Disorders

Caffeine-induced Disorders

305.90   Caffeine Intoxication
292.89   Caffeine-Induced Anxiety Disorder[I]
292.89   Caffeine-Induced Sleep Disorder[I]
292.9   Caffeine-Related Disorder NOS

Cannabis-related Disorders
Cannabis Use Disorders
304.30   Cannabis Dependence[a]
305.20   Cannabis Abuse

Cannabis-induced Disorders
292.89   Cannabis Intoxication
          Specify if: With Perceptual Disturbances
292.81   Cannabis Intoxication Delirium
292.xx   Cannabis-Induced Psychotic Disorder
  .11   With Delusions[I]
  .12   With Hallucinations[I]
292.89   Cannabis-Induced Anxiety Disorder[I]
292.9   Cannabis-Related Disorder NOS

Cocaine-related Disorders
Cocaine Use Disorders
304.20   Cocaine Dependence[a]
305.60   Cocaine Abuse

Cocaine-induced Disorders
292.89   Cocaine Intoxication
          Specify if: With Perceptual Disturbances
292.0   Cocaine Withdrawal
292.81   Cocaine Intoxication Delirium
292.xx   Cocaine-Induced Psychotic Disorder
  .11   With Delusions[I]
  .12   With Hallucinations[I]
292.84   Cocaine-Induced Mood Disorder[I,W]
292.89   Cocaine-Induced Anxiety Disorder[I,W]
292.89   Cocaine-Induced Sexual Dysfunction[I]
292.89   Cocaine-Induced Sleep Disorder[I,W]
292.9   Cocaine-Related Disorder NOS

Hallucinogen-related Disorders
Hallucinogen Use Disorders
304.50   Hallucinogen Dependence[a]
305.30   Hallucinogen Abuse

Hallucinogen-induced Disorders
292.89   Hallucinogen Intoxication
292.89   Hallucinogen Persisting Perception Disorder (Flashbacks)
292.81   Hallucinogen Intoxication Delirium

292.xx Hallucinogen-Induced Psychotic Disorder
   .11   With Delusions[I]
   .12   With Hallucinations[I]
292.84 Hallucinogen-Induced Mood Disorder[I]
292.89 Hallucinogen-Induced Anxiety Disorder[I]
292.9   Hallucinogen-Related Disorder NOS

Inhalant-related Disorders
Inhalant Use Disorders
304.60 Inhalant Dependence[a]
305.90 Inhalant Abuse

Inhalant-induced Disorders
292.89 Inhalant Intoxication
292.81 Inhalant Intoxication Delirium
292.82 Inhalant-Induced Persisting Dementia
292.xx Inhalant-Induced Psychotic Disorder
   .11   With Delusions[I]
   .12   With Hallucinations[I]
292.84 Inhalant-Induced Mood Disorder[I]
292.89 Inhalant-Induced Anxiety Disorder[I]
292.9   Inhalant-Related Disorder NOS

Nicotine-related Disorders
Nicotine Use Disorder
305.10 Nicotine Dependence[a]

Nicotine-induced Disorder
292.0   Nicotine Withdrawal
292.9   Nicotine-Related Disorder NOS

Opioid-related Disorders
Opioid Use Disorders
304.00 Opioid Dependence[a]
305.50 Opioid Abuse

Opioid-induced Disorders
292.89 Opioid Intoxication
       Specify if: With Perceptual Disturbances
292.0   Opioid Withdrawal
292.81 Opioid Intoxication Delirium

292.xx   Opioid-Induced Psychotic Disorder
   .11   With Delusions[I]
   .12   With Hallucinations[I]
292.84   Opioid-Induced Mood Disorder[I]
292.89   Opioid-Induced Sexual Dysfunction[I]
292.89   Opioid-Induced Sleep Disorder[I,W]
292.9   Opioid-Related Disorder NOS

Phencyclidine (or Phencyclidine-like)–related Disorders
Phencyclidine Use Disorders
304.60   Phencyclidine Dependence[a]
305.90   Phencyclidine Abuse

Phencyclidine-induced Disorders
292.89   Phencyclidine Intoxication
            Specify if: With Perceptual Disturbances
292.81   Phencyclidine Intoxication Delirium
292.xx   Phencyclidine-Induced Psychotic Disorder
   .11   With Delusions[I]
   .12   With Hallucinations[I]
292.84   Phencyclidine-Induced Mood Disorder[I]
292.89   Phencyclidine-Induced Anxiety Disorder[I]
292.9   Phencyclidine-Related Disorder NOS

Sedative-, Hypnotic-, or Anxiolytic-related Disorders
Sedative, Hypnotic, or Anxiolytic Use Disorders
304.10   Sedative, Hypnotic, or Anxiolytic Dependence[a]
305.40   Sedative, Hypnotic, or Anxiolytic Abuse

Sedative-, Hypnotic-, or Anxiolytic-induced Disorders
292.89   Sedative, Hypnotic, or Anxiolytic Intoxication
292.0   Sedative, Hypnotic, or Anxiolytic Withdrawal
            Specify if: With Perceptual Disturbances
292.81   Sedative, Hypnotic, or Anxiolytic Intoxication Delirium
292.81   Sedative, Hypnotic, or Anxiolytic Withdrawal Delirium
292.82   Sedative-, Hypnotic-, or Anxiolytic-Induced Persisting Dementia
292.83   Sedative-, Hypnotic-, or Anxiolytic-Induced Persisting Amnestic Disorder
292.xx   Sedative-, Hypnotic-, or Anxiolytic-Induced Psychotic Disorder
   .11   With Delusions[I,W]
   .12   With Hallucinations[I,W]

292.84   Sedative-, Hypnotic-, or Anxiolytic-Induced Mood Disorder[I,W]
292.89   Sedative-, Hypnotic-, or Anxiolytic-Induced Anxiety Disorder[W]
292.89   Sedative-, Hypnotic-, or Anxiolytic-Induced Sexual Dysfunction[I]
292.89   Sedative-, Hypnotic-, or Anxiolytic-Induced Sleep Disorder[I,W]
292.9   Sedative-, Hypnotic-, or Anxiolytic-Related Disorder NOS

Polysubstance-related Disorder
304.80   Polysubstance Dependence[a]

Other (or Unknown) Substance-related Disorders
Other (or Unknown) Substance Use Disorders
304.90   Other (or Unknown) Substance Dependence[a]
305.90   Other (or Unknown) Substance Abuse

Other (or Unknown) Substance-induced Disorders
292.89   Other (or Unknown) Substance Intoxication
         Specify if: With Perceptual Disturbances
292.0   Other (or Unknown) Substance Withdrawal
         Specify if: With Perceptual Disturbances
292.81   Other (or Unknown) Substance-Induced Delirium
292.82   Other (or Unknown) Substance-Induced Persisting Dementia
292.83   Other (or Unknown) Substance-Induced Persisting Amnestic
         Disorder
292.xx   Other (or Unknown) Substance-Induced Psychotic Disorder
   .11   With Delusions[I,W]
   .12   With Hallucinations[I,W]
292.84   Other (or Unknown) Substance-Induced Mood Disorder[I,W]
292.89   Other (or Unknown) Substance-Induced Anxiety Disorder[I,W]
292.89   Other (or Unknown) Substance-Induced Sexual Dysfunction[I]
292.89   Other (or Unknown) Substance-Induced Sleep Disorder[I,W]
292.9   Other (or Unknown) Substance-Related Disorder NOS

Schizophrenia and Other Psychotic Disorders

295.xx   Schizophrenia
The following Classification of Longitudinal Course applies to all subtypes of Schizophrenia:
   Episodic With Interepisode Residual Symptoms
      (*specify if*: With Prominent Negative Symptoms)/Episodic With No
      Interepisode Residual Symptoms
   Continuous
      (*specify if*: With Prominent Negative Symptoms)

Single Episode in Partial Remission
    (*specify if*: With Prominent Negative Symptoms)/Single Episode In Full Remission
Other or Unspecified Pattern
    .30 Paranoid Type
    .10 Disorganized Type
    .20 Catatonic Type
    .90 Undifferentiated Type
    .60 Residual Type
295.40 Schizophreniform Disorder
    Specify if: Without Good Prognostic Features/With Good Prognostic Features
295.70 Schizoaffective Disorder
    Specify type: Bipolar Type/Depressive Type
297.1 Delusional Disorder
    Specify type: Erotomanic Type/Grandiose Type/Jealous Type/Persecutory Type/Somatic Type/Mixed Type/Unspecified Type
298.8 Brief Psychotic Disorder
    Specify if: With Marked Stressor(s)/Without Marked Stressor(s)/With Postpartum Onset
297.3 Shared Psychotic Disorder
293.xx Psychotic Disorder Due to . . . [*Indicate the General Medical Condition*]
    .81   With Delusions
    .82   With Hallucinations
___.__ Substance-Induced Psychotic Disorder (*refer to Substance-Related Disorders for substance-specific codes*)
    Specify if: With Onset During Intoxication/With Onset During Withdrawal
298.9 Psychotic Disorder NOS

❖ Mood Disorders

Code current state of Major Depressive Disorder or Bipolar I Disorder in fifth digit:
    1 = Mild
    2 = Moderate
    3 = Severe Without Psychotic Features
    4 = Severe With Psychotic Features
        Specify: Mood-Congruent Psychotic Features/Mood-Incongruent Psychotic Features

5 = In Partial Remission
6 = In Full Remission
0 = Unspecified

The following specifiers apply (for current or most recent episode) to Mood Disorders as noted:

aSeverity/Psychotic/Remission Specifiers/bChronic/cWith Catatonic Features/ dWith Melancholic Features/eWith Atypical Features/fWith Postpartum Onset

The following specifiers apply to Mood Disorders as noted:

gWith or Without Full Interepisode Recovery/hWith Seasonal Pattern/iWith Rapid Cycling

Depressive Disorders

296.xx Major Depressive Disorder
  .2x Single Episodea,b,c,d,e,f
  .3x Recurrenta,b,c,d,e,f,g,h
300.4 Dysthymic Disorder
    Specify if: Early Onset/Late Onset
    Specify: With Atypical Features
311 Depressive Disorder NOS

Bipolar Disorders

296.xx Bipolar I Disorder
  .0x Single Manic Episodea,c,f
    Specify if: Mixed
  .40 Most Recent Episode Hypomanicg,h,i
  .4x Most Recent Episode Manica,c,f,g,h,i
  .6x Most Recent Episode Mixeda,c,f,g,h,i
  .5x Most Recent Episode Depresseda,b,c,d,e,f,g,h,i
  .7 Most Recent Episode Unspecifiedg,h,i
296.89 Bipolar II Disordera,b,c,d,e,f,g,h,i
    Specify (current or most recent episode): Hypomanic/Depressed
301.13 Cyclothymic Disorder
296.80 Bipolar Disorder NOS
293.83 Mood Disorder Due to . . . [*Indicate the General Medical Condition*]
    Specify type: With Depressive Features/With Major Depressive-Like Episode/With Manic Features/With Mixed Features
___.___ Substance-Induced Mood Disorder (*refer to Substance-Related Disorders for substance-specific codes*)
    Specify type: With Depressive Features/With Manic Features/With Mixed Features
    Specify if: With Onset During Intoxication/With Onset During Withdrawal
296.90 Mood Disorder NOS

Anxiety Disorders

300.01   Panic Disorder Without Agoraphobia
300.21   Panic Disorder With Agoraphobia
300.22   Agoraphobia Without History of Panic Disorder
300.29   Specific Phobia
         Specify type: Animal Type/Natural Environment Type/Blood-Injection-Injury Type/Situational Type/Other Type
300.23   Social Phobia
         Specify if: Generalized
300.3   Obsessive-Compulsive Disorder
         Specify if: With Poor Insight
309.81   Posttraumatic Stress Disorder
         Specify if: Acute/Chronic
         Specify if: With Delayed Onset
308.3   Acute Stress Disorder
300.02   Generalized Anxiety Disorder
293.84   Anxiety Disorder Due to . . . [*Indicate the General Medical Condition*]
         Specify if: With Generalized Anxiety/With Panic Attacks/With Obsessive-Compulsive Symptoms
___.__   Substance-Induced Anxiety Disorder (*refer to Substance-Related Disorders for substance-specific codes*)
         Specify if: With Generalized Anxiety/With Panic Attacks/With Obsessive-Compulsive Symptoms/With Phobic Symptoms
         Specify if: With Onset During Intoxication/With Onset During Withdrawal
300.00   Anxiety Disorder NOS

Somatoform Disorders

300.81   Somatization Disorder
300.82   Undifferentiated Somatoform Disorder
300.11   Conversion Disorder
         Specify type: With Motor Symptom or Deficit/With Sensory Symptom or Deficit/With Seizures or Convulsions/With Mixed Presentation
307.xx   Pain Disorder
    .80   Associated With Psychological Factors
    .89   Associated With Both Psychological Factors and a General Medical Condition
         Specify if: Acute/Chronic
300.7   Hypochondriasis
         Specify if: With Poor Insight

300.7   Body Dysmorphic Disorder
300.82   Somatoform Disorder NOS

✦ Factitious Disorders

300.xx   Factitious Disorder
    .16   With Predominantly Psychological Signs and Symptoms
    .19   With Predominantly Physical Signs and Symptoms
    .19   With Combined Psychological and Physical Signs and Symptoms
300.19   Factitious Disorder NOS

✦ Dissociative Disorders

300.12   Dissociative Amnesia
300.13   Dissociative Fugue
300.14   Dissociative Identity Disorder
300.6   Depersonalization Disorder
300.15   Dissociative Disorder NOS

✦ Sexual and Gender Identity Disorders

Sexual Dysfunctions

The following specifiers apply to all primary Sexual Dysfunctions:
    Lifelong Type/Acquired Type
    Generalized Type/Situational Type
    Due to Psychological Factors/Due to Combined Factors

Sexual Desire Disorders

302.71   Hypoactive Sexual Desire Disorder
302.79   Sexual Aversion Disorder

Sexual Arousal Disorders

302.72   Female Sexual Arousal Disorder
302.72   Male Erectile Disorder

Orgasmic Disorders

302.73   Female Orgasmic Disorder
302.74   Male Orgasmic Disorder
302.75   Premature Ejaculation

Sexual Pain Disorders

302.76 Dyspareunia (Not Due to a General Medical Condition)
306.51 Vaginismus (Not Due to a General Medical Condition)

Sexual Dysfunction Due
to a General Medical Condition

625.8 Female Hypoactive Sexual Desire Disorder Due to . . . [Indicate the General Medical Condition]

608.89 Male Hypoactive Sexual Desire Disorder Due to . . . [Indicate the General Medical Condition]

607.84 Male Erectile Disorder Due to . . . [Indicate the General Medical Condition]

625.0 Female Dyspareunia Due to . . . [Indicate the General Medical Condition]

608.89 Male Dyspareunia Due to . . . [Indicate the General Medical Condition]

625.8 Other Female Sexual Dysfunction Due to . . . [Indicate the General Medical Condition]

608.89 Other Male Sexual Dysfunction Due to . . . [Indicate the General Medical Condition]

___.__ Substance-Induced Sexual Dysfunction (refer to Substance-Related Disorders for substance-specific codes)
Specify if: With Impaired Desire/With Impaired Arousal/With Impaired Orgasm/With Sexual Pain
Specify if: With Onset During Intoxication

302.70 Sexual Dysfunction NOS

Paraphilias

302.4 Exhibitionism
302.81 Fetishism
302.89 Frotteurism
302.2 Pedophilia
Specify if: Sexually Attracted to Males/Sexually Attracted to Females/Sexually Attracted to Both
Specify if: Limited to Incest
Specify type: Exclusive Type/Nonexclusive Type

302.83 Sexual Masochism
302.84 Sexual Sadism
302.3 Transvestic Fetishism
Specify if: With Gender Dysphoria

302.82 Voyeurism
302.9 Paraphilia NOS

Gender Identity Disorders

302.xx Gender Identity Disorder
  .6   in Children
  .85   in Adolescents or Adults
          Specify if: Sexually Attracted to Males/Sexually Attracted to Females/Sexually Attracted to Both/Sexually Attracted to Neither
302.6   Gender Identity Disorder NOS
302.9   Sexual Disorder NOS

✦ Eating Disorders

307.1   Anorexia Nervosa
          Specify type: Restricting Type; Binge-Eating/Purging Type
307.51   Bulimia Nervosa
          Specify type: Purging Type/Nonpurging Type
307.50   Eating Disorder NOS

✦ Sleep Disorders

Primary Sleep Disorders

Dyssomnias

307.42   Primary Insomnia
307.44   Primary Hypersomnia
          Specify if: Recurrent
347   Narcolepsy
780.59   Breathing-Related Sleep Disorder
307.45   Circadian Rhythm Sleep Disorder
          Specify type: Delayed Sleep Phase Type/Jet Lag Type/Shift Work Type/Unspecified Type
307.47   Dyssomnia NOS

Parasomnias

307.47   Nightmare Disorder
307.46   Sleep Terror Disorder
307.46   Sleepwalking Disorder
307.47   Parasomnia NOS

Sleep Disorders Related to Another Mental Disorder

307.42   Insomnia Related to . . . *[Indicate the Axis I or Axis II Disorder]*
307.44   Hypersomnia Related to . . . *[Indicate the Axis I or Axis II Disorder]*

Other Sleep Disorders

780.xx   Sleep Disorder Due to . . . *[Indicate the General Medical Condition]*
   .52   Insomnia Type
   .54   Hypersomnia Type
   .59   Parasomnia Type
   .59   Mixed Type
___.___   Substance-Induced Sleep Disorder *(refer to Substance-Related Disorders for substance-specific codes)*
      Specify type: Insomnia Type/Hypersomnia Type/Parasomnia Type/ Mixed Type
      Specify if: With Onset During Intoxication/With Onset During Withdrawal

❂ Impulse-control Disorders Not Elsewhere Classified

312.34   Intermittent Explosive Disorder
312.32   Kleptomania
312.33   Pyromania
312.31   Pathological Gambling
312.39   Trichotillomania
312.30   Impulse-Control Disorder NOS

❂ Adjustment Disorders

309.xx   Adjustment Disorder
   .0   With Depressed Mood
   .24   With Anxiety
   .28   With Mixed Anxiety and Depressed Mood
   .3   With Disturbance of Conduct
   .4   With Mixed Disturbance of Emotions and Conduct
   .9   Unspecified
      Specify if: Acute/Chronic

❂ Personality Disorders

Note: *These are coded on Axis II.*
301.0   Paranoid Personality Disorder
301.20   Schizoid Personality Disorder
301.22   Schizotypal Personality Disorder

301.7 Antisocial Personality Disorder
301.83 Borderline Personality Disorder
301.50 Histrionic Personality Disorder
301.81 Narcissistic Personality Disorder
301.82 Avoidant Personality Disorder
301.6 Dependent Personality Disorder
301.4 Obsessive-Compulsive Personality Disorder
301.9 Personality Disorder NOS

Other Conditions That May Be a Focus of Clinical Attention

PSYCHOLOGICAL FACTORS AFFECTING MEDICAL CONDITION

316 . . . *[Specified Psychological Factor]* Affecting . . . *[Indicate the General Medical Condition]* Choose name based on nature of factors:
Mental Disorder Affecting Medical Condition
Psychological Symptoms Affecting Medical Condition
Personality Traits or Coping Style Affecting Medical Condition
Maladaptive Health Behaviors Affecting Medical Condition
Stress-Related Physiological Response Affecting Medical Condition
Other or Unspecified Psychological Factors Affecting Medical Condition

Medication-induced Movement Disorders

332.1 Neuroleptic-Induced Parkinsonism
333.92 Neuroleptic Malignant Syndrome
333.7 Neuroleptic-Induced Acute Dystonia
333.99 Neuroleptic-Induced Acute Akathisia
333.82 Neuroleptic-Induced Tardive Dyskinesia
333.1 Medication-Induced Postural Tremor
333.90 Medication-Induced Movement Disorder NOS

Other Medication-induced Disorder

995.2 Adverse Effects of Medication NOS

Relational Problems

V61.9 Relational Problem Related to a Mental Disorder or General Medical Condition
V61.20 Parent-Child Relational Problem

V61.10 Partner Relational Problem

V61.8 Sibling Relational Problem

V62.81 Relational Problem NOS

Problems Related to Abuse or Neglect

995.54 Physical Abuse of Child (*if focus of attention is on victim*)

995.53 Sexual Abuse of Child (*if focus of attention is on victim*)

995.52 Neglect of Child (*if focus of attention is on victim*)

___.___ Physical Abuse of Adult

V61.12 (*if by partner*)

V62.83 (*if by person other than partner*)

___.___ Sexual Abuse of Adult

V61.12 (*if by partner*)

V62.83 (*if by person other than partner*)

995.83 Sexual Abuse of Adult (*if focus of attention is on victim*)

Additional Conditions That May Be a Focus of Clinical Attention

V15.81 Noncompliance With Treatment

V65.2 Malingering

V71.01 Adult Antisocial Behavior

V71.02 Child or Adolescent Antisocial Behavior

V62.89 Borderline Intellectual Functioning

Note: *This is coded on Axis II.*

780.9 Age-Related Cognitive Decline

V62.82 Bereavement

V62.3 Academic Problem

V62.2 Occupational Problem

313.82 Identity Problem

V62.89 Religious or Spiritual Problem

V62.4 Acculturation Problem

V62.89 Phase of Life Problem

Additional Codes

300.9 Unspecified Mental Disorder (nonpsychotic)

V71.09 No Diagnosis or Condition on Axis I

799.9 Diagnosis or Condition Deferred on Axis I

V71.09 No Diagnosis on Axis II

799.9 Diagnosis Deferred on Axis II

Multiaxial System

Axis I   Clinical Disorders
             Other Conditions That May Be a Focus of Clinical Attention
Axis II   Personality Disorders
             Mental Retardation
Axis III   General Medical Conditions
Axis IV   Psychosocial and Environmental Problems
Axis V   Global Assessment of Functioning

APPENDIX C

NORTH AMERICAN NURSING DIAGNOSIS ASSOCIATION (NANDA) LIST OF APPROVED NURSING DIAGNOSES

Activity Intolerance
Activity Intolerance,
    Risk for
Adaptive Capacity:
    Intracranial,
    Decreased
Adjustment, Impaired
Airway Clearance,
    Ineffective
Anxiety
Aspiration, Risk for
Body Image Disturbance
Body Temperature,
    Risk for Altered
Breastfeeding, Effective
Breastfeeding, Ineffective

Breastfeeding,
    Interrupted
Breathing Pattern,
    Ineffective
Caregiver Role Strain
Caregiver Role Strain,
    Risk for
Communication,
    Impaired Verbal
Community Coping,
    Ineffective
Community Coping,
    Potential for
    Enhanced
Confusion, Acute
Confusion, Chronic

Constipation
Constipation, Colonic
Constipation, Perceived
Decisional Conflict
    (Specify)
Decreased Cardiac
    Output
Defensive Coping
Denial, Ineffective
Diarrhea
Disorganized Infant
    Behavior
Disorganized Infant
    Behavior, Risk for
Disuse Syndrome,
    Risk for

North American Nursing Diagnosis Association (1994). NANDA nursing diagnoses: Definitions and classification, 1995–1996. Philadelphia: NANDA.

Diversional Activity
Deficit
Dysfunctional Grieving
Dysfunctional Ventila-
tory Weaning
Response
Dysreflexia
Energy Field Disturbance
Environmental Inter-
pretation Syn-
drome, Impaired
Family Coping: Com-
promised, Ineffective
Family Coping: Dis-
abling, Ineffective
Family Coping: Poten-
tial for Growth
Family Process: Alco-
holism, Altered
Family Processes,
Altered
Fatigue
Fear
Fluid Volume Deficit
Fluid Volume Deficit,
Risk for
Fluid Volume Excess
Functional Incontinence
Gas Exchange, Impaired
Grieving, Anticipatory
Grieving, Dysfunctional
Growth and Develop-
ment, Altered
Health Maintenance,
Altered
Health Seeking Behav-
iors (Specify)
Home Maintenance
Management,
Impaired

Hopelessness
Hyperthermia
Hypothermia
Incontinence, Bowel
Incontinence,
Functional
Incontinence, Reflex
Incontinence, Stress
Incontinence, Total
Incontinence, Urge
Individual Coping,
Ineffective
Infant Feeding Pattern,
Ineffective
Infection, Risk for
Knowledge Deficit
(Specify)
Loneliness, Risk for
Management of Thera-
peutic Regimen:
Community,
Ineffective
Management of Thera-
peutic Regimen:
Families, Ineffective
Management of Thera-
peutic Regimen:
Individual, Effective
Management of Thera-
peutic Regimen
(Individuals), In-
effective Noncom-
pliance (Specify)
Memory, Impaired
Nutrition: Less than
body requirements,
Altered
Nutrition: More than
body requirements,
Altered

Nutrition: Potential for
more than body
requirements,
Altered
Oral Mucous Mem-
brane, Altered
Organized Infant
Behavior, Potential
for Enhanced
Pain
Pain, Chronic
Parent/Infant/Child
Attachment, Risk
for Altered
Parental Role Conflict
Parenting, Altered
Parenting, Risk for
Altered
Perioperative Position-
ing Injury, Risk for
Peripheral Neurovas-
cular Dysfunction,
Risk for
Personal Identity
Disturbance
Physical Mobility,
Impaired
Poisoning, Risk for
Post-Trauma Response
Powerlessness
Protection, Altered
Rape-Trauma Syndrome
Rape-Trauma Syn-
drome: Compound
Reaction
Rape-Trauma
Syndrome: Silent
Reaction
Relocation Stress
Syndrome

Role Performance, Altered
Self Care Deficit
  Bathing/Hygiene
  Feeding
  Dressing/Grooming
  Toileting
Self Esteem, Chronic Low
Self Esteem, Situational Low
Self Esteem Disturbance
Self-Mutilation, Risk for
Sensory/Perceptual Alterations (Specify) (visual, auditory, kinesthetic, gustatory, tactile, olfactory)

Sexual Dysfunction
Sexuality Patterns, Altered
Skin Integrity, Impaired
Skin Integrity, Risk for Impaired
Sleep Pattern Disturbance
Social Interaction, Impaired
Social Isolation
Spiritual Distress
Spiritual Well-Being, Potential for Enhanced
Suffocation, Risk for
Sustain Spontaneous Ventilation, Inability to
Swallowing, Impaired

Thermoregulation, Ineffective
Thought Processes, Altered
Tissue Integrity, Impaired
Tissue Perfusion, Altered (Specify Type) (Renal cerebral, cardiopulmonary, gastrointestinal, peripheral)
Trauma, Risk for
Unilateral Neglect
Urinary Elimination, Altered
Urinary Retention
Violence, Risk for: Self-directed or directed at others

GLOSSARY

Acute dystonic reaction Irregular, involuntary spastic muscle movements; wryneck; facial grimacing; abnormal eye movements or backward rolling of eyes in the sockets. May occur anytime after the first dose of an antipsychotic drug.

Addiction A state of chronic or recurrent intoxication characterized by psychologic dependence, tolerance, and physical dependence. The person is emotionally dependent on a drug, is able to obtain a desired effect from a specific dosage, and experiences withdrawal symptoms after he or she stops taking the drug.

Adjustment disorder A maladaptive reaction in response to an identifiable event or situation that is stress producing and not the result or part of a mental disorder. The reaction generally occurs within three months of the onset of the stressor, manifests itself as impaired social or occupational functioning, and is exaggerated beyond the normal reaction to an identified stressor. Remission of the reaction generally occurs when the stressor diminishes or disappears.

Affect A person's mood, feelings, or tone observable as an outward manifestation. Often referred to as *emotion*. Affect may be referred to as inappropriate, flat, or blunted.

Affective disorder A mental disorder exhibiting prominent and persistent mood changes of elation or depression accompanied by symptoms such as fatigue and insomnia. An abnormality of affect, activity, or thought process is noted. The mood changes appear to be disproportionate to any cause.

Affective disturbance Inappropriate mood. The person lacks the ability to show appropriate emotional response.

Akathisia Motor restlessness. The person experiences a constant state of movement, characterized by restlessness and difficulty sitting still, or a strong urge to move about.

Akinesia Motor retardation or reduced voluntary motor movement.

Alcoholism The inability to stop drinking that seriously alters a normal living pattern. Cessation of drinking or a reduction in intake results in withdrawal symptoms.

649

Alzheimer's disease A presenile brain disease that begins with a slight and easily dismissed flattening of personality characterized by confusion, inability to carry out purposeful movements, and possible hallucinations. Sudden personality changes, violent flashes of anger, episodes of wandering, symptoms of paranoia, a stooped gait, loss of involuntary functions, and seizures may occur.

Ambivalence Contradictory or opposing emotions, attitudes, ideas, or desires for the same person, thing, or situation.

Amnesia Loss of memory that may be organic or emotional in origin.

Anhedonia The inability to experience pleasure while engaged in activities that normally produce pleasurable feelings.

Antidepressant Drug used to treat depressive disorders caused by emotional or environmental stressors, frustrations, or losses.

Antiparkinsonism drugs Drugs used to treat extrapyramidal effects of antipsychotic drugs. Anticholinergic agents are the drugs of choice.

Anxiety A term used to describe feelings of uncertainty, uneasiness, apprehension, or tension that a person experiences in response to an unknown object or situation.

Apathy Lack of emotion, concern, feeling, or interest.

Associative disturbance or looseness An inability to think logically. Ideas expressed have little, if any, connection and shift from one subject to another.

Autism A thought process in which the person retreats from reality. The person may feel unrelated to others or to the environment and appears to be emotionally detached from others.

Barbiturates Drugs that depress the central nervous system and are used for sedative effects.

Behavior therapy Treatment that focuses on modifying observable, quantifiable behavior by manipulation of the environment and behavior.

Bestiality Sexual contact with animals to produce sexual excitement.

Bipolar disorder A major affective disorder characterized by episodes of mania and depression.

Blocking A sudden stoppage in the spontaneous flow or stream of thinking or speaking for no apparent external or environmental reason. May be due to preoccupation, delusional thoughts, or hallucinations.

Bulimia An eating disorder characterized by episodic eating binges or the excessive intake of food or fluids beyond voluntary control.

Catatonia Muscular rigidity and inflexibility, resulting in immobility. A person experiencing catatonia may respond to stimuli and suddenly become extremely agitated.

Child abuse An act of commission in which intentional physical, mental, or emotional harm is inflicted on a child by a parent or other person.

Child neglect An act of omission in which a parent or other person fails to meet a dependent's basic needs, or to provide safe living conditions, physical or emotional care, or supervision, thus leaving the child unattended or abandoned.

Circumstantiality A pattern of speech in which the person gives much unnecessary detail that delays meeting a goal or point.

Clang association Use of rhyming words.

Compensation The act of making up for a real or imagined inability or deficiency with a specific behavior to maintain self-respect or self-esteem.

Compulsion An unwanted, insistent, repetitive urge to perform or engage in an activity contrary to one's wishes or standards.

Conversion The transference of a mental conflict into a physical symptom to release tension or anxiety.

Coping mechanisms Conscious and unconscious methods of adjusting to environmental stress without changing or altering one's goals.

Crisis intervention An attempt to resolve an immediate crisis when a person's life goals are obstructed and usual problem-solving methods fail. The four steps in the process of crisis intervention include assessment, planning therapeutic intervention, implementing techniques of intervention, and resolution of the crisis, including anticipatory planning.

Cyclothymic disorder A disorder characterized by periods of depression and hypomania (a mood somewhere between euphoria and excessive elation). Symptoms of hypomania include rapid or accelerated speech, increased activity, and a decreased need for sleep.

Defense mechanism An intrapsychic reaction to protect oneself from stressful situations, resolve a mental conflict, reduce anxiety or fear, or protect one's self-esteem or sense of security. Common defense mechanisms include compensation, conversion, denial, displacement, rationalization, repression, and suppression. Defense mechanisms are considered unconscious, with the exception of suppression, and are often referred to as *coping mechanisms*.

Déjà vu The sensation of seeing what one has seen in the past.

Delirium An acute brain syndrome that develops rapidly and is characterized by cognitive impairment. Symptoms include clouding of the consciousness, disorientation, memory impairment, and a decreased ability to focus, shift, or sustain attention to environmental stimuli.

Delusion False belief not true to fact and not ordinarily accepted by other members of the person's culture.

Dementia Diffuse brain dysfunction characterized by a gradual, progressive, and chronic deterioration of intellectual function. Judgment, orientation, memory, affect or emotional stability, cognition, and attention all are affected.

Denial Unconscious refusal to face thoughts, feelings, wishes, needs, or reality factors that are consciously intolerable.

Depression A mood state characterized by a feeling of sadness, dejection, despair, discouragement, or hopelessness.

Disorientation A level of consciousness in which a person is unaware of the position of self in relation to time, surroundings, or other persons.

Displacement The transference of feelings such as frustration, hostility, or anxiety from one idea, person, or object to another.

Dissociation The act of separating and detaching a strong emotionally charged conflict from one's consciousness.

Double bind Conflicting demands placed upon an individual resulting in a no-win situation (failure).

Echolalia Pathologic, parrot-like repetition of another person's phrases or words.

Echopraxia Pathologic repetition or imitation of observed movements.

ECT Electroconvulsive therapy. Convulsive seizures are induced by the passage of electrical current through electrodes applied to both temporal areas of the head. Used in the treatment of severe depression.

Ego The part of the personality that meets and interacts with the outside world as an integrator or mediator and is the executive function of the personality that functions at all three levels of consciousness.

Encopresis Fecal incontinence.

Enuresis Urinary incontinence.

Euphoria An exaggerated sense of physical and emotional well-being inconsistent with reality.

Exhibitionism The practice of obtaining sexual gratification by repeatedly exposing the genitals to unsuspecting strangers, such as women and children, who are involuntary observers. The male exhibitionist has a strong need to demonstrate masculinity and potency.

Extrapyramidal side effects Adverse neurologic effects that may occur during the early phase of drug therapy. These effects are classified as parkinsonism, akathisia, and acute dystonic reactions.

Failure to thrive   A syndrome comprised of unexplained weight loss, deterioration in mental status and functional ability, and social isolation.

Family therapy   Treating family members in a modified group therapy is referred to as *family* or *systems* therapy. Such therapy attempts to establish open communication and healthy interactions within the family.

Fantasy   Imagined events or fabricated series of mental pictures such as daydreams. Used to express unconscious conflicts, gratify unconscious wishes, or prepare for anticipated future events.

Fear   The body's physiologic and emotional response to a known or recognized danger.

Fetishism   Sexual contact with an inanimate article such as a piece of clothing (fetish), resulting in sexual gratification. Its occurrence is almost exclusive with men who fear rejection by members of the opposite sex.

Flight of ideas   Overproductivity of talk characterized by verbal skipping from one idea to another. The ideas are fragmentary, and connections between parts of speech often are determined by chance associations.

Folie à deux   Sharing of the same delusion or false belief by two closely related persons.

Free-floating anxiety   Anxiety that is always present and accompanied by a feeling of dread. The person may exhibit ritualistic avoidance or phobic behavior.

Fugue   A rare occurrence in which a person suddenly and unexpectedly leaves home or work and is unable to recall the past or his or her identity. Assumption of a new identity usually occurs after relocation to another geographic area.

Gender identity disorder   A disorder characterized by feelings of discomfort about one's own sexuality due to conflict between anatomic sex and gender identity. The person has difficulty achieving normal heterosexual relations.

Geriatric nursing   Meeting the disease-created needs of older people. Such care is often intuitive and custodial in nature.

Gerontological nursing   The assessment of health care needs of older people, including planning and implementing health care, and evaluating the effectiveness of such care. An effort is made to promote independence, prevent illness, promote health, and maintain life with dignity and comfort.

Grandiosity   An exaggerated belief in one's importance or identity.

Group psychotherapy   Application of psychotherapy techniques in a group setting of approximately six to ten persons. Group therapy provides the opportunity for each member to examine interactions, learn and practice successful interpersonal communication skills, and explore emotional conflicts.

Hallucinations Sensory perceptions that occur in the absence of an actual external stimulus. They may be auditory, visual, olfactory, gustatory, or tactile.

Holistic health care Treatment of the patient's physical, psychological, and spiritual needs. The person receiving holistic health care attempts to identify any stressor(s) related to the present physical condition, discusses ways to modify or eliminate any stressors, and states specific changes that can be made.

Hyperkinesis An attention deficit disorder characterized by restlessness, short attention span, distractibility, overactivity, difficulty in learning, and difficulty with perceptual motor function.

Hypnotic Any drug or agent that induces sleep.

Hypochondriasis A diagnosis used to describe persons who present unrealistic or exaggerated physical complaints. Minor symptoms are of great concern to the person and often result in impairment of social and occupational functioning.

Id That part of the personality that is an unconscious reservoir of primitive drives and instincts dominated by irrational wishing and the pleasure principle.

Ideas of reference A thought process by which a person believes she or he is the object of environmental attention.

Identification A defense mechanism by which a person attempts to be like someone or to resemble the personality and traits of another to preserve his or her ego.

Illusion A false interpretation or perception of a real environmental stimulus that may involve any of the senses.

Intellectualization A defense mechanism by which a person transfers emotional concerns into the sphere of the intellect. Reasoning is used as a means of avoiding confrontation with unconscious conflicts and their stressful emotions.

Introjection A defense mechanism by which a person attributes the good qualities of others to self; symbolically taking on the character traits of another person by "ingesting" the person's philosophy, ideas, and so forth.

Isolation A defense mechanism by which a person separates an unacceptable feeling, idea, or impulse from her or his thoughts.

La belle indifference An inappropriate lack of concern; indifference.

Labile Exhibiting unstable, rapidly shifting emotions; moody.

Libido Emotional energy; psychic drive (often referred to as psychosexual energy).

Lithium A salt that is considered the treatment of choice for the manic phase of a bipolar disorder; also used as maintenance medication to treat recurrent affective episodes.

Major tranquilizer Antipsychotic drug or neuroleptic agent used in the treatment of disorders such as schizophrenia, mania, paranoid disorders, and acute brain syndrome.

Mania A mood disorder characterized by psychomotor overactivity or excitement, insomnia without fatigue, euphoria or a state of elation, distractibility, and pressured speech.

Masochism The act of experiencing pleasure or sexual arousal as a result of emotional or physical pain inflicted by oneself or by others.

Mental health A state of being in which a person is simultaneously successful at working, loving, and resolving conflicts by coping and adjusting to the recurrent stresses of everyday living.

Mental illness A state of being characterized by a disturbance of emotional equilibrium, manifested in maladaptive behavior or impaired functioning due to a biologic, genetic, social, psychological, physical, or chemical disturbance.

Mental retardation A disorder characterized by the onset of subaverage intellectual functioning associated with or resulting in impairments in adaptive behavior before age 18. A person with this disorder is less able to think abstractly, adapt to new situations, learn new information, solve problems, or profit from experience.

Methadone A synthetic narcotic used as a substitute for heroin during detoxification or withdrawal from heroin.

Milieu therapy A therapeutic or structured environment that encourages persons to function within the range of social norms through modification of the person's life circumstances and immediate environment.

Multiple personality A disorder in which a person is dominated by at least one of two or more definitive personalities at one time. Emergence of various personalities occurs suddenly and often is associated with psychosocial stress and conflict.

Münchausen syndrome by proxy A phenomenon in which a parent, usually the mother, fabricates illness in her child and presents the problem to doctors in the hope of gaining attention.

Mutism Refusal to speak even though the person may give indications of being aware of the environment.

Neologism A new word or combination of several words coined or self-invented by an individual and not readily understood by others.

Neuroleptic Major tranquilizer or antipsychotic drug.

Neuroleptic malignant syndrome (NMS) A potentially fatal complication of neuroleptic treatment that may develop within hours of the first dose or after years of continued drug exposure. Symptoms include, but are not limited to, severe muscular rigidity, hyperthermia, deterioration in level of consciousness, and fluctuations in blood pressure.

Neurosis   A descriptive term used to differentiate nonpsychotic clinical symptoms (no longer used as a separate DSM-IV classification).

Nihilism   A viewpoint that existence is senseless and useless.

Obsession   An insistent, painful, intrusive thought, emotion, or urge that arises from within oneself, is considered absurd and meaningless, and cannot be suppressed or ignored.

Occupational therapy   The use of creative techniques and purposeful activities, as well as a therapeutic relationship, to alter the course of an illness. Focuses on vocational skills and activities of daily living to raise self-esteem and promote independence.

Organic mental disorder   A disorder of transient or permanent brain dysfunction caused by a disturbance of physiologic functioning of brain tissue. Causes include mechanical, thermal, or chemical damage to the brain, in addition to aging or physical illness.

Paranoia   A rare condition characterized by a delusional system that develops gradually, becomes fixed, and is based on the misinterpretation of an actual event. The thought process appears clear and orderly, reality testing is intact, affect remains appropriate, sociability is maintained, and delusions are persecutory or grandiose in content.

Paranoid disorder   A psychotic state characterized by moderately impaired reality testing, affect, and sociability. Delusions may be persecutory, grandiose, erotic, or jealous in thought content.

Paraphilia   A disorder in which unusual or bizarre sexual acts or imagery are enacted to achieve sexual excitement.

Parkinsonism   An extrapyramidal side effect characterized by motor retardation or akinesia, a mask-like face, rigidity, tremors, "pill rolling," and salivation. Can occur after the first week of psychotropic drug therapy.

Pedophilia   The use of prepubertal children to achieve sexual gratification.

Personality disorder   A nonpsychotic illness characterized by maladaptive behavior that the person uses to fulfill his or her needs and bring satisfaction to self. As a result of the inability to relate to the environment, the person acts out conflicts socially.

Phobia   An irrational fear of an object, activity, or situation that is out of proportion to the stimulus and results in avoidance of the identified object, activity, or situation. Clinical categories of phobia include agoraphobia, with or without panic attacks; social phobia; and simple phobia.

Play therapy   Used with children between ages 3 and 12. Various toys, puppets, or other materials are used to encourage a child to act out feelings such as anger, hostility, frustration, and fear.

Post-traumatic stress disorder A category reserved for persons who experience a psychologically traumatic event that is considered to be outside the realm of usual human experience. Examples include rape, assault, military combat, and natural disasters.

Premorbid Refers to period of time or state before onset of a disorder (*e.g.*, premorbid personality).

Primary gain Relief from anxiety obtained by using a defense mechanism to keep an internal need or conflict out of awareness.

Projection A defense mechanism in which a person rejects unwanted characteristics of self and assigns them to others.

Psychalgia Psychogenic pain disorder in which severe, prolonged pain is due to psychological factors.

Psychiatric nursing A specialized area of nursing that focuses on the prevention and cure of mental disorders by employing theories of human behavior and the purposeful use of self.

Psychoanalysis A lengthy method of psychotherapy in which the patient talks in an uncontrolled, spontaneous manner termed *free association*. Exploration of repressed anxieties, fears, and childhood images occurs by the interpretation of dreams, emotions, and behaviors.

Psychodrama A form of group therapy by which persons use dramatization to express their own or assigned emotional problems.

Psychosis A mental disorder in which a person experiences an impairment of the ability to remember, think, communicate, respond emotionally, interpret reality, and behave appropriately. Examples include schizophrenia, bipolar depression, and paranoia.

Psychotropic drugs Chemicals that alter feelings, emotions, and consciousness in various ways and are used therapeutically in the practice of psychiatry to treat a broad range of mental and emotional illnesses.

Rape A violent sexual act committed against a person's will, involving the threat or use of force.

Rape trauma syndrome An acute phase of disorganization followed by a longer phase of reorganization experienced by a rape victim. The acute phase is characterized by emotional reactions of anger, guilt, embarrassment, and humiliation; multiple physical or somatic complaints; or a wish for revenge. During the phase of reorganization the victim may change daily life patterns, experience recurring dreams or nightmares, seek support from friends and family, feel the need to discuss the sexual assault, or develop irrational fears of phobias.

Rationalization The act of justifying ideas, actions, or feelings with acceptable reasons or explanations.

Reaction-formation   The act of displaying the exact opposite behavior, attitude, or feeling of that which one would normally show in a given situation.

Regression   Reversion to past levels of behaviors to reduce anxiety and allow one to become dependent on others.

Repression   The inability to recall painful or unpleasant thoughts or feelings, since they are automatically and involuntarily pushed into one's unconsciousness.

Restitution or undoing   The negation of a previous consciously intolerable action or experience to reduce or alleviate feelings of guilt.

Sadism   The act of experiencing sexual gratification while inflicting physical or emotional pain on others.

Scapegoat   Term used to describe the role of a person within a family who is the recipient of angry, hostile, frustrated, or ambivalent emotions experienced by various family members.

Schizophrenia   A serious psychiatric disorder characterized by impaired communication with loss of contact with reality and deterioration from a previous level of functioning in work, social relations, or self-care. Clinical types include disorganized, catatonic, paranoid, residual, and undifferentiated schizophrenia.

Secondary gain   Any benefit or support that a person obtains as a result of being sick, other than relief from anxiety.

Sedative-hypnotic   An agent used to induce a state of natural sleep, reduce periods of involuntary awakenings during the night, and increase total sleep time.

"Shaken baby" syndrome   A sometimes fatal form of abuse that typically occurs when an adult loses control and violently shakes a child who has been crying incessantly.

"Silent rape" syndrome   A maladaptive reaction to rape in which the victim fails to disclose information about the rape, is unable to resolve feelings about the sexual assault, experiences increased anxiety, and may develop a sudden phobic reaction.

Somatoform disorder   A disorder characterized by physiologic complaints or symptoms that are not under voluntary control and do not demonstrate organic findings. Hypochondriasis and conversion disorders are two examples of this disorder.

Stimulant   An agent that directly stimulates the central nervous system and creates a feeling of alertness and self-confidence in the user.

Sublimation The rechanneling of consciously intolerable or socially unacceptable impulses or behaviors into activities that are personally or socially acceptable.

Substitution The act of finding another goal when one is blocked.

Superego The censoring force or conscience of the personality, composed of morals, mores, values, and ethics, largely derived from one's parents.

Suppression The act of willfully or consciously putting a thought or feeling out of one's mind, with the ability to recall the thought or feeling at will.

Symbolization An object, idea, or act represents another through some common aspect and carries the emotional feeling that is associated with the other.

Tardive dyskinesia Most frequent side effect occurring during abrupt termination of an antipsychotic drug, during reduction in dosage, or after long-term, high-dose therapy. Characterized by involuntary rhythmic, stereotyped movements, protrusion of the tongue, puffing of the cheeks, and chewing movements.

Therapeutic community A specific type of milieu therapy using social and interpersonal interactions in the hospital as therapeutic tools to bring about change in the patient by encouraging active participation in treatment. It is democratic, rehabilitative, permissive, and communal in function.

Therapeutic window The serum plasma level of a drug (*e.g.*, tricyclic antidepressants) at which optimal therapeutic response occurs.

Transsexual A type of gender identity disorder in which the person desires to live, dress, and act as a member of the opposite sex because of discomfort with his or her own anatomic sex.

Transvestism A type of paraphilia in which a heterosexual male achieves sexual gratification by wearing the clothing of a woman (cross-dressing).

Undoing See *restitution*.

Verbigeration A severe form of perseveration in which a person repeats the same verbal or motor response to verbal stimuli despite efforts to produce another response.

Voyeurism The achievement of sexual pleasure by looking at unsuspecting persons who are naked, undressing, or engaged in sexual activity.

Waxy flexibility The catatonic person maintains the position in which he or she has been placed.

Word salad Cluster of words without any logical connection.

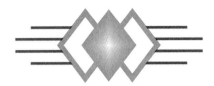

INDEX

transcultural considerations in, 314
treatment of, 316
types of, 313–316
undifferentiated disorder, 316
Somatoform disorders not otherwise specified, 316
Spatial territory, 102
Speaking in tongues, 411
Specificity, in therapeutic relationship, 106
Specific phobia, 290–291
Speech therapist, 125–126
Spiritual care, 137–138
needs of person suffering loss, 270
Splitting, 326
Spontaneous, here-and-now emotions, 10
Spouse abuse. *See also* Abused person
acute beating phase of, 551
forms of, 550
loving phase of, 551
physical, dynamics of, 551–552
tension-building phase of, 551
SSRIs. *See* Selective serotonin reuptake inhibitors
Standards of care, in crisis intervention, 153–154
Standards of Psychiatric and Mental Health Nursing Practice, 26–32
Statement on Psychiatric Nursing Practice, 26
Statutory rape, 562
Stelazine (trifluoperazine), 191, 198, 611
Stereotypic movement disorder, 455
Steroid abuse, 521
STP, 520
Stress
in adolescents, 459
in children, 458
essential hypertension and, 308, 310–311
identification of stressors, 312
psychological factors affecting medical condition, 306–312
Structural approach, to family therapy, 178
Stupor, 77–78
catatonic, 411
Subjective data, 68–69, 81
Sublimation, 14
Substance abuse. *See* Alcoholism; Psychoactive substance abuse
Substance-induced amnestic disorder, 433
Substance-induced anxiety, 331
Substance-induced delirium, 428
Substance-induced dementia, 430
Substance-induced depression, 352–353
Substance-related disorders, DSM-IV classification of, 629–634
Substitution, 13
Succinimides, 213
Suicidal ideation, 375, 381, 383
nursing care plan for, 368–369
patient teaching checklist for, 385
Suicidal intention rating scale (SIRS), 383

Suicide
among adolescents, 374–375, 459
AIDS and, 578
assessing risk of, 379, 381–382
bereaved survivors of, 387
culturally-sanctioned, 378–380
delusional disorders and, 395
among elderly, 375, 594, 598
etiology of, 375–377
individuals at risk for, 377–378
misconceptions about, 380
nurse's feelings about, 383
nursing care plan for, 387–389
nursing diagnoses for, 387–389
nursing interventions for, 382–386, 388–389
outcome criteria for, 388–389
postvention, 387
primary prevention of, 382
psychological autopsy after, 386
secondary prevention of, 382
statistics on, 374–375
"The Suicide Lexicon," 381
tertiary prevention of, 382–383
transcultural considerations regarding, 378–380
warning signs of, 375, 380–382
Suicide precautions, 383–386
Sullivan
interpersonal model of patient care, 128
psychological model of patient care, 127
Superego, 223, 322
Superstition, 23
Superstitiousness, 323
Support group, 162
for AIDS patients, 581
Supportive therapy, 132
Support people, 16–17
Suppression, 12
Surmontil (trimipramine), 205, 209
Suspiciousness, 589
Susto, 331
Suttee, 378
Symbolization, 14
Symmetrel (amantidine), 214–215, 417
Symphonic interaction, 130
Syndrome nursing diagnosis, 88–89
Syphilis, 446
Systematic desensitization, 133, 297
Systems-oriented nursing theory, 129–130
Systems therapy, in childhood disorders, 462

Tactile hallucination, 77
Tagamet (cimetidine), 201
Talwin, 517–518
Tardive dyskinesia, 193, 195
Teacher role, in therapeutic relationship, 107–108
Tegretol (carbamazepine), 201, 212, 214, 330, 464
Telepathy, 323